Comprehensive Virology 13

Comprehensive Virology

Edited by Heinz Fraenkel-Conrat
University of California at Berkeley

and Robert R. Wagner
University of Virginia

Editorial Board

Comprehensive

Edited by

Heinz Fraenkel-Conrat

Department of Molecular Biology and Virus Laboratory
University of California, Berkeley, California

and

Robert R. Wagner

Department of Microbiology
University of Virginia, Charlottesville, Virginia

Virology

13

Structure and Assembly

Primary, Secondary, Tertiary, and Quaternary Structures

PLENUM PRESS · NEW YORK AND LONDON

Library of Congress Cataloging in Publication Data

Fraenkel-Conrat, Heinz, 1910-
  Structure and assembly—primary, secondary, tertiary, and quarternary structures.

  (Their Comprehensive virology; v. 13)
  Includes bibliographies.
  1. Viruses—Morphology. I. Wagner, Robert R., 1923-   II. Title. III. Series.
QR357.F72 vol. 13 [QR450]   576'.64'08s
  ISBN 0-306-40137-1   [576'.64]   79-6

© 1979 Plenum Press, New York
A Division of Plenum Publishing Corporation
227 West 17th Street, New York, N.Y. 10011

Printed in the United States of America

Foreword

The time seems ripe for a critical compendium of that segment of the biological universe we call viruses. Virology, as a science, having passed only recently through its descriptive phase of naming and numbering, has probably reached that stage at which relatively few new—truly new—viruses will be discovered. Triggered by the intellectual probes and techniques of molecular biology, genetics, biochemical cytology, and high resolution microscopy and spectroscopy, the field has experienced a genuine information explosion.

Few serious attempts have been made to chronicle these events. This comprehensive series, which will comprise some 6000 pages in a total of about 18 volumes, represents a commitment by a large group of active investigators to analyze, digest, and expostulate on the great mass of data relating to viruses, much of which is now amorphous and disjointed, and scattered throughout a wide literature. In this way, we hope to place the entire field in perspective, and to develop an invaluable reference and sourcebook for researchers and students at all levels.

This series is designed as a continuum that can be entered anywhere, but which also provides a logical progression of developing facts and integrated concepts.

Volume 1 contains an alphabetical catalogue of almost all viruses of vertebrates, insects, plants, and protists, describing them in general terms. Volumes 2–4 deal primarily, but not exclusively, with the processes of infection and reproduction of the major groups of viruses in their hosts. Volume 2 deals with the simple RNA viruses of bacteria, plants, and animals; the togaviruses (formerly called arboviruses), which share with these only the feature that the virion's RNA is able to act as messenger RNA in the host cell; and the reoviruses of animals and plants, which all share several structurally singular features, the most important being the double-strandedness of their multiple RNA molecules.

Volume 3 addresses itself to the reproduction of all DNA-containing viruses of vertebrates, encompassing the smallest and the largest viruses known. The reproduction of the larger and more complex RNA viruses is the subject matter of Volume 4. These viruses share the property of being enclosed in lipoprotein membranes, as do the togaviruses included in Volume 2. They share as a group, along with the reoviruses, the presence of polymerase enzymes in their virions to satisfy the need for their RNA to become transcribed before it can serve messenger functions.

Volumes 5 and 6 represent the first in a series that focuses primarily on the structure and assembly of virus particles. Volume 5 is devoted to general structural principles involving the relationship and specificity of interaction of viral capsid proteins and their nucleic acids, or host nucleic acids. It deals primarily with helical and the simpler isometric viruses, as well as with the relationship of nucleic acid to protein shell in the T-even phages. Volume 6 is concerned with the structure of the picornaviruses, and with the reconstitution of plant and bacterial RNA viruses.

Volumes 7 and 8 deal with the DNA bacteriophages. Volume 7 concludes the series of volumes on the reproduction of viruses (Volumes 2–4 and Volume 7) and deals particularly with the single- and double-stranded virulent bacteriophages.

Volume 8, the first of the series on regulation and genetics of viruses, covers the biological properties of the lysogenic and defective phages, the phage-satellite system P 2–P 4, and in-depth discussion of the regulatory principles governing the development of selected lytic phages.

Volume 9 provides a truly comprehensive analysis of the genetics of all animal viruses that have been studied to date. These chapters cover the principles and methodology of mutant selection, complementation analysis, gene mapping with restriction endonucleases, etc. Volume 10 also deals with animal cells, covering transcriptional and translational regulation of viral gene expression, defective virions, and integration of tumor virus genomes into host chromosomes.

Volume 11 covers the considerable advances in the molecular understanding of new aspects of virology which have been revealed in recent years through the study of plant viruses. It covers particularly the mode of replication and translation of the multicomponent viruses and others that carry or utilize subdivided genomes; the use of protoplasts in such studies is authoritatively reviewed, as well as the nature of viroids, the smallest replicatable pathogens. Volume 12 deals with special groups of viruses of protists and invertebrates which show properties that set them apart from the main virus families. These are the lipid-containing phages and the viruses of algae, fungi, and invertebrates. These groups will be followed in Volume 14 by special and/or newly characterized vertebrate virus groups (e.g., arena-, corona-, hepatitis, calici-, and bunyaviruses).

The present volume collects chapters on various topics related to the structure and assembly of viruses, dealing in detail with nucleotide and amino acid sequences, as well as with particle morphology and assembly, and the structure of virus membranes and hybrid viruses. The first complete sequence of a viral RNA is represented as a multicolored foldout.

Several subsequent volumes will deal with virus–host relationships and with methodological aspects of virus research.

Contents

Chapter 3

Structure and Function of RNA Bacteriophages

Walter Fiers

Chapter 4

DNA Sequencing of Viral Genomes

Gillian M. Air

Chapter 5

Viral Membranes

Richard W. Compans and Hans-Dieter Klenk

Chapter 6

Adenovirus Structural Proteins

Harold S. Ginsberg

Chapter 7

The Adenovirus-SV40 Hybrid Viruses

Cephas T. Patch, Arthur S. Levine, and Andrew M. Lewis, Jr.

Chapter 8

Bacteriophage Structure

Frederick A. Eiserling

Chapter 9

Genetic Control of Complex Bacteriophage Assembly

William B. Wood and Jonathan King

Amino Acid Sequences of Plant and Animal Viral Proteins

Stephen Oroszlan and Raymond V. Gilden

Biological Carcinogenesis Program
Frederick Cancer Research Center
Frederick, Maryland 21701

1. INTRODUCTION

This chapter will present currently available primary structure data on the proteins of a variety of plant and animal viruses. Excellent descriptions of methods for the determination of amino acid sequences of proteins are found in several review articles and books (Hirs, 1967; Schroeder, 1968; Blackburn, 1970; Needleman, 1970; Starbuck, 1970; Hirs and Timasheff, 1972; Niall, 1973; Perham, 1975) and therefore will not be presented here. Since the pioneering studies on TMV in the early 1960s which contributed to establishing the principle of colinearity of gene and protein, sequencing efforts have contributed to an understanding of evolutionary relationships among other plant and animal viruses. Such data can also provide practical end points such as the design of synthetic vaccines; this may be especially crucial in cases where complete freedom from viral nucleic acids is essential. The continuing development of sensitive automated microsequencing procedures utilizing stepwise Edman degradation, high-sensitivity methods for identification of amino acids, radiolabeled reagents, and proteins with intrinsic radioactivity (Edman and Begg, 1967; Jacobs *et al.*, 1974; McKean *et al.*, 1974; Jacobs and Niall, 1975; Brauer *et al.*, 1975; Oroszlan *et al.*, 1975*a*; Silver and Hood, 1975; Ballou *et al.*, 1976; Bridgen, 1976; Henning *et al.*, 1976; Vitetta *et al.*, 1976; Zimmerman *et al.*, 1976) will allow data gathering on minor (by mass) virion polypeptides, for example, the reverse transcriptases of retroviruses, which until recently would have required the availability of enormous amounts of virus. The concluding section on retrovirus proteins, the major interest of the authors' laboratory, will summarize sequence data and recent evidence of viral groupings based on immunological data.

2. PLANT VIRUSES

2.1. Tobacco Mosaic Virus

Tobacco mosaic virus (TMV), which was the first virus to be identified and crystallized, is a 300-nm-long, rodlike particle with a diameter of 15 nm and an approximate particle weight of 4×10^7. The virion is composed of 5% RNA (single-stranded, single chain) and 95% protein. The protein component representing the viral coat consists of 2130 identical polypeptide subunits, each with an approximate molecular weight of 17,500, consisting of 158 amino acid residues (Fraenkel-Conrat, 1968; Dayhoff, 1972; Benjamini *et al.*, 1972; Smith, 1977). The coat protein of TMV vulgare (common strain) was the first viral protein whose complete amino acid sequence was determined (Tsugita *et al.*, 1960). Now protein sequences of several naturally occurring strains as well as artificially induced mutants are known.

The complete amino acid sequences of six TMV strains—vulgare (V), OM, dahlemense (D), cowpea (CP), U2, and Holmes ribgrass (HR)—are aligned in Fig. 1.

The N termini (serine and alanine) are acetylated in all strains except in U2, which has proline at the N terminus. As pointed out by Fraenkel-Conrat (1968), it appears probable that the acetyl group fulfills a blocking function, protecting the peptide chain against aminopeptidases, and that this function proves redundant in a mutant carrying an N-terminal proline which is not susceptible to cleavage by the known exopeptidases (Hill, 1965).

Those amino acids which are positionally different from the sequence of the common strain (V) protein are underlined in Fig. 1. In order to maintain positional homology (best fit) in the sequence of CP strain protein, which is three residues longer, an insert (glutamic acid) is placed between residues 64 and 65 (Rees and Short, 1975). The HR strain is two residues shorter than the V protein and appears to have a gap consisting of residues 148 and 149. The OM strain has only three amino acid substitutions: in positions 50 (Glu→Gln), 129 (Ile→Val), and 153 (Thr→Asn). The single cysteine appears in position 27 in all strains except CP, where it is substituted by leucine. In general, most of the observed exchanges involve only the smaller and hydrophilic residues, although there are a large number of exceptions. The most variable regions of the protein chain seem to be those from residue 19 to 28, from 49 to 68, from 97 to 101, and from 138 to 158. These regions include a high proportion of hydrophylic residues; therefore, they may represent the positions of the folded protein in the intact virus which may be in contact with the solvent (Fraenkel-Conrat, 1968; Durham and Butler, 1975).

The segments from residue 87 to 94 and from 113 to 122 are identical in all strains except CP. These two regions were thought to be completely conserved sequences until the sequence of the CP strain protein became available just 4 years ago (Rees and Short, 1975). It has been assumed that these regions compose the RNA binding site. They contain four of the six conserved positive charges in the protein (arginine residues 90, 92, 113, 122) which could neutralize the negative charges of the RNA chain–phosphate backbone. The CP strain also has arginine in all the above positions except position 122, where it is substituted by histidine. Apart from the above regions only residues 2, 4, 17, 18, 36–38, 41, 61, 63, 82–83, 88–92, 94, 128, 132, 137, 140, 144–145, 150, and 156 are unchanged in all the six strains for which the complete sequences are given in Fig. 1.

The HR and CP strains appear to be evolutionarily the most distantly related to the other more closely related strains (Dayhoff, 1972). The HR protein has 80 amino acid changes from the common V strain of TMV and CP coat protein has a total of 98 changes (Rees and Short, 1975). The percent differences between the sequences of the above six TMV strains are shown in Table 1. These correspond very well with the previous ordering of TMV strains into groups based on amino acid compositional differences (Fraenkel-Conrat, 1974). The results of nucleic acid hybridization experiments, however, did not reveal a quantitative relationship similar to that shown by amino acid sequence data. Even those strains among the various classes which differ least in primary structure of coat protein (vulgare and dahlemense, representing classes A and B, respectively) were found to show no apparent nucleotide sequence homology. A possible explanation is that

```
        |—T—|—r—|    |—T—|    |—T—|    |—r—|        α
        1       5       10   β  15       20      25

V    Ser-Tyr-Ser-Ile-Thr-Thr-Pro-Ser-Gln-Phe-Val-Phe-Leu-Ser-Ser-Ala-Trp-Ala-Asp-Pro-Ile-Glu-Leu-Ile-Asn-
OM   Ser-Tyr-Ser-Ile-Thr-Thr-Pro-Ser-Gln-Phe-Val-Phe-Leu-Ser-Ser-Ala-Trp-Ala-Asp-Pro-Ile-Glu-Leu-Ile-Asn-
D    Ser-Tyr-Ser-Ile-Thr-Thr-Pro-Ser-Gln-Phe-Val-Phe-Leu-Ser-Ser-Val-Trp-Ala-Asp-Pro-Ile-Glu-Leu-Leu-Asn-
CP   Ala-Tyr-Ser-Ile-Pro-Thr-Pro-Ser-Gln-Leu-Val-Tyr-Phe-Glu-Asn-Tyr-Ile-Asp-Tyr-Ile-Pro-Phe-Val-Asn-
U2   Pro-Tyr-Thr-Ile-Thr-Ile-Asn-Ser-Pro-Ser-Gln-Phe-Val-Tyr-Leu-Ser-Ser-Ala-Tyr-Ala-Asp-Pro-Val-Glu-Leu-Ile-Asn-
HR   Ser-Tyr-Asn-Ile-Thr-Asn-Ser-Asn-Gln-Tyr-Gln-Trp-Phe-Ala-Ala-Val-Trp-Ala-Glu-Pro-Tyr-Pro-Met-Leu-Asn-


        |—T—|        |        β            |        |
        30      35       40        45      50

V    Leu-Cys-Thr-Asn-Ala-Leu-Gly-Asn-Phe-Gln-Phe-Gln-Thr-Gln-Arg-Gln-Phe-Ser-Gln-Glu-
OM   Leu-Cys-Thr-Asn-Ala-Leu-Gly-Asn-Phe-Gln-Gln-Thr-Gln-Gln-Arg-Gln-Phe-Ser-Gln-Gln-
D    Val-Cys-Thr-Ser-Leu-Gly-Asn-Gly-Asn-Gln-Thr-Gln-Gln-Gln-Gln-Gln-Phe-Ser-Gln-Glu-
CP   Arg-Leu-Ile-Asn-Ala-Ser-Ala-Arg-Ser-Phe-Gln-Ser-Gly-Arg-Asp-Gly-Leu-Arg-Glu-Ile-Leu-Ile-Lys-
U2   Leu-Cys-Thr-Asn-Ala-Leu-Gly-Asn-Gln-Phe-Gln-Thr-Gln-Ala-Gly-Thr-Val-Gln-Gln-Phe-Ala-Asp-
HR   Gln-Cys-Ser-Ala-Leu-Ser-Gln-Ser-Gln-Thr-Gln-Ser-Thr-Gln-Ala-Gly-Arg-Asp-Thr-Val-Arg-Gln-Gln-Phe-Ala-Asn-


        |—r—|—T—|        |        β            |—T—|        |—T—|
        55      60            65              70       75

V    Val-Trp-Lys-Pro-Ser-Pro-Gln-Val-Thr-Val-Arg-Phe-Pro-Asp-Ser-Asp-Phe-Lys-Val-Tyr-Arg-Tyr-Asn-Ala-Val-
OM   Val-Trp-Lys-Pro-Ser-Pro-Gln-Val-Thr-Val-Arg-Phe-Pro-Asp-Ser-Asp-Phe-Lys-Val-Tyr-Arg-Tyr-Asn-Ala-Val-
D    Val-Trp-Lys-Pro-Ser-Pro-Gln-Val-Thr-Val-Arg-Phe-Pro-Asp-Ser-Asp-Phe-Lys-Val-Tyr-Arg-Tyr-Asn-Ala-Val-
CP   Ser-Gln-Val-Ser-Val-Ser-Pro-Ile-Ser-Arg-Phe-Pro-Ala-Tyr-Tyr-Ile-Tyr-Leu-Arg-Asp-Pro-Ser-
                                        Glu
U2   Ala-Trp-Lys-Pro-Ser-Pro-Val-Met-Thr-Val-Arg-Pro-Ala-Ser-Asp-Phe-Tyr-Arg-Tyr-Val-Tyr-Arg-Tyr-Asn-Thr-
HR   Leu-Leu-Ser-Thr-Ile-Ala-Pro-Asn-Arg-Pro-Asp-Thr-Gly-Phe-Arg-Val-Tyr-Asn-Ser-Ala-Val-


        |        |        β            |—T—|        α
        80      85            90       95      100

V    Leu-Asp-Pro-Leu-Val-Thr-Ala-Leu-Leu-Gly-Ala-Phe-Asp-Thr-Arg-Asn-Arg-Ile-Ile-Glu-Val-Glu-Asn-Gln-Ala-
OM   Leu-Asp-Pro-Leu-Val-Thr-Ala-Leu-Leu-Gly-Ala-Phe-Asp-Thr-Arg-Asn-Arg-Ile-Ile-Glu-Val-Glu-Asn-Gln-Ala-
D    Leu-Asp-Pro-Leu-Ile-Thr-Ala-Leu-Leu-Gly-Ala-Phe-Asp-Thr-Arg-Asn-Arg-Ile-Ile-Glu-Val-Glu-Asn-Gln-Ala-
CP   Ile-Leu-Thr-Val-Leu-Thr-Ala-Leu-Leu-Gly-Ala-Gln-Asp-Thr-Arg-Asn-Arg-Val-Glu-Ile-Glu-Val-Asn-Gln-Thr-
U2   Leu-Asp-Pro-Leu-Ile-Thr-Ala-Leu-Leu-Asn-Leu-Ser-Asn-Ser-Phe-Asp-Asp-Thr-Arg-Asn-Arg-Ile-Ile-Glx-Val-Asx-Asx-Glx-Ala-
HR   Ile-Ile-Lys-Pro-Leu-Tyr-Leu-Glu-Ala-Leu-Met-Lys-Ser-Phe-Asp-Asp-Thr-Arg-Asn-Arg-Ile-Ile-Glu-Thr-Gln-Glu-Gln-Ser-
```

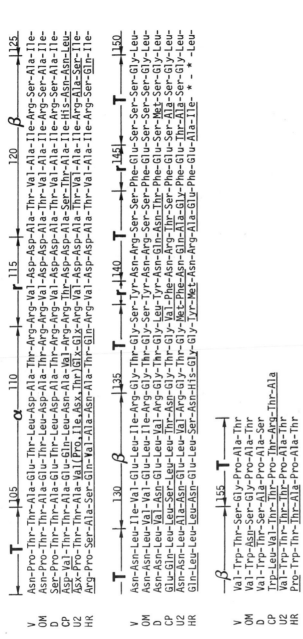

	—————T—— |105 ——————α—— 110 ——————— |115 ———————————r———— |120 ——β——|125 ————
V	Asn-Pro-Thr-Thr-Ala-Glu-Thr-Leu-Asp-Ala-Thr-Arg-Arg-Val-Asp-Asp-Ala-Thr-Val-Ala-Ile-Arg-Ser-Ala-Ile-
OM	Asn-Pro-Thr-Thr-Ala-Glu-Thr-Leu-Asp-Ala-Thr-Arg-Arg-Val-Asp-Asp-Ala-Thr-Val-Ala-Ile-Arg-Ser-Ala-Ile-
D	Ser-Pro-Thr-Thr-Ala-Glu-Thr-Leu-Asp-Ala-Thr-Arg-Arg-Val-Asp-Asp-Ala-Thr-Val-Ala-Ile-Arg-Ser-Ala-Ile-
CP	Asp-Val-Thr-Thr-Ala-Glu-Gln-Leu-Asn-Ala-Val-Arg-Arg-Thr-Asp-Asp-Ala-Ser-Thr-Ala-Ile-His-Asn-Asn-Leu-
U2	Asx-Pro-Thr-Thr-Ala-Val(Pro,Ile,Asx,Thr)Glx-Glx-Arg-Val-Asp-Asp-Val-Ala-Ile-Arg-Ser-Ala-Ile-
HR	Arg-Pro-Ser-Ala-Ser-Gln-Ala-Ala-Thr-Gln-Arg-Val-Asp-Asp-Ala-Thr-Val-Ala-Ile-Arg-Ser-Gln-Ile-

	————T————|130 ——β——|135 ————T———|140 ——r—|145 ————T————|150 ———
V	Asn-Asn-Leu-Ile-Val-Glu-Leu-Ile-Arg-Gly-Thr-Gly-Ser-Tyr-Asn-Arg-Ser-Ser-Phe-Glu-Ser-Ser-Ser-Gly-Leu-
OM	Asn-Asn-Leu-Val-Val-Glu-Leu-Ile-Arg-Gly-Thr-Gly-Ser-Tyr-Asn-Arg-Ser-Ser-Phe-Glu-Ser-Ser-Ser-Gly-Leu-
D	Asn-Asn-Leu-Val-Asn-Glu-Leu-Val-Arg-Gly-Thr-Gly-Leu-Tyr-Asn-Gln-Asn-Thr-Phe-Glu-Ser-Met-Ser-Gly-Leu-
CP	Glu-Gln-Leu-Ser-Leu-Leu-Thr-Asn-Gly-Thr-Gly-Val-Phe-Asn-Arg-Thr-Ser-Phe-Glu-Ser-Ala-Ser-Gly-Leu-
U2	Asn-Asn-Leu-Ala-Asn-Glu-Leu-Val-Arg-Gly-Thr-Gly-Met-Phe-Asn-Gln-Ala-Gly-Phe-Glu-Thr-Ala-Ser-Gly-Leu-
HR	Gln-Leu-Leu-Asn-Glu-Leu-Ser-Asn-His-Gly-Gly-Tyr-Met-Asn-Arg-Ala-Glu-Phe-Glu-Ala-Ile- * - * -Leu-

	——β——|155 ——T——
V	Val-Trp-Thr-Thr-Ser-Gly-Pro-Ala-Thr
OM	Val-Trp-Asn-Ser-Gly-Pro-Ala-Thr
D	Val-Trp-Thr-Ser-Ala-Pro-Ala-Ser
CP	Trp-Leu-Val-Thr-Pro-Thr-Arg-Thr-Ala
U2	Val-Trp-Thr-Thr-Pro-Ala-Thr
HR	Pro-Trp-Thr-Thr-Ala-Pro-Ala-Thr

Fig. 1. Alignment of amino acid sequences of six strains of TMV coat proteins: vulgare (V), OM, dahlemense (D), cowpea (CP), U2, and Holmes ribgrass (HR). Amino acids positionally different from V are underlined. Secondary structure predictions for the V strain are indicated by arrows and symbols α, β, T, and r (see text). The sequences except CP (Rees and Short, 1975) were taken from a monograph by Fraenkel-Conrat (1968) and the *Atlas of Protein Sequence and Structure* by Dayhoff (1972). See these publications for original references.

the coat protein gene, which is located at the 3'-terminal region, comprises less than 10% of the total TMV RNA, and this gene segment may be evolutionarily more preserved than the rest of the virion RNA (Vandevalle and Siegel, 1976).

Based on amino acid sequences, secondary structure predictions for the V strain protein were made by Durham and Butler (1975) using the rules of Chou and Fasman (1974). The symbols ($\alpha = \alpha$ helix; $\beta = \beta$ structure; $T = \beta$ turn; r = random structure) above the sequence of V protein in Fig. 1 indicate these structure assignments. The authors, however, overruled the "native secondary structure predictions" in three places for the following reasons: "From 78 to 88 the choice between α and β structure is marginal and the opportunity for hydrogen bonding to other β regions suggests that β is the more reasonable assignment. Likewise from 23 to 30 we choose β structure which also enables cysteine 27 to lie at its correct radius. From 125 to 128 there is a weakly predicted turn which must be overruled to allow the necessary extensions between carboxyls 116 and 131." With these modifications, Durham and Butler were able to fit the whole secondary structure predictions for the TMV vulgare protein into the chain path (Fig. 2), deduced from X-ray crystallographic data, electron microscopy, and the results from studies of the chemical, enzymatic, and immunological reactivity of various amino acid residues.

Studies have been carried out to localize antigenic determinants in the TMV (vulgare) coat protein sequence. The subject has been reviewed by Benjamini *et al.* (1972). The shortest peptide capable of binding to antibody against the coat protein was a synthetic penta-peptide Leu-Asp-Ala-Thr-Arg, corresponding to residues 108–112.

TABLE 1

Percent Difference between Sequences of TMV Coat Proteins[a]

	V	OM	D	CP	U2	HR
TMV vulgare	0	2	18	58	27	55
TMV OM	2	0	18	58	27	56
TMV dahlemense	18	18	0	59	30	54
TMV cowpea	58	58	59	0	60	63
TMV U2	27	27	30	60	0	55
TMV HR	55	56	54	63	55	0

[a] The data (from Dayhoff, 1972; except data for cowpea) are based on alignment in Fig. 1.

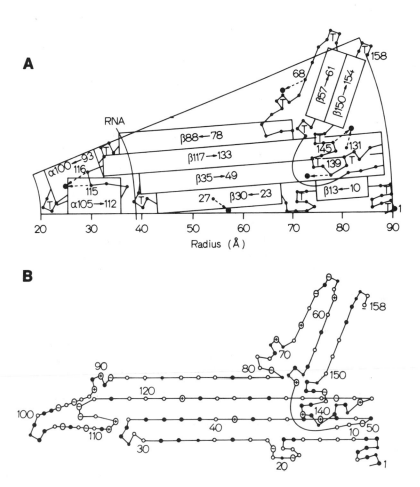

Fig. 2.   Final prediction of TMV polypeptide chain folding, with secondary structure assignments. Radial positions of residues are probably reliable, but azimuthal arrangements were chosen arbitrarily to illustrate the space available for the chain. Some compromises have been necessary to represent the three-dimensional structure in two dimensions. A: Block diagram of assignments and locations, with heavy atom positions represented by heavy dots and amino acid side chains extending toward these indicated by broken lines. B: Nature of the individual amino acid residues. Open circles represent hydrophobic residues (Ala, Ile, Leu, Phe, Trp, Val), and filled circles represent hydrophilic residues (Asn, Gln, Ser, Thr). Charged residues are indicated. Note the localization of the charged residues on the aqueous surfaces of the RNA-binding site and the hydrophobic nature of the protein between 4 nm and 6 nm, where the few hydrophilic residues present are largely amides. From Durham and Butler (1975) with the permission of the authors. [*Note added in proof:* More recent X-ray structures indicate α-helix, not β-sheet, for the four radial arrows (Durham, personal communication).]

2.2. Alfalfa Mosaic Virus

Alfalfa mosaic virus (AMV) has a bacilliform structure with the following dimensions: length 36–58 nm, diameter 18 nm (Smith, 1972). The RNA content ranges from 14% to 21% of total virion mass and the rest is protein. AMV has a multipartite genome (Jaspars, 1974) and the viral capsids of four different lengths contain four nucleoproteins consisting of one single species of protein subunit (Moed and Veldstra, 1968). A large number of antigenically related strains have been isolated and described. They can be differentiated on the basis of pathology of the disease and host range and by serological techniques (Hull, 1969). In addition, amino acid composition and C-terminal amino acid sequence data (Table 2) have been recommended to be used for strain characterization and differentiation. Based on differences in amino acid content and C-terminal sequences, Kraal (1975) divided the best-characterized AMV strains into three subgroups: (1) YSMV, P, A, S, AA-1; (2) 425, Tb-*ts1*; and (3) VRU, 15/64 (see Table 2).

TABLE 2

Comparison between the Amino Acid Compositions and C-Terminal Sequences of Coat Proteins from Nine Different AMV Strains[a]

Amino acid	AMV strain								
	425	Tb-*ts1*	15/64	VRU	YSMV	AA-1	S	P	A
Aspartic acid	211	21	23	22	20	20	20	20	20
Threonine	13	14	12	12	13	13	13	13	13
Serine	15	15	18	18	15	15	15	15	16
Glutamic acid	20	20	19	19	19	20	20	20	20
Proline	17	17	16	16	16	17	17	18	18
Glycine	17	17	16	16	17	18	17	17	17
Alanine	20	19	23	24	21	20	21	21	21
Cysteine	3	3	3	3	3	3	3	3	3
Valine	13	13	12	11	12	14	13	12	12
Methionine	3	3	3	3	3	3	3	3	3
Isoleucine	5	5	5	5	5	5	5	5	5
Leucine	21	21	23	23	22	22	23	21	21
Tyrosine	4	5	4	3	5	5	5	5	5
Phenylalanine	18	18	17	17	16	16	16	16	15
Tryptophan	2	2	2	2	2	2	2	2	2
Lysine	14	14	15	14	14	14	14	14	14
Histidine	7	6	6	7	6	6	6	6	6
Arginine	11	11	11	12	11	10	10	10	10
Total number of residues	224	224	228	227	220	223	223	221	221
C-terminal sequence	Arg-His	Arg-His	Ser-His	Ser-His					

[a] From Kraal (1975).

The complete amino acid sequences of the coat proteins of strain 425 (Kraal *et al.*, 1976) and strain S (Collot *et al.*, 1976) have been determined. The alignment of the sequences is given in Fig. 3. The coat-protein chain of the S strain is three residues shorter and contains only 11 amino acid substitutions, most of which may be explained by single point mutations in the respective RNA triplets. The most important structural features can be summarized as follows:

a. The N-terminal region is rich in basic amino acids and contains no dicarboxylic acids. The first acidic amino acid (Asp) appears at position 67 of the S strain sequence and at position 80 of the strain 425 coat protein. It has been suggested that this highly basic region may be involved in RNA binding.

b. The C-terminal region of the protein from both strains is strongly acidic.

c. A strongly hydrophobic region appears between residues 29 and 42.

It has been postulated (Kraal *et al.*, 1976) for the coat protein of strain 425 that α-helical regions represent 39% of the total protein chain (these appear between residues 22 and 31, 85 and 90, 116 and 123, 127 and 156, 164 and 175, 186 and 196, and 212 and 220) and β-sheet structures occupy approximately 23% (between residues 36 and 41, 49 and 57, 71 and 78, 91 and 100, 105 and 115, and 204 and 211).

2.3. Bromoviruses

The two serologically related members of the bromovirus group, brome mosaic virus (BMV) and cowpea chlorotic mottle virus (CCMV), are small spherical (icosahedron) viruses with a diameter (dry particle) of 25–26 nm and a particle weight of 4.6×10^6. The RNA content of both is approximately 22%, and the rest of the virion mass is protein. The virion is easily dissociated in the presence of 1 M NaCl at pH 7.0 to yield RNA and protein subunits. The single protein subunit has an approximate molecular weight of 19,000–20,000 (Bancroft, 1970; Fraenkel-Conrat, 1974; Smith, 1977).

The N terminus of both BMV and CCMV protein is acetylated. The C terminus is arginine for BMV and tyrosine for CCMV. The N-terminal amino acid sequences of both proteins as reported by Tremaine *et al.* (1972, 1977) are given in Fig. 4. Extensive sequence homology is apparent.

Strain 425:

Strain S:

```
        1                 5                  10                 15                 20                 25
AcSer-Ser-Ser-Gln-Lys-Lys-Ala-Gly-Gly-Lys-Pro-Thr-Lys-Arg-Ser-Gln-Asn-Tyr-Ala-Ala-Leu-Arg

        30                 35                 40                 45                 50
Lys-Ala-Gln-Leu-Pro-Lys-Pro-Ala-Leu-Lys-Val-Pro-Val-Lys-Pro-Thr-Asn-Thr-Ile-Leu-Pro-Gln-Thr-
                                                    Ala-

        55                 60                 65                 70                 75
Gly-Cys-Val-Trp-Gln-Ser-Leu-Gly-Thr-Pro-Leu-Ser-Ser-Phe-Asn-Gly-Leu-Gly-Ala-Arg-Phe-Leu-Thr-
     Ala-Val                                              Val

        80                 85                 90                 95                 100
Ser-Phe-Leu-Lys-Asp-Phe-Val-Gly-Pro-Arg-Ile-Leu-Glu-Glu-Asp-Leu-Ile-Tyr-Arg-Met-Val-Phe-Ser-Ile-Thr
              Thr

        105                110                115                120                125
Pro-Ser-His-Ala-Gly-Thr-Phe-Cys-Leu-Thr-Asp-Asp-Val-Thr-Glu-Asp-Gly-Arg-Ala-Val-Ala-His-Gly-Asn-
                                                                        Asp

        130                135                140                145                150
Pro-Met-Gln-Glu-Phe-Pro-His-Gly-Ala-Phe-His-Ala-Asn-Glu-Lys-Gly-Phe-Gly-Phe-Glu-Leu-Val-Phe-Thr-Ala-Pro-

        155                160                165                170                175
Thr-His-Ala-Gly-Met-Gln-Asn-Gln-Asn-Phe-Lys-His-Ser-Tyr-Ala-Val-Ala-Leu-Cys-Leu-Asp-Phe-Asp-Ala-Gln-
              Ser-                                                                           Glu

        180                185                190                195                200
Pro-Glu-Gly-Ser-Lys-Asn-Pro-Ser-Phe-Arg-Phe-Asn-Glu-Val-Trp-Val-Glu-Arg-Lys-Ala-Phe-Pro-Arg-Ala-Gly-
     Asp-

        205                210                215                220
Pro-Leu-Arg-Ser-Leu-Ile-Thr-Val-Gly-Leu-Phe-Asp-Glu-Ala-Asp-Asp-Leu-Asp-Arg-His
                        Leu-
```

Fig. 3. Complete amino acid sequences of alfalfa mosaic virus coat proteins (strains 425 and S).

```
              5                 10                 15                 20                 25
CCMV Ac-Ser-Thr-Val-Gly-Thr-Gly-Lys-Leu-Thr-Arg-Ala-Gln-Arg-Arg-Ala-Ala-Ala-Arg-Lys-Asn-Lys-Arg-Asn-Thr-Arg-

BMV  Ac-Ser-Thr-Ser-Gly-Thr-Gly-Lys-Met-Thr-Arg-Ala-Gln-Arg-Arg-Ala-Ala-Ala-Arg-Arg-Asn-Arg-Arg-Thr-Ala-Arg-
```

Fig. 4.   N-terminal sequences of bromovirus proteins.

2.4.   Turnip Yellow Mosaic Virus

Turnip yellow mosaic virus (TYMV) is a spherical particle with an average diameter of 28 nm. It contains 40% RNA. Little is known about number and location of genes on the RNA, except that the coat protein gene is at the 3′-terminal region of TYMV as well as of TMV RNA (see Chapter 4, Volume 2 of this series). The complete sequence of the single protein subunit of TYMV was determined by Stehelin *et al.* (1973) and is given in Fig. 5. The N-terminal methionine is acetylated.

3.   ANIMAL VIRUSES

3.1.   Influenza Virus

The hemagglutinin, which is the major protein component of the influenza virus envelope and represents about 30% of the total virus protein (Laver, 1973), has been one of the most thoroughly studied viral antigens among animal virus proteins and glycoproteins. The extensive serological studies were necessitated by antigenic drifts and shifts occurring in this family of viruses and causing difficulties in controlling human influenza by vaccination. The subject of antigenic variation has been reviewed in detail by Webster and Laver (1971). Influenza virus hemagglutinin is composed of two different glycosylated subunits with approximate molecular weights of 58,000 (heavy chain) and 26,000 (light chain). The subunits are generated by proteolytic cleavage from the primary gene product, a glycosylated precursor polypeptide, having an approximate molecular weight of 80,000 (Lazarowitz *et al.*, 1971; Skehel, 1972; Klenk *et al.*, 1972; Hay, 1974) and linked by disulfide bonds (Skehel and Schild, 1971; Laver, 1971) in the molecule. In addition to the immunological investigations, comparative primary structure studies were carried out primarily by Laver and Webster (1968, 1972, 1973; Laver *et al.*, 1974), who utilized peptide mapping in order to detect amino acid sequence differences and/or homology among

```
    1              5              10             15             20             25
Ac-Met-Glu-Ile-Asp-Lys-Glu-Leu-Ala-Pro-Gln-Asp-Arg-Thr-Val-Thr-Val-Ala-Thr-Val-Leu-Pro-Ala-Val-Pro-Gly-

                   30             35             40             45             50
Pro-Ser-Pro-Leu-Thr-Ile-Lys-Gln-Pro-Phe-Gln-Ser-Glu-Val-Leu-Phe-Ala-Gly-Thr-Lys-Asp-Ala-Glu-Ala-Ser-

                   55             60             65             70             75
Leu-Thr-Ile-Ala-Asn-Ile-Asp-Ser-Val-Ser-Thr-Leu-Thr-Thr-Phe-Tyr-Arg-His-Ala-Ser-Leu-Glu-Ser-Leu-Trp-

                   80             85             90             95             100
Val-Thr-Ile-His-Pro-Thr-Leu-Gln-Ala-Pro-Thr-Phe-Pro-Thr-Val-Gly-Val-Cys-Trp-Val-Pro-Ala-Asn-Ser-

                   105            110            115            120            125
Pro-Val-Thr-Pro-Ala-Gln-Ile-Thr-Lys-Thr-Tyr-Gly-Gly-Gln-Ile-Phe-Cys-Ile-Gly-Gly-Ala-Ile-Asn-Thr-Leu-

                   130            135            140            145            150
Ser-Pro-Leu-Ile-Val-Lys-Cys-Pro-Leu-Glu-Met-Met-Asn-Pro-Arg-Val-Lys-Asp-Ser-Ile-Gln-Tyr-Leu-Asp-Ser-

                   155            160            165            170            175
Pro-Lys-Leu-Leu-Ile-Ser-Ile-Thr-Ala-Gln-Pro-Thr-Ala-Pro-Ala-Ser-Thr-Cys-Ile-Ile-Thr-Val-Ser-Gly-

                   180            185
Tnr-Leu-Ser-Met-His-Ser-Pro-Leu-Ile-Thr-Asp-Thr-Ser-Thr
```

Fig. 5.   Complete sequence of turnip yellow mosaic virus.

existing and newly isolated strains of influenza virus. The results of fingerprint analyses were generally in good agreement with immunological findings indicating relationship. In addition, peptide mapping provided clear-cut evidence for recombination events leading to the appearance of new pandemic strains of human influenza. Laver and Webster (1973) showed, for example, that the heavy and light chains of the HA subunits of the Hong Kong strain, which differed greatly from those of three A2/Asian strains isolated before Hong Kong influenza appeared (Laver and Webster, 1972), had amino acid sequences similar to those of influenza virus strains isolated from horses and ducks. While the heavy chains showed some differences, the light polypeptide chains of those three viruses were found to be almost identical. These authors were able to conclude that the Hong Kong strain of human influenza arose by genetic recombination under natural conditions probably between A2/Asian human influena virus and a mammalian or avian strain (Laver and Webster, 1973).

Short N-terminal amino acid sequences for the HA subunits of several strains of influenza virus (including both types A and B) were determined by Skehel and Waterfield (1975). The data shown in Fig. 6 clearly indicate that a high degree of sequence homology between the HA2 (light-chain) subunits of the major subgroups of human type A influenza viruses exists at the N-terminal region. Only a single amino acid substitution is shown in position 12 of the sequence of HA2

Subunit HA2

```
                             1              5              10
Type A   0/Bel/42        Gly-Leu-Phe-Gly-Ala-Ile-Ala-Gly-Phe-Ile-Glx-Gly-Gly-
         1/Weiss/57      Gly-Leu-Phe-Gly-Ala-Ile-Ala-Gly-Phe-Ile-Glx-Gly-Gly-
         2/Singapore/57  Gly-Leu-Phe-Gly-Ala-Ile-Ala-Gly-Phe-Ile-Glx-Gly-
         X-31            Gly-Leu-Phe-Gly-Ala-Ile-Ala-Gly-Phe-Ile- ? -Asx-
         MRC-11          Gly-Leu-Phe-Gly-Ala-Ile-Ala-Gly-Phe-Ile-Glx-Asx-
                                  └─────────→      ←────────────┘

                                        PALINDROME
                                         ──→  ←──
Type B/Lee               Gly-Phe-Phe-Gly-Ala-Ile-Ala-Gly-Phe-Leu-Glx-Gly-Gly-
```

Subunit HA1

```
Type A   0/Bel/42        Asp-Thr-Ile-Ser-Ile-Gly-Tyr-His-Ala-Asx-
         1/Weiss/57      Asn-Thr-Ile-Ser-Ile-Gly-Tyr-His-Ala-Asx-
         2/Singapore/57  Asn-Glu-Ile-Ser-Ile-Gly-Tyr-His-Ala-Asx-
```

Precursor

```
Type A   0/Bel/42        Asx-Thr-Ile-
```

Fig. 6.   N-terminal amino acid sequences of influenza virus hemagglutinin subunits and precursor. Amino acid residues that differ from those of type AO are underlined.

subunit of X-31 and MRC-11 strains. Similarly, the N terminus of the HA2 of type B virus is highly homologous, showing only two conservative substitutions, positions 2 (leucine to phenylalanine) and 10 (isoleucine for leucine), when compared with sequences of type A. The sequence of HA1 (heavy-chain) subunits of the three type A viruses are also almost identical at least up to residue 10, and only a single substitution occurs in position 2 of A2/Singapore/57 where threonine is exchanged to glutamic acid. The sequences of the heavy- and light-chain subunits are unique. The sequence of the hemagglutinin precursor is the same as that of HA1. Thus the gene order and the order of biosynthesis of the precursor is NH_2-HA1-HA2-COOH.

Two additional interesting features of the HA2 sequences have been pointed out by Skehel and Waterfield: (1) "The first 10 residues are all uncharged and apart from the glycine residues are hydrophobic" and (2) "The sequence forms a palindrome of seven residues centered on the isoleucine residue at position 6" (types A and B both). In the sequences of type A HA2 subunits "this structure can be extended to nine residues if the conservative substitution of leucine for isoleucine at positions 2 and 10 is included." The authors have speculated that this hydrophobic palindrome sequence may represent a specific recognition site for the enzyme responsible for the cleavage of the precursor to generate the two subunits.

Bucher *et al.* (1976) determined the N-terminal sequence of hemagglutinin subunits of the recombinant influenza virus strain Heq1N2. The sequence of HA_2 through the first ten residues was identical to that given in Fig. 6 for other type A influenza viruses. Between residues 11 and 24 the sequence was found to be as follows:

11   24
-Glu-Asn-Gly-Trp-Glu-Gly-Leu-Ile-Asp-Gly-X-Tyr-Gly-Tyr-

The HA_1 polypeptide sequence

1   10
Asp-Lys-Ile-Ser-Leu-Gly-Tyr-His-Ala-Val-

shows only three or four different amino acids out of the first ten residues when compared to HA_1 from 0, 1, and 2 subtypes (see Fig. 6).

3.2. Picornaviruses

In the mammalian picornavirus group amino acid sequences (both N-terminal and C-terminal) for the proteins of mengovirus and of several serotypes of foot-and-mouth disease virus (FMDV) were determined.

The four major capsid polypeptides of mengovirus, α (MW 32,500), β (MW 29,600), γ (MW 23,700), and δ (MW 7,350), which are generated by posttranslational cleavage of a larger precursor polyprotein, were studied by Ziola and Scraba (1976). The N- and C-terminal sequences of these proteins as determined by these authors are given in Table 3.

Based on the sequence of events involved in the posttranslational processing of mengovirus polypeptides previously elucidated by Paucha *et al.* (1974) and the amino acid sequence data, Ziola and Scraba suggested that a virus-coded protease with specificity for peptide bonds involving the carbonyl function of glutamine may cleave the precursor polyprotein to yield γ and α capsid polypeptides and an intermediate product, ϵ (MW 39,000), which is subsequently cleaved by another enzyme at the alanylasparagine bond to yield capsid polypeptides δ and β. The following scheme was proposed for the peptide order in the precursor and for the hypothetical cleavage sites (the N-terminal end is blocked):

$$HN-\delta-Ala-Asp-\beta-Gln-Ser-\gamma-Gln-Gly-\alpha-LeuOH$$

Matheka and Bachrach (1975) studied three serotypes of FMDV. The N-terminal sequences of the three major proteins VP1, VP2, and VP3 of types A_{12}, O_1, and C_3 are given in Table 4. Proteins VP1 and VP3 of each virus type show common initial sequences and VP2 of each strain has asparagine as its N terminus.

The C-terminal sequences of the proteins of FMDV A_{12} were found to be -Ser-Gln for VP1 and -Glu-Ala-Leu for VP3 (Bachrach *et al.*, 1973).

TABLE 3
N- and C-Terminal Amino Acid Sequences of the Major Capsid Polypeptides of Mengovirus

Polypeptide	N-terminal sequence	C-terminal sequence
δ	Blocked	-Leu-Leu-Ala
β	Asp-Gln-Asn-Thr-Glu-Glu-Met-Glu-Asn-Leu	-(Val,Leu)-Arg-Gln
γ	Ser-Pro-Ile-Pro-Val-Thr-Ile-Arg-Glu-His	-(Gln)
α	Gly-Val-Glu-Asn-Ala-Glu-Lys-Gly-Val-Thr-	-(Val,Gly,Ala)-Val-Leu

TABLE 4

N-Terminal Amino Acid Sequences of FMDV Proteins

Virus type	VP1	VP2	VP3
A_{12} strain 119	Gly-Ile-(Phe,Pro,Val)-	(Asp,X,Met)-	Thr-Thr-Ala-Thr-
O_1 brugge	Gly-(Ile,Phe)-	Asp-	Thr-Thr-Ser-
C_3	Gly-Ile-Phe-	Asp-Leu-	Thr-Thr-

The nature and uniformity of the N termini among picornavirus structural proteins (glycine, asparagine, aspartic acid, serine, and threonine were commonly found) allowed Bachrach to postulate that posttranslational cleavages of the viral precursor polyproteins occur most frequently at protease-sensitive β bends (1977).

3.3. Reovirus

Attempts have been made to obtain sequence information on reovirus capsids, which were shown to contain seven polypeptides. Three of them are present in the outer shell: $\mu2$ (MW 72,000), $\delta1$ (MW 43,000), and $\delta3$ (MW 34,000). The core itself is composed of four polypeptides: $\lambda1$ (MW 155,000), $\lambda2$ (MW 140,000), $\mu1$ (MW 80,000), and $\delta2$ (MW 36,000). It appears that all these proteins are primary gene products except $\mu2$, which has been shown to be derived from $\mu1$ by proteolytic cleavage (Smith *et al.*, 1969). All but $\mu2$ were found to have a blocked N terminus. The N-terminal sequence of $\mu2$ was found to be Pro-Gly-Gly-Val-Pro (Pett *et al.*, 1973), again an illustration that N-terminal proline can simulate N-terminal (acetyl?-) blocking (see TMV).

3.4. Nuclear Polyhedrosis Virus

The partial amino acid sequences of tryptic peptides of the polyhedral protein of the nuclear polyhedrosis virus of mulberry silkworm (*Bombyx mori*) have been determined by Levitina *et al.* (1974). They found 28 peptides with unique sequence which could account for the 240 amino acid residues of the protein having a molecular weight of ~28,000. The order of the tryptic peptides in the protein, however, was not determined.

3.5. Hepatitis B Virus

Partial N- and C-terminal sequences of the two major component polypeptides of hepatitis B surface antigen (HBSAg) have been reported by Peterson *et al.* (1977). HBSAg, which appears in the electron microscope as a 20-nm spherical particle (one of the three possible forms) and is composed of lipid, carbohydrate, and protein, was dissociated in the presence of sodium dodecylsulfate and 2-mercaptoethanol. Two major components, polypeptides I (MW 22,000) and II (MW 28,000), were resolved subsequently by polyacrylamide gel electrophoresis. These subunits were shown to have identical amino acid composition (same as the intact antigen; see Table 5) and identical C-terminal sequences: -Val-Tyr-Ile. The N-terminal regions of the protein chains were also found to be identical, at least up to nine residues, with the following amino acid sequence:

Met-Glu-Asn-Ile-Thr-Ser(Cys)-Gly-Phe-Leu-

Only polypeptide II, the larger subunit, contained carbohydrate. Based on the above chemical data, the authors concluded that the glycosylated

TABLE 5

**Amino Acid Composition of HBSAg and Its
Subunits**

Amino acid	HBSAg (mol %)	Polypeptides (mol %)	
		I	II
Aspartic acid	5.0	5.6	5.7
Threonine	7.8	8.4	8.6
Serine	11.7	11.9	13.0
Glutamic acid	5.0	5.8	5.7
Proline	12.8	12.5	10.6
Glycine	7.2	6.1	6.6
Alanine	3.4	3.5	3.3
Half-cystine	6.8	7.2	7.0
Valine	4.7	4.1	3.9
Methionine	3.2	3.0	3.1
Isoleucine	5.6	5.7	5.1
Leucine	11.9	11.2	10.9
Tyrosine	2.2	2.4	2.3
Phenylalanine	5.1	4.9	5.1
Lysine	2.2	2.2	2.0
Histidine	0.6	0.7	0.6
Arginine	2.4	2.2	2.1

and unglycosylated protein subunits of HBSAg contain a homologous if not identical polypeptide chain and suggested the possibility that the same gene of the hepatitis B virus genome may code for the protein chain of both subunits. These results are in contrast to previous reports assuming that HBSAg consists of two structurally completely different protein subunits (Gerin *et al.*, 1971; Vyas *et al.*, 1972).

3.6.   Papovaviruses

Papovaviruses have been isolated from mice, rabbits, rhesus and stumptail macaques, and humans. The primate isolates show genetic relationship inferred from cross-reactivity between the nonstructural T antigens (Shah *et al.*, 1975; Takemoto and Martin, 1976; Walker *et al.*, 1973). No such cross-reactivity has been detected between nonprimate and primate groups, and conventional nucleic acid hybridization has not revealed any relationships between groups. More recently, Shah *et al.* (1977) have shown that antisera to disrupted virus or the denatured purified major polypeptide designated VP1 were capable of detecting relationship between SV40 (rhesus origin) and polyoma (mouse origin). The cross-reactivity extended to other members of the papova group, including the human BK virus, the rabbit vacuolating virus, and the stumptail macaque virus.

Among the three major capsid proteins of simian virus 40 (SV40), VP1 (MW 48,000) was found to have the following N-terminal sequence:

Ala-Pro-Thr-Lys-Arg-Lys-Gly-

VP3 (MW 30,000) is probably blocked at the N terminus. VP1 of polyoma virus also starts with the Ala-Pro- sequence. This may be indicative of sequence homology around the cleavage site of a hypothetical precursor (Lazarides *et al.*, 1974). More extensive homology is likely, based on the immunological data described above.

3.7.   Adenovirus

The N-terminal amino acid sequence of adenovirus type 2 hexon protein was determined by Jörnvall *et al.* (1974*a*), who used purified ^{14}C-labeled protein and found that the N terminus is acetylated. The sequence of the radioactive N-terminal peptide obtained by cleaving the

protein with chymotrypsin and thermolysin was determined by mass spectrometry to be acetyl-Ala-Thr-Pro-Ser-.

The C-terminal peptide of the hexon subunit was found to have the following sequence (Jörnvall *et al.*, 1974*b*):

-Thr-Pro-Phe-Ser-Ala-Gly-Asn-Ala-Thr-Thr

The sequences of additional tryptic and chymotryptic peptides corresponding to more than one-tenth of the total length of the hexon subunit (MW 100,000–120,000) were also determined by Jörnvall *et al.* (1974*b*).

A basic, histonelike polypeptide of adenovirus type 2, core protein VII, has been sequenced by Lischwe and Sung (1977). The N-terminal sequence obtained by automated Edman degradation is shown in Fig. 7. The authors pointed out that, similarly to histones, especially to H4, this highly basic viral core protein also has a region at the amino end which is rich in basic amino acids. The sequence shows two clusters of basic residues, the first extending from residues 2 to 5 and the second from positions 23 to 27. It was also noted that between these two clusters the basic residues, histidine and arginine, are placed at nearly regular intervals (see Fig. 7, positions 8, 11, 13, 15, and 17), resulting in an apparently nonrandom distribution of basic amino acids. Similar basic cluster and nonrandom distribution of cationic residues has been observed in H4, an arginine-rich, highly "sequence-conserved" histone and component of eukaryotic chromatin. On the basis of these findings the authors suggested the possibility that the basic N-terminal region of core protein VII may also serve as a DNA combining site in the adenovirus chromatin.

3.8. Retroviruses

The RNA-containing viruses which replicate via a DNA intermediate and contain a virion-bound RNA-dependent DNA polymerase

```
1              5                10                15                20
Ala-Lys-Lys-Arg-Ser-Asp-Glu-His-Pro-Val-Arg-Val-Arg-Gly-His-Tyr-Arg-Ala-Pro-Trp
               25                30                35                40
Gly- x -His-Ly -Arg-Gly-Arg-Thr-Gly-Arg-Thr-Thr-Val-Asx-Asx- x -Ile-Asx- x -Val-
```

Fig. 7. N-terminal amino acid sequence of human adenovirus type 2 core protein VII. x Represents Ala or Ser.

(reverse transcriptase) are grouped together in the family Retroviridae. Members of this family are responsible for a wide variety of pathogenic effects in their natural hosts, ranging from leukemia/sarcoma (type C viruses), carcinoma (type B viruses), neurological disorders (visna, maedi), anemia (equine infectious anemia virus), to no known disease (foamy viruses, type D viruses which include langur, squirrel monkey, and Mason-Pfizer virus). Another unclassified retrovirus, the bovine leukemia virus, is associated with the adult form of lymphosarcoma in cattle. Some of these viruses can exist both as endogenous inherited genomes in their natural hosts and as conventional horizontally transmitted viruses with no evidence of representation in host cell DNA. There are also examples of DNA sequences partially related to those of a normally horizontally transmitted virus in the host of origin (e.g., feline leukemia virus in cats). Thus, taken as a family, this is an extremely diverse group with multiple host–virus relationships and few general principles in terms of pathogenic potential. Accumulating evidence indicates that type C viruses recombine with host cell genes to form pathogenic variants. Whether this will prove to be a generality for the other retroviruses remains to be established. Thus this family of viruses is important in terms both of association with disease in known systems and of providing model systems for study of malignant transformation. (See Chapter 8, Volume 9, and Chapter 5, Volume 10 of this series for in-depth discussions of this topic.)

With increased emphasis on these viruses generated by the discovery of reverse transcriptase (Baltimore, 1970; Temin and Mizutani, 1970), a number of laboratories have conducted studies on interviral relationships using immunological methods (see reviews by Gilden, 1975; Oroszlan and Gilden, 1978a; Stephenson et al., 1978). Such studies have delineated relationships among the mammalian type C viruses and most recently a group designated type D (Colcher et al., 1977; Hino et al., 1977). The availability of purified structural components of virions and appropriate antisera has allowed the development of "interspecies" test systems which intrinsically can detect more diverse relationships than possible in single homologous assays. This approach has detected some unexpected relationships crossing genera in the case of an envelope glycoprotein relationship between gp70s of baboon type C virus, RD114, and the group D retroviruses (Stephenson et al., 1976). Since immunological cross-reactivity is a composite of conformational and sequence-specific determinants, without precise information on the nature of the cross-reactive components one has no clear information on the degree of genetic relationship underlying these reactions. While some general rules of the relationship of primary structure to immunological cross-reactivity have been derived from studies of model proteins (Sarich and Wilson, 1967), these generalities are subject to great variation depending on the particular system studied and the availability of appropriate reagents.

To place relationships inferred from immunological studies on a firm basis, one obviously needs primary structure information. In addition to establishing quantitative relationships among related (or suspected related) proteins in various viruses, the data obtained by sequence analysis are potentially useful in the design of specific probes for immunoassays with the possibility of detecting distantly related molecules. The logic for this is that conserved regions are often internal and not antigenic in the native molecule. Forced antibody production against highly conserved regions of protein homologues could thus provide a reagent of much broader utility than that produced with the native molecule. This approach is currently under study with the type C virus structural proteins (Oroszlan and Gilden, 1978a).

The type C RNA tumor virus genome has a capacity of coding for an approximately 3×10^5-dalton protein sequence. Virion component translational products have been identified for three viral genes designated *gag* (group-specific antigen), *env* (envelope glycoprotein), and *pol* (RNA-dependent DNA polymerase) (Baltimore, 1975). The *gag* gene of a type C virus isolate of mouse origin has been shown to code for a precursor polyprotein which is subsequently cleaved by proteolytic enzymes, giving rise to four internal structural proteins (see reviews by Oroszlan and Gilden, 1978a; Stephenson *et al.*, 1978). Based on approximate molecular weights (in thousands), these antigenically distinct proteins have been designated p30, p15, p12, and p10 (August *et al.*, 1974). The gene order has been shown to be NH_2-p15-p12-p30-p10-COOH (Barbacid *et al.*, 1976; Reynolds and Stephenson, 1977).

Studies of primary structure relationships by sequencing techniques have until recently been restricted to a single protein homologue of the mammalian type C viruses, the ~30,000-dalton protein designated p30. Previous to studies from the authors' laboratory, partial sequences (Fig. 8) of two avian type C viral proteins designated

```
          1          5              10             15             20
p27    Pro-Val-Val-Ile-Lys-Thr-Glu-Gly-Pro-Ala-Trp-Thr-Pro-Leu-Glu-Pro-Lys-Leu-Ile-Thr-Arg-Leu-Ala

                         Glu
p15    Leu-Ala-Met-Thr-Met-Thr-His-Lys-Asp-Arg-Pro-Leu-Val-Arg-Val-Ile-Leu-Thr-Ser-Thr-Gly-Ser-His-Pro-Val
```

Fig. 8.   N-terminal sequence of avian type C virus internal proteins.

gsa and gsb (p27 and p15, respectively, by current terminology) had been obtained by Niall *et al.* (1970). The mammalian type C virus p30s had shown cross-reactive determinants as established by both immunodiffusion and radioimmunoassays, and they have been found to be compositionally similar (Oroszlan *et al.*, 1975*b*). The amino acid compositional data are shown in Table 6. The primary sequence data of the N-terminal regions (Oroszlan *et al.*, 1975*b*, 1977) clearly provided support for the immunological findings. For example, comparison of 25–30 residues of the p30s of a variety of murine leukemia virus (MuLV) serotypes showed only a single residue difference (Fig. 9). This is consistent with the high degree of relationship seen in immunoassays where MuLV p30 is essentially group specific in reactivity. Yet differences may be seen in appropriate tests, and these slight differences are also revealed by peptide mapping techniques (Oroszlan *et al.*, 1974). In contrast to the near identity among the MuLV p30s, this homology in other mammalian viruses shows considerable variation, yet with strong evidence of homology with MuLV p30. As shown in Fig. 9, following the initial tripeptide Pro-Leu-Arg, common to all mammalian type C virus p30s, the region of residues 4–10 is highly variable, containing as many as five differences between viruses from different species. At position 11 and beyond, all the p30s show a region of homology, the length of which has not yet been determined. The sequence data in Fig. 9 also show evidence of three subgroupings of the p30s based on alignment to MuLV p30. The baboon and RD114 (endogenous cat) viruses show a single gap occurring as indicated and delineating these p30s as distinct from all others. The sequence identity is consistent with all other evidence indicating a close relationship between these two viruses and the potential origin of RD114 from an Old World monkey progenitor in the remote past (Benveniste *et al.*, 1974; Sherr *et al.*, 1975; Stephenson and Aaronson, 1977). The p30s of gibbon ape and woolly monkey viruses form another distinctive group based on the requirement for two insertions totaling seven residues (our hypothesis) to align with MuLV p30 (Oroszlan *et al.*, 1977). Note that when this alignment is made the GaLV group of viruses shows more homology to MuLV than to FeLV or other p30s. This is consistent with the hybridization data of Benveniste *et al.* (1974), suggesting origin from a *Mus* progenitor in the remote past. The p30s of mouse (MuLV), rat (RaLV), and cat (FeLV) seem to align without evidence for insertions or deletions in the N-terminal region. Thus, based on the data of the baboon and GaLV groups, these seem to constitute a distinctive subgrouping. In this regard, immunological data obtained by radioim-

TABLE 6

Amino Acid Composition of Mammalian Type C Virus p30s

Amino acid	Number of residues per 30,000 MW[a]								
	R-MuLV[c]	AKR[c]	G-MuLV[f]	WMuLV[e]	RadLV[e]	M-MuLV[c]	FeLV[a]	RD114[d]	SSAV[g]
Lysine	15	16	16	16	16	16	13	17	14
Histidine	4	3	3	3	3	4	4	4	4
Arginine	29	27	31	27	28	25	22	22	29
Aspartic acid	31	28	30	30	28	30	23	22	30
Threonine	14[b]	16[b]	17	13[b]	15	16[b]	14[b]	19[b]	13
Serine	12[b]	12[b]	14	13[b]	15	13[b]	14[b]	13[b]	14
Glutamic acid	44	48	49	47	46	48	50	46	46
Proline	19	18	17	19	17	17	23	22	17
Glycine	17	17	18	17	17	17	11	14	17
Alanine	13	14	14	14	13	16	20	21	15
Half-cystine	1[h]	1[h]	—	1[h]	—	1[h]	1[h]	1[h]	—
Valine	8	9	10	8	9	9	10	9	7
Methionine	2[i]	2[i]	2	2[h]	2	2[h]	2[h]	4[h]	2
Isoleucine	7	5	5	7	6	7	7	9	6
Leucine	32	33	33	33	35	30	37	31	35
Tyrosine	7	7	7	7	7	7	6	6	7
Phenylalanine	6	6	5	6	7	6	7	8	6
Total	261	262	271	264	263	264	264	268	262

[a] Abbreviations as in caption of Fig. 9. Also RadLV, radiation leukemia virus; SSAV, simian sarcoma associated virus (woolly monkey).

[b] Corrected for hydrolytic losses by extrapolation to zero time.

[c] Based on a single complete analysis.

[d] Based on a duplicate complete analysis.

[e] Based on a single analysis without performic acid oxidation.

[f] Based on a single 24-hr hydrolysis. THR and SER corrected by 5% and 10%, respectively, to account for hydrolytic losses.

[g] Based on a duplicate 24-hr hydrolysis. THR and SER corrected by 5% and 10%, respectively, to account for hydrolytic losses.

[h] Determined as cysteic acid.

[i] Determined as methionine sulfone.

```
                      1                 5                  10                 15                 20                 25
CAT
FeLV       Pro-Leu-Arg-Glu-Gly-Pro-Asn-Asn-Arg-Pro-Gln-Tyr-Trp-Pro-Phe-Ser-Ala-Ser-Asp-Leu-Tyr-Tyr-Asn-Trp-Lys-Ser-
RD114      Pro-Leu-Arg-Thr- * -Val-Asn-Arg-Thr-Val-Gln-Tyr-Trp-Pro-Phe-Ser-Ala-Ser-Asp-Leu-Tyr-Asn-Trp-Lys-Thr-

BABOON
BAB8-K     Pro-Leu-Arg-Thr- * -Val-Asn-Arg-Thr-Val-Gln-Tyr-Trp- X -Phe

MOUSE
R-MuLV     Pro-Leu-Arg-Leu-Gly-Asn-Gly-Gly-Leu-Leu-Tyr-Trp-Pro-Phe-Ser-Ser-Asp-Leu-Tyr-Asn-Trp-Lys
AKR        Pro-Leu-Arg-Leu-Gly-Gly-Gly-Gln-Leu-Gln-Tyr-Trp-Pro-Phe-Ser-Ser-Asp-Leu-Tyr
G-MuLV     Pro-Leu-Arg-Leu-Gly-Gly-Gln-Leu-Gln-Tyr-Trp-Pro-Phe-Ser-Ser-Asp-Leu-Tyr
WMuLV      Pro-Leu-Arg-Ser-Gly-Gly-Gln-Leu-Gln-Tyr-Trp-Pro-Phe-Ser-Ser-Asp-Leu-Tyr-Asn-Trp-Lys
SLV        Pro-Leu-Arg-Ala-Gly-Gly-Gln-Leu-Gln-Tyr-Trp-Pro-Phe-Ser-Ser-Asp-Leu-Tyr-Asn-Trp-Lys
M-MuLV     Pro-Leu-Arg-Ala-Gly-Gly-Gln-Leu-Gln-Tyr-Trp-Pro-Phe-Ser-Ser-Asp-Leu-Tyr

RAT
MSV (RaLV) Pro-Leu-Arg-Gln-Gly-Gly-Ala- X -Gly- X -Met-Gln-Tyr-Trp- X -Phe

GIBBON APE
GaLV*      Pro-Leu-Arg-Ala-Ile-Gly-Asn-Gly-Pro-Leu-Gln-Tyr-Trp-Pro-Phe-Ser- X -Ala-Asp-Leu-Tyr
                                              (-Leu-Val-)
                                              (-Pro-Pro-Ala-Glu-Pro-)

                      30
CAT
FeLV       His-Asx-Pro-Pro-Phe
RD114      His-Asn-Pro- X -Phe
```

Fig. 9. N-terminal amino acid sequences of p30s from several type C RNA viruses. Abbreviations: FeLV, feline leukemia virus; RD114, endogenous feline type C virus; BAB8-K, baboon type C virus; R-MuLV, Rauscher murine leukemia virus; AKR, AKR mouse leukemia virus; G-MuLV, Gross leukemia virus; WMuLV, wild mouse leukemia virus; SLV, Scripps leukemia virus; M-MuLV, Moloney murine leukemia virus; MSV (RaLV), rat type C virus; and GaLV, gibbon ape type C virus. *, The sequence of woolly monkey type C virus (SSAV) is identical. X, Unidentified.

munoassay procedures are consistent with these p30s forming a distinctive subgroup. To date only short sequences are available for the expected p30 homologue in non-type C viruses. These are given in Table 7. The distinguishing feature of these sequences is the common N-terminal proline, followed by a nonpolar residue (valine, leucine, isoleucine). This could indicate conservation of a progenitor cleavage site utilized in the generation of the component polypeptides from the *gag* gene polyprotein precursor. Thus, as a generality, the p30 sequences give good support to grouping based on the immunological or morphological criteria for grouping viruses. Insufficient data are available at present to test the hypothesis that the major proteins of non-type C retroviruses in the 25,000–30,000 range are related to the type C p30s. The immunological data showing lack of relationship are not conclusive based on inherent limitations of sensitivity of these techniques. The sequence similarity of the suspected cleavage site (see below) leads us to suspect such a relationship.

In addition to p30, the p10s apparently form a clearly related group, similar to the p30s, based on immunological cross-reactivity and binding to single-stranded DNA (Long *et al.*, 1977). Thus no distinction among MuLV serotypes could be made either in gel diffusion or immunoassays. To date N-terminal sequences are available for the three MuLV serotypes AKR, R-MuLV, and M-MuLV (Oroszlan *et al.*, 1978). As shown in Fig. 10, these sequences are identical through the initial 10–18 residues.

The p12 component of the *gag* gene of MuLV is highly type specific in immunoassays (see review by Stephenson *et al.*, 1978) and

TABLE 7

N-Terminal Sequences of the Major Internal Proteins (p24-p30) of Several Retroviruses

Virus[a]	Sequence of
Type C	
avian	Pro-Val-Val-
mammalian	Pro-Leu-Arg-
MMTV	Pro-Val-Val-
MPMV	Pro-Val-Thr-
BLV	Pro-Ile-Ile
Visna	Pro-Ile-Val-

[a] Abbreviations: MMTV, mouse mammary tumor virus; MPMV, Mason-Pfizer monkey virus; BLV, bovine leukemia virus.

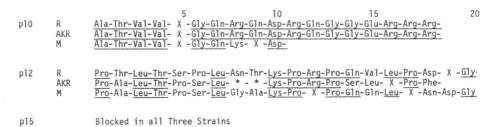

Fig. 10. N-terminal amino acid sequences of R-MuLV, AKR-MuLV, and M-MuLV *gag*-gene-coded proteins. The sequences for p30, the fourth *gag* gene product, are given in Fig. 9.

has the important property of binding to homologous viral RNA in a highly specific manner (Sen *et al.*, 1976, 1977). Sequence analysis of three MuLV serotypes has revealed clear evidence of homology but also a high degree of individuality (Fig. 10). The differences seen among the AKR, R-MuLV, and M-MuLV sequences show a 50% difference in the N-terminal region. Such a difference easily accounts for the type specificity seen in the function and immunoassay. One future plan is to determine if a synthetic region of p12 will substitute for the whole molecule in RNA binding studies. The p12s are phosphoproteins in most type C viruses, with the exception of the baboon and RD114 viruses, where a component of 15,000 daltons exhibits this property (Pal *et al.*, 1975), and the other properties of MuLV p12. Since p15 in MuLV and p12 in baboon viruses both have blocked N termini (Oroszlan *et al.*, 1978), the differences in molecular weight appear to be based on shifts in cleavage sites. The *gag* gene components thus show substantial agreement between immunoassays and primary sequence data in a qualitative sense.

The C-terminal amino acid sequences of MuLV proteins derived from the *gag*-gene-coded precursor polyprotein have also been determined (Oroszlan *et al.*, 1978) and are shown in Table 8. These findings combined with the N-terminal sequence data and the reported peptide order in the precursor permitted us to postulate possible proteolytic cleavage sites (Oroszlan *et al.*, 1978) for the posttranslational processing of this precursor (Fig. 11). This model is based on the assumption that proteolytic cleavage of the polyprotein between the C terminus of p15 and the N terminus of p10 occurs only at three sites to yield the four final *gag* gene products, p15, p12, p30, and p10, and that excision of any amino acid residues does not occur during processing. It is further assumed that the cleaved gene products are not altered by proteolytic enzymes during their purification. The peptide bond

TABLE 8
C-Terminal Amino Acid Sequences of R-MuLV and AKR-MuLV *gag* Gene Products

Protein		
R-MuLV	AKR-MuLV	C-terminal sequence[a]
p30		-Lys-Leu-Leu
	p30	-Leu
p15		-Leu-Tyr
	p15	-(Ala,X)-Phe
p12		-Ala- X -Phe
	p12	-(Ala,X)-Phe

[a] In the sequences the letter "X" indicates the presence of one out of three possible amino acid residues, i.e., Ser, Asn, or Gln.

hydrolyzed between MuLV p15 and p12 is tyrosylproline, between p12 and p30, phenylalanylproline, and between p30 and p10, leucylalanine, according to the scheme proposed in Fig. 11.

Thus far, significant sequence data are available for the envelope gene products of one serotype of MuLV, namely R-MuLV. The sequence of 46 residues (Fig. 12) was obtained by Dr. L. Hood (personal communication) on a preparation from this laboratory. We had previously determined approximately 20 residues of this glycoprotein (gp70) with identical results (Henderson *et al.*, 1978). For comparative purposes only a short sequence of the AKR virus has been determined

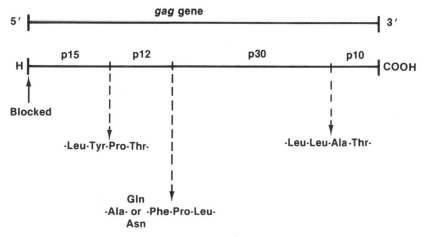

Fig. 11. Proposed order of *gag* gene products in R-MuLV precursor polyprotein and possible cleavage sites.

```
                     5                  i0                15               20              25
gp70    Ala-Ala-Pro-Gly-Ser-Ser-Pro-His-Gln-Val-Tyr- X -Ile-Thr-Trp-Glu-Val-Thr-Asn-Gly-Asp- ? -Glu-Thr-Val-

gp45    Ala-Ala-Pro-Gly-Ser-Ser-Pro-His-Gln-Val-Tyr- X -Ile-Thr-Trp-Glu-Val

                    30                 35                40               45
gp70    Trp-Ala-Ile-Ser-Gly-Asn(His)Pro-Leu(Trp)Thr-Gly-Phe-Ser-Val(Glu)Tyr-Pro-Asp-Ser(Ala)
```

Fig. 12. N-terminal amino acid sequences of R-MuLV *env* gene products, glycoproteins gp70 and gp45.

which gave identical results through only five residues determined with RLV gp70. A minor glycoprotein component of approximately 45,000 molecular weight has also been noted in certain type C virions. Based on immunological data we concluded that for R-MuLV this was highly related to gp70 (Marquardt *et al.* 1977; Charman *et al.*, 1977). In fact, the N-terminal sequence is identical to gp70 (Fig. 12); however, amino

TABLE 9

Amino Acid Analysis of gp45 and gp70

	gp45[a]		gp70[b]	
Amino acid	Residues per protein	Nearest integer	Residues per protein	Nearest integer
Aspartic acid	33.73	34	38.50	39
Threonine	28.44	28	44.77	45
Serine	32.66	33	37.05	37
Glutamic acid	23.81	24	30.09	30
Proline	47.23	47	53.68	54
Glycine	31.99	32	37.72	38
Alanine	17.93	18	24.57	25
Valine	17.01	17	28.33	28
Methionine	2.12	2	2.12	2
Isoleucine	9.17	9	8.70	9
Leucine	29.11	29	40.71	41
Threonine	11.72	12	20.02	20
Phenylalanine	5.81	6	6.64	7
Histidine	8.13	8	11.00	11
Lysine	10.53	11	15.16	15
Arginine	14.21	14	17.32	17
Total[c]		324		418

[a] Normalized results from four independent analyses of samples hydrolyzed for 24, 48, and 72 hr.
[b] Normalized results from duplicate samples hydrolyzed for 24, 48, and 72 hr.
[c] Without cysteine and tryptophan.

acid composition (Table 9) and determination of the C termini revealed differences (Tyr for gp70 and Leu for gp45) consistent with the generation of gp45 from gp70 by proteolytic cleavage of the C-terminal region (Henderson *et al.*, 1978). The other *env* gene product of MuLVs (Karshin *et al.*, 1977) has been designated p15 (E). This component has a virion surface localization and is immunologically unrelated to gp70 (Ikeda *et al.*, 1975; Ihle *et al.*, 1975; Oroszlan and Gilden, 1978*b*). Thus far no sequence data are available for this component. Similarly, the virion reverse transcriptases have not been available in sufficient quantity for sequence analysis.

This brief sketch of sequence data of retrovirus proteins indicates the scarcity of data available for comparative purposes. With the development of newer micromethods for sequencing and sensitive methods for analysis, one would expect a radical change in this situation over the next few years. This should provide information critical for design of new reagents for both immunological and functional studies. The recent description of potential transforming proteins associated with avian and feline sarcoma viruses (Brugge and Erikson, 1977; Stephenson *et al.*, 1977) obviously makes these prime candidates for primary structural analysis.

ACKNOWLEDGMENTS

The authors are indebted to Ms. M. A. Morgan for help in the survey of the literature pertaining to certain parts of this review and to Ms. D. L. Whiten for typing the manuscript. The chemical analyses and sequence determinations carried out in the authors' laboratory were primarily done by Dr. L. E. Henderson, Mr. T. D. Copeland, and Mr. G. W. Smythers. Dr. J. Olpin, Mr. D. J. Bova, and Mr. R. C. Sowder helped in protein purification. Some of the purified proteins analyzed were obtained from Drs. J. N. Ihle, C. W. Long, and J. R. Stephenson.

The studies conducted in the author's laboratory were supported by the Virus Cancer Program, Contract NO1-CO-75380 with the National Cancer Institute, National Institutes of Health, Bethesda, Maryland 20014.

4. REFERENCES

August, J. T., Bolognesi, D. P., Fleissner, E., Gilden, R. V., and Nowinski, R. C., 1974, A proposed nomenclature for the virion proteins of oncogenic RNA viruses, *Virology* **60**:595.

Bachrach, H. L., 1977, Foot-and-mouth disease virus: Properties, molecular biology, and immunogenicity, in: *Beltsville Symposia in Agricultural Research I: Virology in Agriculture* (J. A. Romberger, ed.), pp. 3–31, Allanheld, Osmun and Co., Montclair, N.J.

Bachrach, H. L., Swaney, J. B., and Vande Woude, G. F., 1973, Isolation of the structural polypeptides of foot-and-mouth disease virus and analysis of their C-terminal sequences, *Virology* **52**:520.

Ballou, B., McKean, D. J., Freedlender, E. F., and Smithies, O., 1976, HLA membrane antigens: Sequencing by intrinsic radioactivity, *Proc. Natl. Acad. Sci. USA* **73**:4487.

Baltimore, D., 1970, Viral RNA-dependent polymerase, *Nature (London)* **226**:1209.

Baltimore, D., 1975, Tumor viruses: 1974, *Cold Spring Harbor Symp. Quant. Biol.* **39(2)**:1187.

Bancroft, J. B., 1970, The self-assembly of spherical plant viruses, *Adv. Virus Res.* **16**:99.

Barbacid, M., Stephenson, J. R., and Aaronson, S. A., 1976, *Gag* gene of mammalian type-C RNA tumor viruses, *Nature (London)* **262**:554.

Benjamini, E., Michaeli, D., and Young, J. T., 1972, Antigenic determinants of proteins of defined sequences, *Current Topics in Microbiol. Immunol.* **58**:85.

Benveniste, R. E., Heinemann, R., Wilson, G. L., Callahan, R., and Todaro, G. J., 1974, Detection of baboon type C viral sequences in various primate tissues by molecular hybridization, *J. Virol.* **14**:56.

Blackburn, S., 1970, *Protein Sequence Determination*, Marcel Dekker, New York.

Brauer, A. W., Margolies, M. N., and Haber, E., 1975, The application of 0.1 M quardrol to the microsequence of proteins and the sequence of tryptic peptides, *Biochemistry* **14**:3029.

Bridgen, J., 1976, High sensitivity amino acid sequence determination: Application to proteins eluted from polyacrylamine gels, *Biochemistry* **16**:3600.

Brugge, J. S., and Erikson, R. L., 1977, Identification of a transformation-specific antigen induced by an avian sarcoma virus, *Nature (London)* **269**:346.

Bucher, D. J., Li, S. S.-L., Kehoe, J. M., and Kilbourne, E. D., 1976, Chromatographic isolation of the hemagglutinin polypeptides from influenza virus vaccine and determination of their amino-terminal sequences, *Proc. Natl. Acad. Sci. USA* **73**:238.

Charman, H. P., Marquardt, H., Gilden, R. V., and Oroszlan, S., 1977, Immunologic characterization of gp70 and gp45 from Rauscher murine leukemia virus, *Virology* **83**:163.

Chou, P. Y., and Fasman, G. D., 1974, Prediction of protein conformation, *Biochemistry* **13**:222.

Colcher, Y., Termoto, Y., and Schlom, J., 1977, An interspecies radioimmunoassay for the major structural proteins of primate type-D retroviruses, *Proc. Natl. Acad. Sci. USA* **74**:5739.

Collot, D., Peter, R., Das, B., Wolff, B., and Duranton, H., 1976, Primary structure of alfalfa mosaic virus coat protein (strain S), *Virology* **74**:236.

Dayhoff, M. (ed.), 1972, *Atlas of Protein Sequence and Structure*, Vol. 5., National Biomedical Research Foundation, Washington, D.C.

Durham, A. C. H., and Butler, P. J. G., 1975, A prediction of the structure of tobacco-mosaic-virus protein, *Eur. J. Biochem.* **53**:397.

Edman, P., and Begg, G., 1967, A protein sequenator, *Eur. J. Biochem.* **1**:80.

Fraenkel-Conrat, H., 1968, The small RNA viruses of plants, animals and bacteria, in: *Molecular Basis of Virology* (H. Fraenkel-Conrat, ed.), pp. 134–168, Reinhold, New York.

Fraenkel-Conrat, H., 1974, Descriptive catalogue of viruses, *Comprehensive Virology*, Vol. 1 (H. Fraenkel-Conrat and R. R. Wagner, eds.), Plenum, New York.

Fraenkel-Conrat, H., Salvato, M., and Hirth, L., 1977, The translation of large plant viral RNAs, in: *Comprehensive Virology*, Vol. 11 (H. Fraenkel-Conrat and R. R. Wagner, eds.), p. 201, Plenum, New York.

Gerin, J. L., Holland, P. V., and Purcell, R. H., 1971, Australia antigen: Large-scale purification from human serum and biochemical studies of its proteins, *J. Virol.* 7:569.

Gilden, R. V., 1975, Interrelationships among RNA tumor viruses and host cells, *Adv. Cancer Res.* 22:157.

Hay, A. J., 1974, Studies on the formation of the influenza virus envelope, *Virology* 60:398.

Henderson, L. E., Copeland, T. D., Smythers, G. W., Marquardt, H., and Oroszlan, S., 1978, Amino-terminal amino acid sequence and carboxyl-terminal analysis of Rauscher murine leukemia virus glycoproteins, *Virology* 85:319.

Henning, R., Milner, R. J., Reske, K., Cunningham, B. A., and Edelman, G. M., 1976, Subunit structure, cell surface orientation, and partial amino acid sequences of murine histocompatibility antigens, *Proc. Natl. Acad. Sci. USA* 73:118.

Hill, R. L., 1965, Hydrolysis of proteins, *Adv. Protein Chem.* 20:37.

Hino, S., Tronick, S. R., Heberling, R. L., Kalter, S. S., Hellman, A., and Aaronson, S. A., 1977, Endogenous new world primate retrovirus: Interspecies antigenic determinants shared with the major structural protein of type D RNA viruses of Old World monkeys, *Proc. Natl. Acad. Sci. USA* 74:5734.

Hirs, C. H. W. (ed.), 1967, Enzyme structure, in: *Methods in Enzymology 11*, Academic Press, New York.

Hirs, C. H. W., and Timasheff, S. N. (eds.), 1972, Enzyme structure, Part B, in: *Methods in Enzymology 25*, Academic Press, New York.

Hull, R., 1969, Alfalfa mosaic virus, *Adv. Virus Res.* 15:365.

Ihle, J. N., Hanna, M. G., Jr., Schafer, W., Hunsmann, G., Bolognesi, D. P., and Hyper, G., 1975, Polypeptides of mammalian oncornaviruses, *Virology* 63:60.

Ikeda, H., Hardy, Jr., W., Tress, E., and Fleissner, E., 1975, Chromatographic separation and antigenic analysis of proteins of the oncornaviruses, *J. Virol.* 16:53.

Jacobs, J. W., and Niall, H. D., 1975, HIgh sensitivity automated sequence determination of polypeptides, *J. Biol. Chem.* 250:3629.

Jacobs, J. W., Kemper, B., Niall, H. D., Habener, J. F., and Potts, Jr. J. T., 1974, Structural analysis of human proparathyroid hormone by a new microsequencing approach, *Nature (London)* 249:155.

Jaspars, E. M. J., 1974, Plant viruses with a multipartite genome, *Adv. Virus Res.* 19:37.

Jörnvall, H., Ohlsson, H., and Philipson, L., 1974*a*, An acetylated N-terminus of adenovirus type 2 hexon protein, *Biochem. Biophys. Res. Commun.* 56:304.

Jörnvall, H., Pettersson, U., and Philipson, L., 1974*b*, Structural studies of adenovirus type-2 hexon protein, *Eur. J. Biochem.* 48:179.

Karshin, W. L., Arcement, L. J., Naso, R. B., and Arlinghaus, R. B., 1977, Common precursor for Rauscher leukemia virus gp69/71, p15(E), and p12(E), *J. Virol.* 23:787.

Klenk, H.-D., Scholtissek, C., and Rott, R., 1972, Inhibition of glycoprotein biosynthesis of influenza virus by D-glucosamine and 2-deoxy-D-glucose, *Virology* **49**:723.

Kraal, B., 1975, Amino acid analysis of alfalfa mosaic virus coat proteins: An aid for viral strain identification, *Virology* **66**:336.

Kraal, B., Van Beynum, G. M. A., De Graaf, J. M., Castel, A., and Bosch, L., 1976, The primary structure of the coat protein of alfalfa mosaic virus (strain 425), *Virology* **74**:232.

Laver, W. G., 1971, Separation of two polypeptide chains from the hemagglutin subunit of influenza virus, *Virology* **45**:275.

Laver, W. G., 1973, The polypeptides of influenza viruses, *Adv. Virus Res.* **18**:57.

Laver, W. G., and Webster, R. G., 1968, Selection of antigenic mutants of influenza viruses. Isolation and peptide mapping of their hemagglutinating proteins, *Virology* **34**:193.

Laver, W. G., and Webster, R. G., 1972, Studies on the origin of pandemic influenza. II. Peptide maps of the light and heavy polypeptide chains from the hemagglutinin subunits of A2 influenza viruses isolated before and after the appearance of Hong Kong influenza, *Virology* **48**:445.

Laver, W. G., and Webster, R. G., 1973, Studies on the origin of pandemic influenza. III. Evidence implicating duck and equine influenza viruses as possible progenitors of the Hong Kong strain of human influenza, *Virology* **51**:383.

Laver, W. G., Downie, J. C., and Webster, R. G., 1974, Studies on antigenic variation in influenza virus. Evidence for multiple antigenic determinants on the hemagglutinin subunits of A/Hong Kong/68 (H3 N2) virus and the A/England/72 strains, *Virology* **59**:230.

Lazarides, E., Files, J. G., and Weber, K., 1974, Simian virus 40 structural proteins: Amino-terminal sequence of the major capsid protein, *Virology* **60**:584.

Lazarowitz, S. G., Compans, R. W., and Choppin, P. W., 1971, Influenza virus structural and nonstructural proteins in infected cells and their plasma membranes, *Virology* **46**:830.

Levitina, T. L., Kozlov, E. A., and Serebryani, S. B., 1974, Amino acid sequence of some tryptic peptides of polyhedral protein of nuclear polyhedrosis virus of *B. mori, Biokhimiya* **39**:303.

Lischwe, M. A., and Sung, M. T., 1977, A histone-like protein from adenovirus chromatin, *Nature (London)* **267**:552.

Long, C. W., Berzinski, R., and Gilden, R. V., 1977, Immunologic studies of the low molecular weight DNA binding protein of murine oncornaviruses, *Int. J. Cancer* **19**:843.

Marquardt, H., Gilden, R. V., and Oroszlan, S., 1977, Envelope glycoproteins of Rauscher murine leukemia virus: Isolation and chemical characterization, *Biochemistry* **16**:710.

Matheka, H. D., and Bachrach, H. L., 1975, N-terminal amino acid sequences in the major capsid proteins of foot-and-mouth disease virus types A, O, and C, *J. Virol.* **16**:1248.

McKean, D. J., Peters, E. H., Waldby, J. L., and Smithies, O., 1974, Amino acid sequence determination with radioactive proteins, *Biochemistry* **13**:3048.

Moed, J. R., and Veldstra, H., 1968, Alfalfa mosaic virus: Comparative investigation of top component a and bottom component by means of fingerprinting and immunological techniques, *Virology* **36**:459.

Needleman, S. B. (ed.), 1970, *Protein Sequence Determination*, Springer, New York.

Niall, H. D., 1973, Automated Edman degradation: The protein sequenator, in: *Methods of Enzymology*, Vol. 27 (C. H. W. Hirs and S. N. Timasheff, eds.), p. 942, Part D, Academic Press, New York.

Niall, H. D., Sauer, R., and Allen, D. W., 1970, The N-terminal amino acid sequence of two avian leukosis group specific antigens, *Proc. Natl. Acad. Sci. USA* **67**:1804.

Oroszlan, S., and Gilden, R. V., 1978a, RNA tumor virus antigens, *Scand. J. Immunol.* **7**(Suppl. **6**):81.

Oroszlan, S., and Gilden, R. V., 1978b, Immune lysis of type C viruses by antisera to purified viral subunits, in: *Comparative Leukemia Research 1977* (P. Bentvelzen, J. Hilgers, and D. S. Yohn, eds.), pp. 90–93, Elsevier/North-Holland, Amsterdam.

Oroszlan, S., Summers, M. R., Foreman, C., and Gilden, R. V., 1974, Murine type-C group-specific antigens: Interstrain immunochemical, biophysical, and amino acid sequence differences, *J. Virol.* **14**:1559.

Oroszlan, S., Copeland, T., Summers, M., and Smythers, G., 1975a, Automated microsequence analysis in the presence of double carrier: Application to viral structural proteins, in: *Solid-Phase Methods in Protein Sequence Analysis* (R. A. Laursen, ed.), pp. 179–192, Pierce Chemical Co., Rockford, Ill.

Oroszlan, S., Copeland, T., Summers, M. R., Smythers, G., and Gilden, R. V., 1975b, Amino acid sequence homology of mammalian type C RNA virus major internal proteins, *J. Biol. Chem.* **250**:6232.

Oroszlan, S., Copeland, T., Smythers, G., Summers, M. R., and Gilden, R. V., 1977, Comparative primary structure analysis of the p30 protein of woolly monkey and gibbon type C viruses, *Virology* **77**:413.

Oroszlan, S., Henderson, L. E., Stephenson, J. R., Copeland, T. D., Long, C. W., Ihle, J. N., and Gilden, R. V., 1978, Amino- and carboxy-terminal amino acid sequences of murine leukemia virus *gag* gene coded proteins, *Proc. Natl. Acad. Sci. USA* **75**:1404.

Pal, B. K., McAllister, R. M., Gardner, M. B., and Roy-Burman, P., 1975, Comparative studies on the structural phosphoproteins of mammalian type C viruses, *J. Virol.* **16**:123.

Paucha, E., Seehafer, J., and Colter, J. S., 1974, Synthesis of viral-specific polypeptides in mengo virus-infected L cells: Evidence for asymmetric translation of the viral genome, *Virology* **61**:315.

Perham, R. N. (ed.), 1975, *Instrumentation in Amino Acid Sequence Analysis*, Academic Press, New York.

Peterson, D. L., Roberts, I. M., and Vyas, G. N., 1977, Partial amino acid sequence of two major component polypeptides of hepatitis B surface antigen, *Proc. Natl. Acad. Sci. USA* **74**:1530.

Pett, D. M., Vanaman, T. C., and Joklik, W. K., 1973, Studies on the amino and carboxyl terminal amino acid sequences of reovirus capsid polypeptides, *Virology* **52**:174.

Rees, M. W., and Short, M. N., 1975, The amino acid sequence of the cowpea strain of tobacco mosaic virus protein, *Biochim. Biophys. Acta* **393**:15.

Reynolds, R. K., and Stephenson, J. R., 1977, Intracistronic mapping of the murine type C viral *gag* gene by use of conditional lethal replication mutants, *Virology* **81**:328.

Sarich, V. M., and Wilson, H. C., 1967, Rates of albumin evolution in primates, *Proc. Natl. Acad. Sci. USA* **58**:142.

Schroeder, W. A., 1968, *The Primary Structure of Proteins*, Harper and Row, New York.

Sen, A., and Todaro, G. J., 1977, The genome-associated, specific RNA binding proteins of avian and mammalian type C viruses, *Cell* **10**:91.

Sen, A., Sherr, C. J., and Todaro, G. J., 1976, Specific binding of the type C viral core protein p12 with purified viral RNA, *Cell* **7**:21.

Shah, K. V., Daniel, R. W., and Strandberg. J. D., 1975, Sarcoma in a hamster inoculated with BK virus, a human papovavirus, *J. Natl. Cancer Inst.* **54**:945.

Shah, K. V., Ozer, H. L., Ghazey, H. N., and Kelly, Jr., T. J., 1977, Common structural antigen of papovaviruses of the simian virus 40-polyoma subgroup, *J. Virol.* **21**:179.

Sherr, C. J., Fedele, L. A., Benveniste, R. E., and Todaro, G. J., 1975, Interspecies antigenic determinants of the reverse transcriptases and p30 proteins of mammalian type C viruses, *J. Virol.* **15**:1440.

Silver, J., and Hood, L., 1975, Automated microsequence analysis by use of radioactive phenylisothiocyanate, *Anal. Biochem.* **67**:392.

Skehel, J. J., 1972, Polypeptide synthesis in influenza virus-infected cells, *Virology* **49**:23.

Skehel, J. J., and Schild, G. C., 1971, The polypeptide composition of influenza A viruses, *Virology* **44**:396.

Skehel, J. J., and Waterfield, M. D., 1975, Studies on the primary structure of the influenza virus hemagglutinin, *Proc. Natl. Acad. Sci. USA* **72**:93.

Smith, K. M., 1972, *Plant Virus Diseases*, Academic Press, New York.

Smith, K. M., 1977, *Plant Viruses*, 6th ed., p. 78, Chapman and Hall, London.

Smith, R. E., Zweerink, H. J., and Joklik, W. K., 1969, Polypeptide components of virions, top component and cores of reovirus type 3, *Virology* **39**:791.

Starbuck, W. C., 1970, The determination of the sequence of amino acids in proteins, in: *Methods in Cancer Research*, Vol. 5 (H. Busch, ed.), pp. 251–351, Academic Press, New York.

Stehelin, D., and Duranton, P. et H., 1973, III. Séquence des peptides chymotrypsiques de la protéine aminoethylée et enchaînement des peptides trypsiques, *Biochim. Biophys. Acta* **317**:253.

Stephenson, J. R., and Aaronson, S. A., 1977, Endogenous C-type viral expression in primates, *Nature (London)* **266**:469.

Stephenson, J. R., Hino, S., Garrett, E. W., and Aaronson, S. A., 1976, Immunological cross reactivity of Mason-Pfizer monkey virus with type C RNA viruses.

Stephenson, J. R., Khan, A. S., Sliski, A. H., and Essex, M., 1977, Feline oncornavirus-associated cell membrane antigen: Evidence for an immunologically crossreactive feline sarcoma virus-coded protein, *Proc. Natl. Acad. Sci. USA* **74**:5608.

Stephenson, J. R., Devare, S. G., and Reynolds, Jr. F. H., 1978, Translational products of type-C RNA tumor viruses, *Adv. Cancer Res.* **27**:1.

Takemoto, K., and Martin, M. A., 1976, Transformation of hamster kidney cells by BK papovavirus DNA, *J. Virol.* **17**:247.

Temin, H., and Mizutani, S., 1970, RNA-dependent DNA polymerase in virions of Rous sarcoma virus, *Nature (London)* **226**:1211.

Tremaine, J. H., Agrawal, H. O., and Childlow, J., 1972, Partial sequence of the N-terminal portion of the protein of cowpea chlorotic mottle virus, *Virology* **48**:245.

Tremaine, J. H., Ronald, W. P., and Agrawal, H. O., 1977, Some tryptic peptides of bromovirus proteins, *Virology* **83**:404.

Tsugita, A., Gish, D. T., Young, J., Fraenkel-Conrat, H., Knight, C. A., and Stanley, W. M., 1960, The complete amino acid sequence of the protein of tobacco mosaic virus, *Proc. Natl. Acad. Sci. USA* **46**:1463.

Vandevalle, M. J., and Siegel, A., 1976, A study of nucleotide sequence homology between strains of tobacco mosaic virus, *Virology* **73**:413.

Vitetta, E. S., Capra, J. D., Klapper, D. G., Klein, J., and Uhr, J. W., 1976, The partial amino acid sequence of an H-2K molecule, *Proc. Natl. Acad. Sci. USA* **73**:905.

Vyas, G. N., Williams, E. W., Klaus, G. G. B., and Bond, H. E., 1972, Hepatitis-associated Australia antigen: Protein, peptides and amino acid composition of purified antigen with its use in determining sensitivity of the hemagglutination test, *J. Immunol.* **108**:1114.

Walker, D. L., Padgett, B. L., ZuRhein, G. M., Albert, A. E., and Marsh, R. F., 1973, Human papovavirus JC: Induction of brain tumours in hamsters, *Science* **181**:674.

Webster, R. G., and Laver, W. G., 1971, Antigenic variation in influenza virus biology and chemistry, *Progr. Med. Virol.* **13**:271.

Ziola, B. R., and Scraba, D. G., 1976, Structure of the mengo virion, *Virology* **71**:111.

Zimmerman, C. L., Appella, E., and Pisano, J. J., 1976, Advances in the analysis of amino acid phenylthiohydantoins by high performance liquid chromatography, *Anal. Biochem.* **75**:77.

CHAPTER 2

Structure of the RNA of Eukaryotic Viruses

H. Fraenkel-Conrat

Department of Molecular Biology and Virus Laboratory
University of California
Berkeley, California 94720

1. INTRODUCTION

The first natural homodisperse polyribonucleotides to become available for chemical characterization were the virion RNAs of plant viruses and certain animal viruses. The finding that the infectivity of many viruses, first of tobacco mosaic virus, was a property of their RNAs (Fraenkel-Conrat, 1956; Gierer and Schramm, 1956; Fraenkel-Conrat *et al.*, 1957; Colter *et al.*, 1957), and that these thus represented the first pure genes as well as mRNAs to become available, made studies of their nucleotide sequences obviously of great interest. The later and gradual realization that the virions of many other virus families, e.g., the rhabdo-, myxo-, paramyxo- and reoviridae, carried minus-strand or double-stranded RNAs which had to be transcribed before they could serve as messenger did not diminish the intrinsic importance and interest in their nucleotide sequence.

As in the chemical studies of other polymeric substances and particularly of proteins, methods of end-group analysis were first developed and represented important tools in RNA sequence studies. Also, as with proteins, the development of methods for the selective cleavage of the long RNA molecules into sets of manageable fragments of various lengths represented the second requirement. Methods for the

separation and purification of these fragments were the third requirement; and methods for sequence analysis of these often still large fragments were obviously the ultimate key to RNA sequencing. We will
here briefly illustrate the development of the principles of this
methodology as used first with TMV RNA and other plant viral
RNAs. The enormous advances made when the RNA phages became
available for such studies represent the subject of the following chapter
by Dr. Fiers. These improved techniques are now being applied to plant
and animal viral RNAs, and the main results of these current studies on
eukaryotic viral RNAs will here be summarized. We will not list long
sequences, some of which can be found in Volume 1 of this series, but
rather point out their general significance in terms of RNA conformation, location of genes and untranslated segments, specific protein-bind-
ing capabilities, and transcription and translation strategies.

2. GENERAL FEATURES OF RNA SEQUENCING

2.1.   End-Group Analysis and Stepwise Degradation of RNA

    RNA chains can carry one or several phosphates at either the ter-
minal 5'-hydroxyl (formerly called "3'-linked," but now generally
termed the "5' end") or the terminal 3'-hydroxyl, 5'-linked, or 3' end,
or both. Such phosphates can represent help or hindrance in sequence
analysis, as illustrated in Fig. 1. Since phosphatase (phospho-
monoesterase, PME) treatment selectively removes such terminal phosphates, their hindrance can easily be overcome. The principle of
several RNA end-group methods lies in complete degradation of the
RNA to either 3' nucleotides or 5' nucleotides and separation from
those of one or the other terminal residue either as a nucleoside or as a
nucleoside di-, tri-, or tetraphosphate. Chromatographic and particularly electrophoretic methods are available to separate these species of
different charges. If degradation by alkali yields a single nucleoside
residue without phosphatase pretreatment, then this represents an
unphosphorylated 3' terminus. The identification of adenosine as the 3'
end group of TMV RNA by this method (Sugiyama and Fraenkel-
Conrat, 1961) was the first bit of chemical information about a large
natural RNA, and the first evidence that such an RNA represents a
population of identical molecules. The separation of one nucleoside
from 6400 nucleotides without dephosphorylation of a single one of the
latter represented initial problems which were overcome. This and most
other end-group methods require that the RNA be highly, generally,

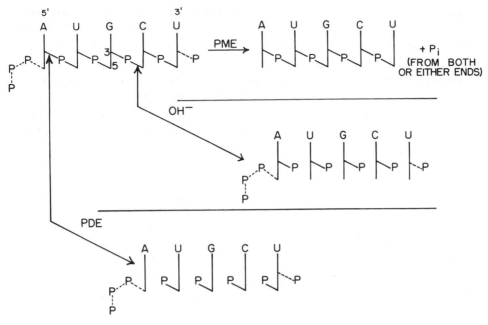

Fig. 1.   Schematic presentation of a polynucleotide chain with potential 5′ mono-, -di-, or -triphosphate and 3′ phosphate groups. PME, treatment with phospho*mono*esterase or phosphatase; OH⁻, treatment with MKOH; PDE, treatment with snake venom phospho*die*sterase. It is obvious that with or without phosphatase pretreatment the 5′- and 3′-terminal residues will be released with different negative charges than the internal nucleotides.

and equally labeled by a radioactive atom. When nucleosides are to be determined, the label is usually ^{14}C or ^{3}H. In the early experiments plants were grown in a ^{14}CO$_2$-containing atmosphere. Now the use of ^{3}H-labeled nucleosides is more common and advantageous. When the products are phosphorylated, ^{32}P introduced into the plants in the form of inorganic phosphate is the most convenient useful label.

The presented end-group method, and its variants in which ribonucleases are used instead of alkali to degrade the RNA, has proven of great usefulness. Since in TMV RNA pancreatic ribonuclease A, which splits only after pyrimidines, also released adenosine, evidence was at hand that the 3′-terminal sequence was -Py-p-A (Whitfeld, 1965). These same results were obtained also with MS2 phage RNA (Sugiyama, 1965).

The mode of biosynthesis of RNA from 5′ triphosphates would lead one to expect the presence of pppXp in alkaline digests of an RNA as an indication of the nature of its 5′ end. To our surprise, no di-, or tri-, or tetraphosphate (pXp, ppXp, pppXp) was found in alkaline

TMV RNA digests, suggesting that the 5' end was unphosphorylated (Fraenkel-Conrat and Singer, 1962). As a corollary to the methods for determining the nature of the 3' ends, unphosphorylated 5' ends should become identifiable by degrading RNA with snake venom phosphodiesterase (PDE, see Fig. 1), which, while attacking a chain from the 3' end, yields on complete digestion 5' nucleotides and a single nucleoside from an unphosphorylated 5' end. This method has not found much usage with large RNAs, probably because of the difficulty of obtaining the diesterase free from traces of phosphatases; as will be shown below, it has given an erroneous result with TMV RNA.

An alternate method to characterize a 5' end is by introducing a ^{32}P-labeled 5'-terminal phosphate in the nonradioactive RNA by means of *Escherichia coli* polynucleotide kinase (Richardson, 1965) and then identifying the [^{32}P]-pXp after alkaline or ribonuclease digestion. This method has found extensive use in recent years as a means of secondary labeling of RNA fragments (e.g., Gross *et al.*, 1978), but with TMV RNA and several other large RNAs erroneous results were obtained, probably because of the frequent presence of small amounts of degradation products in such RNAs. Both the snake venom diesterase and the polynucleotide kinase method indicated adenosine as the predominant 5'-terminal residue of TMV RNA and the latter method gave the same results in several laboratories and with several other RNAs (e.g., see p. 58), all of which we now know to be "capped" (see below). As an explanation of these false results it was suggested that random fragments of a large RNA might mainly terminate in adenosine because C-p-A has been shown to be the most easily split bond in an RNA.

While the proper identification of the 5' ends of several viral RNAs by the methodology outlined in Fig. 1 has presented technical problems due to their unexpected nature (see below), those of the bacteriophages (see following chapter), certain plant viruses, and influenza virus were found to yield the expected and identifiable di- or triphosphates. In such cases the corresponding 5'-terminal oligonucleotides in ribonuclease digests could also be identified and characterized by secondary phosphatase treatment of oligonucleotide fractions of a certain number of negative charges; internal fragments would under such circumstances lose only their 3' phosphate, while the terminal ones would lose, depending on the level of their 5'-terminal phosphorylation, one to three additional phosphates.

The problems encountered with RNA chains seemingly lacking terminal 5' positions, phosphorylated or not, were resolved only in recent years when it became evident that the eukaryotic cell tended to attach a new type of blocking group to the 5' end of cellular and many viral mRNAs (Furuichi and Miura, 1975; Shatkin, 1976). These so-called caps generally consist of a 7-methylguanosine 5'-linked to the terminal 5' triphosphate. Most animal (viral) mRNAs carry one or several additional methyl groups on the 5'-terminal purines and riboses, but these are lacking in plant viral caps. Such caps were often also found in plus-strand virion RNAs, first in reo- and RNA tumor viruses and then in several plant viruses (Keith and Fraenkel-Conrat, 1975a,b; Zimmern, 1975; Dasgupta et al., 1976), although never in bacteriophages.

While it was at first believed that the cap was an essential feature for eukaryotic mRNAs, it soon became evident that certain eukaryotic viral RNAs lack caps and yet are good messengers in vitro and in vivo. Among these are the picornaviridae (poliovirus, etc.), tobacco necrosis virus and its satellite, cowpea mosaic virus, and one of the two components of tobacco rattle virus.

Modification of the 3'-terminal glycol group of RNA chains has supplied an additional tool for 3'-terminal analysis as well as for step-wise degradation of an RNA. The glycol group can selectively be oxidized by means of periodate. The resulting dialdehyde can be condensed with labeled aldehyde reagents and thus yield a quantitative measure of completeness of oxidation, and of chain length (Steinschneider and Fraenkel-Conrat, 1966a). It can be labeled more stably by reduction with [³H]sodium borohydride (RajBhandary, 1968). The terminal base can then after degradation by alkali or ribonucleases be identified by comparison with correspondingly modified nucleoside markers. This again is a method that has yielded some erroneous results with large viral RNAs for not clearly understood reasons. However, when used to label with ³H the chain end, which after nuclease degradation was isolated as an oligonucleotide, this methodology has proven must useful, often also with ³²P-labeled RNA (e.g., Glitz et al., 1968).

Valid results for the 3' terminus of intact RNA were obtained by utilizing the lability of the 5' phosphate linkage of the terminal periodate-oxidized nucleoside, i.e., without blocking or reducing the aldehyde groups, a so-called β-elimination reaction. It was found that the result of the classical procedure of releasing that terminal residue with alkali (e.g., Whitfeld, 1965) could be achieved at pH 5, thus under conditions applicable to RNA, by the addition of aniline (Steinschneider and Fraenkel-Conrat, 1966b). The released modified nucleoside could be identified. The remaining chain was 3'-phosphorylated; it could then be treated with phosphatase, the resulting glycol oxidized, the oxidized residue eliminated, and this procedure continued until the increasing heterogeneity of the released nucleoside derivative made sequential identification impossible. Five nucleosides were in that manner stepwise released from the 3' end of TMV RNA and identified, and the resultant sequence (-G-C-C-C-A) was later confirmed by other methods (Mandeles, 1967; Glitz *et al.*, 1968). However, more recently it was recognized that the cap on the 5' end of TMV RNA, since it contained another glycol group, would also be attacked by periodate and that the 7-methylguanosine would thus also be split off. The presence of twice as many aldehyde groups in periodate-treated TMV RNA, as compared to phage RNA, was noted but not understood in 1966 (Steinschneider and Fraenkel-Conrat, 1966*a*). This now serves to explain why TMV RNA was inactivated by one step of elimination and phage RNA was not (Kamen, 1969). The 3'-terminal adenosine probably is unessential in both types of viruses, and it seems that it may be added by posttranscriptional enzyme action. The cap, however, that was removed at the same time from the 5' end of TMV RNA has recently been shown by its enzymatic removal to be essential for the viral infectivity (Ohno *et al.*, 1976). The 5' end of the phage RNA, not being capped, was unaffected by the oxidative reaction; apparently removal of 5'-terminal phosphates from that RNA by the phosphatase treatment was not *per se* inactivating.

One other technique of sequence analysis of RNA that must be mentioned, although not advocated, is the use of exonucleases. Snake venom phosphodiesterase and polynucleotide phosphorylase attack chains mainly from the 3' end, and spleen phosphodiesterase from the 5' end. Both diesterases have been used successfully to obtain sequence information for oligonucleotides. Both have consistently given erroneous sequence results, probably due to insufficient terminal specificity, when used with RNAs of the size of viral RNA.

2.2. Internal Sequences of Viral RNAs and Structural Considerations

Pancreatic ribonuclease A splits RNA after the pyrimidines, and T1 ribonuclease after guanine residues. The action of ribonuclease A can be made more specific by blocking its action on either of the two pyrimidines (Gilham, 1962; Mazo and Kisselev, 1975). Carboxymethylation of the enzyme has also been reported to render it more selective in that it then attacks almost only A-Py bonds (see next chapter). The first step in structural analyses of viral RNAs has usually been the isolation of large fragments resulting from and thus resistant to complete digestion by either of these enzymes, particularly after the more selective T1 digestion. At first, characteristic large fragments were separated from the smaller ones by column chromatography on DEAE-cellulose in the presence of urea (Sinha *et al.*, 1965; Mandeles, 1968) or by hydroxylapatite column chromatography (Mundry, 1969). Later the various paper electrophoretic and chromatographic methods of Sanger and co-workers (Sanger *et al.*, 1965; Brownlee *et al.*, 1968; Brownlee and Sanger, 1969; Barrell, 1971) became the methods of choice. By such two-dimensional methods it was possible to obtain very characteristic autoradiograms of ^{32}P-labeled oligonucleotide patterns, so-called fingerprints, clearly differentiating and identifying different viruses (Horst *et al.*, 1972a,b). Structural information about each of these spots in terms of ribonuclease-A-resistant fragments and total nucleotide composition is easily obtained (Barrell, 1971). Quite apart from their usefulness as a first step in sequence analysis, these methods have supplied most important information concerning relationships, mutational events, deletions, complexity and thus molecular weight of RNAs, etc.

But even before the development of this high-resolution methodology (which is described in some detail in the following chapters), the existence of characteristic nucleotide sequences allowed chemical differentiation of strains and relationships of viruses. Thus TMV (wild-type) RNA contains a 72-residues-long sequence lacking internal guanosine (Mandeles, 1968), a sequence that is absent or shorter in other strains (Mundry, 1969). Several other T1 nuclease fragments of 14–26 nucleotides were also separated, and were sequenced (Garfin and Mandeles, 1975). The approximate location of these fragments on the RNA chain was studied by gradual stripping of the protein coat off the virus rod (Mandeles, 1968) by means of detergents. Since then stripping has been recognized to begin at the 5′ rather than the 3′ end of the RNA, but the validity of the principle of that technique was confirmed when the longest (72 nucleotides) first released piece (Ω) was recently found to be located next to the 5′ cap (Richards *et al.*, 1978a). In a similar manner tracts of purines terminating in a pyrimidine can be obtained by ribonuclease A digestion of viral RNA, and can be used to detect differences among closely related viruses.

As progressively longer sequences, both terminal and internal, became known, their potential code equivalents in amino acid sequences were compared with known virus protein sequences, at first only of the respective coat proteins. The general conclusions were negative, an easily explained result in view of the fact that only a small fraction of the viral RNAs were required for coat protein information. Certainly, translation to coat protein did not start at the 5′ nor finish at the 3′ end of plant viral RNAs. Instead it became evident that the terminal sequences were often quite similar even among unrelated viral RNAs. The plus-strand animal viral RNAs (picorna- and togaviridae), as well as a very few plant viral RNAs, had 3′-terminal RNase-A- and T1-resistant poly(A) sequences, resembling in this regard most eukaryotic mRNAs and the more complex animal virion RNAs and mRNAs. All those plant viral RNAs that did not carry 3′-terminal poly(A) resembled the bacterial viruses in carrying several (two or three) cytidines with or without an adenosine at the end; the latter then seemed to be added, like the poly(A) of the others, by a nontranscriptive mechanism, and not to be essential for viral infectivity.

The caps at the 5′ end were evidently very similar except that the simple plus-strand plant virus caps carried only one methyl group on the external 5′-linked guanosine (type 0), while the RNA caps of the more complex viruses belonged to type 1 or 2 carrying one or two adjacent ribose- and also often base-methylated residues. A study of the uncapped ends also showed great similarities; for example, influenza viral RNAs, of both types A and B, each consisting of eight components, showed the identical 5′ sequence for all [(p)ppApGpUp-] (Moss *et al.*, 1978), and the uncapped ends of all reovirus minus strands were ppGpApUp- (Furuichi *et al.*, 1975*a*; Furuichi and Miura, 1975).

As longer 5′ and 3′-terminal sequences became established for a group of related RNAs, such as the four RNAs representing four different genes of the brome mosaic virus, those showed almost identical 5′ and 3′ terminal sequences for the first 56 and the last 161 nucleotides (Dasgupta *et al.*, 1975; Dasgupta and Kaesberg, 1977). The latter polynucleotide fragments, from all four BMV RNA components, were relatively enzyme resistant and therefore split off *in toto* on gentle T1 ribonuclease digestion, which indicates extensive H-bonded interaction. Furthermore, these fragments were said to retain the capability of the intact RNAs of becoming charged with tyrosine by the appropriate enzyme.

As longer 5′-terminal sequences were worked on, it became evident that the first AUG initiation codon was variably distant from the 5′ end and that subsequent nucleotide sequences after this or another AUG further downstream corresponded to the N-terminal sequences of the gene products, if known. The first exact gene locations were thus identified. It also became evident that most viral RNA plus strands carried only this one functional gene and that, if they were polycistronic, special mechanisms had to be invoked to render subsequent initiation site(s) operative (see Chapter 4, Volume 11 of this series). No recurring features were identified in the sequence preceding the initiation signal that would account for its recognition (Briand *et al.*, 1978).

At this stage in the development of RNA sequencing technology, the work on the RNA phages made enormous and rapid progress, culminating in the first complete sequences first of a gene and then of a genome. This represents the subject matter of the following chapter.

Attention might here be drawn in this general discussion of the methods and achievements in this field to an extraordinary development in the technology of sequencing of macromolecules. Protein sequencing techniques were very laborious in the 1950s and 1960s, and continue to be so, with only minor addition of techniques and equipment. RNA sequencing has until quite recently been similarly laborious. DNA sequencing, which 5 years ago was impossible, is now easy; long sequences can be established in a few days by a variety of methods.

Thus the sequence of an RNA can now be obtained most easily, as already mentioned, by transcribing it to complementary DNA(cDNA), and protein sequences can be read off the RNA. It may therefore be surmised that direct sequencing of RNA and proteins may have a limited future. On the other hand, posttranscriptional features such as the caps of viral mRNAs, as well as posttranslational modifications of proteins, can only be ascertained by the classical methods. This is true also for the nature of readthrough translation which leads to the A1 protein of Qβ (see following chapter) and similar situations for proteins resulting from readthrough translation of TMV RNA (Pelham, 1978) and most probably many other plant viral RNAs. The amino acids inserted at such termination sites must be established by protein methodology. Thus it appears important to continue the search for more facile methods of protein and RNA sequence analysis, undeterred by the stream of long ribonucleotide and amino acid sequences that are being published all the time by molecular biologists equipped with reverse transcriptase, polyacrylamide, ^{32}P, and a codon dictionary. It appears that the adaptation of DNA sequencing technology to RNA is becoming feasible (e.g., Donis-Keller *et al.*, 1977) and that the possibility of sequencing minimal amounts of nonradioactive RNA will represent a great stimulus to this activity (Gross *et al.*, 1978). However, no easy and reliable methods to sequence long peptide chains are as yet in sight.

3. ELUCIDATION OF PLANT VIRUS RNA SEQUENCES

3.1. Bromovirus and Cucumovirus Group

The genomes of the bromovirus group, whose prototype is the brome mosaic virus, are all distributed over four RNA molecules, the preparative separation of which continues to be difficult. It appears that components 1 and 2 of 1.1 and 1.0×10^6 daltons each carry a single gene, component 3 of 0.7×10^6 daltons carries two genes of which only the first (from the 5' end) is directly translated, and component 4 of 0.28×10^6 daltons carries one gene, the coat protein gene, which also occurs as the second one on component 3 (see Chapter 1, Volume 11 of this series). All four RNA molecules carry type 0 caps (only one methyl group, 7MeG) (Dasgupta et al., 1976). The preceding statements are true also for cucumber mosaic virus (Symons, 1975).

In BMV4 the cap is followed by nine nucleotides before the first AUG, which represents the initiation site of this gene. This is the shortest untranslated leader sequence now known for any mRNA. The subsequent 13 triplets, sequenced for BMV4, correspond to the expected coat protein N-terminal sequence (Dasgupta et al., 1975, 1976).

Another characteristic fragment of all four BMV RNA components that has been elucidated is their 3'-terminal 161-nucleotide sequence (Dasgupta and Kaesberg, 1977). This part of these molecules has apparently much conformational stability, since it remains intact during gentle T1 nuclease treatment. The four RNAs are almost identical in this sequence, with one or two nucleotide replacements in components 1 and 2, compared to 3 and 4. The fact that these fragments end in -CCA and are all able to become charged with tyrosine, i.e., act like tRNAs, probably accounts for their tight conformation and enzyme resistance. In view of the tRNA-like activity of this part of the BMV RNA molecules, it appeared significant that two sequences of eight to ten nucleotides were found to be identical to sequences in the Tyr tRNAs of *T. utilis* and *S. cerevisiae*, including their anticodon (GUA). However, these BMV sequences were not located in a manner corresponding to their location in the Tyr tRNA. A structure with some resemblance to a cloverleaf could nevertheless be postulated for the last 107 nucleotides of the BMV components. Such folding would bring an AUA at residues 65–68 into the anticodon position, which is definitely in line with the tyrosine binding capability of these RNAs and fragments. The fact that the four different BMV genes are as good as identical in their last 161 nucleotides obviously proves that these are not translated.

There has recently been much interest in an RNA component of many but not all cucumber mosaic virus (CMV) strains, because this RNA greatly affects the pathogenicity of the virus without representing part of its tripartite genome (Kaper *et al.*, 1976). This satellite RNA of about 10^5 daltons, termed "CARNA 5," has been found to have little if any sequence homology to CMV genomic RNAs (Lot *et al.*, 1977). Its 335 nucleotides have now been sequenced (Richards *et al.*, 1978*b*). CARNA 5 is capped, and judging by potential initiation and termination triplets it could code for two small peptide chains (2800 and 4800 daltons) in reasonable accord with *in vitro* translation data (Owens and Kaper, 1977). When isolated from different strains of CMV, CARNA 5 showed similar oligonucleotide patterns, but several differences were detected, and some of these occurred also as variants in different preparations derived from the same inoculum, again an illustration of the ready mutability of RNA sequences (see Domingo *et al.*, 1978).

3.2. Alfalfa Mosaic Virus

Alfalfa mosaic virus shows many similarities to the bromo- and cucumoviruses, including the four-component nature of its genome. The nucleotide sequences of these RNAs have been studied to a lesser extent, but one study of the smallest component which represents the mRNA for the coat protein has given a 74-nucleotide 5'-terminal sequence. The typical cap (Pinck, 1975) is followed by G and 35 untranslated nucleotides lacking G, then an AUG, and a sequence corresponding to the known amino acid sequence of that protein (Koper-Zwarthoff *et al.*, 1977).

3.3. Tobacco Mosaic Virus

When the properties of the cap in mRNAs became known, a cap of type 0 was quickly found in TMV RNA (Keith and Fraenkel-Conrat, 1975*a*; Zimmern, 1975). Recently evidence was adduced that the first long G-lacking sequence that was isolated from TMV RNA (Mandeles, 1968) actually is located 5'-terminal immediately after the cap (Richards *et al.*, 1977, 1978) and that it ends in AUG which on the basis of ribosome binding and other studies represents an initiation site, most probably for a long protein (about 110,000 daltons).

This long G-lacking 5′-terminal sequence, termed "Ω" by Mandeles (1968), has recently been sequenced also in two strains of TMV, dahlemense and U2 (B. Kukla, 1978, thesis at Université Louis Pasteur, Strasbourg). Of these strains, dahlemense is known to be related much more closely to TMV vulgare than U2 (classes B and C, respectively, according to Fraenkel-Conrat's terminology; see Volume 1 of this series, p. 113); these relationships are borne out by a much greater resemblance of this 5′-terminal sequence in dahlemense than in U2 when compared to common TMV. Actually the U2 sequence shows very little resemblance to that of common TMV, a surprising finding in view of the fact that in all other groups of related RNA viruses studied the untranslated 5′-terminal sequences are highly conserved (see also the following chapter). Searching for identity near the initiating AUG we find in all three strains the following sequence: A-C-A-A-Py-N-A-C-A-AUG.

In common TMV the following 164 nucleotides have now been sequenced, and we have thus the beginning amino acid sequence of this not yet isolated protein of unknown function. It is comforting to note that no in-phase termination codon occurs in this 164-nucleotide sequence, or, it is to be hoped, among the following 1000 triplets. At the end of this series of about 3000 nucleotides a single UAG is apparently read through with relative ease (Pelham, 1978), yielding in that case a yet larger protein (about 165,000 daltons). The function of these proteins is not known, nor whether there exists a second initiation site for a 35,000-dalton protein (see Chapter 4, Volume 11 of this series, for a discussion of this question), prior to that for the coat protein which begins about 750 nucleotides from the 3′ end and is not translated from the intact RNA, but only after processing or partial degradation. The coat protein gene occurs as a separate molecule in certain strains of TMV, as well as intracellulary (see Chapter 4, Volume 11 of this series); it has not yet been studied in chemical detail, beyond establishing that it is capped.

Earlier studies were aimed at isolating the segment of TMV RNA that had a particular affinity for the coat protein in the belief that virus assembly, and thus this RNA segment, would define one end of the molecule. When partial T1 digests of TMV RNA were treated with TMV protein under conditions favoring virus reconstitution, three nucleoprotein complexes were detected and isolated. Surprisingly their RNA sequence of 232 nucleotides turned out to correspond consecutively to the amino acids 53–130 of the 158 making up the coat protein (Richard *et al.*, 1974; Guilley *et al.*, 1975*b,c*). Thus these RNA fragments were obviously not derived from either end of the RNA. When similar experiments were done with partial ribonuclease A digests, other RNA sequences became protected, unrelated to the known RNA chain ends and not carrying coat protein information (Jonard *et al.*, 1977).

At that time attempts were under way at the MRC Laboratory of Cambridge to isolate the virus assembly initiation site starting with intact TMV RNA and minimal amounts of coat protein (Zimmern and Butler, 1977; Zimmern, 1977). This approach differs from that used at Strasbourg as quoted above, since that focused on the coat protein affinity of fragments in partial nuclease digests. To summarize the principal result: the RNase A fragments of Jonard *et al.* (1977) were partly within the range of intact virus assembly, while the T1 fragments of Guilley *et al.* (1975*b,c*), part of the coat protein gene, were not.

The binding of coat protein and protection of limited segments of the RNA of TMV were altogether less stoichiometric and less sharply defined than the binding by phage RNAs of coat protein, ribosomes, or RNA polymerase (see the following chapter). At all early stages of TMV reconstitution variable-length rods were seen and the nuclease-protected area of the RNA was also quite variable (Zimmern, 1977). Analysis of that protected RNA after deproteination and complete nuclease digestion led the authors to conclude that the "complexity of the fingerprints is substantially greater than we expected, and certainly represents more RNA than could be bound to a single disk (maximally 150 nucleotides)." That this "nucleation site" was not more sharply delineated rendered its analysis much more difficult and the interpretation of the assembly mechanism more ambiguous. That the nucleation site was functionally genuine and competent was confirmed by the ease and completeness of rebinding of stripped-off protein to that population of RNA segments ranging in length from 50 to 500 nucleotides.

Of the 250–300 nucleotide stretch representing the nucleation region, a sequence of 149 was largely established which showed the following features: (1) assembly proceeds in the then unexpected direction toward the 5′ end of the RNA; (2) the sequence, as stated, overlaps 110 nucleotides of the region isolated by its protein binding affinity from partial ribonuclease A digests of TMV RNA by Jonard *et al.* (1977); (3) there is partial homology between the assembly nucleation and the coat protein gene sequence, although the translation product of the former is not the coat protein; (4) no simple sequence periodicity accounting for binding of a single initiating disk can be detected, although attention is drawn to the absence of C from a 50-nucleotide sequence (= 1 disk equivalent), and the presence of several purine-rich sequences (G-A-G-A-G-A, A-G-A, etc.). There is also a row of ten trip-lets of which eight start with G and six have A as the next base. Nevertheless, it seems that nucleation must involve several disks and must be more a consequence of RNA conformation than of nucleotide sequence.

Of particular interest appear the sequence similarities between the nucleation region and those T1 fragments that have affinity for coat protein. The biological significance of the existence of two such areas showing considerable sequence homology and specific protein binding affinity, yet different messenger activity, and only one now functional in virus assembly, represents another interesting puzzle. According to Jonard et al., "possibly T1 [the protein binding T1 fragments] repre-sents the remnant of the initiation site of an ancestral form of TMV."

It has long been suspected, and recently conclusively proven (Do-mingo et al., 1978), that RNA viruses continuously undergo frequent spontaneous mutations. This is also borne out by sequence differences detected between the Cambridge and Strasbourg stocks of so-called TMV vulgare. It may well be that evolution is fast enough in these viruses for structural and functional changes to become established and detectable in the course of a single research period. If this occurs it may also, although indirectly and only phenotypically, lead to changes in the hair color of the investigator.

We have surveyed the known facts about the structure of TMV RNA from the 5' end through the assembly nucleation area about 5400 nucleotides downstream, and into the coat protein gene located in the last 750 nucleotides. From the rest of the molecule was isolated and sequenced a 71-nucleotide segment (Guilley et al., 1975a) terminating with the previously established 3'-terminal -G-C-C-C-A (Steinschneider and Fraenkel-Conrat, 1966b). TMV RNA is able to accept histidine when treated with the aminoacyl-tRNA synthetase under proper condi-tions, although less efficiently, than other plant viruses that bind specific amino acids. The 3'-terminal nucleotide sequence of TMV RNA was therefore expected to form a cloverleaflike structure that would account for this activity. This, however, is not the case. Only two hairpin loops, somewhat similar to such structures at the 3' ends of the phage RNAs, are suggested by that sequence. Thus the mechanism of histidine binding by this RNA remains obscure. There are at least three termination codons in this 3'-terminal sequence, including U-A-A-U-A-A.

Yet the preceding sequence fails to correspond to the carboxyl end of TMV coat protein. Since there is strong evidence against any other gene being carried by the last 1000 nucleotides of the RNA, one must surmise that this fragment represents part of a longer untranslated, possibly polymerase-binding, sequence. Although a considerable amount of work on TMV RNA has been done, it has as yet revealed less than one-tenth of the entire sequence.

3.4. Tymoviruses

Another plant viral RNA which has in small part been sequenced is that of the turnip yellow mosaic virus (TYMV). This RNA of 2×10^6 daltons is apparently associated in the virion with a shorter RNA molecule which has been found to represent the coat protein gene and to be also present as the 3'-terminal segment of the large RNA (Klein *et al.*, 1976; Pleji *et al.*, 1976). Both RNAs are typically capped. The first 110 nucleotides of the large RNA have recently been sequenced (Briand *et al.*, 1978). There are two AUG codons near one another, the second of which, 94 nucleotides from the cap, appears to be functional in terms of ribosome binding. The "rule" derived from the previously discussed plant viral RNAs, that the first G after the cap (7MeGpppG) is part of the initiation codon, breaks down with TYMV, although the number of Gs in the untranslated 94-nucleotide sequence is also low here (eight until the first AUG in position 88–90). Little, i.e., nothing definite, is known about the gene(s) translated from the subsequent long sequence. What is known is only the 3'-terminal 159-nucleotide sequence (Briand *et al.*, 1977; Silberklang *et al.*, 1977) and a longer 3'-terminal sequence on the grounds that that part of the molecule is believed to be identical to the recently elucidated sequence of 695 nucleotides of the small RNA (Guilley and Briand, 1978). This latter carries a typical cap, with A as the first internal nucleotide (all other plant viral caps are 7MeGpppG), followed by 18 nucleotides including two Gs, and the initiation codon for the previously known (see Chapter 1) viral coat protein of 189 amino acids (567 nucleotides).

This sequence is followed by an untranslated 109-nucleotide sequence containing four in-phase termination codons in the next 40 nucleotides. What makes this sequence of particular interest is the fact that the TYMV RNAs, long and short, are able to bind valine with high efficiency when treated with yeast valyl tRNA synthetase and nucleotidyl transferase, which attaches a terminal A to the largely -C-C-terminated RNAs (Pinck *et al.*, 1970; Klein *et al.*, 1976; Giegé *et al.*, 1978). Thus further structural similarities between the TYMV 3'-terminal structures and tRNAs were expected and sought. There is obviously no close similarity since this like all viral RNAs lacks all modified bases. However, various cloverleaf conformations can be postulated which generally permit hydrogen-bonded stems of similar relative location and length as in typical tRNAs and result in a valine anticodon (CAC) in the proper place. Thus there is some structural basis for the unexpected property of TYMV RNA of simulating tRNA in being able to become charged with valine; the same is true for eggplant mosaic virus, a virus related to TYMV, of which 59 3'-terminal nucleotides are known (Briand *et al.*, 1976) and which is also capable of binding valine. As previously stated, similar structural suggestions have been made to account for BMV's tyrosine binding capability, but no reasonable evidence for any such structure was found for TMV RNA to account for its histidine-binding capability.

An intriguing observation made by Briand *et al.* (1978) is that region 95–103 of the 5'-terminal sequence of TYMV RNA which includes the presumed initiation codon can form nine neighboring base pairs with a sequence near the 3' end of the same molecule as well as of the homologous coat protein messenger.

3.5. Viroids

Of particular interest is the recent sequencing of a 359-nucleotide-long cyclical viroid molecule (Gross *et al.*, 1978). This highly pathogenic RNA represents many challenges to virologists and molecular biologists in general, because its mode of action remains unclear. Probably because of their small size (one-tenth that of the smallest virus genome) and compact conformation, viroids, which are strictly and only infectious RNA molecules, not protein-coated particles, appear not to become translated. This, however, is not necessarily true for a viroid-complementary RNA (Matthews, 1978). The recent realization that plants contain RNA replicases (see Ikegami and Fraenkel-Conrat, 1978) could account for the replication of viroids, but there are strong indications that viroid replication occurs in the nucleus and may utilize DNA replication or template activities. This subject is dealt with in detail in Chapter 6, Volume 11 of this series.

As far as the nucleotide sequence of the prototype viroid, potato spindle tuber "virus," is concerned, nothing unusual was observed except for the high level of possible pairing involving about 60% of all bases which may shape this cyclic molecule into a rod, in agreement with its appearance on electron micrographs. Oligonucleotide patterns ("fingerprints") have been obtained for several viroids (Gross *et al.*, 1977) usually infecting different hosts, and while only the potato spindle tuber viroid has as yet been sequenced, the comparison of the various fingerprint patterns clearly shows that at least three different species of viroids exist.

It should be noted that the viroid sequence was established entirely by 5'-terminal ^{32}P labeling, by means of *E. coli* polynucleotide kinase (Richardson, 1965), of oligonucleotides derived from unlabeled viroid RNA by partial nuclease digestions. The sequences of these terminally labeled fragments were then determined by the new methods derived from the techniques of DNA sequencing (Donis-Keller *et al.*, 1977).

3.6. Other Plant Virus RNA Sequences

Cowpea mosaic virus, a two-component covirus, has been found to contain the only plant viral RNAs with terminal poly(A) (El Manna and Bruening, 1973). It was found, however, to lack a cap as well as a free or phosphorylated 5' terminus (Klootwijk *et al.*, 1977). This mystery was recently resolved when Daubert *et al.* (1978) found that this RNA carried a 5'-linked protein of approximately 5000 daltons. It seems quite intriguing that this plant viral RNA resembles that of the animal picornaviruses and differs from all plant virus RNAs at both ends, as well as in its translation strategy (see Chapters 2 and 4, Volume 11 of this series). This appears to point to an unusual evolutionary origin for this group of viruses.

Tobacco necrosis virus (TNV) and its satellite (STNV) also do not fit the pattern of typical plant viruses. While cowpea mosaic resembles the animal picornaviridae in several respects, TNV and STNV show similarities to the RNA phages both structurally and in their translation strategy (see Chapter 4, Volume 11 of this series). As far as terminal sequences are concerned, of TNV only the 5'-terminal (p)ppA-G-U is known (Lesnaw and Reichmann, 1970).

The 5' end of STNV RNA is also uncapped, while being an excellent mRNA; that it is partly di- and partly triphosphorylated is not so uncommon and is usually attributed to the action of phosphatases; however, the finding that its 3' end is in part phosphorylated is a singular feature that remains to be explained in terms of origin and function. Thus what is known of its sequence can be summarized as follows (Horst *et al.*, 1971): (p)ppA-G-U——G-A-C-U-A-C-C-C(p). A ribosome binding oligonucleotide from STNV RNA contains AUG and a di- and trinucleotide consistent with the N-terminal sequence of the STNV coat protein (Leung *et al.*, 1976).

Tobacco rattle virus is also a two-component covirus but with a large infective component (see Chapter 2, Volume 11 of this series). Only the smaller of the two components which codes for the coat protein carries a cap. The 3' end of both components resembles most plant (and bacterial) RNA viruses in being -G-C-C-C (Minson and Darby, 1973*a,b*; Abou Haidar and Hirth, 1977). These two RNAs have about 600 common nucleotides (Darby and Minson, 1973) but these are not located near the 3' end, although the fingerprints of 3'-^{3}H-labeled oligonucleotides appear identical (Gugerli *et al.*, 1978).

Plant reoviruses (e.g., rice dwarf and wound tumor viruses) and plant rhabdoviruses (e.g., wheat striate mosaic and lettuce necrotic yellow virus) closely resemble their respective insect (cytoplasmic polyhedrosis virus) and mammalian (reovirus and vesicular stomatitis virus) counterparts in all respects, and the reader is referred to the discussion of the latter (Sections 4.3 and 4.4) for indications about what is known or may be assumed about the corresponding plant viruses.

4. ELUCIDATION OF ANIMAL VIRUS RNA SEQUENCES

Since sequence analysis usually starts with end-group analysis, and is often greatly assisted by characteristic terminal features, we will survey the present state of knowledge of animal viral RNA structures with primary and particular reference to the end groups of the main RNA virus families. Another reason for doing so is the scarcity of data on nonterminal sequences. We will concern ourselves here only with virion RNAs, not with the intracellularly formed mRNAs. The latter are quite generally, for RNA as for DNA viruses, 5'-capped and 3'-polyadenylated. We will also restrict this discussion to chemical studies, excluding results obtained by hybridization techniques. In general it appears that these latter are less discriminating in terms of detecting limited variations between related RNAs than are the chemical methods.

4.1. Picornaviridae

The RNA of the picornaviridae, though plus strand mRNAs, are uncapped. To the extent that their 5' ends have been critically examined, their 5'-phosphorylated terminal nucleotide, apparently always uridylic acid, is covalently linked to a small protein. This was definitely demonstrated for the polio, encephalomyocarditis, and foot-and-mouth disease viruses (Lee *et al.*, 1977; Nomoto *et al.*, 1977; Sangar *et al.*, 1977; Hruby and Roberts, 1978). The subsequent sequence in polio RNA is -U-A-A-A-A-C-A-G (Flanegan *et al.*, 1977). At least the first ten nucleotides are not translated in polio (Pettersson *et al.*, 1977*a*) and bovine enterovirus RNA (Frisby, 1977).

The 3' ends of the picornaviridae carry poly(A) tracts of apparently variable lengths. It now appears probable that these may range from 15 for EMC (Giron *et al.*, 1976; Burness *et al.*, 1977) to 90 for polio (Yogo and Wimmer, 1972; Spector and Baltimore, 1975) and possibly somewhat longer for rhinovirus (Nair and Panicali, 1976). A sequence of nucleotides next to the poly(A) of EMC has been established, in part by classical methods (Merregaert *et al.*, 1978), and more extensively (up to 166 residues) by new variations on cDNA methodology (Zimmern and Kaesberg, 1978; Porter *et al.*, 1978). This sequence is not translated for at least the last 26 residues and shows little indication of potential secondary structure. According to these data, polio RNA terminates with two Gs, and EMC RNA with one G before the poly(A). Mengo virus and foot-and-mouth disease virus have a characteristic tract of 100–200 cytidylic acids (Porter *et al.*, 1974; Brown *et al.*, 1974), about 400 nucleotides from the 5' end (Chumakov and Agol, 1976; Harris and Brown, 1976). The comparison of oligonucleotide "fingerprints" of many picornaviruses has given useful data concerning their interrelationships (Frisby *et al.*, 1976; Lee and Wimmer, 1976; Frisby, 1977).

4.2. Toga- and Coronaviridae

Of the togaviridae, also containing plus-strand RNAs, only the alfaviruses, Sindbis and Semliki Forest virus, appear to have been studied with regard to nucleic acid chemistry. These RNAs carry caps of type 0, i.e., without internal methylation, A-U-G being the following nucleotides (Hefti *et al.*, 1976; Dubin *et al.*, 1977). Semliki Forest virus has been shown to terminate in about 100 As (Wengler and Wengler, 1976). The coronaviruses are only beginning to be studied. Their RNA is a plus strand of 5.5×10^6 daltons; it is infectious. This RNA carries poly(A) of about 4 S (70 nucleotides long) (Schochetman *et al.*, 1977; MacNaughton and Madge, 1978).

4.3. Minus-Strand RNA Viruses

The rhabdo-, myxo-, and paramyxoviruses carry minus-strand
RNAs. They thus all lack caps and poly(A). The prototype
rhabdovirus, vesicular stomatitis virus (VSV), begins with pppACG
(Hefti and Bishop, 1975; Colonno and Banerjee, 1976) and ends with
PyGU (Banerjee and Rhodes, 1976; Keene et al., 1977). These are also
the sequences of the RNAs of defective interfering particles. Actually
the 3' termini, determined by a novel technique, are the same for residues
1–8 and 13–17 from that end and then diverge (Keene et al., 1978). It
must obviously be assumed that the complementarity of the two ends of
all VSV genome components, noted in these studies, as well as by
Colonno and Banerjee (1978), plays an important role in their replication. A comparison of the oligonucleotide patterns of many strains of
VSV has given an interesting insight into structural relationships (Clewly
et al., 1977).

The RNAs of the flu viruses are generally present in eight minus-
strand segments. The first definitive evidence that these were different
genomic components, and not the smaller ones degradation products of
the larger, was presented by Horst et al. (1972a). This resulted from the
first applications to eukaryotic viral RNA of the technique of comparing T1 oligonucleotide fingerprints obtained by the Brownlee and
Sanger (1969) method. The 5' and 3' end groups were found to be pppA
for most if not all components (Young and Content, 1971), and -U, the
latter by a method that has frequently given erroneous results
(Lewandowski et al., 1971). All eight genome segments of both type A
and B influenza virus start with pppA-G-U (Moss et al., 1978). In fowl
plague and X31, both type A viruses, this is followed by the sequence
A-G-A-A-A-U-U^{10}-A-G-G; after a variable triplet the common
sequence continues with U-U-U-U^{20}-U-U-A (Skehel and Hay, 1978a).
In B-Hong Kong virus, residues 10–16 differ from type A and residue 15
differs in the different segments. The sequence of in vitro transcripts of
several of these were also studied and potential initiation sites were
detected between the 20th and 30th residues (Skehel and Hay, 1978b).

Sendai virus, a typical paramyxovirus, also starts with pppA-, and
both the plus and minus strands (Leppert and Kolakofsky, 1978) and
the various defective interfering particles studied show the same terminus (Leppert et al., 1977).

A typical bunyavirus, Uukuniemi virus, contains three different
segments of RNA about 8000, 3500, and 1900 nucleotides long, with
inverted complementary 3' and 5' ends, which leads to their forming

circular molecules under nondenaturing conditions. They all start with pppA- and obviously are cap- and poly(A)-less (Pettersson *et al.*, 1977*b*).

4.4. Double-Stranded Viruses

The reoviruses, particularly the insect cytoplasmic polyhedrosis virus, were the material in which the existence and the structure of the cap were first detected and elaborated (Furuichi and Miura, 1975). These viruses contain 10–12 double-stranded RNA segments, each representing a single gene. The intracellular mRNAs are transcribed by the RNA polymerase contained in the virion from the (by definition) minus strand of the virion RNA. Since these mRNAs become capped and the progeny genome of the virus is again double-stranded, the virion's plus strand is also likely to be capped. Thus the reoviruses follow the general rule that plus strands are frequently capped, while minus strands are not, be they in virions or intracellular.

The terminal sequences for the various reoviruses that have been studied are

Mammalian	− strand, 5′	ppGAU———(A)GC		(Furuichi *et al.*, 1975*a*;
(reov.)	+ strand, 3′	CUA———UCG^m cap		Faust *et al.*, 1975)
Insect (CPV)	−	ppGGC———ACU		(Miura *et al.*, 1974;
	+	CCG———UGA^m cap		Furuichi and Miura, 1975)
Plant (rice	−	ppGGC———GAU		(Miura *et al.*, 1975)
dwarf v.)	+	CCG———CUA (no cap)		
Plant and insect		———U		(Rhodes *et al.*, 1977)
(wound tumor v.)	+	C———A^m cap		

4.5. Retroviridae

The RNAs of the RNA tumor viruses have been studied more intensely than other viral RNAs in recent years, as a consequence of the war-on-cancer psychology of research funding. Until 1973 these viruses were believed to carry one 70 S RNA molecule of about 10^7 daltons although its dissociation under nucleic acid denaturing conditions to subunits of 35 S was recognized (Duesberg and Vogt, 1973). At that time the use of oligonucleotide patterns ("fingerprints") (Horst *et al.*, 1972*a,b*) began to become applied to the study of the complexity of RNA digests, and these gave chemical indications of the molecular or possibly repeating unit weights of the RNAs (Beemon *et al.*, 1974; Billeter *et al.*, 1974). The resultant value of about 3.4×10^6 for RSV RNA was unexpected. However, the end-group analyses of Keith *et al.* (1974) showed that there was one 3'-terminal adenosine per 3×10^6 daltons and thus definitely established this as the approximate chain length of RSV RNA. Several earlier reports of 3'-terminal uridine, as well as the report of an equal number of 5'-terminal unphosphorylated adenosines, again illustrated the fallibility of the methods used (see pp. 40, 41) (Maruyama *et al.*, 1971; Erikson *et al.*, 1971; Lewandowski *et al.*, 1971; Silber *et al.*, 1973).

The actual 5'-terminal situation was established by the demonstration of the presence of a typical type 1 cap (7-methyl-GpppG^m), also 1 per 3×10^6 daltons (Keith and Fraenkel-Conrat, 1975*b*). This appears to be the only virion RNA cap of type 1 known at present. The retroviruses also seem to be the only virions containing additional methylated bases within their RNA chain, a feature so common for eukaryotic and viral mRNAs. The distribution of the twelve 6-methyl-A residues over the viral genome has been studied, and the fact noted that a transformation-defective deletion mutant had only seven methylated As (Beemon and Keith, 1977). Similar results were reported with B77 avian sarcoma virus where twelve 6-methyl-As were reported to be located between G and C and one or two between A and C (Dimock and Stoltzfuss, 1977).

That RSV, as well as mouse leukemia virus, contained poly(A) had been shown in 1972, although a variable fraction of the molecules were found to lack poly(A) (Lai and Duesberg, 1972; Keith *et al.*, 1974); this study indicated about 200 as its length, but the end-group analysis method (Keith *et al.*, 1974) gave a ratio of Ap/A of about 130, and furthermore proved that the poly(A) was located at the 3' end.

The discrepancy between the molecular weights of 10×10^6 and 3×10^6 for RSV RNA remained to be explained. Electron microscopy suggested a compromise of about 6×10^6 for the 70 S component (Mangel *et al.*, 1974), and it now appears that there are two identical chains in the virion and that the original higher molecular weight value assigned to the 70 S component must be attributed to the difficulties frequently encountered in obtaining definitive values for the molecular weights of RNA by physicochemical methods. Similar to the situation with proteins and other macromolecules, the molecular weight of an RNA is definitively established only at the time that the complete nucleotide sequence has been determined.

This has not yet been achieved, although progress is being made. The first step was the sequencing of a T1 fragment carrying the cap, thus 5'-terminal, 23 nucleotides long (Beemon and Keith, 1977). This sequence later required a minor correction based on the results obtained by the cDNA technique of RNA sequencing. This technique first suggested itself with the RNA tumor viruses, since they contributed the necessary reverse transcriptase to the biochemical toolkit. The sequence most easily established by this type of study was the 5'-terminal one from the tryptophan tRNA primer to the cap, the transcript of which has been termed "strong spot DNA" (Haseltine et al., 1977; Shine et al., 1977; Collett et al., 1977). The characteristic length of strong spot DNA, ranging from 101 nucleotides for RSV RNA to 135 for murine leukemia virus, and its definite sequence differences among different retroviruses have recently been proposed as a basis of classification of this virus family (Haseltine and Kleid, 1978). There are several potential initiation sites in the 5'-terminal nucleotide sequence of RSV RNA, two of which are not in phase with nearby termination triplets. Of these the AUG centered at position 83 is the one most likely to initiate a protein, with the sequence Met-Lys-Gln-Lys-Ala-.

The possibility of extensive intermolecular H-bonding within the 5'-terminal sections of about 60 nucleotides of RSV RNA are also pointed out and two models for the interaction of two 5'-terminal segments are proposed (Haseltine et al., 1977), which could account for the dimerization of that RNA to the usually observed 70 S state. Such interaction accords well with electron microscopic observations (Bender and Davidson, 1976).

Another segment that became available by this method of cDNA transcription was the 3'-terminal sequence adjacent to the poly(A). At first it was established that the heteropolynucleotide chain terminated with C, and then its upstream neighbors were transcribed by reverse transcriptase to the first G using $(dT)_9$ riboG as primer; the presence of a single ribonucleotide made it possible to remove the oligo(dT) handle by alkali treatment of the transcription product. Three products were obtained 15, 18, and 20 nucleotides long, but identical in the sequence of the first 15 before the first G (Schwartz et al., 1977). The most important result of the availability of these 3'-terminal sequences adjacent to the poly(A) is the fact that they proved to be identical to the 5'-terminal ones. The same general conclusion was reached for mouse leukemia virus, avian myeloblastosis virus, and all other retroviruses that were studied in this regard (Rose et al., 1976; Stoll et al., 1977; Coffin et al., 1978). Such terminal redundancy must obviously play an important role in the replication of and/or transformation by the RNA tumor viruses. Various mechanisms and pathways are discussed by Haseltine et al. (1977) and others. Thus "the nascent DNA chain (strong-spot DNA) could float away from its template at the 5' end and pair with a new template at the 3' end for further elongation." If the nascent chain "jumps" to the sister molecule, transcripts of great length could result. Formation of cyclic transcripts could also be easily envisaged which would be favorable intermediates in the integration of the viral into the chromosomal DNA.

It seems that sequence analysis, particularly of terminal regions, has been and will continue to be fruitful in elucidating the modes of replication, transcription and translation of these, as of many other virus groups. That research proposals to continue work along these lines were not looked upon favorably a few years ago* appears in retrospect a misjudgment.

5. REFERENCES

Abou Haidar, M., and Hirth, L., 1977, 5'-Terminal structure of tobacco rattle virus RNA: Evidence for polarity of reconstitution, *Virology* **76**:173.

Banerjee, A. K., and Rhodes, D. P., 1976, 3'-Terminal sequence of vesicular stomatitis virus genome RNA, *Biochem. Biophys. Res. Commun.* **68**:1387.

Barrell, B. G., 1971, Fractionation and sequence analysis of radioactive nucleotides, in: *Procedures in Nucleic Acid Research*, Vol. 2 (G. L. Cantoni, and D. R. Davies, eds.), p. 751, Harper and Row, New York.

Beemon, K., and Keith, J., 1977, Localization of N^6-methyladenosine in the Rous sarcoma virus genome, *J. Mol. Biol.* **113**:165.

Beemon, K., Duesberg, P., and Vogt, P., 1974, Evidence for crossing-over between avian tumor viruses based on analysis of viral RNAs, *Proc. Natl. Acad. Sci. USA* **71**:4254.

Bender, W., and Davidson, N., 1976, Mapping of poly(A) sequences in the electron microscope reveals unusual structure of type C oncornavirus RNA molecules, *Cell* **7**:595.

Billeter, M. A., Parsons, J. T., and Coffin, J. M., 1974, The nucleotide sequence complexity of avian tumor virus RNA, *Proc. Natl. Acad. Sci. USA* **71**:3560.

Briand, J.-P., Richards, K. E., Bouley, J. P., Witz, J., and Hirth, L., 1976, Structure of the amino-acid accepting 3'-end of high-molecular-weight eggplant mosaic virus RNA, *Proc. Natl. Acad. Sci. USA* **73**:737.

Briand, J.-P., Jonard, G., Guilley, H., Richards, K., and Hirth, L., 1977, Nucleotide sequence (*n*-159) of the amino-acid-accepting 3'-OH extremity of turnip-yellow-mosaic-virus RNA and the last portion of its coat-protein cistron, *Eur. J. Biochem.* **72**:453.

Briand, J.-P., Keith, G., and Guilley, H., 1978, Nucleotide sequence at the 5' extremity of TYMV genome RNA, *Proc. Natl. Acad. Sci. USA* **75**:3168.

---

* The author's repeated attempts to obtain continuing support for the rather successful RNA tumor virus research of his laboratory (Horst, Keith, and co-workers) failed, and this work was discontinued in 1976 for lack of funds; this may just be one more illustration of the fallibility of the peer review system.

Brown, F., Newman, J., Stott, J., Porter, A., Frisby, D., Newton, C., Carey, N. and Feller, P., 1974, Poly(C) in animal viral RNAs, *Nature* (*London*) **251**:342.

Brownlee, G. G., and Sanger, F., 1969, Chromatography of ^{32}P-labeled oligonucleotide on thin layers of DEAE-cellulose, *Eur. J. Biochem.* **11**:395.

Brownlee, G. G., Sanger, F., and Barrell, B. G., 1968, The sequence of 5 S ribosomal ribonucleic acid, *J. Mol. Biol.* **34**:379.

Burness, A. T. H., Pardoe, I. U., Duffy, E. M., Bhalla, R. B., and Goldstein, N. O., 1977, The size and location of the poly(A) tract in EMC virus RNA, *J. Gen. Virol.* **34**:331.

Chumakov, K. M., and Agol, V. I., 1976, Poly(C) sequence is located near the 5'-end of encephalomyocarditis virus RNA, *Biochem. Biophys. Res. Commun.* **71**:551.

Clewly, J. P., Bishop, D. H. L., Kang, C.-Y., Coffin, J., Schnitzlein, W. M., Reichmann, M. E., and Shope, R. E., 1977, Oligonucleotide fingerprints of RNA species obtained from Rhabdoviruses belonging to the vesicular stomatitis virus subgroups, *J. Virol.* **23**:152.

Coffin, J. M., Hageman, T. C., Maxam, A. M., and Haseltine, W. A., 1978, Structure of the genome of Moloney murine leukemia virus: A terminally redundant sequence, *Cell* **13**:761.

Collett, M. S., Dierks, P., Cahill, J. F., Faras, A. J., and Parsons, J. T., 1977, Terminally repeated sequences in the avian sarcoma virus RNA genome, *Proc. Natl. Acad. Sci. USA* **74**:2389.

Colonno, R. J., and Banerjee, A. K., 1976, A unique RNA species involved in initiation of vesicular stomatitis virus RNA transcription *in vitro*, *Cell* **8**:197.

Colonno, R. J., and Banerjee, A. K., 1978, Complete nucleotide sequence of the leader RNA synthesized *in vitro* by vesicular stomatitis virus, *Cell* **15**:93.

Colter, J. S., Bird, H. H., Moyer, A. W., and Brown R. A., 1957, Infectivity of ribonucleic acid isolated from virus-infected tissues, *Virology* **4**:522.

Darby, G., and Minson, A. C., 1973, The structure of tobacco rattle virus ribonucleic acids: Common nucleotide sequences in the RNA species, *J. Gen. Virol.* **21**:285.

Dasgupta, R., and Kaesberg, P., 1977, Sequence of an oligonucleotide derived from the 3' end of each of the four brome mosaic viral RNAs, *Proc. Natl. Acad. Sci. USA* **74**:4900.

Dasgupta, R., Shih, D. S., Saris, C., and Kaesberg, P., 1975, Nucleotide sequence of a viral RNA fragment that binds to eukaryotic ribosomes, *Nature* (*London*) **256**:624.

Dasgupta, R., Harad, F., and Kaesberg, P., 1976, Blocked 5' termini in brome mosaic virus RNA, *J. Virol.* **18**:260.

Daubert, S. D., Bruening, G., and Najarian, R. C., 1978, Protein blocks the 5'-end of cowpea mosaic virus RNAs, *Eur. J. Biochem.* **92**:45.

Dimock, K., and Stoltzfus, C. M., 1977, Sequence specificity of internal methylation in B77 avian sarcoma virus RNA subunits, *Biochemistry* **16**:471.

Domingo, E., Sabo, D., Taniguchi, T., and Weissmann, C., 1978, Nucleotide sequence heterogeneity of an RNA phage population, *Cell* **13**:735.

Donis-Keller, H., Maxam, A. M., and Gilbert, W., 1977, Mapping adenines, guanines, and pyrimidines in RNA, *Nucleic Acids Res.* **4**:2527.

Dubin, D. T., Stollar, V., Hsuchen, C.-C., Timko, K., and Guild, G. M., 1977, Sindbis virus messenger RNA: The 5'-termini and methylated residues of 26 and 42 S RNA, *Virology* **77**:457.

Duesberg, P. H., and Vogt, P. K., 1973, Gel electrophoresis of avian leukosis and sarcoma viral RNA in formamide: Comparison with other viral and cellular RNA species, *J. Virol.* **12:**594.

El Manna, M., and Bruening, G., 1973, Polyadenylate sequences in the ribonucleic acids of cowpea mosaic virus, *Virology* **56:**198.

Erikson, R. L., Erikson, E., and Walker, T. A., 1971, The identification of the 3'-hydroxyl nucleoside terminus of avian myeloblastosis virus RNA, *Virology* **45:**527.

Faust, M., Hastings, K. E. M., and Millward, S., 1975, m⁷G⁵' ppp⁵' GmpCpUp at the 5' terminus of reovirus messenger RNA, *Nucleic Acids Res.* **2:**1329.

Flanegan, J. B., Pettersson, R. F., Ambros, V., Hewlett, M. J., and Baltimore, D., 1977, Covalent linkage of a protein to a defined nucleotide sequence at the 5'-terminus of virion and replicative intermediate RNAs of polio virus, *Proc. Natl. Acad. Sci. USA* **74:**961.

Fraenkel-Conrat, H., 1956, The role of the nucleic acid in the reconstitution of active tobacco mosaic virus, *J. Am. Chem. Soc.* **78:**882.

Fraenkel-Conrat, H., and Singer, B., 1962, The absence of phosphorylated chain ends in tobacco mosaic virus ribonucleic acid, *Biochemistry* **1:**120.

Fraenkel-Conrat, H., Singer, B., and Williams, R. C., 1957, Infectivity of viral nucleic acid, *Biochim. Biophys. Acta* **25:**87.

Frisby, D., 1977, Oligonucleotide mapping of non-radioactive virus and messenger RNAs, *Nucleic Acids Res.* **4:**2975.

Frisby, D. P., Newton, C., Carey, N. H., and Fellner, P., 1976, Oligonucleotide mapping of picornavirus RNAs by two-dimensional electrophoresis, *Virology* **71:**379.

Furuichi, Y., and Miura, K.-I., 1975, A blocked structure at the 5' terminus of mRNA from cytoplasmic polyhedrosis virus. *Nature (London)* **253:**374.

Furuichi, Y., Morgan, M., Muthukrishnan, and Shatkin, A. J., 1975*a*, Reovirus messenger RNA contains a methylated, blocked 5'-terminal structure: m⁷G(5')ppp(5')GᵐpCp-, *Proc. Natl. Acad. Sci. USA* **72:**362.

Furuichi, Y., Shatkin, A. J., Stavnezer, E., and Bishop, J. M., 1975*b*, Blocked, methylated 5'-terminal sequence in avian sarcoma virus RNA, *Nature (London)* **257:**618.

Garfin, D. E., and Mandeles, S., 1975, Sequences of oligonucleotides prepared from tobacco mosaic virus ribonucleic acid, *Virology* **64:**388.

Giegé, R., Briand, J.-P., Mengual, R., Ebel, J.-P., and Hirth, L., 1978, Valylation of the two RNA components of turnip-yellow mosaic virus and specificity of the tRNA amino acylation reaction, *Eur. J. Biochem.* **84:**251.

Gierer, A., and Schramm, G., 1956, Die Infektiosität der Ribonukleinsäure des Tabakmosaikvirus, *Z. Naturforsch.* **11b:**138 [also *Nature (London)* **177:**702].

Gilham, P. T., 1962, An addition reaction specific for uridine and guanosine nucleotides and its application to the modification of ribonuclease action, *J. Am. Chem. Soc.* **84:**687.

Giron, M.-L., Logeat, F., Hanania, N., Fossar, N., and Huppert, J., 1976, Size of the poly(A) sequences in encephalomyocarditis virus RNA, *Intervirology* **6:**367.

Glitz, D. G., Bradley, A., and Fraenkel-Conrat, H., 1968, Nucleotide sequences at the 5'-linked ends of viral RNAs, *Biochim. Biophys. Acta* **161:**1.

Gross, H. J., Domdey, H., and Sanger, H. L., 1977, Comparative oligonucleotide fingerprints of three plant viroids, *Nucleic Acids Res.* **4:**2021.

Gross, H. J., Domdey, H., Lossow, C., Jank, P., Raba, M., Alberty, H., and Sänger, H. L., 1978, Nucleotide sequence and secondary structure of potato spindle tuber viroid, *Nature (London)* **273:**203.

Gugerli, P., Darby, G., and Minson, A. C., 1978, The structure of tobacco rattle virus ribonucleic acids: Comparison of large oligonucleotides derived from the 3' ends, *J. Gen. Virol.* **38**:273.

Guilley, H., and Briand, J. P., 1978, Nucleotide sequence of turnip yellow mosaic virus coat protein messenger RNA, *Cell* **15**:113.

Guilley, H., Jonard, G., and Hirth, L., 1975*a*, Sequence of 71 nucleotides at the 3'-end of tobacco mosaic virus RNA, *Proc. Natl. Acad. Sci. USA* **72**:864.

Guilley, H., Jonard, G., Richards, K. E., and Hirth, L., 1975*b*, Sequence of a specifically encapsidated RNA fragment originating from the tobacco-mosaic-virus coat-protein cistron, *Eur. J. Biochem.* **54**:135.

Guilley, H., Jonard, G., Richards, K. E., and Hirth, L., 1975*c*, Observations concerning the sequence of two additional specifically encapsidated RNA fragments originating from the tobacco-mosaic-virus coat-protein cistron, *Eur. J. Biochem*, **54**:145.

Harris, T. J. R., and Brown, F., 1976, The location of the poly(C) tract in the RNA of foot-and-mouth disease virus, *J. Gen. Virol.* **33**:493.

Haseltine, W. A., and Kleid, D. G., 1978, A method for classification of 5' termini of retroviruses, *Nature (London)* **273**:358.

Haseltine, W. A., Maxam, A. M., and Gilbert, W., 1977, Rous sarcoma virus genome is terminally redundant: The 5' sequence, *Proc. Natl. Acad. Sci. USA* **74**:989.

Hefti, E., and Bishop, D. H. L., 1975, The 5' nucleotide sequence of vesicular stomatitis viral RNA, *J. Virol.* **15**:90.

Hefti, E., Bishop, D. H. L., Dubin, D. T., and Stollar, V., 1976, 5' Nucleotide sequence of Sindbis viral RNA, *J. Virol.* **17**:149.

Horst, J., Fraenkel-Conrat, H., and Mandeles, S., 1971, Sequence heterogeneity at both ends of STNV RNA, *Biochemistry* **10**:4748.

Horst, J., Content, J., Mandeles, S., Fraenkel-Conrat, H., and Duesberg, P., 1972*a*, Distinct oligonucleotide patterns of distinct influenza virus RNAs, *J. Mol. Biol.* **69**:209.

Horst, J., Keith, J., and Fraenkel-Conrat, H., 1972*b*, Characteristic two-dimensional patterns of enzymatic digests of oncorna and other viral RNAs, *Nature (London) New Biol.* **240**:105.

Hruby, D. E., and Roberts, W. K., 1978, Encephalomyocarditis virus RNA III. Presence of a genome-associated protein, *J. Virol.* **25**:413.

Ikegami, M., and Fraenkel-Conrat, H., 1978, RNA-dependent RNA polymerase of tobacco plants, *Proc. Natl. Acad. Sci. USA* **75**:2122.

Jonard, G., Richards, K. E., Guilley, H., and Hirth, L., 1977, Sequence from the assembly nucleation region of TMV RNA, *Cell* **11**:483.

Jonard, G., Richards, K., Mohier, E., and Gerlinger, P., 1978, Nucleotide sequence at the 5' extremity of tobacco-mosaic-virus RNA 2: The coding region (nucleotides 69–236), *Eur. J. Biochem.* **84**:521.

Kamen, R., 1969, Infectivity of bacteriophage R17 RNA after sequential removal of 3' terminal nucleotides, *Nature (London)* **221**:321.

Kaper, J. M., Tousignant, M. E., and Lot, H., 1976, A low-molecular-weight replicating RNA associated with a divided genome plant virus: Defective or satellite RNA? *Biochem. Biophys. Res. Commun.* **72**:1237.

Keene, J. D., Rosenberg, M., and Lazzarini, R. A., 1977, Characterization of the 3' terminus of RNA isolated from vesicular stomatitis virus and from its defective interfering particles, *Proc. Natl. Acad. Sci. USA* **74**:1353.

Keene, J. D., Schubert, M., Lazzarini, R. A., and Rosenberg, M., 1978, Nucleotide sequence homology at the 3' termini of RNA from vesicular stomatitis virus and its defective interfering particles, *Proc. Natl. Acad. Sci. USA* **75**:3225.

Keith, J., and Fraenkel-Conrat, H., 1975a, Tobacco mosaic virus RNA carries 5'-terminal triphosphorylated guanosine blocked by 5'-linked 7-methylguanosine, *FEBS Lett.* **57**:31.

Keith, J., and Fraenkel-Conrat, H., 1975b, Identification of the 5' end of Rous sarcoma virus RNA, *Proc. Natl. Acad. Sci. USA* **72**:3347.

Keith, J., Gleason, M., and Fraenkel-Conrat, H., 1974, Characterization of the end groups of RNA of Rous sarcoma virus, *Proc. Natl. Acad. Sci. USA* **71**:4371.

Klein, C., Fritsch, C., Briand, J. P., Richards, K. E., Jonard, G., and Hirth, L., 1976, Physical and functional heterogeneity in TYMV RNA: Evidence for the existence of an independent messenger coding for coat protein, *Nucleic Acids Res.* **3**:3043.

Klootwijk, J., Klein, I., Zabel, P., and van Kammen, A., 1977, Cowpea mosaic virus RNAs have neither m^{7}GpppN . . . nor mono-, di-, or triphosphates at their 5' ends, *Cell* **11**:73.

Koper-Zwarthoff, E. C., Lockard, R. E., Alzner-deWeerd, B., RajBhandary, U. L., and Bol. J. F., 1977, Nucleotide sequence of 5' terminus of alfalfa mosaic virus RNA 4 leading into coat protein cistron, *Proc. Natl. Acad. Sci. USA* **74**:5504.

Lai, M. M. C., and Duesberg, P. H., 1972, Adenylic acid-rich sequence in RNAs of Rous sarcoma virus and Rauscher mouse leukaemia virus, *Nature (London)* **235**:383.

Lee, Y. F., and Wimmer, E., 1976, "Fingerprinting" high molecular weight RNA by two-dimensional gel electrophoresis: Application to poliovirus RNA, *Nucleic Acids Res.* **3**:1647.

Lee, Y. F., Nomoto, A., Detjen, B. M., and Wimmer, E., 1977, A protein covalently linked to poliovirus genome RNA, *Proc. Natl. Acad. Sci. USA* **74**:59.

Leppert, M., and Kolakofsky, D., 1978, 5'-Terminus of defective and nondefective Sendai viral genomes if pppAp, *J. Virol.* **25**:427.

Leppert, M., Kort, L., and Kolakofsky, D., 1977, Further characterization of Sendai virus D1-RNAs: A model for their generation, *Cell* **12**:539.

Lesnaw, J. A., and Reichmann, M. E., 1970, Identity of the 5'-terminal RNA nucleotide sequence of the satellite tobacco necrosis virus and its helper virus: Possible role of the 5'-terminus in the recognition by virus-specific RNA replicase, *Proc. Natl. Acad. Sci. USA* **66**:140.

Leung, D. W., Gilbert, C. W., Smith, R. E., Sasavage, N. L., and Clark, J. M., Jr., 1976, Translation of satellite tobacco necrosis virus ribonucleic acid by an *in vitro* system from wheat germ, *Biochemistry* **15**:4943.

Lewandowski, L. J., Content, J., and Leppla, S. H., 1971, Characterization of the subunit structure of the ribonucleic acid genome of influenza virus, *J. Virol.* **8**:701.

Lot, H., Jonard, G., and Richards, K. E., 1977, Cucumber mosaic virus RNA t: Partial characterization and evidence for no large sequence homologies with genomic RNAs, *FEBS Lett.* **80**:395.

MacNaughton, M. R., and Madge, M. H., 1978, The genome of human coronavirus strain 229E, *J. Gen. Virol.* **39**:497.

Mandeles, S., 1967, Base sequence at the 5'-linked terminus of TMV-RNA, *J. Biol. Chem.* **242**:3103.

Mandeles, S., 1968, Location of unique sequences in TMV-RNA, *J. Biol. Chem.* **243**:3671.

Mangel, W. F., Delius, H., and Duesberg, P. H., 1974, Structure and molecular weight of the 60–70 S RNA and the 30–40 S RNA of the Rous sarcoma virus, *Proc. Natl. Acad. Sci. USA* **71**:4541.

Maruyama, H. B., Hatanaka, M., and Gilden, R. V., 1971, The 3'-terminal nucleosides of the high molecular weight RNA of C-type viruses, *Proc. Natl. Acad. Sci. USA* **68**:1999.

Matthews, R. E. F., 1978, Are viroids negative-strand viruses? *Nature* **276**:850.

Mazo, A. M., and Kisselev, L. L., 1975, Ribopolynucleotides modified at pyrimidine residues are cleaved selectively by T_2 ribonuclease at purine residues, *FEBS Lett.* **59**:177.

Merregaert, J., van Emmelo, J., Devos, R., Porter, A., Fellner, P., and Fiers, W., 1978, The 3'-terminal nucleotide sequence of encephalomyocarditis virus RNA, *Eur. J. Biochem.* **82**:55.

Minson, A. C., and Darby, G., 1973a, 3'-Terminal oligonucleotide fragments of tobacco rattle virus ribonucleic acids, *J. Mol. Biol.* **77**:337.

Minson, A. C., and Darby, G., 1973b, A study of sequence homology between tobacco rattle virus ribonucleic acids, *J. Gen. Virol.* **19**:253.

Moss, B., Keith, J. M., Gershowitz, A., Ritchey, M. B., and Palese, P., 1978, Common sequence at the 5' ends of the segmented RNA genomes of influenza A and B viruses, *J. Virol.* **25**:312.

Miura, K.-I., Watanabe, K., and Sugiura, M., 1974, 5'-Terminal nucleotide sequences of the double-stranded RNA of silkworm cytoplasmic polyhedrosis virus, *J. Mol. Biol.* **86**:31.

Miura, K., Furuichi, Y., Shimotohno, K., Urushibara, T., and Sugiura, M., 1975, Structure of the termini of the RNAs of reoviridae, *Inserm.* **47**:153.

Mundry, K. W., 1969, Structural elements of viral ribonucleic acid and their variation. I. An adenine-rich and strain-specific segment in tobacco mosaic virus ribonucleic acid, *Mol. Gen. Genet.* **105**:361.

Nair, C. N., and Panicali, D. L., 1976, Polyadenylate sequences of human rhinovirus and poliovirus RNA and cordycepin sensitivity of virus replication, *J. Virol.* **20**:170.

Nomoto, A., Kitamura, N., Golini, F., and Wimmer, E., 1977, The 5'-terminal structures of poliovirion RNA and poliovirus mRNA differ only in the genome-linked protein VPg, *Proc. Natl. Acad. Sci. USA* **74**:5345.

Ohno, T., Okada, Y., Shimotohno, K., Miura, K.-I., Shinshi, H., Miwa, M., and Sugimura, T., 1976, Enzymatic removal of the 5'-terminal methylated blocked structure of tobacco mosaic virus RNA and its effect on infectivity and reconstitution with coat protein, *FEBS Lett.* **67**:209.

Owens, R. A., and Kaper, J. M., 1977, Cucumber mosaic virus associated RNA 5. II. In vitro translation in a wheat germ protein-synthesis system, *Virology* **80**:196.

Pelham, H. R. B., 1978, Leaky UAG termination codon in tobacco mosaic virus RNA, *Nature (London)* **272**:469.

Pettersson, R. F., Flanegan, J. B., Rose, J. K., and Baltimore D., 1977a, 5' Terminal nucleotide sequences of polio virus polyribosomal RNA and virion RNA are identical, *Nature* **268**:270.

Pettersson, R. F., Hewlett, M. J., and Baltimore, D., 1977b, The genome of Uukuniemi virus consists of three unique RNA segments, *Cell* **11**:51.

Pinck, L., 1975, The 5'-end groups of alfalfa mosaic virus RNAs are m⁷G⁵′ppp⁵′Gp, *FEBS Lett.* **59**:24.

Pinck, M., Yot, P., Chapeville, F., and Duranton, H. M., 1970, Enzymatic binding of valine to the 3' end of TYMV-RNA, *Nature (London)* **226**:954.

Pleji, C. W. A., Neeleman, A., van Vloten-Doting, L., and Bosch, L., 1976, Translation of turnip yellow mosaic virus RNA *in vitro:* A closed and an open coat protein cistron, *Proc. Natl. Acad. Sci. USA* **73**:4437.

Porter, A., Carey, N., and Fellner, P., 1974, Presence of a large poly(rC) tract within the RNA of encephalomyocarditis virus, *Nature (London)* **248**:675.

Porter, A. G., Merregaert, J., van Emmelo, J., and Fiers, W., 1978, Sequence of 129 nucleotides at the 3'-terminus of encephalomyocarditis virus RNA, *Eur. J. Biochem.* **87**:551.

RajBhandary, U. L., 1968, The labeling of end groups in polynucleotides: The selective modification of diol groups in RNA, *J. Biol. Chem.* **243**:556.

Rhodes, D. P., Reddy, D. V. R., MacLeod, R., Black, L. M., and Banerjee, A. K., 1977, *In vitro* synthesis of RNA containing 5'-terminal structure mG(5')ppp(5')Apᵐ by purified wound tumor virus, *Virology* **76**:554.

Richards, K. E., Guilley, H., Jonard, G., and Hirth, L., 1974, A specifically encapsidated fragment from the RNA of tobacco mosaic virus: Sequence homology with the coat protein cistron, *FEBS Lett.* **43**:31.

Richards, K., Guilley, H., Jonard, G., and Hirth, L., 1978a, Nucleotide sequence at the 5' extremity of tobacco-mosaic-virus RNA 1. The noncoding region (nucleotides 1–68), *Eur. J. Biochem.* **84**:513.

Richards, K., Jonard, G., Guilley, H., and Keith, G., 1977, Leader sequence of 71 nucleotides devoid of G in tobacco mosaic virus RNA, *Nature (London)* **267**:548.

Richards, K. E., Jonard, G., Jacquemond, M., and Lot, H., 1978b, Nucleotide sequence of cucumber mosaic virus-associated RNA 5, *Virology* **89**:395.

Richardson, C. C., 1965, Phosphorylation of nucleic acid by an enzyme from T4 bacteriophage-infected Escherichia coli, *Proc. Natl. Acad. Sci. USA* **54**:158.

Rose, J. K., Haseltine, W. A., and Baltimore, D., 1976, 5'-Terminus of Moloney murine leukemia virus 35 S RNA is m⁷G⁵′ppp⁵′GmpCp, *J. Virol.* **20**:324.

Sangar, D. V., Rowlands, D. J., Harris, T. J. R., and Brown F., 1977, Protein covalently linked to foot-and-mouth disease virus RNA, *Nature (London)* **268**:648.

Sanger, F., Brownlee, G. G., and Barrell, B. G., 1965, A two-dimensional fractionation procedure for radioactive nucleotides, *J. Mol. Biol.* **13**:373.

Schochetman, G. Stevens, R. H., and Simpson, R. W., 1977, Presence of infectious polyadenylated RNA in the coronavirus avian bronchitis virus, *Virology* **77**:772.

Schwartz, D. E., Zamecnik, P. C., and Weith, H. L., 1977, Rous sarcoma virus genome is terminally redundant: The 3' sequence, *Proc. Natl. Acad. Sci. USA* **74**:994.

Shatkin, A. J., 1976, Capping of eukaryotic mRNAs, *Cell* **9**:645.

Shine, J., Czernilofsky, A. P., Friedrich, R., Bishop, J. M., and Goodman, H. M., 1977, Nucleotide sequence at the 5' terminus of the avian sarcoma virus genome, *Proc. Natl. Acad. Sci. USA* **74**:1473.

Silber, R., Malathi, V. G., Schulman, L. H., and Hurwitz, J., 1973, Studies of the Rous sarcoma virus RNA: Characterization of the 5'-terminus, *Biochem. Biophys. Res. Commun.* **50**:467.

Silberklang, M., Prochiantz, A., Haenni, A.-L., and RajBhandary, U. L., 1977, Studies on the sequence of the 3'-terminal region of turnip-yellow-mosaic-virus RNA, *Eur. J. Biochem.* **72**:465.

Sinha, N. K., Enger, M. D., and Kaesberg, P., 1965, Comparison of pancreatic RNase digestion products of R17 viral RNA and M12 viral RNA, *J. Mol. Biol.* **12**:299.

Skehel, J. J., and Hay, A. J., 1978*a*, Influenza virus transcription, *J. Gen. Virol.* **39**:1.

Skehel, J. J., and Hay, A. J., 1978*b*, Nucleotide sequences at the 5' termini of influenza virus RNAs and their transcripts, *Nucleic Acids Res.* **5**:1207.

Spector, D. H., and Baltimore, D., 1975, Polyadenylic acid in poliovirus RNA. II. Poly(A) on intracellular RNA's, *J. Virol.* **15**:1418.

Steinschneider, A., and Fraenkel-Conrat, H., 1966*a*, Studies of nucleotide sequences in tobacco mosaic virus ribonucleic acid. III. Periodate oxidation and semicarbazone formation, *Biochemistry* **5**:2729.

Steinschneider, A., and Fraenkel-Conrat, H., 1966*b*, Studies of nucleotide sequences in tobacco mosaic virus ribonucleic acid. IV. Use of aniline in step-wise degradation, *Biochemistry* **5**:2735.

Stephenson, M. L., Scott, J. F., and Zamecnik, P. C., 1973, Evidence that polyadenylic acid segment of "35 S" RNA of avian myeloblastosis virus is located at the 3'-OH terminus, *Biochem. Biophys. Res. Commun.* **55**:8.

Stoll, E., Billeter, M. A., Palmenberg, A., and Weissmann, C., 1977, Avian myeloblastosis virus RNA is terminally redundant: Implications for the mechanism of retrovirus replication, *Cell* **12**:57.

Sugiyama, T., 1965, 5'-Linked end group of RNA from bacteriophage MS2, *J. Mol. Biol.* **11**:856.

Sugiyama, T., and Fraenkle-Conrat, H., 1961, Identification of 5'-linked adenosine as end-group of TMV-RNA, *Proc. Natl. Acad. Sci. USA* **47**:1393.

Symons, R. H., 1975, Cucumber mosaic virus RNA contains 7-methylguanosine at the 5'-terminus of all four RNA species, *Mol. Biol. Rep.* **2**:277.

Wengler, G., and Wengler, G., 1976, Localization of the 26-S RNA sequences on the viral genome type 42-S RNA isolated from SFV-infected cells, *Virology* **73**:190.

Whitfeld, P. R., 1965, Application of the periodate method for the analysis of nucleotide sequence to tobacco mosaic virus RNA, *Biochim. Biophys. Acta* **108**:202.

Wimmer, E., Chang, A. Y., Clark, J. M., Jr., and Reichmann, M. E., 1968, Sequence studies of satellite tobacco necrosis virus RNA, *J. Mol. Biol.* **38**:59.

Yogo, Y., and Wimmer, E., 1972, Polyadenylic acid at the 3'-terminus of poliovirus RNA, *Proc. Natl. Acad. Sci. USA* **69**:1877.

Young, R. J., and Content, J., 1971, 5'-Terminus of influenza virus RNA, *Nature (London) New Biol.* **230**:140.

Zimmern, D., 1975, The 5' end group of tobacco mosaic virus RNA is m^{7}G$^{5'}$ppp$^{5'}$Gp, *Nucleic Acids Res.* **2**:1189.

Zimmern, D., 1977, The nucleotide sequence at the origin for assembly on tobacco mosaic virus RNA, *Cell* **11**:463.

Zimmern, D., and Butler, J. G., 1977, The isolation of tobacco mosaic virus RNA fragments containing the origin for viral assembly, *Cell* **11**:455.

Zimmern, D., and Kaesberg, P., 1978, 3'-Terminal nucleotide sequences of encephalomyocarditis virus and poliovirus RNAs determined by use of reverse transcriptase and chain terminating inhibitors, *Proc. Natl. Acad. Sci. USA* **75**:4257.

CHAPTER 3

Structure and Function of RNA Bacteriophages

Walter Fiers

Laboratory of Molecular Biology
University of Ghent
Ghent, Belgium

1. INTRODUCTION

Although RNA bacteriophages were discovered only relatively recently (Loeb and Zinder, 1961), they have attracted considerable attention ever since. Because of their small size, one could hope that these would be the first viruses whose complete structure would be elucidated, and for which all biological events constituting the infection cycle would be understood in molecular and biophysical detail. These biological events include phage adsorption and penetration, expression of the viral genetic information, interference with the host cell metabolism, replication of the viral genome, assembly, and virus release through lysis. Although these aims have certainly not yet been completely fulfilled, today the molecular biology of the RNA bacteriophages is undoubtedly the most advanced of that for any living organism (assuming of course that a virus is considered an "organism," which is a question of definition). Another reason for the interest in RNA phages is that they constitute a convenient model system whose molecular biology may contribute considerably to the understanding of RNA viruses in general. The versatility of a microbial system for biochemical and genetic experimentation, combined with the short infection cycle (less than 30 min) and high yields (more than 2×10^{12}

pfu/ml),* offer obvious practical advantages. Last but not least, the phage RNAs have played a crucial role in our understanding of the mechanism of translation, such as initiation, elongation, and termination (Bosch, 1972; Capecchi and Webster, 1975; Lodish, 1976). The expression of the three viral genes is intricately regulated, and although in other systems a wide variety of translational controls may exist, it is nevertheless likely that the mechanism operative in the expression of the RNA phage genome will contribute considerably to the understanding of other systems.

In Volume 2 of *Comprehensive Virology*, Eoyang and August (1974) have presented a thorough description of the RNA bacteriophages, with special emphasis on their replication. References to review articles dealing with specific aspects of the RNA bacteriophages are also given in the aforementioned chapter. In addition, the book *RNA Phages*, edited by N. D. Zinder (1975), deserves special attention; it is a compilation of review articles concerning all facets of the molecular biology of RNA phages.

The present chapter deals mainly with the structure of the viral genome and of the virus-induced proteins, and with the biological events that can be partly understood on the basis of this structural information.

2. CLASSIFICATION OF RNA PHAGES

2.1. RNA Coliphages

Loeb and Zinder (1961) searched for viruses which would plate on male *Escherichia coli* cells (F^+ or Hfr) and not on female cells. Actually they found two types, represented by the prototypes f1 and f2, and so named in reference to the fertility (F) factor present in the host cell. The former turned out to be a filamentous, single-stranded DNA phage. It forms turbid plaques as the progeny viruses are released without cell lysis and without blocking of cell division. Bacteriophage f1, together with the closely related fd and M13 phages, has also been intensively studied both in its own right and as a model system for the investigation of DNA replication in general.

The f2-type phage forms clear plaques, has a sedimentation constant of around 80 S, and demonstrates plaque formation that is sensitive to ribonuclease (it is not the particle, but rather a phase

---

* pfu, Plaque-forming unit.

following virus adsorption that is sensitive to ribonuclease). Using specificity for male *E. coli* cells and any of the latter properties for selection, a large number of RNA phages were soon isolated, mostly from sewage. Although they were obtained in widely different locations, they turned out to be remarkably similar (see below) and are now classified as group I phages. Besides f2 and f4, isolated in New York, other typical examples are MS2 (for male specific) in San Francisco (A. Clark, cited in Davis *et al.*, 1961), R17 in Philadelphia (Paranchych and Graham, 1962), fr in Heidelberg (Marvin and Hoffmann-Berling, 1963), and M12 in Munich (Hofschneider, 1963). It became clear that RNA coliphages are present in fairly high concentration in nearly all sewage samples tested, and they have been isolated on all continents.

A first comparative study based on immunological cross-reactivity was made by Scott (1965). He found that all phages of his collection were clearly related, albeit none of them were identical by the criteria used. The order of relatedness as tested by anti-f2 serum was f2 > R17 > FH5 > M12 > MS2 > β > fr > f4. Detection of these small but real differences is remarkable, as the amino acid sequences of the coat protein of MS2 and of R17 are identical (Weber and Konigsberg, 1975), and also the amino acid composition of the f4 coat protein is the same as that of the former two (Modak and Notani, 1969)* (amino acid sequences will be further discussed in Section 3.2). Therefore, either some nucleic acid bases may be accessible near the surface and codetermine the immunological response, or the A protein, which is a minor virion component (Section 3.3), also plays a role. That the A protein is not the main antigenic determinant, however, is shown by the fact that immune precipitation of lysates from cells infected with amber mutants is specific for the presence of coat protein, not of A protein (Zinder and Cooper, 1964; Horiuchi, 1975). Also, similar results were obtained when relatedness was tested by serological inactivation rate or by complement fixation (Scott, 1965), and there is a close correlation between inactivation rate and quantitative immunoprecipitation (Rappaport, 1970). Moreover, mutants resistant to anti-wild-type serum are always affected in the amino acid sequences of the coat protein (Vandekerckhove *et al.*, 1975). Up to 80–112 antibody molecules can combine with one MS2 particle, i.e., about one per coat protein dimer (Rohrmann and Krueger, 1970; Rappaport, 1970). The immuno-

---

* In the absence of unambiguous tests, it is difficult to work in the same laboratory with different types of these highly infectious RNA phages; therefore, the data of Modak and Notani (1969) may perhaps not refer to the same f4 as used by Scott (1965) and by Krueger (1969).

genic response is related to the quaternary structure of the virus shell, as the dissociated protein subunits are antigenically distinct (Rohrmann and Krueger, 1970; Hirata *et al.*, 1972). An infective complex of A protein with viral RNA (Section 3.3) is not inhibited by antiphage serum (Shiba and Miyake, 1975).

A large number of RNA coliphages were isolated by I. Watanabe *et al.* (1967*a,b*) from sewage and from feces in Japan. They could be classified in three non-cross-reacting groups (Table 1). Later a fourth group was added (Sakurai *et al.*, 1968; Miyake *et al.*, 1969). $Q\beta$, which is the prototype of group III, has been immensely useful as the virus-induced RNA polymerase can readily be obtained in a specific template-dependent (Haruna and Spiegelman, 1965*a*) and biochemically pure (Kamen, 1970; Kondo *et al.*, 1970; Eoyang and Ausust, 1971) form. Also, the molecular biology of $Q\beta$ differs in important ways from

TABLE 1

Serological Groups of RNA Coliphages[a]

		Other distinctive properties[b]				
		Phage particle			Coat protein[c]	
	Serotypes	Buoyant density in CsCl(g/cm³)	$s_{20,w}$ value (S)	RNA A/U ratio[d]	Amino acids absent	C-terminal
Group	Types					
I	Main: f2, MS2, R17, fr, M12 Others: f4, μ2, FH5, β, ZR, GR, MY, SN, f can 1, R23, R40	1.46	79	0.95–0.98	His	-Ile-Tyr
II	Main: GA Others: EI, KJ, SW, SS, SD, SB, MC, SK	1.44	76	0.84–0.86	His, Met, Cys	-(Tyr, Phe)-Ala
III	Main: $Q\beta$ Others: CF, HI, NH, NM, SG, VK, ST, SO	1.47[e]	83	0.78–0.79	His, Met, Trp	-Ala-Tyr
IV[f]	Main: SP, FI	—[g]	—	—	—	—

[a] Main references: Scott (1965), Watanabe *et al.* (1967*a,b*), Krueger (1969).
[b] Nishihara *et al.* (1969), Nishihara and Watanabe (1969).
[c] The N-terminal is Ala for all groups analyzed.
[d] Ratio of A and U bases in the viral RNA.
[e] The phage precipitates out in the band.
[f] References: Sakurai *et al.* (1968), Miyake *et al.* (1969).
[g] Not distinguishable from $Q\beta$.

TABLE 2
Relative Rates of Neutralization of the RNA Coliphages[a]

Phage	K' values with antiserum to phage				
	MS2	R17	f2	fr	Qβ
MS2	1.00	0.68	0.58	0.21	<0.01
M12	0.84	0.84	0.70	0.38	<0.01
R17	0.68	1.00	0.86	0.54	0.03
f2	0.52	0.50	1.00	0.72	0.08
β	0.41	0.40	0.40	0.85	0.22
fr	0.20	0.24	0.22	1.00	0.50
f4	0.10	0.12	0.10	0.20	0.70
Qβ	0.02	0.03	0.03	0.11	1.00

[a] From Krueger (1969).

that of the group I phages, as will be discussed in a later section. The serological classification is a reflection of the difference in capsid structure, and it is not surprising that the three main groups can also be differentiated by their amino acid composition and by their C-terminal end as revealed by carboxypeptidase A treatment (Table 1). Krueger (1969) confirmed the aforementioned results of Scott (1965) that all group I phages are distinct but related (Table 2). Moreover, he observed that Qβ showed a weak but significant cross-reactivity with some anti-group I sera; more specifically, f4 and fr appeared to be clearly related to Qβ. This finding is most remarkable because although the fr coat protein contains 22 substitutions relative to the MS2 coat protein it is still quite obviously related (83% homology), while the Qβ coat sequence requires nine deletions and substitutions to be somewhat comparable and even then the homology is only 30 identical residues out of 132, i.e., on the borderline of statistical significance (cf. Section 3.2). Other investigators, however, did not find any immunological cross-reaction whatsoever between MS2 and Qβ (Overby et al., 1966b). In the author's laboratory, no inactivation of fr phage by Qβ antiserum was observed, nor was Qβ phage inactivated by fr antiserum (Fiers and co-workers, unpublished observations). Other criteria which have been used to distinguish the three main phage groups are buoyant density in CsCl, inactivation rate by UV irradiation, sedimentation rate, base ratios of the RNA, electrophoretic mobility, adsorption on membrane filters, and sensitivity to high or low pH (Watanabe et al., 1967a,b; Miyake et al., 1967; cf. also Table 1). In a separate study, Bradley characterized six independently isolated coliphages (Bradley, 1964;

Bishop and Bradley, 1965). Although they were all serologically related, they fell into two groups differing up to 200-fold in immunological inactivation rate. Their relationship to the three groups of Watanabe (Table 1) is unknown, and they have apparently not been further investigated.

A series of crude sewage samples derived from urban and rural regions all showed RNA coliphage titers of around 10^2–10^3 pfu/ml; all phages were of either the MS2 type or the $Q\beta$ type, and most samples contained only phage of one type, not both (Dhillon and Dhillon, 1974).

The immunological properties discussed above are dependent on the structural proteins of the virions. A completely different criterion for classification is the interaction between the viral replicase and the viral RNA in a heterologous system. Spiegelman and co-workers (Haruna *et al.*, 1963) first isolated the replicases from MS2-infected cells and from $Q\beta$-infected cells. Both enzymes responded specifically to their homologous viral RNA as template, while the activity was negligible in either heterologous system. The replicase induced by group I phages, however, is notoriously difficult to purify. But it can be shown in an *in vivo* system that amber mutants of the viral replicase subunit of phage MS2, f2, or R17 complement with amber mutants in any of the other two cistrons (P. Model, cited in Horiuchi, 1975; M. van Montagu, personal communication). As replication is needed to provide the helper function, these results mean that at least the replicases of MS2, f2, and R17 are not functionally distinct. Although group III can be further divided into three subgroups by serological criteria, the replicases induced by $Q\beta$, by VK, or by ST, which represent these different subdivisions, can effectively accept any group III viral RNA as template but not group I or group II viral RNAs (Haruna *et al.*, 1967; Miyake *et al.*, 1971). Also, group IV can be further divided into two subdivisions, and the representative phages SP and FI differ more than tenfold in inactivation rate by serum (Miyake *et al.*, 1969). The corresponding viral replicases, however, are fully active with a heterologous group IV viral RNA; there is even a low activity with $Q\beta$ RNA (about 20% efficiency), indicating that group III and group IV phages are related (Haruna *et al.*, 1971; Miyake *et al.*, 1971).

The specificity of RNA coliphages for male cells concerns only the adsorption and injection steps. If these are circumvented by infection of spheroplasts by free viral RNA, then a normal life cycle can also take place in female cells (Davis *et al.*, 1961; Engelhardt and Zinder, 1964; Strauss and Sinsheimer, 1967). There is no evidence for restriction or modification. Variations in the relative efficiency of plaque formation or in size of plaques between male strains usually reflect differences in derepression of F factor or in metabolic activity, and do not allow discrimination between phages. An interesting and useful exception, however, is the *E. coli* mutant M27 isolated by Silverman *et al.* (1967). Group I phages do not plate at all on this strain, while Qβ (and male-specific DNA phages) give almost normal plaque counts. Amber mutants in *traD*, one of the F-factor genes required for conjugational transfer, exhibit the same phenotype as M27 (Achtman *et al.*, 1971). Miyake *et al.* (1969) also reported a difference in host range between group IV phages which were serologically closely related. Another discriminative property is the ability of the phage to interfere with the metabolism of its host during the infection cycle. R23 phage, which is serologically closely related to f2, is apparently much more efficient in shutting off host RNA and protein synthesis (Watanabe *et al.*, 1968; Watanabe and Watanabe, 1970).

To conclude, all RNA coliphages form a homogeneous class which share many biophysical, biochemical, and biological properties. They can all be distinguished serologically, even some which have an identical coat protein amino acid sequence. The inactivation rates by antisera and some other criteria allow a subdivision into at least four groups, but it is possible that all RNA coliphages are related, albeit distantly. Two types have mainly been studied and differ in important aspects: on the one hand, the group I phages f2-MS2-R17, which are so closely related that for most purposes results obtained with one are also valid for the others; on the other hand, the phage Qβ, which belongs to group III.

In this section a comparison was made of properties, such as the immunological cross-reactivity, which are directly dependent on the structure of the viral proteins. These will be further dealt with in Section 3. But ultimately the comparative analysis should be based on the genetic information itself, i.e., on the RNA nucleotide sequence. To a limited extent this is already possible, as will be discussed later in this chapter.

2.2. RNA Bacteriophages of Other Genera

The aforementioned RNA phages are all specific for the F pilus of *E. coli* male cells, which they need for adsorption and penetration. But if the F factor is introduced in some other members of Enterobacteriaceae, such as *Shigella*, *Proteus*, and *Salmonella*, then these genera also become susceptible to the above phages, although the initiation or the infection cycle is not always fast or efficient enough to lead to plaque formation on plates (Brinton *et al.*, 1964; Horiuchi and Adelberg, 1965; Kitano, 1966*a,b*). In fact, the real host in nature of all the so-called RNA coliphages is not known for certain.

RNA phages specific for other bacterial genera have also been described, namely for *Pseudomonas* and for *Caulobacter*. Another isolate infects specifically cells that harbor the drug resistance factor RP1 (Table 3). It is remarkable that all these phages closely resemble the RNA phages of *E. coli* and thus form a very homogeneous virus group. They all adsorb on special pili on the host, they all have a ribonuclease-sensitive step following adsorption, they all are icosahedral viruses with a sedimentation rate in the range of 70–88 S and a diameter of 21–25 nm, and—where investigated—contain a major coat protein of $12–15 \times 10^3$ daltons and a minor structural protein of $38–45 \times 10^3$ daltons corresponding to the A protein of the RNA coliphages.

7S and PP7 are two serologically related phages which infect *Pseudomonas aeruginosa* (Feary *et al.*, 1963, 1964; Bradley, 1966; Lin and Schmidt, 1972). They adsorb on polar pili which are not determined by the *Pseudomonas* sex factor FP. The diameter of these receptor pili is only 4.5 nm compared to 8.5–9.5 nm for the *E. coli* F pilus (Bradley, 1966; Brinton, 1971). Bacterial mutants which lack these specific pili are resistant to the RNA phages, but become susceptible to the viral RNA after conversion to spheroplasts (Weppelman and Brinton, 1971). PP7 specifies three viral polypeptides of similar size as the gene products of the coliphages (Davies and Benike, 1974). The viral RNA is estimated to be about 20% smaller than Qβ RNA and therefore PP7 resembles more closely the group I coliphages (Benike *et al.*, 1975).

Phages which specifically infect one of the *Caulobacter* species *crescentus*, *bacteroides*, or *fusiformis* have been described (Table 3). These phages are also serologically distinguishable. The life cycle of *Caulobacter* involves some sort of primitive form of differentiation, and the Cb phage can be used to distinguish different phases (Shapiro and Agabian-Keshishian, 1970; Shapiro *et al.*, 1971). The stalked bacterium develops into a predivisional form, in which a flagellum appears on the polar end as well as pili. Then asymmetrical division occurs, which results in a stalked cell and a swarmer cell; the latter subsequently loses its flagellum and the pili and develops also into a stalked cell. As the Cb phage requires the pili for adsorption, only the predivisional form and the swarmer cells are susceptible to infection. The structure of the virion is very similar to that of the coliphages: the major component is

TABLE 3
Properties of ssRNA Bacteriophages[a]

Host	Phage	Morphology	$s_{20,w}$ (S)	Diameter (nm)	Host receptor site	Coat (daltons)	A protein (daltons)
Escherichia coli	MS2-R17-f2	Icosahedral	79–80	26.0–26.6	F pili	13,731	43,988[b]
Escherichia coli	Qβ	Icosahedral	83–84	26.0	F pili	14,125	41,000[c]
Pseudomonas aeruginosa	7 S[d,e]	Icosahedral	88	25.0	Polar pili	+[h,i]	+[h,i]
	PP7[f,g]	Icosahedral		25.0	Polar pili		
Caulobacter crescentus	Cb5[j]	Icosahedral	70–71	23.0	Polar pili	12,000	40,000
	Cb12r[k,l]	Icosahedral		22.0–23.0	Polar pili		
Caulobacter bacteroides	Cb8r[k,l]	Icosahedral	—	22.0–23.0	Polar pili		
Caulobacter fusiformis	Cb23r[k,l]	Icosahedral	—	21.0–23.0	Polar pili		
RP plasmid[m]	PRR1[n]	Icosahedral	80	25.0	RP pili	+[h,o]	+[h,o]

[a] Adapted from Shapiro and Bendis (1975).
[b] Fiers et al. (1975).
[c] Weber and Konigsberg (1975).
[d] Feary et al. (1963).
[e] Feary et al. (1964).
[f] Bradley (1966).
[g] Lin and Schmidt (1972).
[h] +, Present and similar in size to the group I coliphages (MS2-R17-f2).
[i] Davies and Benike (1974).
[j] Bendis and Shapiro (1970).
[k] Schmidt and Stanier (1965).
[l] Schmidt (1966).
[m] This plasmid has a wide host range (see text).
[n] Olsen and Thomas (1973).
[o] Dhaese et al. (1977).

the coat component with a molecular weight of 12,000, whereas a minor component corresponding to the A protein has a molecular weight of 40,000. Unlike the coliphages the Cb5 coat protein contains histidine but no methionine (cysteine and tryptophan were not measured) (Bendis and Shapiro, 1970). Purification of this phage presents some problems, as it is unusually sensitive to high ionic strength (Bendis and Shapiro, 1970; Leffler *et al.*, 1971).

A recent and very interesting addition to the list of RNA phages is PRR1 (Olsen and Thomas, 1973). This phage is specific for bacteria in which the drug resistance P plasmid has been introduced (P compatibility group, e.g., R1822 or RP4). The latter was originally described in *Pseudomonas aeruginosa* but has a remarkably broad host range and can be transferred to most gram-negative bacteria (Datta *et al.*, 1971; Olsen and Shipley, 1973). Although the burst sizes and efficiencies of plating are generally rather low, plaques were observed on P-containing *Pseudomonas aeruginosa*, *P. fluorescens*, *P. putida*, *Escherichia coli* Hfr, *E. coli* F⁻, *Salmonella typhimurium*, and *Vibrio cholerae* (Olsen and Thomas, 1973). Other genera, which also expressed the P plasmid functions, were killed by high multiplicities of phage but did not propagate them (*Acinetobacter calco-aceticus*, *Neisseria perflava*, *Azotobacter vinlandii*, and *Proteus mirabilis*). Still others, like *Shigella boydii*, were not affected at all. A successful infection cycle requires at least correct translation of all viral genes and replication of the viral genome, processes which involve intimate interactions and cooperation between viral and crucial host components. Therefore, studies with the PRR1 phage can provide important information on the functional relationship of these systems in different genera. It is unlikely that the P plasmid itself contributes a gene product to the translation or replication of the viral genome, as tested by a spheroplast system (P. Dhaese, personal communication). The main and presumably only reason that the PRR1 phage is specific for P-containing bacteria is that they specifically adsorb to and penetrate via a plasmid-induced P pilus. They also closely resemble the coliphages and other RNA phages in many other properties, such as morphology, diameter, sedimentation rate, and buoyant density (Olsen and Thomas, 1973). They contain a main coat protein and a minor A protein of similar size as those of MS2; the former is 131 amino acids long and like the Cb5 phage contains histidine but no cysteine or tryptophan (Dhaese *et al.*, 1977). RPP1 differs mainly from the RNA coliphage in its susceptibility to high concentrations of ribonuclease and to EDTA. This does not necessarily indicate any fundamental difference in architecture compared to the coliphages, as under appropriate physical conditions removal of divalent cations also labilizes MS2 (Verbraeken and Fiers, 1972a).

We have seen in this section that RNA bacteriophages have been isolated from quite different bacterial genera, so far all gram negative. All these RNA phages constitute a physically very homogeneous group and they all penetrate into their host via specific pili. No extensive hunts for RNA phages in the bacterial world have yet been carried out, and therefore it is likely that many remain to be discovered. New species of RNA phages are of considerable interest for studying their evolutionary relationship and for the investigation of the species specificity of the translational processes. The latter aspect has also been studied in *in vitro* systems, as will be discussed in Section 4.3.1.

For completeness I should mention here the RNA bacteriophage $\phi6$, which infects *Pseudomonas phaseolicola* (Semancik *et al.*, 1973; Vidaver *et al.*, 1973; van Etten *et al.*, 1974). This phage, dealt with in detail in Chapter 5 of Volume 12 of this series, is much larger than the RNA phages hitherto discussed as the diameter amounts to 65 to 75 nm (Bamford *et al.*, 1976). It is remarkably rich in lipid (25%). The genome is composed of three double-stranded RNA molecules with a combined molecular weight of 9.5×10^6 (vs. 1.24×10^6 for MS2 RNA). In these properties it resembles more the diplornaviruses (animal and plant viruses with a segmented, double-stranded RNA genome), like reovirus and clover wound tumor virus. However, there is one analogy with the preceding group of RNA phages—$\phi6$ also infects its host via adsorption on specific pili. But the bacterial cell wall constitutes a complex barrier, and there may exist only a limited number of ways to penetrate the cell for a phage which does not possess a complicated tail structure. Therefore, the fact that both the single-stranded RNA phages and $\phi6$ use special pili as receptor sites may not be indicative of a distant evolutionary relatedness but may rather represent an example of convergent evolution.

3. ARCHITECTURE OF THE VIRION

3.1. General Properties

A schematic map of the genome of MS2 is shown in Fig. 1A (MS2 is taken as a prototype of the group I phages). The three genes have been characterized genetically, biochemically, and chemically, and they code for the A protein (also called "maturation protein"), the coat pro-

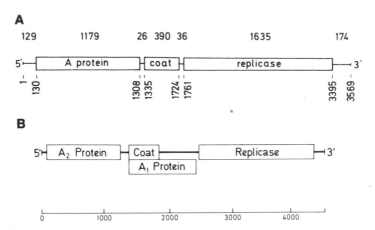

Fig. 1. Genetic map of the RNA bacteriophages. A: The genome of MS2. The nucleotides in the viral RNA are numbered from the 5' end to the 3' end and the positions of some important signals are indicated underneath (Fiers *et al.*, 1976) (the initiation codon is considered part of the genes and the termination codon, part of the untranslated region). The length of the different regions, expressed in number of nucleotides, is shown above the diagram. B: The genome of Qβ. The different genes are represented in blocks, and their position can be estimated on the basis of the nucleotide scale shown below.

tein, and the viral replicase subunit. Likewise, for Qβ genetic analysis indicated only three complementation groups. Biochemical and chemical studies, however, revealed the presence of a fourth gene product, the A1 protein or readthrough protein (protein IIb in the nomenclature of Garwes *et al.*, 1969) (Fig. 1B). Some properties of the virus-coded proteins are listed in Table 4.

An MS2 virion contains a single, 3569-nucleotide-long RNA molecule, a shell composed of 180 copies of the coat protein, and one molecule of A protein. It has recently been recognized that each particle also contains nearly 1000 molecules of spermidine; this is sufficient to neutralize a large proportion of all negative charges on the viral RNA (Fukuma and Cohen, 1975). The main physicochemical parameters of the virus particle are summarized in Table 5. Camerini-Otero *et al.* (1974) have evaluated various hydrodynamic and optical methods which can be used to estimate the particle weight of the virions. The average of five different procedures is 3.85×10^6.

The diameter of the particle is about 26.3 nm and the protein shell is only 2–3 nm thick, as determined both by X-ray scattering (Zipper *et al.*, 1971) and by electron microscopy (Crowther *et al.*, 1975). There may be a slight penetration of the RNA into the protein shell (Zipper *et*

TABLE 4
Virus-Coded Proteins

	Molecular weight	Number of amino acids	Number of molecules per virion	Function
MS2-R17-f2				
Coat	13,731	129[a]	180[b]	Main capsid protein
A protein	43,988[c,d]	393[c]	1	Assembly and adsorption; penetrates together with the infecting RNA into the host cell[e,f]
Replicase	60,692[g]	544[g]	—	Responsible, together with host proteins, for viral RNA replication
Qβ				
Coat	14,125	132[h,p]	180[b]	Main capsid protein
A1 (or IIb) protein	38,000[i,j]	350 ± 20	3–14[k]	Readthrough product of the coat gene[i,k,l], required for the formation of infectious phage particles[m]
A2 (or IIa) protein	44,000[i,j]	410 ± 20	1	Assembly and adsorption
Replicase	67,000 ±2,000[n,o]	610 ± 20	—	Responsible, together with host proteins, for viral RNA replication

[a] Weber and Konigsberg (1967).
[b] This number is based on symmetry considerations (triangulation number $T = 3$); as a few coat molecules may be replaced by the A protein, or as a few coat proteins may be preferentially bound (Sugiyama et al., 1967), the real number may be slightly less or slightly more.
[c] Fiers et al. (1975).
[d] Remaut and Fiers (1972).
[e] Kozak and Nathans (1972).
[f] Krahn et al. (1972).
[g] Fiers et al. (1976).
[h] Maita and Konigsberg (1971).
[i] Moore et al. (1971).
[j] These values may be underestimated as A1 moves slightly faster and A2 slightly slower relative to A protein of MS2 in a sodium dodecylsulfate–polyacrylamide gel electrophoresis system (Remaut and Fiers, unpublished).
[k] Weiner and Weber (1971).
[l] Horiuchi et al. (1971).
[m] Hofstetter et al. (1974).
[n] Kondo et al. (1970).
[o] Kamen (1970).
[p] Stoll et al. (1977).

TABLE 5

Physical Properties of the Virions[a]

Property	MS2-R17-f2	Qβ
Molecular weight	$3.6 \times 10^{6b,c}$–3.85×10^{6d}	4.2×10^{6e}
$s_{20,w}$, S	79–80[c]	83–84[e]
Density, g/cm³	1.46[b]	1.47[f]
Partial specific volume, $\bar{v}$, ml/g	0.690–0.703[b,e]	0.695[e]
Diffusion coefficient, $D_{20,w}$, cm²/sec	1.64×10^{-7d}	1.55×10^{-7e}
Diameter, nm	26.0–26.6[b,g]	—
Inner diameter, nm	21.0[h]	—
Radius of gyration, R_G	105.2[h]–128[g]	—
RNA content, %	31–34[b,i]	—
Specific absorbancy, $A_{260\ nm}^{1\ mg/ml}$	7.66–8.03[b,c]	8.02[e]
Ratio $A_{260\ nm}/A_{280\ nm}$	1.79[j]	—
Water content, g H_2O/g	0.9–1.0[g,h]	—
Isoelectric point, pH	3.9[e]	5.3[e]–4.1[k]
Refractive increment at 546 nm, cm³/g	0.174[d]–0.199[e]	0.198[e]

[a] Usually only a single typical reference is given, but often concurrent results have been obtained.
[b] Strauss and Sinsheimer (1963).
[c] Gesteland and Boedtker (1964).
[d] Camerini-Otero et al. (1974).
[e] Overby et al. (1966a).
[f] Watanabe et al. (1967a).
[g] Fischbach et al. (1965).
[h] Zipper et al. (1971).
[i] Enger et al. (1963).
[j] Vasquez et al. (1966).
[k] Rice and Horst (1972).

al., 1971; Jacrot et al., 1977). Recent studies by neutron scattering have suggested the presence of a central hole, with a radius of about 6 nm (Jacrot et al., 1977). As indicated by the low isoelectric point, there are many negative charges on the surface, and these seem to occur in clusters (Matthews and Cole, 1972b). Presumably these correspond to carboxyl groups of the coat protein, but some contribution by negative charges of the RNA has not been excluded. The protein shell is rather porous as even relatively bulky molecules like ethidium bromide readily penetrate into the particle (Wong et al., 1974).

The icosahedral shell has a $T = 3$ surface lattice, but electron microscopy does not reveal very characteristic morphological subunits. Presumably the coat protein molecules associate as dimers, which then form rings of five about the 5-fold axes and rings of six about the 3-fold (quasi 6-fold) axes (Crowther et al., 1975). The holes, and hence penetration of EM stain, are more in evidence at the 3-fold position than at the 5-fold positions. A superficially similar but actually different bonding scheme was proposed by Dunker and Paranchych (1975). The much-quoted capsid model proposed by Vasquez et al. (1966), involving 32 morphological subunits, is not compatible with the newer, higher-resolution data.

The virion particles in a purified virus population are physicochemically completely homogeneous. Yet there is evidence for functional heterogeneity (Paranchych, 1975); the defect at the molecular level in the noninfectious particles is unknown. Various physically deviant particles, related to the virion, are worth mentioning. Empty particles correspond to the coat protein shells of the virus and lack both the total RNA complement and the A protein. They can be obtained by limited alkaline degradation of the virus (Samuelson and Kaesberg, 1970) or by assembly of coat protein subunits under appropriate ionic conditions (Matthews and Cole, 1972a; Knolle and Hohn, 1975), or—in the most natural way—by addition of phage to susceptible cells, a process which releases the empty shells into solution (Paranchych et al., 1970). These empty particles sediment at 42–45 S, and, according to the physicochemical characterization of Samuelson and Kaesberg (1970), their diameter amounts to 26.2 nm, which proves that they really correspond to the virion protein shell.

Infection of nonpermissive cells with mutant virus that has an amber mutation in the A gene leads to an almost normal infection cycle concluded by lysis of the cell, but with production of noninfectious, so-called defective particles (Lodish et al., 1965; Heisenberg, 1966; Argetsinger and Gussin, 1966). These can only be obtained in an undegraded form from mutants of E. coli deficient in ribonuclease I (Gesteland, 1966). The "defective" particles have the same buoyant density as normal virions and contain the same components, except for the missing A protein. An intact molecule of RNA is present, which is infectious when assayed in an amber suppressor-containing spheroplast system (Argetsinger and Gussin, 1966). "Defective" particles sediment at 69 S as a slightly broadened band; this decreased sedimentation rate for particles which have about the same molecular weight as intact phage must be explained by a higher frictional coefficient. Presumably the capsid shell is assembled in the normal way, but the viral RNA partly dangles out at one or more sites. Indeed, these particles are very sensitive to ribonuclease, and although the latter enzyme decreases the total weight by digestion, the sedimentation rate may actually go up to 74 S as a result of the reduction in frictional drag (Heisenberg, 1966). The A protein can also be removed from complete virions by treatment in high salt, e.g., as occurs during prolonged CsCl centrifugation. This selective loss of the A protein does not change the quaternary structure of the particles and they still sediment at 80 S, although they have become noninfectious (Verbraeken and Fiers, 1972b).

Still other virus-related particles were first described by Argetsinger (1968), viz. infective, expanded forms. These are generated by incubation of phage in low ionic strength buffer at moderate temperature (e.g., 46°C). The expanded particles sediment at 55–56 S; they contain all the components of the virion and their lowered sedimentation rate is again due to an increase in frictional coefficient (Verbraeken and Fiers, 1972*a*). Undoubtedly they are formed by extrusion of RNA loops through the pores of the virus shell; this process is irreversible. The particles are nearly as infectious as intact virions but extremely sensitive to ribonuclease. This enzyme removes about two-thirds of the RNA, while the A protein remains associated with the core particle. The expansion is an all-or-none, highly cooperative process; presumably it is due either to the melting of weak bonds between the RNA and the inner side of the protein shell or to loss of a specific tertiary structure of the viral RNA (Verbraeken and Fiers, 1972*a*). As one would expect from the low temperature at which the transition occurs, the secondary structure of the RNA is nearly unaffected by the expansion process (Thomas *et al.*, 1976).

3.2. Coat Protein

The coat protein of the group I phages contains 129 amino acids and that of Qβ, 132. The amino acid composition of some RNA phages is summarized in Table 6, and we have already noted in Section 2.1 that the main serological groups of RNA coliphages can also be distinguished by the absence of certain amino acids (Nishihara *et al.*, 1969). All the RNA coliphages lack histidine, but there is apparently no absolute block against the presence of this amino acid as van Assche *et al.* (1974) have characterized a phenotypically neutral mutant which does contain histidine (in position 42).

The first complete amino acid sequences were established for f2 by Weber and Konigsberg (1967) and for fr by Wittman-Liebold and Wittman (1967). The sequence of the R17 protein and MS2 protein differs only from f2 by a Met residue in position 88 instead of Leu (Weber, 1967; Lin *et al.*, 1967). When the nucleotide sequence of the MS2 coat gene was established (Min Jou *et al.*, 1972), it became possible to correct three errors in the amino acid sequence; all three involved Asn $\leftrightarrow$ Asp interchanges, namely at positions 11, 12, and 17. These corrections were confirmed by direct amino acid sequencing (Vandekerckhove, 1973; Weber and Konigsberg, 1975). The two cysteine residues are present in the reduced form (Lin *et al.*, 1967; Thomas *et al.*, 1976). The amino acid sequences of MS2 and fr are compared with each other and with that of Qβ in Fig. 2. As already mentioned in Sec-

TABLE 6

Amino Acid Composition of RNA Phage Coat Proteins[a]

	MS2-R17[b]	f2	GA[c]	Qβ	φCb5[d]	PRR1[e]
Ala	14	14	15	15	7	6
Arg	4	4	5	7	5	9
Asp + Asn	14	14	13	15	7	17
Cys	2	2	0	2	N.D.[f]	0
Glu + Gln	11	11	7	13	12	11
Gly	9	9	9	7	11	7
His	0	0	0	0	2	2
Ile	8	8	8	4	3	6
Leu	7	8	8	12	9	9
Lys	6	6	7	7	7	7
Met	2	1	0	0	0	2
Phe	4	4	4	3	4	4
Pro	6	6	5	8	3	5
Ser	13	13	13	10	9	7
Thr	9	9	9	12	9	13
Trp	2	2	2	0	N.D.	0
Tyr	4	4	5	4	6	4
Val	14	14	16	13	9	22
Total	129	129	(126)[g]	132	(103)[g]	131

[a] Values are rounded off to nearest integers.
[b] The phage M12 is presumably identical, except for a Lys to Glx change (Enger and Kaesberg, 1965).
[c] Nishihara *et al.* (1969).
[d] Bendis and Shapiro (1970).
[e] Dhaese and Van Montagu (personal communication).
[f] N.D., Not determined.
[g] Values in parentheses are very approximate and are not supported by any sequence data.

tion 2.1, MS2–R17 show an 83% homology with the serologically distantly related fr; most of the 22 amino acid changes can be explained by a single nucleotide mutation in the genome. It is of interest that there is a long segment going from position 20 to position 70 which is identical in the two phages except for two conservative mutations (an Asn ↔ Gln and a Val ↔ Ile change). Presumably this part plays an important role in the establishment of the overall structure. On the other hand, the Qβ sequence, established by Konigsberg *et al.* (1970; Maita and Konigsberg, 1971), is hardly similar to the group I phages. Several insertions and deletions have to be invoked in order to reveal some homologies and even then a claim to evolutionary relationship on this evidence alone would hardly be convincing. Recently, a corrected version of the amino acid sequence of the Qβ coat protein has been published; this reinvestiga-

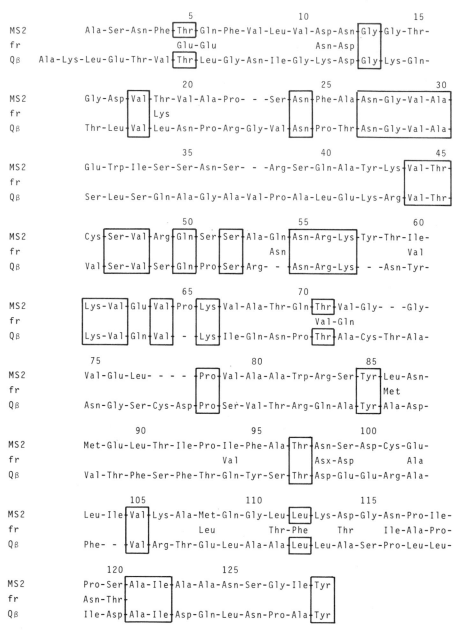

Fig. 2.   Amino acid sequence of the coat protein of phage MS2 (or R17), of phage fr, and of phage Qβ. Only the residues in the fr sequence which are different or possibly different from MS2-R17 are shown. Identical residues in MS2 and Qβ (after optimal alignment by some insertions and deletions) are enclosed in boxes. The f2 coat protein has a Leu at position 88 instead of Met (references are given in the text).

tion was again prompted by discordant nucleic acid sequence data (Stoll *et al.*, 1977).

From symmetry considerations one would conclude that there are exactly 180 coat protein subunits per viral particle. This number could be too high if a few coat monomers on an apex are replaced by a single A protein; this is perhaps not too likely as the A protein can be located in one of the surface holes revealed by electron microscopy (Section 3.1). Alternatively, one (Spahr *et al.*, 1969) or a few (Sugiyama *et al.*, 1967; Sugiyama, 1971) extra coat proteins could bind to the repressor site in the viral RNA (Section 4.3.6) and be present inside the virion; also, this hypothesis is not too likely as the viral RNA must be free of repressor when it penetrates into the host cell.

Pure coat protein can be obtained by treatment of a virus preparation with 66% acetic acid (Fraenkel-Conrat, 1957; Hohn, 1967; Sugiyama *et al.*, 1967) or with 66% 2-chloroethanol (Schubert and Frank, 1970). It is monomeric only under well-defined ionic conditions (e.g., 10^{-2} M acetic acid) or in the presence of ionic detergents such as sodium dodecylsulfate. Outside the boundary conditions of monomer stability, the coat protein readily forms dimers and higher aggregates.

Several physical methods indicate that the native coat protein in the virion has little or no α helicity. This is in contrast to the single-stranded, F^+-specific DNA phages, where the coat protein is largely α helical. Isenberg *et al.* (1971) found neither α-helix nor β structure by circular dichroism and by infrared spectrophotometry, while optical rotatory dispersion results did not permit reaching unambiguous conclusions about the coat protein conformation (Oriel and Koenig, 1968). More recent studies by means of laser–Raman spectroscopy, however, reveal about 60% ($\pm 20\%$) β-sheet conformation in the native protein and again virtually no α helicity (0% $\pm$ 20%) (Thomas *et al.*, 1976).

So far little is known concerning the relation between the primary amino acid sequence and its conformation in the native particle. Cross-linking studies with bisulfite indicate that only a limited number of the coat monomers can react with an appropriately positioned cytidylate residue (Turchinsky *et al.*, 1974). This would suggest that not all coat monomers are in equivalent positions or else that the viral RNA has a rigid internal configuration such that only a limited number of C residues are available for the cross-linking reaction to the protein. Further studies may allow the identification of the nucleotide and amino acid positions involved. Characterization of MS2 mutants that are affected in presumptive surface properties, such as serum resistance or electrophoretic mobility, has suggested that the amino acid positions

13, 16, 17, 70, 76, and 102 are exposed (Vandekerckhove *et al.*, 1975). A study by Langbeheim *et al.* (1976) points in the same direction. These authors cleaved MS2 coat protein into three peptide fragments 1–88 (P₁), 89–108 (P₂), and 109–129 (P₃). Not only could the first fragment, P₁, be used to raise neutralizing antibodies against MS2 virus, but also synthetic P₂, linked to an appropriate carrier, did induce an active antiserum against the phage. These results hold great promise as in principle they open up the possibility of vaccination by means of relatively short, synthetic peptides.

3.3.   A Protein

Zinder and co-workers (Lodish *et al.*, 1965) identified a gene in f2 which, if not functional, resulted in the production of a normal burst of noninfectious particles; as these virions were not correctly assembled, the function of this missing gene must be involved in proper maturation (cf. Section 3.1).

Nathans *et al.* (1966) could then show that the aforementioned gene product was in fact present in the virus particle as a minor structural component. The coat protein does not contain histidine, and Argetsinger-Steitz (1968*a*) took advantage of this property to label specifically the minor structural component by adding radioactive histidine to growing infected cultures. In this way she could isolate and characterize this protein, now called the "maturation protein" or "A protein."* This product is required not only for *A*ssembly but also for *A*dsorption of the phage on its host cell. The original molecular weight estimate was around 38,000; we now know that the exact value is 43,988 (Fiers *et al.*, 1975). On the basis of an amino acid analysis on a 90% purified product, Argetsinger-Steitz (1968*b*) determined that the A protein contained five histidine residues (later confirmed). By measuring the histidine content of the phage, she could then conclude that each virion particle contains only one A protein molecule. The ratio of one A protein molecule per particle was later confirmed using uniformly labeled viral protein; furthermore, it was shown that the A protein could be selectively leached out by high salt solutions, e.g., during centrifugation in CsCl (Verbraeken and Fiers, 1972*b*). The removal of A protein is strictly correlated with loss of biological activity, indicating that it is required not only for proper assembly but also for adsorption

---

* The name "A protein" was originally given because the protein corresponded to the A cistron as defined by the genetic analysis of Gussin (1966).

on susceptible host cells. The A-less particles are normal in all physical aspects and still sediment at about 80 S (Section 3.1). The fact that the A protein can be so readily removed by high salt treatment strongly suggests that it is located at the outside of the particle (or in a hole of the porous capsid shell; see above). This is supported by iodination and immunological studies, which show that the A protein is indeed very reactive and hence exposed to the solvent (Curtiss and Krueger, 1974).

As mentioned above, the A protein (of R17) was first purified and characterized by Argetsinger-Steitz (1968b), starting from virus preparations specifically labeled with tritiated histidine. Subsequently the isolation was considerably simplified by taking advantage of the rather selective precipitation of the A protein–viral RNA complex on treatment of a phage solution with 2 vol glacial acetic acid (Osborn *et al.*, 1970b). Isolated A protein is insoluble in aqueous solution, unless denaturing agents, such as ionic detergents or urea, are present. It has the annoying tendency to adhere to nearly all kinds of surfaces, including dialysis tubing, and hence is very cumbersome to work with. The N-terminal sequence of R17 A protein was determined as Met-Arg-Ala-Phe-Ser-Ala-Leu-Asx by Weiner *et al.* (1972). Hence the initiating methionine is not removed after biosynthesis, as is also true for the analogous N-terminal sequence Met-Arg-Val of UDP-galactose-4-epimerase (Musso *et al.*, 1974). The resistance of the methionine residue is not complete, however, as also some A protein with N-terminal arginine is present (quoted in Weber and Konigsberg, 1975). In the case of Qβ A protein (protein IIa, see below), the N-terminal sequence is Pro-Lys-Leu-Pro and hence the initiating methionine has been removed (Weiner and Weber, 1971).

On the basis of the complete nucleotide sequence of MS2 RNA, discussed in Section 4.4.7, the total amino acid sequence of the A protein of MS2 can of course be deduced (Fiers *et al.*, 1975) (Fig. 3). Independently, the A protein of MS2 itself has largely been sequenced by Vandekerckhove *et al.* (1977). It differs from the R17 sequence by an Ala → Thr change at position 6 and a Lys → Arg change at the C terminus. An overall comparison between the corresponding viral RNAs, as far as the information is available, will be given in Section 5.7.2. From an inspection of the amino acid sequence no clues emerge as to its structure–function relationship. Compared with the coat protein, the A protein has a higher leucine-to-isoleucine ratio (factor 2.6), a higher tryptophan content (factor 2.0), and in particular a higher arginine content (factor 2.4). A direct interaction between the A protein and the viral RNA is suggested by the complex obtained after acetic acid treat-

```
130
GUG·CGA·GCU·UUU·AGU·ACU·CUC·GAU·AGG·GAG·AAC·GAG·ACC·UUC·GUC·CCC·UCC·GUU·CGC·GUU
Met Arg Ala Phe Ser Thr Leu Asp Arg Glu Asn Glu Thr Phe Val Pro Ser Val Arg Val
                                                                               20

190
UAC·GCG·GAC·GGU·GAG·ACU·GAA·GAU·AAC·UCA·UUC·UCU·UUA·AAA·UAU·CGU·UCG·AAC·UGG·ACU
Tyr Ala Asp Gly Glu Thr Glu Asp Asn Ser Phe Ser Leu Lys Tyr Arg Ser Asn Trp Thr
                                                                               40

250
CCC·GGU·CGU·UUU·AAC·UCG·ACU·GGG·GCC·AAA·ACG·AAA·CAG·UGG·CAC·UAC·CCC·UCU·CCG·UAU
Pro Gly Arg Phe Asn Ser Thr Gly Ala Lys Thr Lys Gln Trp His Tyr Pro Ser Pro Tyr
                                                                               60

310
UCA·CGG·GGG·GCG·UUA·AGU·GUC·ACA·UCG·AUA·GAU·CAA·GGU·GCC·UAC·AAG·CGA·AGU·GGG·UCA
Ser Arg Gly Ala Leu Ser Val Thr Ser Ile Asp Gln Gly Ala Tyr Lys Arg Ser Gly Ser
                                                                               80

370
UCG·UGG·GGU·CGC·CCG·UAC·GAG·GAG·AAA·GCC·GGU·UUC·GGC·UUC·UCC·CUC·GAC·GCA·CGC·UCC
Ser Trp Gly Arg Pro Tyr Glu Glu Lys Ala Gly Phe Gly Phe Ser Leu Asp Ala Arg Ser
                                                                               100

430
UGC·UAC·AGC·CUC·UUC·CCU·GUA·AGC·CAA·AAC·UUG·ACU·UAC·AUC·GAA·GUG·CCG·CAG·AAC·GUU
Cys Tyr Ser Leu Phe Pro Val Ser Gln Asn Leu Thr Tyr Ile Glu Val Pro Gln Asn Val
                                                                               120

490
GCG·AAC·CGG·GCG·UCG·ACC·GAA·GUC·CUG·CAA·AAG·GUC·ACC·CAG·GGU·AAU·UUU·AAC·CUU·GGU
Ala Asn Arg Ala Ser Thr Glu Val Leu Gln Lys Val Thr Gln Gly Asn Phe Asn Leu Gly
                                                                               140

550
GUU·GCU·UUA·GCA·GAG·GCC·AGG·UCG·ACA·GCC·UCA·CAA·CUC·GCG·ACG·CAA·ACC·AUU·GCG·CUC
Val Ala Leu Ala Glu Ala Arg Ser Thr Ala Ser Gln Leu Ala Thr Gln Thr Ile Ala Leu
                                                                               160

610
GUG·AAG·GCG·UAC·ACU·GCC·GCU·CGU·CGC·GGU·AAU·UGG·CGC·CAG·GCG·CUC·CGC·UAC·CUU·GCC
Val Lys Ala Tyr Thr Ala Ala Arg Arg Gly Asn Trp Arg Gln Ala Leu Arg Tyr Leu Ala
                                                                               180

670
CUA·AAC·GAA·GAU·CGA·AAG·UUU·CGA·UCA·AAA·CAC·GUG·GCC·GGC·AGG·UGG·UUG·GAG·UUG·CAG
Leu Asn Glu Asp Arg Lys Phe Arg Ser Lys His Val Ala Gly Arg Trp Leu Glu Leu Gln
                                                                               200

730
UUC·GGU·UGG·UUA·CCA·CUA·AUG·AGU·GAU·AUC·CAG·GGU·GCA·UAU·GAG·AUG·CUU·ACG·AAG·GUU
Phe Gly Trp Leu Pro Leu Met Ser Asp Ile Gln Gly Ala Tyr Glu Met Leu Thr Lys Val
                                                                               220

790
CAC·CUU·CAA·GAG·UUU·CUU·CCU·AUG·AGA·GCC·GUA·CGU·CAG·GUC·GGU·ACU·AAC·AUC·AAG·UUA
His Leu Gln Glu Phe Leu Pro Met Arg Ala Val Arg Gln Val Gly Thr Asn Ile Lys Leu
                                                                               240

850
GAU·GGC·CGU·CUG·UCG·UAU·CCA·GCU·GCA·AAC·UUC·CAG·ACA·ACG·UGC·AAC·AUA·UCG·CGA·CGU
Asp Gly Arg Leu Ser Tyr Pro Ala Ala Asn Phe Gln Thr Thr Cys Asn Ile Ser Arg Arg
                                                                               260

910
AUC·GUG·AUA·UGG·UUU·UAC·AUA·AAC·GAU·GCA·CGU·UUG·GCA·UGG·UUG·UCG·UCU·CUA·GGU·AUC
Ile Val Ile Trp Phe Tyr Ile Asn Asp Ala Arg Leu Ala Trp Leu Ser Ser Leu Gly Ile
                                                                               280

970
UUG·AAC·CCA·CUA·GGU·AUA·GUG·UGG·GAA·AAG·GUG·CCU·UUC·UCA·UUC·GUU·GUC·GAC·UGG·CUC
Leu Asn Pro Leu Gly Ile Val Trp Glu Lys Val Pro Phe Ser Phe Val Val Asp Trp Leu
                                                                               300

1030
CUA·CCU·GUA·GGU·AAC·AUG·CUC·GAG·GGC·CUU·ACG·GCC·CCC·GUG·GGA·UGC·UCC·UAC·AUG·UCA
Leu Pro Val Gly Asn Met Leu Glu Gly Leu Thr Ala Pro Val Gly Cys Ser Tyr Met Ser
                                                                               320

1090
GGA·ACA·GUU·ACU·GAC·GUA·AUA·ACG·GGU·GAG·UCC·AUC·AUA·AGC·GUU·GAC·GCU·CCC·UAC·GGG
Gly Thr Val Thr Asp Val Ile Thr Gly Glu Ser Ile Ile Ser Val Asp Ala Pro Tyr Gly
                                                                               340

1150
UGG·ACU·GUG·GAG·AGA·CAG·GGC·ACU·GCU·AAG·GCC·CAA·AUC·UCA·GCC·AUG·CAU·CGA·GGG·GUA
Trp Thr Val Glu Arg Gln Gly Thr Ala Lys Ala Gln Ile Ser Ala Met His Arg Gly Val
                                                                               360

1210
CAA·UCC·GUA·UGG·CCA·ACA·ACU·GGC·GCG·UAC·GUA·AAG·UCU·CCU·UUC·UCG·AUG·GUC·CAU·ACC
Gln Ser Val Trp Pro Thr Thr Gly Ala Tyr Val Lys Ser Pro Phe Ser Met Val His Thr
                                                                               380

1270
UUA·GAU·GCG·UUA·GCA·UUA·AUC·AGG·CAA·CGG·CUC·UCU·AGA·UAG
Leu Asp Ala Leu Ala Leu Ile Arg Gln Arg Leu Ser Arg
                                                     393
```

ment, as discussed above; also, the salt sensitivity of the A protein binding in the particle indicates the involvement of ionic bonds, presumably to the RNA. The abundant arginine residues (e.g., in regions 168–177, 185–195, and 388–393) may well be involved in this strong binding to the RNA. Also, some clustering of hydrophobic amino acids is observed (e.g., the regions 196–206, 261–267, and 272–303), and this may explain the general stickiness of this protein. Although it is conceivable that during the formation of the viral capsid a single coat protein molecule out of the 180 is replaced by an A protein molecule, there are no regions of extensive sequence homology in these two proteins. The amino acid sequence of the A protein is apparently less rigid than that of the other two viral genes. On one hand, all known amber mutants in the *A* gene can be suppressed by any suppressor strain, irrespective of the nature of the inserted amino acid. On the other hand, the number of conserved spontaneous mutations is slightly higher in this gene (Min Jou and Fiers, 1976*b*). Nevertheless, neither a polypeptide which is too short nor a polypeptide which is too long is incorporated in the viral particles (Remaut and Fiers, 1972); a polypeptide which is only 88% of full length is synthesized by one class of amber mutants under nonpermissive conditions (Vandamme *et al.*, 1972). A too long A protein is synthesized in various amber suppressor strains infected with wild-type MS2; the prolonged polypeptide contains an additional 27 amino acids at the C terminus (Remaut and Fiers, 1972; Contreras *et al.*, 1973) (cf. also Section 4.4.6).

As mentioned above, it is likely that there is a direct interaction between the A protein and the viral RNA. This is further supported by the observation that, following adsorption, the A protein penetrates together with the viral RNA into the host cell (Kozak and Nathans, 1971; Krahn *et al.*, 1972). It is clear that the A protein specifically interacts with the F receptor sites; after binding, the A protein may promote active penetration of the viral RNA. Whether it also plays a role inside the cell, e.g., in directing the first steps in translation, is not known. However, its necessity can obviously not be absolute as pure viral RNA is infectious in a spheroplast system, albeit at low efficiency. Interestingly, the A protein while promoting RNA penetration is cleaved by a specific cell surface protease into a 24,000-dalton and a 15,000-dalton fragment (Krahn *et al.*, 1972). Possibly, the A protein

Fig. 3. The A protein of bacteriophage MS2. The total nucleotide sequence of the A protein gene is given, and the nucleotide numbering on the left refers to the viral RNA (cf. Fig. 1A). The deduced amino acid sequence of the A protein is indicated below the nucleotide sequence (note that the initiating methionine is conserved). From Fiers *et al.* (1975).

may interact with sites far apart on the viral RNA, and in this way promote condensation required for proper packaging; cleavage of the protein then allows some loosening of the three-dimensional structure, such that translational processes can start. It is amusing to reflect that highly specific proteases are also present at the surface of eukaryotic cells and play there an important role in some cellular responses (Reich, 1974).

The A protein–viral RNA complex can be directly isolated from the phage by the acetic acid method (Leipold and Hofschneider, 1975) or it can be reconstituted from purified A protein and viral RNA (Shiba and Mizake, 1975). The complex infects male *E. coli* cells via the F^+ pili, sediments almost like viral RNA, and is highly sensitive to ribonucleases; the infectivity is resistant to antiphage serum. The coat protein and ribosomes interact with specific regions of the RNA; the RNA segment involved in this binding is protected against nuclease degradation and can be isolated (Section 4.3). We have been unable, however, to protect in a similar way a specific segment of the viral RNA by A protein (unpublished experiments in collaboration with B. Leipold, P. Hofschneider, and W. Min Jou). Perhaps the A protein interacts with local features of the specifically folded viral RNA, which are far apart in the primary sequence. Nevertheless, the interaction must be very specific, as Shiba (1975) found only activity if the A protein of MS2 was added to MS2 RNA and not if added to Qβ RNA, and vice versa.

Garwes *et al.* (1969) made the observation that the phage Qβ contains two A-type proteins. This is remarkable as only three complementation groups have been found, just as in the group I phages (Section 5). The larger polypeptide is called A2 or IIa and has a molecular weight of about 44,000. It is coded by the bona fide A protein gene and is present in a ratio of one molecule per virion (Table 4). The other A protein, A1 or IIb, has a molecular weight of 38,000 and is a readthrough product of the coat gene (Weiner and Weber, 1971; Moore *et al.*, 1971; Horiuchi *et al.*, 1971). The latter conclusion is based on the following findings: The sequence of eight N-terminal amino acids was established and turned out to be identical to those of the coat protein. Furthermore, amber mutants in the coat gene grown under nonpermissive conditions fail to synthesize not only coat proteins but also IIb polypeptides. As it is known that the termination signal UGA is rather leaky in normally used *E. coli* strains (i.e., there is a weak suppressor activity), this triplet is the most likely candidate as a stop signal of the coat gene. Qβ wild-type virus grown on an UGA suppressor strain contains indeed up to 13–14 IIb molecules per virus particle compared to only three to five when grown on standard *E. coli* strains (Weiner and Weber, 1971). Direct analysis of the viral polypeptides made in the infected cell confirms the strong enhancement of the amount of IIb protein in a UGA-suppressor strain; the actual degree of readthrough in a normal *E. coli* K12 strain, expressed on a molar basis, is around 2.5% while it amounts to 11% in the suppressor strain (Remaut and Fiers, 1972; Weiner and Weber, 1973); it must be noted that some other *E. coli* strains are less leaky than K12. Final proof that the termination of the Qβ coat gene is a *single* UGA codon was provided by Weiner and Weber (1973). They isolated a 55-amino-acid-long peptide from IIb protein and showed that it overlapped over more than 20 amino acids with the C-terminal part of the coat protein, then came a single tryptophan residue (inserted by the suppression) followed by another sequence of around 25 residues. The higher ratio of readthrough protein to coat protein in infected cells relative to virus particles suggests that during assembly there is some bias against the incorporation of IIb protein. That the virus population is heterogeneous in respect to its IIb protein content was directly shown by Radloff and Kaesberg (1973).

The readthrough of the coat gene could *a priori* be just a coincidence, or it could represent an ingenious way to code for four proteins with a minimum of genetic material. It turned out that IIb is in fact an essential component as in order to reconstitute *in vitro* infectious phage, viral RNA, coat protein, A protein (IIa), and readthrough (IIb) protein are needed (Hofstetter *et al.*, 1974). Also, the tripartite complex A protein–readthrough protein–viral RNA is infectious, while other combinations are not (Shiba, 1975). Qβ needs about an extra 600 nucleotides to code for the readthrough segment, but the other genes are similar in length to those of the group I phages (Table 4 and Fig. 1); consequently, the Qβ genome is about 4500 nucleotides in length while MS2 contains 3569 nucleotides (Section 4.4.7). One can speculate whether Qβ is an evolutionary ancestor of the group I phages, which have progressed to a simpler form (downhill evolution) or whether Qβ is in fact a more advanced form and has already expanded its genetic library (uphill evolution) (cf. Hofstetter *et al.*, 1974). RNA phages have little genetic versatility; they cannot recombine and any damage to their genome is never repaired in the cell; the error frequency per nucleotide during replication is indeed very high (Section 5.7.1). Under these conditions it would seem that a smaller genome constitutes indeed an advantage, but of course the true evolutionary relationship between MS2 and Qβ may never be known.

3.4. Viral RNA

The chemical structure of viral RNA will be discussed in detail in Section 4. The most important physical parameters are summarized in Table 7; the values for some of these vary considerably. To some extent this is due to the fact that parameters which reflect shape or secondary structure are highly dependent on the solvent composition, not only the ionic strength but also the nature of the cations present. Viral RNA preparations undoubtedly also vary in the amount of bound spermidine

TABLE 7
Physical Properties of the Viral RNA

Property	MS2-R17-f2	Qβ
Molecular weight	1.23×10^{6a}	1.5×10^{6b}
Number of nucleotides	3569^a	± 4500
$s_{20,w}$, S		
in 0.1 M NaCl	26^d–$27^{c,d}$	29^e
in 0.01 M NaCl	16.5^d	
Specific absorbancy, $E_{260\,nm}^{1\,mg/ml}$	22.6–$25.1^{f,g}$	25.5^e
ϵ_P	7400–$8600^{g,h}$	
Ratio $A_{260\,nm}/A_{280\,nm}$	$2.09 \pm 0.1^{i,j,k}$	
Hypochromicity, %	26–27	
T_m, °C		
in 0.1 M NaCl–0.01 M EDTA	59.5^d	
in 0.01 M NaCl–0.001 M EDTA	41^d	
Helicity, %		
by spectrophotometry	73–$82^{c,k}$	
by IR	63 ± 5^h	
Buoyant density in Cs_2SO_4, g/cm³	1.63^j	1.63^e
Partial specific volume, $\bar{v}$, cm³/g	0.495^l	
R_G, nm		
in 0.1 M NaCl	18.3–19.6^d	
in 0.08 M phosphate	21.0^l	
in 0.01 M NaCl	48.5^d	
Solvation water, g H_2O/g RNA	5.5^l	
Base composition[e,g,l]		
A	$23.3 \pm 0.26(23.4)$	22.1 ± 0.05
U	$24.8 \pm 0.23(24.5)$	29.5 ± 0.15
G	$26.4 \pm 0.83(26.0)$	23.7 ± 0.23
C	$25.5 \pm 0.86(26.1)$	24.7 ± 0.35

[a] Fiers *et al.* (1976), Fiers (unpublished).
[b] Boedtker (1971).
[c] Mitra *et al.* (1963).
[d] Gesteland and Boedtker (1964).
[e] Overby *et al.* (1966b).
[f] Slegers *et al.* (1973).
[g] Strauss and Sinsheimer (1963).

[h] Isenberg *et al.* (1971).
[i] Fiers *et al.* (1965).
[j] Billeter *et al.* (1966).
[k] Boedtker (1967).
[l] Values in parentheses are derived from the complete MS2 RNA sequence.

TABLE 8
Molecular Weight of Group I Viral RNA

Phage	Molecular weight	Number of nucleotides	Method	Reference
MS2	1.05–1.15 $\times 10^6$		Light scattering	Strauss and Sinsheimer (1963)
R17	1.0–1.4 $\times 10^6$		Sedimentation-viscosity	Mitra et al. (1963)
fr	1.3 $\times 10^6$		Sedimentation-viscosity	Marvin and Hoffmann-Berling (1963)
R17	1.1 ± 0.1 $\times 10^6$		Light scattering	Gesteland and Boedtker (1964)
MS2	1.0–1.12 $\times 10^6$		Purine tract analysis	Fiers et al. (1965)
R17	1.1 ± 0.1 $\times 10^6$		Purine tract analysis	Sinha et al. (1965b)
MS2	1.0 $\times 10^6$		Light scattering	Overby et al. (1966)
R17	1.3 $\times 10^6$		Relative electrophoretic mobility	Boedtker (1971)
MS2		3500 ± 200	Purine tract analysis	Haegeman et al. (1971)
MS2	1.15 $\times 10^6$		Light scattering	Slegers et al. (1973)
	1.09–1.35 $\times 10^6$		Sedimentation-viscosity	Slegers et al. (1973)
MS2	1.23 $\times 10^6$	3569	Complete primary structure	Fiers (1976), Fiers and Min Jou (unpublished)

and Mg^{2+}. Furthermore, macromolecular RNA is very labile, and not all measurements have really been carried out on intact material.

One of the most important parameters is of course the molecular weight, and it is of interest to compare the various estimates, based on physical or chemical approaches, with the exact value deduced from the complete chemical structure, viz. 1.23×10^6 for the Na^+ salt of MS2 RNA (Table 8). As an example of the uncertainties inherent in the determination of a physical parameter, we may take the partial specific volume ($\bar{v}$). This value should be rather independent of solvent composition or intactness of the RNA. Yet $\bar{v}$ was taken as 0.53 ml/g by Mitra et al. (1963) (an average of published values determined by pycnometry) and as 0.55 ml/g by Marvin and Hoffmann-Berling (1963) (based on Haselkorn, 1962). More recent determinations made by a digital density meter give $\bar{v}$ as only 0.495 ml/g (Slegers et al., 1973) or even 0.457 ml/g (Zipper et al., 1975) (the latter value was determined at 4°C).

Another important characteristic is the volume and shape of the viral RNA, as reflected by the sedimentation constant. At neutral pH and moderate to high ionic strength the molecule sediments at about 27 S. It is of interest that TMV RNA, which has almost twice the molecular weight of MS2 RNA, also sediments at approximately 27 S (Boedtker, 1960). TMV RNA has a considerably more extended and looser configuration; presumably this is related to the virus structure, as the RNA in TMV particles is totally embedded between the protein subunits and then has no secondary structure of its own (Stubbs *et al.*, 1977). MS2 RNA can be expanded by decreasing the salt concentration and especially by removal of divalent ions. Moderate expansion leads to a sedimentation constant of 20–22 S and under these conditions no loss of hypochromicity is observed (Strauss and Sinsheimer, 1968; Slegers and Fiers, 1973a). This suggests that the tertiary structure of the molecule has been unfolded, but without appreciable loss of secondary structure. A similar partial unfolding of tRNA superstructure has been reported (Crothers *et al.*, 1974; Hilbers and Schulman, 1974; Wong *et al.*, 1975). Complete removal of divalent counterions and further decrease of the salt concentration lead to an extended random coil. For example, in 0.01 M NaCl group I phage RNA sediments at 13–16.5 S (Franklin, 1967; Gesteland and Boedtker, 1964). But even under the latter conditions the molecule is not fully denatured and after moderate heating in 1 mM EDTA a sedimentation rate as low as 11.7 S has been observed (Slegers and Fiers, 1973a).

The secondary structure in RNA can largely be eliminated by treatment with formaldehyde (Fraenkel-Conrat, 1954). After a standard reaction which involves brief, moderate heating in phosphate buffer in the presence of 1.8% formaldehyde, most base-pair interactions are eliminated, although base stacking is still present. The treated MS2 RNA sediments at 14 S (Strauss and Sinsheimer, 1963). This procedure has been developed into a method to estimate the molecular weight of RNA molecules independently of conformation by measuring the sedimentation rate relative to known standards such as group I phage RNA (Boedtker, 1968). In the same vein, but using an organic solvent instead of formaldehyde, Strauss *et al.* (1968) have worked out a procedure to estimate the molecular weight by measuring the sedimentation rate in 99% dimethylsulfoxide relative to known standards, and they showed that under these conditions the remaining secondary structure was negligible. Similar methods to estimate the molecular weight of fully denatured RNA molecules by comparison with known standards can be based on relative mobility in polyacrylamide gel electrophoresis, either after treatment with formaldehyde (Boedtker, 1971) or in the presence of formamide (Pinder *et al.*, 1974; Spahr *et al.*, 1976).

The native 27 S viral RNA can not only expand, but also shrink. At low pH, in the presence of small concentrations of Mg^{2+} ions, and at low ionic strength, the conformation of MS2 RNA fairly abruptly changes to a 57 S form (e.g., at pH 3.8 and 6×10^{-5} M $MgCl_2$; high NaCl concentrations interfere because they displace the Mg^{2+} ions) (Slegers and Fiers, 1973*a*). The nature of the interactions involved has not yet been solved, but the effect is not specific for viral RNA as similar transitions can be observed with ribosomal RNA (Slegers and Fiers, 1972). It is most remarkable that notwithstanding the compactness of this "acidic" 57 S conformation—its volume is about 7 times smaller than that of native 27 S RNA—more than 50% of the secondary structure has been lost. The "acidic" conformation can be fixed with formaldehyde, which forms methylene cross-links upon prolonged reaction (Slegers and Fiers, 1973*b*). This "fixed" species still sediments at 37–46 S (depending on the pretreatment) in the same neutral buffer wherein the native form sediments at 27 S. At least half of the bound formaldehyde can be removed again, and, remarkably, this does not affect the sedimentation rate of the contracted molecule. Neither is there an appreciable regain of secondary structure, presumably because the cross-links prevent the required conformational rearrangements.

Although a physical parameter such as the radius of gyration (R_G) depends on the shape of the macromolecule under consideration, it is not possible on this basis alone to derive unambiguously the axial ratio and the hydrodynamic volume of the equivalent ellipsoid. The uncertainty can be solved, however, if several shape-dependent parameters are compared, such as R_G, the intrinsic viscosity, and the sedimentation constant. In this way it is found that native (27 S) MS2 RNA behaves hydrodynamically as a prolate ellipsoid with an axial ratio of 5.9 and a volume of 11.4×10^3 nm³ (Slegers *et al.*, 1973). The model was further refined by Zipper *et al.* (1975), who carried out small-angle X-ray scattering measurements on MS2 RNA solutions. They come to a flattened prolate ellipsoid with semiaxes of 30.9, 16.0, and 4.7 nm in the three dimensions. Such a body has a volume of 10.6×10^3 nm³, which is in remarkably good agreement with the value given above, especially considering the completely different approach. It is worth noting that the "native" viral RNA in solution is not so compact as is perhaps often thought. Only 8.2% of the hydrodynamic volume is actually occupied by the RNA, the rest being water. The volume in the virus particle enclosed by the protein shell amounts to 4.85×10^3 nm³. As apparently there is not much interpenetration of the viral RNA into the protein shell, it means that the virus assembly involves a shrinking of the volume from approximately 11.4×10^3 to 4.85×10^3 nm³. This loss of water is brought about either by a more specific and compact tertiary structure, which has been irreversibly lost during extraction, or by binding of protein, or both. Furthermore, the RNA does not fill evenly the central volume of the virus particle, but apparently leaves an empty central hole of about 6 nm radius (Jacrot *et al.*, 1977).

Optical studies have revealed a high degree of secondary structure in phage RNA. In 0.1 M phosphate buffer the hypochromicity amounts to 21–23% and the T_m is 58°C; the latter is further enhanced by addition of Mg^{2+} (Gesteland and Boedtker, 1964; Boedtker, 1967; Slegers and Fiers, 1973*a*). The increase in chromicity starts only on reaching a temperature above 40°C, which means that there are few regions of marginal stability (see below for a discussion on the specificity of the secondary structure). An early estimate, based on the hypochromicity, indicated that approximately 76% of the nucleotides are in a helical configuration (Mitra *et al.*, 1963). Inside the virion, the value may perhaps amount to 82%. Hypochromicity, however, is due not only to base pairing but also to stacking of bases in single-stranded regions. By measuring the temperature profile of RNA after complete reaction with formaldehyde, Boedtker (1967) was able to estimate the contribution of unstacking to the hyperchromic increase. The minimum value she obtained for the percent nucleotides involved in base-pair interactions was 73% ± 5%. Isenberg *et al.* (1971) determined the helicity by an entirely different method, viz. the infrared spectrum of the deuterated species in H_2O buffer. They find only 63%, but this lower estimate may perhaps be due to some denaturation during their sample preparation. A-U and G-C base pairs contributed about equally, namely 33% ± 5% and 30% ± 5%, respectively. More recent results by laser Raman spectroscopy confirm the high degree of secondary structure; about 85% of the bases are either paired or stacked, both inside the virion and in the isolated viral RNA (Thomas *et al.*, 1976). The degree of secondary structure is quantitatively very similar to that found in tRNA (Thomas and Hartman, 1973).

Gralla and Delisi (1974) reported that even random polynucleotides fold into some kind of secondary structure and the percent base-paired nucleotides may run up to 60% for longer chains. This, however, is still far below the value of 73% observed in the viral RNA as well as the similar values found in ribosomal RNA, tRNA, and perhaps some (prokaryotic) messenger RNAs. Moreover, the secondary structure in a random heteropolymer is not only less extensive, it is also far less stable, as is evident from a comparison of the melting profiles (Ricard and Salzer, 1975; cf. also discussion above). As the secondary structure is not due to chance, it must be genetically coded. This conclusion not only rests on the aforementioned experimental observations but also is supported by a statistical analysis of the primary nucleotide sequence. This reveals that nearly adjacent complementary sequences, which form the basis of the (often imperfect) hairpins in the secondary structure, occur with a frequency far exceeding the probability of chance events. These complementary sequences correspond of course to (imperfect) palindromes in a hypothetical duplex RNA molecule. The secondary structure is specific and homogeneous, i.e. the same for all molecules in the population, as will be discussed in Section 4.4.2, on the basis of experimental findings. Strauss and Sinsheimer (1968), however, detected by analytical ultracentrifugation some evidence of conformational heterogeneity. This is not unexpected, in view of the considerable expansion of the RNA molecule following the deproteinization step.

The secondary structure and the overall conformation of the viral RNA are intrinsically interesting, but far more important is its direct role and involvement in crucial biological processes, such as the control of translational expression (Section 5.4.3), as well as other activities which are at present less understood, such as replication and survival in a cytoplasm loaded with nucleases and RNA-processing enzymes.

4. STRUCTURE OF THE VIRAL RNA

4.1. Terminal Sequences

4.1.1. The 5'-Terminal Sequence

If the viral RNA chain is synthesized in the direction 5' to 3', one might expect that the 5' end would still be phosphorylated. Therefore, Takanami (1966) separated an alkaline hydrolysate of f2 RNA on a DEAE-Sephadex column in the presence of urea and could indeed isolate a 5'-triphosphoryl-3'(2')-monophosphorylnucleoside or pppNp (this end group represents only 0.1% of the radioactivity applied on the column). The latter residue was correctly identified as pppGp by Roblin (1968), who worked with R17 RNA. Similar results were soon obtained for the genomes of MS2 (De Wachter et al., 1968a), f2 (Dahlberg, 1968), and Qβ and R23 (Watanabe and August, 1968). In the case of MS2 RNA, the identification could be based on a direct comparison with the pppNp derivatives of the four nucleosides, which had been chemically synthesized for this purpose (Messens and van Montagu, 1968).

The next step was to isolate an oligonucleotide derived from the 5′ end (De Wachter *et al.*, 1968*b*). The most obvious approach was to digest MS2 RNA with pancreatic ribonuclease (RNase A) and to search for the terminal segment by assaying for release of pppGp after alkaline digestion. The enzymatic hydrolysate was first fractionated according to net negative charge on a DEAE-cellulose column, and in this system the 5′-terminal sequence was found to coincide with the heptanucleotide peak, suggesting a structure of the form pppG-Pu-Pu-Py.

A special procedure was then developed which allowed to obtain the oligonucleotide in an absolutely pure form. It consists of gradient chromatography in the presence of 8 M formamide on a sheet of DEAE paper. When the aforementioned heptanucleotide peak was run in this system, the terminal sequence moved well ahead of the bona fide heptanucleotides and its structure could be unambiguously identified as pppG-G-G-U (De Wachter *et al.*, 1968*b*). It may be noted that such oligonucleotides, containing a row of G residues and moreover polyphosphorylated, easily aggregate and adsorb tenaciously on various materials, and therefore are hard to characterize. The same 5′-terminal sequence was subsequently isolated by different procedures from R17 RNA (Cory *et al.*, 1970; Adams and Cory, 1970), from f2 RNA (Ling, 1971), and again from MS2 RNA (Haegeman *et al.*, 1971) (Table 9).

The major conclusion that could be drawn from these results was that the viral RNA does not start with an initiation codon for protein synthesis. This was the first evidence for an untranslated 5′-leader sequence, a feature which subsequently became well established not only for viral RNAs but also for prokaryotic and eukaryotic messenger RNAs (the only known exception so far is the mRNA for bacteriophage λ c_I repressor synthesis, initiated at the Prm promotor; Pirotta *et al.*, 1976). The first nucleotides in the viral RNA presumably play an essential role in the initiation of a new round of synthesis. The high stacking tendency between G residues may perhaps be of special significance in this process.

The same methodology, worked out for the identification of the 5′-terminal oligonucleotide of MS2 RNA, was also applied to Qβ RNA. Remarkably, two sequences were obtained in approximately equal amounts, namely pppG-G-G-G-A-A-C and pppG-G-G-G-G-A-A-C, even in a series of independent preparations derived from single plaques (De Wachter and Fiers, 1969). Presumably some slippage occurs at the initiation step by the RNA-dependent RNA polymerase (or replicase) complex. Billeter *et al.* (1969) found a slightly different sequence,

TABLE 9

Terminal Nucleotide Sequences

Phage	Nucleotide sequence		References	
	5'-Terminal	3'-Terminal	5'-Terminal	3'-Terminal
MS2	pppG-G-U ...	... G-U-U-A-C-C-A-C-C-C-A	De Wachter et al. (1968b)	De Wachter and Fiers (1967)
f2	pppG-G-U ...	... G-U-U-A-C-C-A-C-C-C-A	Ling (1971)	Weith and Gilham (1967)
R17	pppG-G-U ...	... G-U-U-A-C-C-A-C-C-C-A	Cory et al. (1970)	Dahlberg (1968)
Qβ	{ pppG-G-G-A-A-C[a] ... pppG-G-G-G-A-A-C ... pppG-G(G)₁₋₂A-C[a] ...	... G-C-C-C-U-C-U-C-U-C-C-A	De Wachter and Fiers (1969) Billeter et al. (1969)	Weith and Gilham (1969)

[a] The difference between the sequence containing A-A-C and A-C is the result of the Qβ strain used (our unpublished results).

containing (G)-A-C instead of (G)-A-A-C, but this is due to the use of a different virus stock (our unpublished results) (Table 9).

The method worked out for the identification and the quantitative determination of the 5′ pppNp residue could also be applied to obtain some information on the mechanism of *in vivo* RNA replication. This process involves the synthesis of complementary (negative or minus strand) copies of the parental RNA, which in turn are used for the synthesis of progeny (positive or plus) strands (Eoyang and August, 1974). The negative and positive strands anneal to each other during deproteinization of the cell extract (Borst and Weissmann, 1965). Two structures have been identified. The first, called "replicative form" or RF (in analogy to the RF first identified in φX174-infected cells) consists of a complete positive and a complete negative strand (Ammann *et al.*, 1964; Francke and Hofschneider, 1966). The second structure is only partially double stranded and is called "replicative intermediate" or RI (Fenwick *et al.*, 1964; Erikson and Franklin, 1966). It contains, in addition to a full-length positive and negative strand, one or more nascent positive strands. It may be noted that translation proceeds already on these nascent strands (Hotham-Iglewski *et al.*, 1968; Engelhardt *et al.*, 1968; Konings *et al.*, 1970). The RF and RI structures can conveniently be separated either by gel electrophoresis (Bishop *et al.*, 1967) or— on a more preparative scale—by salt fractionation, followed by chromatography on cellulose in the presence of ethanol (Franklin, 1966) and finally centrifugation in a sucrose gradient.

Analysis of the pppNp released on alkaline hydrolysis of RF revealed only pppGp in the expected amount of one terminal group per chain of approximately 3500 residues (Fiers *et al.*, 1968; Vandenberghe *et al.*, 1969). As 50% of the end groups must be derived from the negative strands, this result meant that the latter also start with pppGp. Banerjee *et al.* (1969a), who studied the *in vitro* replication of Qβ RNA, showed that also in this system negative strands start with a pppGp residue.

Similar identification and quantitative analyses were carried out on the 5′-phosphorylated end group of the RI structures (Fiers *et al.*, 1968; Vandenberghe *et al.*, 1969; Robertson and Zinder, 1968, 1969). Again only pppGp was found and none of the other three nucleoside tetraphosphates. Considering that these structures contain a heterogeneous population of growing strands and hence of growing points, it was concluded that the unique nucleoside tetraphosphate could not be derived from a growing point. This means that progeny viral RNA chains grow in the direction 5′ to 3′, as indeed is true for all other known systems of polynucleotide synthesis. On the basis of the pppGp content, it was calculated that each RI structure contains on the average 2.5 growing chains (Vandenberghe *et al.*, 1969). Other authors, using either a similar technique (Robertson and Zinder, 1969) or electron microscopy (Granboulan and Franklin, 1968), obtained a lower estimate, viz. one nascent strand or less per negative strand template. It should be noted, however, that the fragile nascent strands are easily detached during manipulations, and especially that displacement may occur during the deproteinization step. Therefore, the higher value is more likely to be correct, and we conclude that several progeny RNA strands can be simultaneously synthesized from the same template, just as several messenger RNA copies can be transcribed from one operon.

4.1.2. The 3'-Terminal Sequence

The first observation on the 3'-terminal end of a bacteriophage RNA was made by Sugiyama (1965), who showed that alkaline hydrolysis of MS2 RNA released a single nucleoside, identified as adenosine. He also found that the penultimate was a pyrimidine nucleotide. The next step then consisted in the isolation of an oligonucleotide derived from the 3' end. For this purpose, De Wachter and Fiers (1967) specifically labeled the 3'-terminal residue by periodate oxidation followed by reduction with tritiated borohydride, a labeling procedure developed by RajBhandary (1968). In order to monitor the purification of this 3'-terminal oligonucleotide, the specifically 3'-^{3}H-labeled MS2 RNA was mixed with uniformly ^{32}P-labeled MS2 RNA. The viral RNA preparation was digested with ribonuclease T1, and this hydrolysate was fractionated. After three successive column chromatographic steps under different conditions, a pure T1 oligonucleotide was obtained, which represented 85% of the original ^{3}H counts. Its nucleotide sequence was established as U-U-A-C-C-A-C-C-C-A_{OH} (De Wachter and Fiers, 1967). It is worthwhile mentioning that one of the approaches used in the nucleotide sequence determination of this purified oligonucleotide was partial degradation (from the 3' end) with snake venom exonuclease, followed by labeling of the newly created 3' ends with tritium by the periodate oxidation–borohydride reduction method and separation of the partially degraded products according to their chain length. Identification of the ^{3}H-labeled 3' end group in each successive peak then directly allowed deduction of the aforementioned nucleotide sequence. The possibilities of such nucleotide sequencing approaches by partial degradation followed by labeling of the newly generated end groups have been further explored by Randerath *et al.* (1974).

Weith and Gilham (1967) treated a ribonuclease T1 digest of f2 RNA with periodate, and they could selectively retain the 3'-terminal oligonucleotide (now oxidized to a terminal dialdehyde) on an amino-ethylcellulose column. By stepwise degradation, involving cycles of periodate oxidation, β elimination, and phosphatase treatment, they came independently to the same nucleotide sequence. Dahlberg (1968) developed still another method to isolate the 3'-terminal oligonucleotide from a T1 digest of uniformly ^{32}P-labeled phage RNA. It was based on the fact that all oligonucleotides except the 3'-terminal one contain a 3'-phosphomonoester group. On two-dimensional electrophoresis, but with a phosphatase treatment applied between the first and second dimensions, the 3'-terminal oligonucleotide is the only one which moves identically in both dimensions and hence can be found on the diagonal. In this way the same nucleotide sequence was again confirmed, this time on the phage R17 RNA (Table 9). He also isolated the 3'-terminal oligonucleotide of Qβ RNA in this way. The sequence of the latter was correctly established as C-C-C-U-C-U-C-U-C-C-U-C-C-C-A$_{OH}$ (Weith and Gilham, 1969).

It may be noted that analyses of the 3'-terminal residue of phage RNA preparations very often indicate some cytidine. This is especially true for *in vitro* synthesized Qβ RNA (Rensing and August, 1969; Weber and Weissman, 1970). In our later studies, however, in which the 3'-terminal decanucleotide was often isolated in high yield (Section 4.4.6), we never found a trace of the corresponding oligonucleotide lacking the terminal adenosine. Therefore, there is no strong reason to doubt—at least for the group I phages—that all RNA molecules encapsidated in virus particles indeed end with -C-C-A.

Perhaps the most important conclusion which could be drawn from these 3'-terminal sequences was that neither of them contained a termination codon for polypeptide synthesis (UAA, UAG, or UGA). As a 3' physical end of a polyribonucleotide chain is in itself not sufficient for polypeptide chain release from the ribosome, it followed that a stretch of genetic information is present at the 3' end of the genome which is not translated into protein and which, undoubtedly, must serve another important function. This situation is thus completely analogous to the untranslated 5' leader sequence (preceding section).

Another interesting feature is that the last three nucleotides present in all phage RNAs analyzed, namely -C-C-A, are the same as found in all tRNAs. In addition, this terminal sequence had already been identified as the 3′ end of tobacco mosaic virus (TMV) RNA by Steinschneider and Fraenkel-Conrat (1966) and was later also found at the 3′ end of many other plant viruses (Glitz and Eichler, 1971; Bastin *et al.*, 1976; Briand *et al.*, 1976, 1977; Silberklang *et al.*, 1977). Remarkably, the last A residue is not part of the direct genetic information. Indeed, we have seen in the preceding section that the negative strand of MS2 RNA starts with a pppGp residue. Especially in the case of Qβ RNA, whose negative strand is initiated likewise with pppGp, it has been clearly proven that the latter residue (the 5′ end of the minus strand) is coded by the 3′-penultimate C residue of the plus strand (Eoyang and August, 1974). In agreement with this replication model was the finding that the last A residue can be removed from the viral RNA without damaging its infectivity as tested in a spheroplast system (Kamen, 1969). Removal of the penultimate 3′ C residue, however, was lethal. Qβ RNA from which the terminal A had been removed still functioned effectively as a template for *in vitro* RNA replication (Rensing and August, 1969; Weber and Weissmann, 1970). As the progeny molecules contained again a 3′-terminal A residue, it follows that the latter must be added by a different mechanism. Possibly this adenylation event is part of the mechanism to release the fully synthesized RNA progeny molecule from the replication complex. The Qβ replicase, however, was unable to add back an A residue to Qβ RNA chains from which the 3′-terminal A had been chemically removed (Weber and Weissmann, 1970).

Possibly, the fact that the ... C-C-A end of RNA phages is identical to that of tRNAs and many plant viral RNAs is a coincidence.* The last A residue of tRNAs may or may not be genetically coded, but this residue as well as the preceding Cs are readily restored by the tRNA adenylyl- and cytidylyltransferase, which at least in *E. coli* is an essential enzyme. Phage RNA from which one or two nucleotides have been removed, however, cannot be repaired by this enzyme (Gross *et al.*, 1970). The 3′ ... C-C-A end of several plant viral RNAs may be related to the finding that the latter can often become aminoacylated (Pinck *et al.*, 1970; Litvak *et al.*, 1973), but no intact phage RNA has ever been shown to be chargeable with an activated amino acid.

All phage RNAs start with three G residues (or more in the case of

---

* *Editor's comment:* See the preceding chapter for further discussion of the role of the terminal A in TMV RNA.

$Q\beta$ RNA) (preceding section) and the results on the 3' end of the plus strands show that the same is true for the negative (minus) chains. Possibly a series of G residues, which are known to have a high stacking energy, is an energetic requirement in order to initiate RNA-dependent RNA synthesis.

4.2. Internal Oligonucleotides

4.2.1. Fractionation by Column Chromatography

Pancreatic ribonuclease A cleaves RNA only after pyrimidine residues. Hence all products present in a complete digest of phage RNA with this enzyme have the general structure $(Pup)_nPyp$, i.e., a series of n purine nucleotides followed by a 3'-terminal pyrimidine nucleotide. These can be separated according to chain length $(n + 1)$ on a DEAE-cellulose column in the presence of 7 M urea (Sinha *et al.*, 1965*b*; Fiers *et al.*, 1965). For small values of n all possible sequence isomers are present in each peak (on isopleth) but for larger n values the number of different oligonucleotides becomes small, and the individual components can be resolved by a second chromatography at an acidic pH value. In this way two undecanucleotides, one decanucleotide, two nonanucleotides, and three octanucleotides were individually isolated from an MS2 RNA digest and sequenced (Min Jou and Fiers, 1969). As a unique oligonucleotide is present in one molar equivalent per viral chain, it is possible to calculate the molecular weight of the latter on the basis of the fraction of radioactivity recovered in the characterized oligonucleotide. Special precautions have to be taken to avoid losses; e.g., even pure ribonuclease A has a tendency to cleave A-A bonds if the ionic strength is too low. But under optimal conditions it is possible to obtain by this chemical approach a molecular weight estimate of the total viral RNA which is at least as accurate as the physical measurements (Table 8). The first phage-coded proteins whose complete primary amino acid sequence became known were the coat protein of bacteriophage f2 (Weber and Konigsberg, 1967) and of fr (Wittman-Liebold and Liebold, 1967) followed by that of R17 (Weber, 1967) (Section 3.2). On this basis, and with the knowledge of the genetic code dictionary, one can write possible nucleotide sequences for the coat gene and compare these with the nucleotide sequence of the polypurine tracts. Unfortunately, it turned out that none of the latter could be derived from the coat gene (Min Jou and Fiers, 1969). A number of unique ribonuclease A oligonucleotides from R17 RNA and from M12

RNA have likewise been sequenced (Thirion and Kaesberg, 1968*a,b*, 1970). Some of the sequences turned out to be identical in the three phages, while others were quite different. These results extended the serological comparisons (Section 2.1) and showed that although these phages are evidently related, they are far from identical. Subsequently more data became available, which allowed expression of the relationships in quantitative terms (Robertson and Jeppesen, 1972; Min Jou and Fiers, 1976*b*) (Section 5.7.2).

Bacteriophage MS2 RNA can be split enzymatically into a one-third piece or 15 S component and a two-thirds piece or 21 S component (Fiers, 1967). This remarkable reaction must be related to the overall folding of the viral RNA and has been observed for different group I phages and also for Qβ RNA (Bassel and Spiegelman, 1967). Spahr and Gesteland (1968) partially purified an enzyme called ribonuclease IV from a ribonuclease-I-negative *E. coli* strain. This ribonuclease IV has the peculiar property of readily cleaving phage RNA into one third-two thirds fragments, while further degradation is very slow. Furthermore, they showed that the 15 S fragment is derived from the 5′ end. Bacteriophage MS2 RNA was thus cleaved into the 15 S and 21 S fragments, and each was analyzed by complete digestion with ribonuclease A. In this way all the longer polypurine tracts could be assigned either to the left one-third or the right two-thirds of the genome (Min Jou *et al.*, 1969).

Aspergillus oryzae ribonuclease T1 cleaves specifically after G residues, and complete digestion of RNA produces a mixture of T1 oligonucleotides of the type $(Up)_m(Cp)_n(Ap)_oGp$. These products could initially not be separated so readily according to chain length by column chromatography, although improved procedures were worked out subsequently (Kelley *et al.*, 1971).

One particular experiment is worth mentioning: It was known that some amber mutants of f2 map in position 6 of the coat protein. On the basis of the amino acid sequence and the genetic code dictionary, one can deduce that there is a 75% probability that this mutation (a CAG to UAG transition) would be present in a T1 oligonucleotide containing 12 or more residues. By comparing the appropriate column chromatographic profiles of T1 digests from wild-type and amber mutant RNA, Robinson *et al.* (1969) could indeed isolate a 17-residue-long T1 oligonucleotide, whose sequence matched the amino acid sequence of positions 1–6 of the coat protein. In this way a direct correlation between nucleotide sequence and primary structure of the gene product was made.

4.2.2. Two-Dimensional Fractionation (Fingerprinting)

In 1965, Sanger, Brownlee, and Barrell introduced a new method that had a considerable impact on molecular biology. In this procedure ^{32}P-labeled oligonucleotides, e.g., those present in a ribonuclease T1 digest, are resolved in a first dimension according to base composition by electrophoresis on cellulose acetate at pH 3.5. The material is then quantitatively transferred to DEAE-cellulose paper and the second dimension is carried out again by electrophoresis at pH 1.9 or pH 1.7 in formic acid solution. The procedure is fast and sensitive, and the resolution is excellent, at least for not too complex mixtures (e.g., for ribonuclease T1 digests of tRNA or 5 S RNA). Oligonucleotides containing three or more Up residues, however, hardly move in the second dimension. This can be improved by dephosphorylation, such that now only oligonucleotides containing four or more Up residues remain near the start of the second dimension (Brownlee, 1972). Alternatively, gradient chromatography on a DEAE-cellulose sheet can be carried out as a second dimension (De Wachter et al., 1968b, 1971). Later a more versatile system was developed by Brownlee and Sanger (1969) and is called "homochromatography." The nucleotide material, separated as before by electrophoresis at pH 3.5 on cellulose acetate, is now transferred to a thin-layer plate made up from an appropriate mixture of DEAE-cellulose and cellulose. The second dimension, however, involves chromatographic elution at 60°C with a "homomixture," consisting of partially degraded RNA and 7 M urea. In this way resolution is achieved by partial displacement chromatography. The separation, especially of the longer T1 oligonucleotides, is excellent, and the experimental condition (ratio of DEAE-cellulose to cellulose and composition of the "homomixture") can easily be adapted to the problems at hand. Improved procedures were later introduced for transfer of the material after the first dimension (Southern, 1974) and for preparing appropriate "homomixtures" (Jay et al., 1974). Instead of DEAE-cellulose one can also use polyethyleneimine (PEI)-impregnated cellulose for coating the thin layer plates. The latter system gives sharper spots but is not suitable for oligonucleotides containing tracts of G residues as occur in ribonuclease A digests. Not too complex mixtures can be conveniently fingerprinted using a polyethyleneimine thin-layer plate and elution with a salt solution in the second dimension (Southern and Mitchell, 1971; Griffin, 1971; Contreras et al., 1971). Like the electrophoresis on DEAE paper in formic acid, this system mainly separates according to the content of Up residues but has the advantage that oligonucleotides containing three and more Up residues can still be mobilized. Many of these improvements were incorporated into a procedure, referred to as "minifingerprinting," which allows separation of all components present in an enzymatic digest of MS2 RNA according to base composition and chain length in the first and second dimensions, respectively (Volckaert *et al.*, 1976). The second dimension involves an appropriate "homomixture" as solvent and a polyethyleneimine thin-layer plate for a ribonuclease T1 digest while a DEAE-cellulose plate is used for ribonuclease A digests. All the longer oligonucleotides (more than 30 in the case of the T1 digest) are clearly resolved and can be used for nucleotide sequence determination or for comparative purposes (Fig. 4). It may be noted that a complex ribonuclease T1 or A digest can also be resolved by two-dimensional electrophoresis in polyacrylamide gel (De Wachter and Fiers, 1972). This method presents the advantages that the load can be quite high (while for electrophoresis on cellulose acetate not more than about 60 μg should be used), the fractionation is very reproducible (important for comparative studies) and resolution of the longer oligonucleotides is excellent. This method has been most useful for the analysis of very complex T1 digests, e.g., those derived from oncorna- or picornaviral RNAs (Billeter *et al.*, 1974; Fisby *et al.*, 1976; Lee and Wimmer, 1976).

Prior to the development of these techniques, Adams *et al.* (1969) analyzed a total ribonuclease T1 digest of R17 RNA by the electrophoresis–DEAE-cellulose–thin-layer "homochromatographic" system. The second-largest T1 oligonucleotide turned out to be 21 residues long and its structure was determined (Section 4.4.6). This nucleotide sequence can be "translated" in three possible reading frames on the basis of the potential code word dictionary. Fortunately, one of the three alternatives, a segment of seven amino acids, matched exactly with a segment of the known coat protein. In this way, they could for the first time make a direct correlation between a genetically coded nucleotide sequence and a corresponding amino acid sequence.

The nucleotide sequence of a number of the longer T1 oligonucleotides present in a digest of R17 RNA was reported by Jeppesen (1971). This study was followed by a comparison of T1 oligonucleotides of R17, f2, and MS2 (Robertson and Jeppesen, 1972). We have mentioned in the preceding section that phage RNA can be cleaved by ribonuclease IV into a one-third piece derived from the 5′ end and a two-thirds piece corresponding to the 3′-terminal fragment (Spahr and Gesteland, 1968). These two fragments were then used as messenger RNA in a cell-free protein synthesizing system. As A protein is not

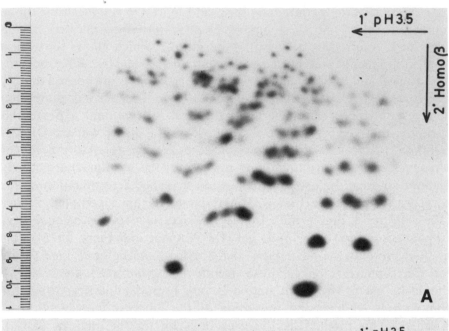

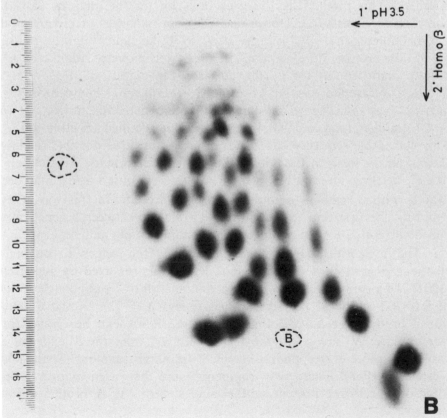

made under such conditions and as neither fragment is very active in forming the coat protein, these two genes could not be localized (it was later shown in fact that ribonuclease IV cuts in the beginning of the coat protein gene). The two-thirds fragment, however, was active in directing the synthesis of the virus-specified replicase protein (Spahr and Gesteland, 1968). Jeppesen *et al.* (1970) then characterized the two pieces by T1 fingerprinting, and as they knew already the genetic function corresponding to some large T1 oligonucleotides (see above), they could establish that the gene order in the bacteriophage R17 RNA is 5'-A protein–coat protein–replicase–3'. The same gene order was established independently by Konings *et al.* (1970), who prepared nascent strands from replicative intermediates, fractionated these according to increasing chain length, and determined the genetic information content of the different size classes by using these as messenger RNA in a cell-free protein-synthesizing system.

4.3. Specifically Protected Regions

4.3.1. Ribosome Binding Sites

Early studies on the mechanism of protein synthesis had indicated that the formation of an initiation complex required a messenger RNA, the 30 S ribosomal subunit, formylmethionine tRNA, and three initiation factors IF1, IF2, and IF3 present in a ribosomal wash (Lucas-Lenard and Lipmann, 1971). Binding of formylmethionine tRNA to the ribosome could be stimulated not only by AUG but also by GUG and UUG (Clark and Marcker, 1966; Ghosh *et al.*, 1967). As neither of these signals is present at the extreme 5' physical end of the phage

---

Fig. 4.   Minifingerprints of ^{32}P-labeled bacteriophage MS2 RNA digests. A: Autoradiograph of a minifingerprint of a ribonuclease T1 hydrolysate of ^{32}P-labeled bacteriophage MS2 RNA. The digest was separated in the first dimension on cellulose acetate, blotted over on a polyethyleneimine thin-layer plate according to Southern (1974), and developed with a modified "homomixture" in the second dimension. Note that the scale on the left is in centimeters. The separation in the first dimension is according to charge, and in the second according to chain length. Nearly all the spots in the upper part of the fingerprint are unique, i.e., occur once in the total viral RNA chain. From Volckaert *et al.* (1976). B: Autoradiograph of a minifingerprint of a pancreatic ribonuclease A hydrolysate of ^{32}P-labeled bacteriophage MS2 RNA. The digest was separated as in A, except that the thin-layer plate was DEAE-cellulose. The scale on the left is in centimeters. Note again the separation according to chain length in the second dimension and the resolution of individual, unique oligonucleotides in the top part of the fingerprint. From Volckaert *et al.* (1976).

RNA (cf. Section 4.1.1), it follows that the initiating ribosomal subunit complex must recognize an internal feature on the molecule, such as a primary and/or secondary nucleotide sequence, which would correspond to the start of a gene. Takanami *et al.* (1965) could show that a single ribosome binds indeed to an f2 RNA molecule. After treatment with ribonuclease they obtained a specific fragment, about 25–30 nucleotides long, which was protected from digestion by the ribosome. The conditions for isolating a specifically protected ribosomal binding site were improved by Steitz (1969). Using intact phage RNA she obtained one major product which was about 30 nucleotides long (the complex was trimmed with ribonuclease A) and established its nucleotide sequence (Table 10). It contains an AUG signal at about the middle, and the following triplets correspond exactly to the N-terminal sequence of the R17 coat protein, thus proving that this region is derived indeed from the beginning of the coat gene. Interestingly, this region can fold into a hairpin structure with the AUG exposed in the loop (Fig. 5). When instead of intact phage RNA slightly degraded preparations were used, two other ribosome binding regions could be characterized; these were shown to be derived from the A protein gene and the replicase gene respectively (Table 10). Similar approaches were followed for the isolation and nucleotide sequence determination of the ribosome binding site corresponding to the phage f2 coat gene and the three Qβ genes (Gupta *et al.*, 1970; Hindley and Staples, 1969; Table 10 and references therein).

Although all these regions contained an AUG signal at about the middle, followed by triplets which indicated that these were really the initiation regions of the respective phage genes, no clearly identifiable common features were at first apparent. Remarkably, not even the AUG was constant, as Volckaert and Fiers (1973) found that the A protein gene of MS2 starts with GUG. The nucleotide sequence preceding and following this initiation codon is identical to that of R17 RNA (Table 10). As the respective A proteins are made *in vivo* about as efficiently with the two phages, it follows that AUG and GUG must be functionally equivalent. Another natural gene initiated with a GUG codon has recently been identified, viz. the repressor gene *i* of the *lac* operon (Steege, 1977). This degeneracy in the first position of the initiation codon involves an interaction of A and G, respectively, with the U residue of the formyl methionine tRNA anticodon.

An important breakthrough in our understanding how ribosomes can recognize specific regions of the mRNA and initiate polypeptides correctly was made by Shine and Dalgarno (1974). They established

TABLE 10
Ribosome Binding Sites[a]

Phage gene	Binding Sites	Reference
R17 A protein	CAU UCC UAG GAG GUU UGA CCU AUG CGA GCU UUU AGU G	Steitz (1969)
MS2 A protein	CAU UCC UAG GAG GUU UGA CCU GUG CGA GCU UUU AGU G	Volckaert and Fiers (1973)
Qβ A protein	UCA CUG AGU AUA AGA GGA CAU AUG CCU AAA UUA CCG CGU	Staples et al. (1971)
R17 coat	CC UCA ACC GGG GUU UGA AGC AUG GCU UCU AAC UUU	Steitz (1969)
f2, MS2 coat	CC UCA ACC GGA GUU UGA AGC AUG GCU UCC AAC UUU ACU	Gupta et al. (1970) Min Jou et al. (1972)
Qβ coat	AAA CUU UGG GUC AAU UUG AUC AUG GCA AAA UUA GAG ACU	Hindley and Staples (1969)
R17, MS2 replicase	AA ACA UGA GGA UUA CCC AUG UCG AAG ACA ACA AAG	Steitz (1969) Min Jou et al. (1972)
Qβ replicase	AG UAA CUA AGG AUG AAA UGC AUG UCU AAG ACA G	Staples and Hindley (1971) Steitz (1972)

[a] The underlined segment is complementary to part of the 3'-terminal sequence of *E. coli* 16 S RNA: (G)A-U-C-A-C-C-U-C-C-U-U-A$_{OH}$ (dots indicate a G-U base pair; the f2 and MS2 coat sequence imply a looped-out base). This interaction is presumably involved in ribosome binding (Shine and Dalgarno, 1974; Sprague and Steitz, 1975). A noninitiating AUG present in the replicase ribosome binding region of all the phages analyzed is shown in box.

the sequence of the 3′-terminal segment of *E. coli* 16 S RNA as
. . . (G)A-U-C-A-C-C-U-C-C-U-U-A$_3$′ and hypothesized that this part
of the 30 S ribosomal subunit might be functionally involved in mRNA
recognition on the basis of direct RNA-RNA complementarity. Indeed,
all known ribosome binding sites contain a purine-rich sequence six to
ten nucleotides before the initiation codon, which is complementary to
the aforementioned 3′ end of 16 S RNA (Table 10). Direct experimental evidence for the Shine and Dalgarno hypothesis was obtained by
Steitz and Jakes (1975). They made ingenious use of an earlier
observation that colicin E3 inactivates the ribosome by cleavage of the
16 S mRNA 49 nucleotides from the 3′ end. After treatment of a 70 S
ribosome bound to the A protein initiation region of R17 with colicin
E1 and mild dissociation of the products, Steitz and Jakes could isolate
a base-paired complex between the 49-nucleotide-long 3′-terminal segment of the 16 S RNA and the A protein ribosome binding site.
Further experiments confirmed that the interaction indeed involves the
polypurine segment A-G-G-A-G-G-U (Table 10) and its complement
near the 3′ end of the colicin-produced 16 S RNA fragment (Steitz *et al.*,
1977; Steitz and Steege, 1977; Steitz, 1979). It should be stressed that
this interaction alone is not sufficient to explain the ribosome binding; it
occurs as part of a more complex process, in which the ribosome
superstructure and several proteins are also involved (cf. interaction
between codon and anticodon).

In discussing the role of the polypurine sequence in specific
ribosome binding, three aspects should be considered: (1) the stability
of the interaction with the rRNA 3′ terminus (this depends on the
number and the nature of contiguous complementary base pairs), (2)
the distance from the initiation codon, and (3) the masking of the complementary region by secondary and tertiary structure effects.

An estimate of the relative interaction efficiencies of the different
phage ribosome binding regions can be obtained by isolating these
ribosome-protected fragments and testing their efficiency in rebinding
(Steitz, 1973*b*). It turned out that the ribosomes preferred by far the A
initiator fragment; its binding was fortyfold higher than the coat initiator fragment and elevenfold higher than the replicase fragment. This is
in excellent agreement with the strong base complementarity present in
the A protein initiator fragment (Table 10), although the poor reactivity
of the coat fragment can also be explained by the fact that the latter
forms a rather stable hairpin (at one time it was believed that this
hairpin formation promoted strong ribosome binding). It is not known
whether the higher affinity for the ribosome also means that initiation

at the A gene is most efficient. This may be so and is not necessarily in contradiction with the relative efficiencies of gene expression *in vivo*, which are about in the ratio 0.05:1:0.30 for the A protein, the coat protein, and the replicase, respectively. Indeed, the latter ratios depend on complex regulatory systems, e.g., the A protein is translated from nascent chains while the coat protein is made mostly, if not exclusively, from mature viral RNA (further discussed in Section 5.4.3).

One naturally arisen mutation in the complementary polypurine sequence is known (Table 10). It occurs in the coat gene initiation region; Steitz (1969) found the sequence G-G-G-G-U for R17 RNA, while both MS2 RNA and another R17 strain (used in Geneva) have G-G-A-G-U at this position (Min Jou *et al.*, 1972; Adams *et al.*, 1972*a*). This mutation certainly must affect the interaction with the 3′ end of 16 S RNA (although in what way is more difficult to predict, depending on whether a looped-out C residue is allowed in the interaction stem). This mutation is not known to affect the translation efficiency and its effect must certainly be minor. However, initiation at the coat gene is unusual in several respects (see below) and therefore is atypical.

Little information is available on the allowable distance between the polypurine interaction region and the initiation codon. Some flexibility is obvious from the list of ribosome binding sites so far characterized (Steitz, 1979). But it may be noted that the Qβ replicase initiator region contains another, nonfunctional AUG triplet immediately following the complementary polypurine sequence (Table 10). This suggests that there are topological constraints and presumably there is an optimal distance between the complementary polypurine sequence and the initiation codon.

It is not only the Shine–Dalgarno interaction that determines ribosome binding; the AUG (or GUG) initiation codon is also important. Its role in correct phasing of the translation has long been recognized (Stanley *et al.*, 1969). Direct evidence for the importance of this interaction has recently been obtained by Taniguchi and Weissmann (1978). These authors succeeded in obtaining site-specific mutants in this region by the following procedure. Qβ minus strand was synthesized *in vitro* on a Qβ plus strand to which a ribosome was bound. The replicase proceeded until it was blocked at the coat initiator sequence by the ribosome. The latter was removed and limited further synthesis was allowed in the presence of the mutagen N^4-hydroxy-CTP. The minus strand was then completed with normal precursors and used as a template for *in vitro* synthesis of progeny plus strands. In this way a mixture of viral RNAs was obtained, which consisted not only of wild-type molecules with an A-U-G-G sequence at the beginning of the coat gene but also of mutant molecules in which the latter sequence was replaced by A-U-A-G, A-U-G-A, or A-U-A-A. This mixture was then used in a ribosome binding assay and the following binding efficiencies were derived relative to the wild-type sequence: <0.1 for A-U-A-G, 3.2 for A-U-G-A, and 0.3 for A-U-A-A. These results strikingly illustrate that the interaction between the initiating AUG and the anticodon CAU of the formylmethionine tRNA is important for ribosome binding. Elimination of the G-C base pair (in the mutant containing A-U-A-G) nearly abolished binding. Most remarkably, the residue immediately following the initiation triplet can also affect the binding. It is strongly enhanced when the latter is an A residue; this can be explained by the formation of an additional base pair, involving the U which precedes the CAU in the anticodon loop (Taniguchi and Weissmann, 1978). Whether such an additional interaction would interfere with proper translation of the phage gene is not known, but there are several examples of naturally occurring ribosome binding regions in which the initiating AUG is followed by an A residue (Steitz, 1979).

As we have discussed above, the specific recognition of the beginning region of the phage genes by the ribosomes presumably involves an interaction between a purine-rich segment (Shine–Dalgarno sequence) and a complementary segment near the 3' end of 16 S rRNA, as well as an interaction between the initiating AUG (or GUG) and the anticodon of formylmethionyl tRNA. But it should be stressed that these RNA-RNA interactions, although essential, are only part of a more elaborate recognition system, involving of course the ribosome matrix but also specific proteins. Two of the latter are of special relevance, namely IF3 and S1. Both can be removed from the active ribosome subunit by washing in high salt, and both are normally bound in the neighborhood of the 3' end of 16 S rRNA (Czernilofsky *et al.*, 1975; van Duin *et al.*, 1975; Steitz, 1979). Both are required for translation of all three phage genes. The role of the initiation factor IF3 in the formation of an active ribosome subunit and in mRNA binding has been well documented. S1 is the largest protein of the 30 S particle. It has a high affinity for single-stranded, especially pyrimidine-rich regions, and this property may be involved in altering the folding of the 3'-terminal region of 16 S rRNA such that the appropriate region becomes available for interaction (Dahlberg and Dahlberg, 1975). Addition of excess S1 to an *in vitro* translation system actually inhibits protein synthesis [this has been interpreted as a specific interference with the expression of the coat gene by Groner *et al.* (1972), but in later studies no clear discrimination between the genes was observed (Senear and Steitz, 1976)]. Salt-washed ribosomes can still recognize the specific ribosome binding regions on the messenger, but at much reduced efficiency. Stimulation of binding by addition of IF3 and S1 is twofold for the A protein gene, tenfold for the coat gene and five- to eightfold for the replicase gene (Steitz *et al.*, 1977). This result illustrates that the stronger Shine–Dalgarno interaction for the A protein gene leads to less dependency on supplementary protein factors.

Protein synthesis in the living cell is expected to be a very accurate process, starting only at the beginning of the genes. Yet it is surprising how strictly this accuracy of initiation is maintained in an *in vitro* system. Even when the latter is programmed with partially degraded phage RNA, almost only accurate proteins (coat protein and replicase) are made. One has to fragment the phage RNA to pieces smaller than 100 nucleotides before appreciable synthesis of new formylmethionine dipeptides is observed (Steitz, 1979) (synthesis of such a dipeptide is an assay for a functional ribosome-mRNA interaction). Yet if one scans the complete MS2 RNA sequence one finds numerous AUG or GUG triplets which are preceded at an appropriate distance by a polypurine-rich sequence capable, on paper at least, of interacting with the 3' end of 16 S rRNA (Fiers *et al.*, 1976) (Table 11). Clearly, these potential sites must be masked by the secondary (and to some extent perhaps tertiary) structure of the viral RNA. Direct evidence for such cryptic sites was obtained by Lodish (1970*b*), who treated f2 RNA with formaldehyde and observed that the partially unfolded viral RNA directed the synthesis of a new set of formylmethionine dipeptides (an alternative explanation, however, would be that the new ribosome binding site was not preexisting, but was created as a result of the formaldehyde addition to some specific nucleotides). For a short while immediately after synthesis (or after translation) such an illegitimate ribosome binding site is expected to occur in the accessible form (e.g., before the complement is available). As there is no evidence for spurious initiation *in vivo*, Steitz (1979) introduced the concept of a minimum time during which the region must remain "open" before a ribosome makes a functional interaction.

The superstructure of the viral RNA may be important in other ways than in shielding unwanted potential ribosome binding sites. We have seen above that binding of the ribosome to intact phage RNA is very efficient and is almost exclusively to the coat protein gene. Yet rebinding of the ribosome to the isolated coat initiator fragment is neg-

TABLE 11
Some Examples of Internal Regions in MS2 RNA Similar to Ribosome Binding Sites[a]

HOA-U-U-C-C-U-C-C-A-C-Py . . .	16 S RNA
. . . A-C-G-G-G-G-G-G-C-G-U-U-A-A-G-U-G . . . . . . A-C-G-G-G-G-U-C- -G-C-U-G-A-A-U-G . . . . . . C-C-G-G-G-G-U-U-U-G-A-A-G-C [A-U-G] . .	R17 coat
. . . A-A-G-A-G-U-U-U-C-U-U-C-C-U-A-U-G . . . . . . U-A-G-A-G-A-A-U-A- -A-C-A [A-U-G] . .	trp E
. . . G-U-G-G-G-A-U-G-C-U-C-C-U-A-C-A-U-G . . . . . . A-A-U-G-G-A-A-A-C-U-U-C-C-U-C [A-U-G] . .	f1 coat
. . C-A-A-G-G-U-C-U-C-C-U-A-A-A-A-G-A-U-G . . . . . C-U-A-G-G-A-G-G-U-U-U-G-A-C-C-U [A-U-G] . .	R17 A protein
. . . U-A-A-G-G-A-G-C-C-U-G-A-U-A-U-G . . . . . . A-G-A-G-G-A-A-A-C-A-G-C-U [A-U-G] . .	lac z
. . . A-G-A-A-A-G-G-G-G-U-C-G-G-U-G . . . . . . U-A-A-G-A-G-G-A- -C-A-U [A-U-G] . .	Qβ A protein
. . . C-G-G-G-G-A-C-G-A-U-A-U-U-A-U-A-U-G . . . . . . A-C-C-G-G-A-G-U-U-U-G-A-A-G-C [A-U-G] . .	MS2 coat
. . . U-C-G-A-G-G-U-G-C-C-U-A-A-A-A-G-U-G . . . . . . A-G-A-A-G-G-U-U-U-C-U-U-A-C-A-U-G . . . . . . C-C-C-A-G-G-U-G-C-C-U-U-C-G-A-U-G . . . . . . A-A-A-A-G-G-U-A-A-U-U-C-A-A [A-U-G] . .	f1 gene

[a] A number of bona fide ribosome binding sites are shown indicated by a boxed-in initiator AUG; these correspond to either RNA phage genes, DNA phage genes, or bacterial genes (for references, see Steitz, 1979). Above each true ribosome binding region one or more sequences are shown which are derived from internal regions of the MS2 RNA and which do not normally interact with ribosomes. These sequences share an AUG or GUG triplet, preceded at a suitable distance by a sequence (underlined) complementary to part of the 3' end of 16 S rRNA (shown on top).

ligible. Furthermore, fragmentation of the viral RNA has a drastic effect on the ribosome binding to the coat gene, in the case of both R17 (Adams *et al*., 1972*a*; Steitz, 1973) and Qβ (Porter and Hindley, 1973). This could mean that the ribosome first binds to a sequence some distance away and then transfers to the correct position, but for several reasons this model is unlikely. Presumably, a specific tertiary (and/or secondary) structure is required in order to allow efficient binding; perhaps the formation of the hairpin with the initiation AUG in the top loop (Fig. 5) has to be avoided. When fragmentation of the viral RNA is too extensive, this special three-dimensional conformation would be lost. Possibly, the interaction with the ribosome involves a structural transition of the viral RNA brought about by S1 (van Dieijen *et al.*, 1976). These more stringent requirements for ribosome initiation at the coat gene may even mean that the latter is normally not translated concomitantly with the RNA synthesis, but starts only on mature viral RNA molecules.

Interaction between a ribosome and phage RNA has also been used as a test for exploring species specificity at the translation level. Lodish (1969, 1970*a*) has shown that ribosomes from the thermophilic organism *Bacillus stearothermophilus* initiate quite well at the A protein site but virtually not at the two other phage genes. This effect was later traced to the small subunit proteins S12 and S1 (Held *et al.*, 1974; Steitz *et al.*, 1977). Apparently, *B. stearothermophilus* lacks an S1-like protein because simple addition of *E. coli* S1 to a *B. stearothermophilus in vitro* translation system programmed with f2 RNA is sufficient to obtain synthesis of coat protein and of replicase (Isono and Isono, 1975, 1976). The 3′-terminal sequence of *B. stearothermophilus* 16 S rRNA is the same as for *E. coli*, except that the terminal A is replaced by U-C-U-A$_{OH}$ (Shine and Dalgarno, 1975*a*; Sprague *et al.*, 1977). This suggests that these ribosomes are equally capable of interacting with the polypurine segment present in the region before the initiation codon (Table 10). At 65°C, the *B. stearothermophilus* ribosomes protect only the A gene initiator region, while at 49°C both the A protein and to some extent the replicase initiator region is protected (Goldberg and Steitz, 1974) (the former temperature is optimal for protein synthesis with the thermophile system, while the latter temperature is a compromise which allows direct comparison between *E. coli* and *B. stearothermophilus*). The specificity for the A protein gene then fits nicely with the idea that in this case the complementarity is sufficiently strong in itself, while for the replicase and especially for the coat gene adequate binding requires the supplementary action of proteins, especially S1.

We have mentioned above that numerous potential ribosome binding regions remain silent by being buried in the secondary (and tertiary) structure (cf. Table 11). Even at 65°C no new initiator regions become exposed in R17 RNA. In Qβ RNA, however, no bona fide initiator regions are recognized at this temperature, but two internal segments in the viral RNA are specifically protected by ribosomes (Steitz, 1973*a*; Sprague *et al.*, 1977). Both of these illegitimate binding sites contain a polypurine sequence which shows extensive base complementarity to the 3′ end of the 16 S rRNA, thus again supporting the Shine and Dalgarno hypothesis.

The 3′ end of 16 S rRNA of *Caulobacter crescentus* is almost identical to that of *B. stearothermophilus*, lacking only the terminal A residue (Shine and Dalgarno, 1975*b*). An *in vitro* translation system derived from *C. crescentus*, however, cannot be programmed with MS2 RNA but is active when RNA from the *Caulobacter* phage Cb5 (Section 2.2) is added (Leffler and Szer, 1973). Conversely, the Cb5 RNA is not translated in an *E. coli* system, and this species specificity has again been traced to the 30 S ribosomal subunit. At one time it was thought that the initiation factor was a codeterminant of species specificity, but this is not so. IF3 was isolated from *C. crescentus* and from *E. coli*, and both preparations have similar biochemical properties and are interchangeable in *in vitro* systems (Leffler and Szer, 1973, 1974). Unlike the situation with *B. stearothermophilus*, *C. crescentus* ribosomes do contain an S1 protein, which is able to substitute for its *E. coli* homologue, at least in the MS2 RNA-directed formylmethionine tRNA binding assay (Szer *et al.*, 1975). It was proposed that the ribosomal protein S12 and the 16 S rRNA play a dominant role in imposing the species specificity (compare, however, the *B. stearothermophilus* system as regards the role of the 16 S rRNA). Clearly these comparative studies can be very illuminating for our understanding of the species specificity of translational initiation, but more data are needed on the actual initiator regions recognized and on the specific components involved.

It is remarkable that although the machinery for protein synthesis and the general chemical structure of the messenger RNAs are so different between prokaryotes and eukaryotes, group I phage RNA and even better Qβ RNA can be used to program a mammalian or a wheat germ protein-synthesizing system (Aviv *et al.*, 1972; Morrison and Lodish, 1973; Schreier *et al.*, 1973; Davies and Kaesberg, 1973). Mostly coat protein but also some replicase is made in such systems (Morrison and Lodish, 1974). The fidelity of translation is good, although also some internal initiation occurs and the overall efficiency is rather low. These systems have been exploited to characterize suppressor tRNAs of eukaryotic origin. Amber mutations in the coat or replicase genes of Qβ can be suppressed by tRNA from an amber-suppressing yeast strain, while the normal termination codon UAA of the

$Q\beta$ replicase gene can be suppressed (to give a readthrough protein) if tRNA from an ochre suppressor yeast strain is added to the system (Capecchi *et al.*, 1975; Gesteland *et al.*, 1976).

4.3.2. Regions Protected by the Ribosomal Protein S1

We have seen in the preceding section that the 30 S component S1 is required for translation of all three phage genes. Moreover, the same protein is a constituent of the $Q\beta$ enzymatic complex for RNA replication (Wahba *et al.*, 1974; Inouye *et al.*, 1974) and presumably of the f2 replicase system (Fedoroff, 1975). The isolated S1 protein has a high affinity for single-stranded, pyrimidine-rich regions (Steitz, 1979). Addition of pure S1 protein to $Q\beta$ RNA followed (or preceded) by ribonuclease T1 digestion allows the isolation of a specific nucleoprotein complex which is retained on a nitrocellulose filter (Senear and Steitz, 1976; Goelz and Steitz, 1977). The specifically bound material was further fractionated by gel electrophoresis and two bands were observed. These were characterized as

    I   U-A-U-C-U-U-U-U-U-A-U-U-A-A-C-C-C-A-A-C-G

    II   . A-A-U-A-A-A-U-U-A-U-C-A-C-A-A-U-U-A-C-U-C-U-U-A-C-G

The former oligonucleotide (I) is derived from an intercistronic region preceding the coat gene (Section 4.3.5), while the latter oligonucleotide (II) is derived from a region near the 3' terminus of $Q\beta$ RNA (it corresponds to residues -38 to -63). Both T1 oligonucleotides are very rich in U and A residues and are unlikely to fold into a stable secondary structure. The interaction with oligonucleotide I presumably has a functional significance (cf. Section 4.3.5), but this is not clear for the second binding site. S1 binds also to R17 RNA but apparently to a large number of sites and no specific complex could be isolated.

4.3.3. Regions Protected by the Initiation Factor IF$_3$

IF$_3$ is known to stimulate binding of the 30 S ribosomal subunit to natural messenger RNA, although it has other functions as well (Steitz, 1979). Perhaps its pleiotropic effect is due to a conformational change of the 30 S subunit. Its binding site involves a portion of the 16 S rRNA close to the 3' end (van Duin *et al.*, 1975). Leffler and Szer (1974) observed that purified IF$_3$ binds to MS2 RNA and protects a region against nuclease digestion. This segment was isolated and characterized in more detail by Johnson and Szekely (1977). The fingerprint was relatively simple; by correlating the oligonucleotides with the known sequence of MS2 RNA (Vandenberghe *et al.*, 1975; Fiers *et al.*, 1976), they could conclude that most of the oligonucleotides (but not all) were derived from a region rather close to the 3′ terminus, viz. from nucleotide 3427 to nucleotide 3502 (Fig. 5). But even this segment was apparently not present as an intact piece. It appeared as if the protein had been bound to a specific subregion of the three-dimensional viral RNA structure and that only parts of this subregion were shielded from nuclease digestion. It is doubtful whether this interaction has a functional significance.

4.3.4. Regions Protected by the Host Factor HF

Qβ replicase (Section 4.3.5) requires a host factor (HF) for copying Qβ plus-strand RNA. This HF is not needed when other template RNAs are used such as Qβ minus-strand RNA or 6 S variant Qβ RNA (Eoyang and August, 1974). Neither is the HF apparently involved in replication of group I phage RNA (Fedoroff, 1975). At one time it was believed that in addition a second host factor was required for Qβ RNA replication (Eoyang and August, 1974), but this was later shown to be based on an artifact (Kamen *et al.*, 1974). HF is a hexamer of molecular weight 72,000 (Carmichael *et al.*, 1975). It is a heat-stable protein, normally associated with the ribosomes, from which it can be released by a high-salt wash. Its role in the uninfected cell is unknown. An active HF has also been isolated from *Pseudomonas putida*, a gram-negative organism with a quite different DNA composition (DuBow and Blumenthal, 1975).

HF binds to single-stranded RNA, e.g., Qβ RNA, *E. coli* rRNA, R23 RNA, or f2 RNA (Eoyang and August, 1974). Especially remarkable is its high affinity for poly(A); in fact, HF can be considerably purified by taking advantage of this property (Carmichael *et al.*, 1975). The binding of HF to RNA is specific and strong enough to protect a region against nuclease degradation. These HF binding regions were characterized in molecular detail by Senear and Steitz (1976). With R17 RNA only a single strong binding site was obtained:

C-G-A-A-G-A-A-U-A-A-U-A-A-A-A-U-A-G-A-U-C

This segment corresponds to residues 2350–2370 of MS2 RNA (Fig. 5) and is localized at about the middle of the replicase gene (Fiers *et al.*, 1976). Presumably this interaction has no biological meaning, but it may be noted that the sequence is particularly A rich and moreover the central T1 oligonucleotide A-A-U-A-A-U-A-A-A-A-U-A-G has peculiar and very exceptional properties such as strong sticking tendency to cellulose acetate or DEAE-cellulose.

HF binds to two sites in Qβ RNA, both corresponding to A-rich T1 oligonucleotides (Senear and Steitz, 1976):

Band I: A-C-C-A-A-U-A-C-U-A-A-A-A-A-G
Band II: A-A-U-A-A-A-U-U-A-U-C-A-C-A-A-U-U-A-C-U-C-U-U-A-C-G

Although some related longer segments are also obtained, the two aforementioned T1 oligonucleotides are the main products after treatment of the HF–Qβ RNA complex with ribonuclease T1. Both oligonucleotides, like the one derived from R17 or MS2 RNA, are rich in A tracts, contain several U residues, and are believed to occur largely as single strands in the three-dimensional structure. Band II is derived from near the 3′ end of Qβ RNA, namely residues -63 to -38 (Senear and Steitz, 1976; Weissmann *et al.*, 1973). Possibly this interaction is involved in Qβ RNA replication, e.g., for bringing the 3′ end of the template in an appropriate position relative to the enzymatically active center of the replicase complex.

Band I is located in the Qβ replicase cistron, several hundred residues from the 3′ end of the RNA, and the biological significance of this second HF binding site is obscure.

4.3.5. Regions Protected by the Qβ Replicase

Qβ replicase is the only viral RNA-dependent RNA polymerase which has been obtained in sufficient purity and quantity to carry out binding and protection experiments. The original studies of Haruna and Spiegelman (1965a) had indicated that MS2 replicase accepts only MS2 RNA as a template and not Qβ RNA while the converse was true for the Qβ replicase. This led to the optimistic belief that the study of the interaction between a replicase and its homologous template would lead to a reasonable understanding of the remarkable template specificity of these enzymes. The situation, however, seems to be much more complex than had at first been anticipated.

Qβ replicase is composed of four nonidentical subunits: the largest (70,000 daltons) is the 30 S ribosome protein S1 (cf. Section 4.3.2), the second is the phage-coded replicase subunit (65,000 daltons) and the two small subunits are the protein synthesis elongation factors EF-Tu and EF-Ts (45,000 and 35,000 daltons, respectively) (Kamen, 1970; Kondo *et al.*, 1970; Blumenthal *et al.*, 1972; Wahba *et al.*, 1974; Inouye *et al.*, 1974). As only the 65,000-dalton polypeptide is phage coded, one would normally assume that this component confers the specificity, but there is no direct evidence to prove this. Under appropriate conditions, replicase lacking the largest component S1 can be obtained (Kamen *et al.*, 1972). It is still endowed with enzymatic activity, when $Q\beta$ minus strand or variant "6 S" RNA or poly(C) is used as template, but it can no longer specifically interact with the $Q\beta$ plus strand.

$Q\beta$ replicase binds avidly and rather specifically to $Q\beta$ RNA even in the absence of any other component of the reaction, such as HF, nucleoside triphosphates, or even Mg^{2+} ions (August *et al.*, 1968). That this binding was not (only) to the 3′ end of the template but that the overall conformation of the $Q\beta$ RNA was also important for replication was already known from the early experiments of Haruna and Spiegelman (1965*b*), who showed that even partially degraded $Q\beta$ RNA no longer sustained initiation of RNA synthesis. $Q\beta$ replicase protects a region on the $Q\beta$ RNA against T1 ribonuclease degradation (Weber *et al.*, 1972). In fact, several fragments were obtained, which all came from the same region on the viral RNA. The longest fragment was about 100 nucleotides long. It is to some extent remarkable that the enzyme can protect such a large sequence; the reason may be that the replicase interacts with a number of critical sites on the tertiary structure of the viral RNA rather than tightly binding to a primary nucleotide sequence. The complete nucleotide sequence of the protected region was determined (Weber *et al.*, 1972) (Fig. 6). It turned out that the 3′ end overlapped with the ribosome binding site of the coat gene. Hence this replicase binding region is located at about 1400 nucleotides (31%) from the 5′ terminus. This interaction may have an important physiological role, not only in replication but also in regulation of translation. Indeed, Kolakofsky and Weissmann (1971) showed that replicase can prevent ribosomes from initiating translation of the coat gene, and this repressor activity fits nicely with the specificity of replicase-template interaction (Section 2.1). We mentioned before that replicase which has lost its largest subunit S1 no longer accepts $Q\beta$ plus-strand RNA as a template. Consideration of this, as well as of the role of S1 in binding of the ribosomal subunit to the mRNA, leads to the hypothesis that S1 could be responsible for the specific binding of $Q\beta$ replicase to the region just preceding the coat gene. As the group I phages also induce a specific replicase which contains S1 (Fedoroff and Zinder, 1971; Fedoroff, 1975), one would then suppose—if all processes

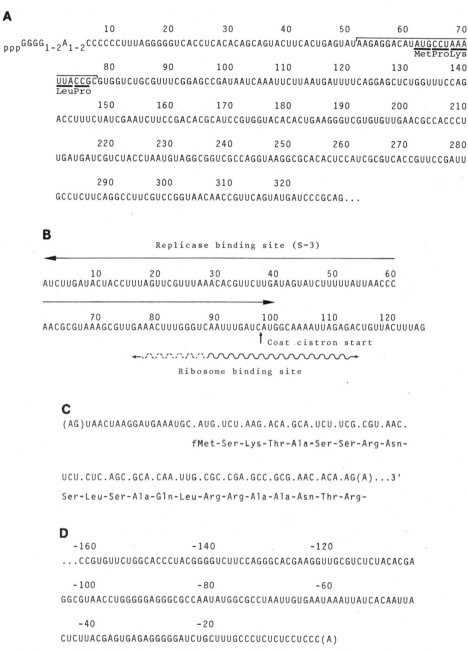

Fig. 6. Nucleotide sequence of some Qβ RNA regions. A: The 5′-terminal region. B: Region around the beginning of the coat gene (ribosome binding site and replicase binding site). C: Region around the beginning of the replicase subunit gene. D: The 3′-terminal region. Details on the 5′ terminus are given in Table 9 and on ribosome binding regions, in Table 10. From Weissmann *et al.* (1973), Porter *et al.* (1974), Weber (1976), Taniguchi and Weissmann (1978), and M. Billeter (personal communication).

proceed analogously—that the region before the coat site in the latter phages would also constitute a binding site for the S1-containing group I phage replicase and hence would show some similarity to the corresponding $Q\beta$ RNA sequence. However, no convincing sequence homology between these corresponding regions could be demonstrated (Contreras *et al.*, 1973).

The interaction between $Q\beta$ replicase and the region just before the coat gene of $Q\beta$ RNA requires incubation at 37°C and addition of monovalent ions, e.g., 0.15 M NaCl, but not Mg^{2+}. Because of this salt dependence, this protected region is called the S site. At 0°C, in the absence of high salt concentration but in the presence of Mg^{2+}, the replicase specifically binds to another region, called the M site (Weber *et al.*, 1974). The M site is located somewhere inside the replicase gene, around nucleotide 2100–2700 (47–60%) from the 5' end. The M site consists of three nonoverlapping sequences of chain length 164, 60, and 21 nucleotides, respectively (Meyer *et al.*, 1975). It is believed that this M interaction may play an important role in forming the initiation complex for replication. Binding of HF to the template is another essential step and perhaps its function is to bring the 3' end of the template in an appropriate position relative to the active center on the enzyme. Striking electron micrographic pictures, showing the interaction between $Q\beta$ replicase and the two sites on the template RNA, have been obtained by Vollenweider *et al.* (1976) (Fig. 7).

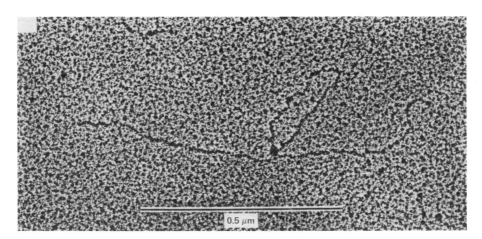

Fig. 7. Electron micrograph of $Q\beta$ replicase bound to two sites on the partially extended $Q\beta$ RNA molecule. The two sites presumably correspond to the S and the M sites (see text). After formation of the complex, a formaldehyde treatment was applied for fixation and extension of the RNA, followed by preparation for electron microscopy. From Vollenweider *et al.* (1976).

4.3.6. Regions Protected by the Coat Protein

We have mentioned already in Section 3.2 that the coat protein interacts specifically with the viral RNA. This interaction plays an important regulatory role, as the coat protein functions like a translational repressor on the expression of the replicase gene (this regulation will be further discussed in Section 5.4.5a). At low concentrations of coat protein to viral RNA a so-called complex I is formed (Sugiyama *et al.*, 1967). Addition of much more coat protein leads cooperatively to complex II, without evidence for intermediary structures. Complex II corresponds to a viruslike capsid but is noninfectious, sediments slower than virus, and contains RNA that remains susceptible to nucleases; cf. Section 3.1).

According to Sugiyama *et al.* (1967), complex I formed in 0.1 M tris buffer, pH 7.4, contains about six molecules of coat protein per viral RNA. Spahr *et al.* (1969), using different ionic conditions—viz., 0.1 M tris buffer, pH 7.5, 0.01 M magnesium acetate, and 0.08 M potassium chloride—find only one coat protein bound per RNA molecule. This 1:1 molar ratio was also confirmed in later studies (Bernardi and Spahr, 1972; Gralla *et al.*, 1974). The formation of complex I is rather specific; MS2 or f2 coat protein does not interact with Qβ RNA and neither does Qβ coat protein interact with MS2 or f2 RNA (Eggen and Nathans, 1969; Robertson *et al.*, 1968; Ward *et al.*, 1968). However, the phage fr, which is less closely related (Fig. 2), still cross-reacts with f2 RNA (Ward *et al.*, 1968).

Bernardi and Spahr (1972) treated R17 complex I with ribonuclease T1 and could isolate a unique, 59-nucleotide-long fragment which was protected by the coat protein against the nuclease treatment. Its nucleotide sequence was determined and it corresponds to residues 1708–1766 in the total MS2 RNA sequence (Fig. 5). This means that the fragment spans the termination region of the coat gene, first sequenced by Nichols (1970), as well as part of the replicase ribosome binding site characterized by Steitz (1969). The specificity of this binding strongly suggests that the coat protein blocks expression of the replicase gene by directly preventing access of ribosomes to this initiator region (Section 5.4.5a). The 59-nucleotide fragment contains two hairpins; the first corresponds to the termination region of the coat gene (the termination signal is in the top of the loop) as was proposed by Nichols (1970) (also shown in Fig. 5); the second hairpin contains the initiating AUG of the replicase in the hydrogen-bonded stem and was first proposed as an alternative conformation for this region of the molecule (Fig. 6 in Min Jou *et al.*, 1972). The former is considerably more stable than the latter, as the T_m values in 8 mM $MgCl_2$ amount to 88°C and to 64°C, respectively (Gralla *et al.*, 1974). Biochemical (Steitz, 1974) as well as physicochemical (Gralla *et al.*, 1974) evidence indicates that the coat protein binds only to the latter hairpin, which contains the initiating codon of the replicase gene. The fact that under the conditions used by Bernardi and Spahr a 59-nucleotide fragment is obtained can be explained by the absence of susceptible G residues in the single-stranded region connecting the first (coat terminator) hairpin to the second ("closed" replicase initiation) hairpin. It was further shown by Gralla *et al.* (1974) that the coat protein actually binds to the hairpin as such, and, as a result, its rate of melting is decreased a hundredfold. Thus the repressor role of the coat protein can be explained by a freezing-in of a particular conformation of the replicase initiator region, in which the initiating AUG is sequestered.

Also, Qβ coat protein protects a region around the replicase initiation site against nuclease degradation (Weber, 1976). Several fragments from this area were obtained, the longest of which was 88 nucleotides and extended some way into the replicase gene (Fig. 6). It is interesting that a very similar hairpin can be drawn as discussed above for R17-MS2, and it is likely that it is this feature which is recognized by the Qβ coat protein. Again, the initiating AUG of the replicase gene is part of the helical stem, and again blocking of this hairpin structure by the Qβ coat protein would explain its repressor activity on the expression of the replicase gene.

4.3.7. Regions Protected by the A Protein

We have discussed in Section 3.3 the direct interaction between the A protein and the viral RNA, the role of this complex in the first phases of the infection cycle, and the reconstitution *in vitro* of a biologically active A protein–viral RNA complex. Hence the obvious question is whether the A protein can also protect a specific region of the viral RNA against nuclease degradation. The binding is clearly not so strong and site restricted as for the coat protein. But under appropriate conditions a number of hairpins derived from a few quite separate regions of MS2 RNA can be protected and selectively isolated by the Millipore filtration assay (B. Leipold, D. Iserentant, W. Min Jou, and W. Fiers, in preparation). It seems as if the A protein interacts with several different sites on the macromolecule and perhaps its role in assembly is to bring these scattered regions together in a more compact, three-dimensional structure.

4.4. Approaches Leading to Partial Sequences of R17 and f2 RNA and to the Total Sequence of MS2 RNA

4.4.1. Introduction

The first primary structure of a nucleic acid was established by Holley *et al.* (1965), namely the total nucleotide sequence of yeast alanine tRNA. The approach followed was straightforward: (1) complete digestion of the RNA with the two known base-specific ribonucleases, T1 RNase and pancreatic RNase A, and separation of the resulting oligonucleotides; (2) sequence determination of all the oligonucleotides present in the RNase T1 and in the RNase A digest; and (3) ordering of the oligonucleotides by partial digestion of the RNA and characterization of these partial products. The analytical fractionations of the oligonucleotides were obtained by column chomatography. This approach, however, lacks speed, resolving power, and sensitivity of detection. The last drawback can be remedied by using ^{32}P-labeled viral RNA of high specific activity, as discussed in Sections 4.1 and 4.2.

A dramatic breakthrough in ease of operation and in resolution was the two-dimensional fractionation procedure worked out by Sanger *et al.* (1965). We have described this fingerprinting technique as well as later improvements such as homochromatography on DEAE–thin-layer plates in Section 4.2.2. These methods have been enormously useful for sequencing small RNA molecules such as tRNA and 5 S RNA (Brownlee *et al.*, 1968). Viral RNAs, however, are more than an order of magnitude larger, and therefore beyond the resolving power of these two-dimensional fingerprinting techniques. The two-dimensional gel system of De Wachter and Fiers (1972) or the minifingerprinting system of Volckaert *et al.* (1976) does allow the separation of all the longer, unique oligonucleotides in a total RNase T1 or RNase A digest of such an RNA, but these methods lack discrimination of the many oligonucleotides of intermediate length in these digests, most of them present many times in the sequence. The difficulty presented by the great length of the viral RNAs was solved by applying two new developments: the realization that ribonucleic acids have a defined three-dimensional structure, such that specific fragments can be

obtained by partial digestion, and the remarkable resolving power
obtainable by electrophoresis in polyacrylamide gel.

4.4.2. Partial Digestion of Viral RNA and Separation of the Fragments by Polyacrylamide Gel Electrophoresis

Through the work of Holley (Holley *et al.*, 1965) and others, it
became clear in the middle 1960s that at least some RNAs must have a
specific secondary (and perhaps tertiary) structure. By specific is meant
that the same conformation is present in all the molecules of the population. Some ribonucleases, such as RNase T1, cleave under appropriate conditions preferentially in single-stranded regions, and this
offers the possibility to obtain a rather limited number of partial fragments.

McPhie *et al.* (1966) and Gould (1966) showed that when ribosomal RNA is treated with nucleases under mild conditions which
preserve secondary structure, a discrete number of partial products is
obtained; furthermore, they introduced the use of polyacrylamide gel
electrophoresis to resolve these RNA fragments. The pattern of partial
products was very reproducible and depended on the type of ribosomal
RNA analyzed. It was then an obvious decision to try the same
approach with the bacteriophage RNAs. Indeed, physicochemical evidence had already indicated that approximately 73% ± 5% of the
nucleotides are involved in base pairing (Section 3.4) (Mitra *et al.*,
1963; Boedtker, 1967). Also, there was evidence from partial degradation that this secondary structure was ordered and specific (Fiers, 1967;
Bassel and Spiegelman, 1967; Spahr and Gesteland, 1968). As one
would expect from these considerations, treatment of bacteriophage
RNA with a low concentration of RNase T1 or RNase A at 0°C and
fractionation of the resulting digest by polyacrylamide gel electrophoresis led to a reproducible, discrete set of bands (Min Jou *et al.*,
1968; Adams *et al.*, 1969); Thach and Boedtker, 1969; Samuelson,
1969). Bacteriophage MS2 RNA contains more than 900 G residues,
and in the absence of secondary structure RNase T1 is little influenced
by the nature of the residues neighboring the G residue cleaved.
Therefore, the number of potential partial products is astronomically
large. The fact then that a discrete series of fragments is obtained
constitutes very clear and direct evidence for a highly ordered secondary and perhaps tertiary structure. Moreover, this procedure provided a
real breakthrough for nucleotide sequence analysis. Indeed, the

chemically enormously complex structure of the more than 3500-monomer-long viral RNA molecule could now be cut into discrete fragments which came within the the realm of the elegant sequencing methods pioneered by Sanger and co-workers (Sanger *et al.*, 1965; Brownlee *et al.*, 1968).

One of the advantages of partial enzymatic digestion as well as of polyacrylamide gel electrophoresis is that these techniques are very versatile. When the digestion is carried out with RNase T1 at 0°C and at an enzyme to substrate ratio of 1 unit per 20 μg bacteriophage RNA, and the partial hydrolysate is fractionated on a 12% polyacrylamide gel, a series of bands are obtained, which vary in chain length from approximately 30 to 260 nucleotides (Adams *et al.*, 1969; De Wachter *et al.*, 1971; De Wachter and Fiers, 1971). Somewhat surprisingly, the presence of Mg^{2+} in the digestion buffer and even the time of incubation are not very important variables. The G residues in single-stranded regions, such as between the hairpins and in the loops of hairpins, are cleaved, but the helical structures are not affected, as is evident from the fact that no loss of hypochromicity occurs under these conditions of partial digestion (Ysebaert, 1975) (Fig. 8).

But of course some segments are present in a single-stranded form, and in order not to lose this important information milder digestion conditions have to be used. By limiting the enzyme to substrate ratio of 1 unit RNase T1 per 100 or 200 μg viral RNA, a series of products are obtained which can be separated on a 6% polyacrylamide gel (De Wachter *et al.*, 1971). Again, these digestion conditions lead to a reproducible pattern of bands, corresponding to products with a chain length of 35–700 nucleotides. The components, which make up these bands, represent one or more hairpins, to which single-stranded regions are still linked. They contain virtually all the original secondary structure, and in fact often correspond to complexes held together by secondary interactions alone.

4.4.3. Fractionation of RNA Fragments

When the partial digestion is rather severe, only the strongly hydrogen-bonded hairpins survive; after polyacrylamide gel electrophoresis of such a digest, some of the bands may represent almost only one component, and this material is then suitable for direct sequence analysis. But more often the material eluted from a band is actually a mixture of many fragments, and further resolution is required. When

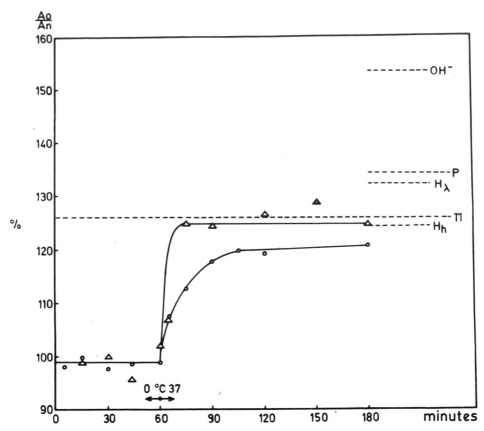

Fig. 8.   Maintenance of secondary structure under conditions of partial digestion of bacteriophage MS2 RNA. The percent increase in absorbancy at 260 nm is used as an index for loss of secondary structure. Ribonuclease T1 was added under conditions of either mild partial digestion (O), i.e., 1 unit T1 enzyme/200 μg MS2 RNA, or more severe partial digestion (Δ), i.e., 1 unit T1 enzyme/20 μg MS2 RNA, and the mixtures were incubated at 0°C. Under normal conditions of partial digestion, viz. 20 min at 0°C, no loss of hypochromicity becomes detectable. Such partial enzymatic digests result in a characteristic and reproducible band pattern, which formed the starting material for all further structural analysis (De Wachter et al., 1971a; Fiers, 1975). After the temperature of the reaction mixture is increased to 37°C, further hydrolysis now accompanied by rapid loss of hypochromicity ensues. Key (each was made with an identical amount of MS2 RNA and corrections for volume changes and salts were applied): T1, absorbancy after complete digestion with ribonuclease T1; P, absorbancy after complete digestion with pancreatic ribonuclease; OH$^-$, absorbancy after complete hydrolysis to mononucleotides by alkali; H$_\lambda$, absorbancy after complete melting by heating; H$_h$, calculated absorbancy after complete loss of secondary structure (the difference H$_\lambda$ – H$_h$ corresponds to base-stacking effects). Similar results were obtained under conditions of partial digestion with CM ribonuclease at 15°C. Reproduced from Ysebaert (1975).

the chain length does not exceed 60–70 nucleotides, this can be achieved by homochromatography according to Brownlee and Sanger (1969). As the first dimension is run in denaturing conditions (pH 3.5 and 7 M urea), the complexes are dissociated, and the net result is that very pure fragments are obtained by this procedure.

However, very often one has to resolve fragments (and complexes) of larger size, e.g., those obtained after milder digestion conditions and which still contain information from single-stranded regions. For this purpose, the two-dimensional polyacrylamide gel electrophoresis was developed by De Wachter and Fiers (1972). The material present in each of the bands of the neutral gel (12% or 6% polyacrylamide; cf. preceding section) is eluted, concentrated, and loaded on a new gel run at pH 3.5 and 7 M urea. Under these conditions, the fragments are denatured and the polynucleotides are resolved according to chain length and nucleotide composition. Then the strip is cut out and inserted in a new gel, which is now run at a perpendicular direction and at neutral pH (the gel concentration and buffer systems are so chosen that stacking occurs such that compact spots are obtained). Under the conditions of the second dimension, the polynucleotides can renature (depending whether the complementary sequence was part of the same molecule or was resolved in the first dimension), and the fractionation depends on chain length and on conformation. The resolution obtainable by this method is excellent (Fig. 9). Moreover, the procedure is very versatile; the percent acrylamide can be adapted according to the problem at hand, and the method has been used to fractionate successfully all the bands present in the primary digests (preceding section). In this way a large number of fragments derived from ^{32}P-labeled MS2 RNA were obtained in pure form, and the procedure has been of crucial importance in the elucidation of the total nucleotide sequence of bacteriophage MS2 RNA. Moreover, the procedure has been widely used for fingerprinting complex viral RNA genomes, as discussed above (Section 4.2.2).

4.4.4. Sequence Determination of Oligonucleotides

Once a fragment of chain length 30–300 is obtained, an RNase T1 and an RNase A fingerprint can be made by one of the procedures mentioned in Section 4.2.2. It may be noted here that although the term "fingerprint" suggests an analytical rather than a preparative procedure, one is in fact dealing with ^{32}P-labeled RNA of high specific

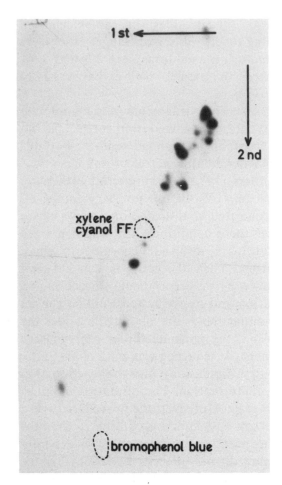

Fig. 9. Fractionation of MS2 RNA fragments by two-dimensional electrophoresis on polyacrylamide gel. ^{32}P-labeled MS2 RNA was partially digested with ribonuclease T1 under mild conditions (see text) and fractionated by electrophoresis on a 6% polyacrylamide gel run at neutral pH (De Wachter *et al.*, 1971*a*). The material present in one particular band (γ5) was eluted, concentrated, and further resolved by two-dimensional electrophoresis (De Wachter and Fiers, 1972). The first dimension was run on an 8% polyacrylamide gel in 0.025 M citric acid–6 M urea, pH 3.5. The strip containing the resolved bands was excised and polymerized in a 16% polyacrylamide gel. The second dimension was then run in 0.4 M tris-acetate buffer, pH 8.0. The spots correspond to pure fragments suitable for detailed structural analysis.

activity. Hence the amounts of material handled are minimal (usually unlabeled "carrier" RNA is added), but the amount of radioactivity is sufficient to carry out further quantitative analyses and characterizations.

The procedures followed to determine the structure of an oligonucleotide are based on the extensive studies on the specificity of various nucleases in the 1950s and early 1960s. In principle, an oligonucleotide can be sequenced by partial exonucleolytic digestion and characterization of the product obtained at each step. Alternatively, an oligonucleotide can be further cleaved to smaller products by endonucleases, and if this is done in various ways the sequence of the original oligonucleotide can be deduced from the overlaps. In reality, each approach has drawbacks and pitfalls, and therefore nearly all oligonucleotides of

MS2 RNA have been sequenced by more than one approach. The characterization of an oligonucleotide by such degradative processes requires a large number of fractionations, and the fast, sensitive, and reliable procedures worked out by Sanger and his colleagues have also been immensely useful for this purpose (reviewed in Brownlee, 1972).

Pancreatic RNase A nucleotides have the form $(A)_m(G)_n U$ or $(A)_m(G)_n Cp$. If they do not contain G residues, the sequence can be derived from the nucleotide composition (e.g., A_5C), but an independent chain length determination is essential. If a single G residue is present, an analysis with RNase T1 provides the sequence (e.g., A-G-A-A-A-U). When several G residues occur, additional sequence information must be obtained by partial exonuclease digestion, using either spleen exonuclease or, after dephosphorylation, snake venom exonuclease. The increase in electrophoretic mobility is larger after exonucleolytic removal of a G residue than after removal of an A residue; on this basis it is possible to tentatively deduce the residue removed at each step of the partial exonucleolytic degradation (Sanger *et al.*, 1965; Sanger and Brownlee, 1967). A more sensitive and simple modification of this method, but based on the increase in chromatographic mobility, was later worked out by Volckaert and Fiers (1974). It is well known that G-rich oligonucleotides have a tendency to aggregate. This problem becomes especially severe when runs of four or more consecutive G residues are present. These are nearly impossible to sequence by the partial exonucleolytic approach, and therefore an alternative procedure was developed (Min Jou and Fiers, 1976*a*). The reagent kethoxal forms an adduct with G residues (Staehelin, 1959) and in this way not only prevents aggregation but moreover makes it resistant to hydrolysis by ribonuclease U2. After treatment, the resulting products consists of the G series followed by A, U, or C. In this way, it could, for example, be shown that both G-A-G-G-G-G-U and G-G-G-G-A-G-U occur in MS2 RNA.

T1 oligonucleotides have the general structure $(A)_m(U)_n(C)_o G$, and obviously they are often much longer than pancreatic RNase A oligonucleotides. Details of the basic sequencing procedures have been described by Brownlee (1972). Partial degradation with spleen exonuclease and characterization of each intermediate product can in principle provide the sequence. However, C residues are only slowly removed and consecutive C residues constitute almost a block to further procession. Alternatively, partial exonucleolytic digestion in the 3' to 5' direction can be applied, e.g., by means of snake venom exonuclease, but the residual endonuclease activity often present in these enzyme preparations constitutes a problem. The exonucleolytic procedures become less valuable when the chain length increases beyond seven to ten residues; indeed, the limited radioactivity is then distributed over too many spots, and the partial products become more difficult to cleanly separate from each other. Some information on the nature of the nucleotide removed at each step can again be obtained by considering the increase in electrophoretic mobility (Sanger et al., 1965; Sanger and Brownlee, 1967; Brownlee, 1972). This method is more reliable and can be extended to longer oligonucleotides if the mobilities in two dimensions are considered (Szekely and Sanger, 1969; Ling, 1972; Rensing and Schoenmakers, 1973).

Most T1 oligonucleotide sequences, however, have mainly been solved by further degradation with endonucleases and overlap analysis. A first step is double digestion analysis with RNase A, which gives the different A tracts, e.g., A-A-C + A-C + A-U + C + G. Hydrolysis with ribonuclease U2 (specific for purines) results in tracts of the structure $(U)_m,(C)_nA$, as well as $(U)_o(C)_pG$. As consecutive A residues are more slowly cleaved, additional information is often obtained, e.g., U2 analysis of the oligonucleotide C-C-U-C-A-C-A-A-C-U-C-G gave $(C_3,U)A$, $(C_2U)G$, and both C-A and C-A-A, thus indicating that the A-A-C was not preceded by a series of pyrimidine nucleotides. Another base-specific degradation consists in blocking the U residues with N-cyclohexyl-N'-β-(4-methylmorpholinium)ethylcarbodiimide p-toluene sulfonate (CMCT) such that now RNase A cleaves only after C residues (Ho and Gilham, 1967; Adams et al., 1969); in this way, tracts of U residues or U and A residues can be characterized; thus, for example, the oligonucleotide U-U-U-C-G gave only the products U-U-U-C and G. The only remaining difficulty now is to characterize pyrimidine series rich in C residues. Fortunately another enzyme, Physarum polycephalum ribonuclease, became available, which cleaves after U and A residues, but virtually not at all after C residues (Contreras and Fiers, 1975). For example, the oligonucleotide C-U-C-C-C-U-A-C-G gave almost exclusively C-U, C-C-C-U, A-C-G, and A + C-G, which were readily ordered on the basis of the additional RNase U2 and CMCT–RNase A results. Longer pyrimidine series could often be sequenced by analysis of partial Physarum RNase products (Contreras and Fiers, 1975). The specificity of this enzyme has been further confirmed by studies on model substrates (Braun and Behrens, 1969; Pilly et al., 1978). The above procedures are often still not sufficient to order unambiguously all the partial segments; in this case the T1 oligonucleotide is partially digested as described for polynucleotides in the following section, and the different fragments are characterized.

4.4.5.   Ordering of Oligonucleotides and Derivation of the Nucleotide Sequence of an RNA Fragment

In the previous sections we have explained how a pure fragment of the phage RNA is obtained, with a chain length 30–300 nucleotides. This fragment is then characterized by making a catalogue of all T1 and of all pancreatic RNase A oligonucleotides whose sequence has been established. Now the problem of ordering these oligonucleotides remains. It is mainly a question of ordering the T1 oligonucleotides; either the RNase A oligonucleotides contain no G residues and are part of a longer T1 oligonucleotide, or those containing G residues constitute the bridges between the T1 oligonucleotides. It is rather seldom that the structure of the oligonucleotides themselves contains enough information to order them unambiguously. For example an RNase A product A-A-G-A-C indicates that a T1 oligonucleotide ending with a Py-A-A-G has to be followed by another one which starts with A-C . . . . G. Most often, the fragment has to be further partially digested, and the subfragments have to be separated and characterized by RNase T1 and A fingerprints.

For partial digestion of the fragment one can again use RNase T1, especially if the product does not contain much residual secondary structure. The presence of the latter does create problems, as in this case further cleavage is rather site specific, so that no overlapping segments are obtained. To avoid this difficulty, one can apply partial T1 digestion in the presence of 70% dimethylsulfoxide (Merregaert, 1975). Under these conditions the polynucleotide is largely denatured, while the enzyme is still active. Hence all G residues can be cleaved with almost equal probability; this method, however, can be used only on rather short oligonucleotides, since otherwise the variety of partial products becomes unmanageable.

Another important step, which has played a decisive role in the determination of the total nucleotide sequence of MS2 RNA, was the introduction of ε-carboxymethyl-lysine-41-pancreatic ribonuclease (CM-RNase) for obtaining specific, partial products (Contreras and Fiers, 1971). Under appropriate conditions, this enzyme cleaves almost exclusively between C-A and U-A sequences, thus generating a different set of subfragments, which in most cases provide enough overlap information to reconstruct the sequence of the polynucleotide. Another useful enzyme is spleen acid endonuclease (Brownlee *et al.*, 1968; Brownlee, 1972). It results in a series of discrete partial products, although the type of internucleotide bond most susceptible to cleavage varies somewhat according to the polynucleotide, and no general conclusions on its specificity can be drawn. This enzyme is also very useful for partial digestion of T1 oligonucleotides (Jeppesen, 1971). Unfortunately, it is not commercially available and it is difficult to prepare.

The subfragments, i.e., the products obtained by partial digestion of the fragments, can be resolved either by an appropriate electrophoresis–homochromatography system (Section 4.2.2) or by two-dimensional polyacrylamide gel electrophoresis (Section 4.4.3). It is not unusual to obtain 10–30 subfragments from a single partial digestion of a fragment, and each of these subfragments has to be characterized by an RNase T1 and an RNase A fingerprint. Since a partial digestion of total phage RNA may produce, after the fractionation procedures described in Sections 4.4.2 and 4.4.3, hundreds of primary fragments, the analysis of all the resulting subfragments is a considerable task. Therefore, fast and inexpensive methods are needed, although the resolution is less of a problem as the composition of the subfragments is rather simple. In the MS2 RNA project, the RNase T1 and RNase A digests of the subfragments were usually analyzed by the two-dimensional fingerprinting method involving electrophoresis at pH 3.5 on cellulose acetate followed by chromatography on a polyethyleneimine thin-layer plate with a formate-pyridine buffer (Section 4.2.2) (Southern and Mitchell, 1971; Griffin, 1971; Contreras *et al.*, 1971). The autoradiograms of these fingerprints of the subfragments can usually be interpreted visually on the basis of the characterized standard fingerprint of the fragment. More recently, a miniversion for the analysis of RNase A digests was introduced (Volckaert and Fiers, 1977).

The purpose of the partial digestion is to order unambiguously the T1 oligonucleotides on the basis of bridging (G-containing) RNase A oligonucleotides. If more than one T1 oligonucleotide starts with the same 5′ sequence, then difficulties may arise. For example, the two oligonucleotides U-A-U-G and U-C-G may be present in the T1 fingerprint, while the RNase A digest indicates a single G-U as the only bridging RNase A oligonucleotide. Obviously, one of the two T1 oligonucleotides must be derived from the 5′ end of the subfragment, but the question is which one. The answer can be obtained by mild exonucleolytic digestion before fingerprinting. If in the above example the subfragment is treated lightly with spleen exonuclease before subsequent characterization, the T1 oligonucleotide which constitutes the 5′ end of the subfragment will disappear and give rise to shorter oligonucleotides in the fingerprint.

4.4.6. Nucleotide Sequence of Fragments of the Group I Phage RNAs

Sanger and his colleagues were the first to establish the nucleotide sequence of a phage RNA fragment (Adams *et al.*, 1969). This was a remarkable achievement, even more so as the 57-nucleotide segment which they reported was actually derived from the coat gene of R17 RNA, and therefore they could for the first time make a direct correlation between the primary chemical structure of the genetic material and the structure of the gene product. A discussion of the biological implications of these RNA sequences will be presented later (Section 5).

Following the realization that protein synthesis cannot initiate immediately at the physical 5′ end of the RNA molecule (De Wachter *et al.*, 1968; Section 4.1.1), it became of interest to know where the first gene actually starts. Cory *et al.* (1970) reported the nucleotide sequence of a 74-nucleotide fragment derived from the 5′ end of R17 (Adams and Cory, 1970). This fragment has a rather stable structure, so that its isolation from partial digests is relatively easy. De Wachter and Fiers (1970) presented at the same time a somewhat less complete but apparently identical sequence derived from MS2 RNA. The same fragment, but isolated from f2 RNA, was subsequently sequenced by Ling (1971). It was known that the A protein was the first gene (Jeppesen *et al.*, 1970) (Fig. 1), and the ribosome binding region of the A gene had been sequenced (Steitz, 1969). De Wachter *et al.* (1971*a*) then worked out procedures to isolate larger fragments, still containing the 5′ terminus. In this way they did find an overlap with the aforementioned A gene initiator region and established that there was a 129-nucleotide-long, untranslated leader sequence preceding the first gene. The nucleotide sequence of this leader segment was reported in detail both for MS2 RNA (De Wachter *et al.*, 1971) and for R17 RNA (Adams *et al.*, 1972*b*). It turned out that the first gene in MS2 RNA starts with GUG rather than AUG as in R17 RNA (Volckaert and Fiers, 1973); this was the first time that a naturally occurring GUG-initiation codon was identified.

The 3′-terminal T1 oligonucleotide of group I RNA bacteriophages is U-U-A-C-C-A-C-C-C-A$_{OH}$ (Section 4.1.2). By screening for this oligonucleotide, fragments derived from the 3′ end could be identified in a partial T1 digest. The polyacrylamide gel bands were analyzed, and those of interest were further purified by homochromatography. The 3'-terminal sequence was first elongated to 16 nucleotides (Min Jou *et al.*, 1970), then to 51 for R17 RNA (Corey *et al.*, 1970, 1972), and to 70 for MS2 RNA (Fiers *et al.*, 1971). Using the more powerful two-dimensional electrophoresis method for obtaining longer fragments (Section 4.4.3) the former sequence was rapidly elongated to 104 nucleotides (Contreras *et al.*, 1971) and further (following section).

Another region which forms a rather strong hairpin structure occurs around the termination of the coat protein gene (cf. Section 4.3.6). A 44-nucleotide segment was characterized by Nichols (1970). It coded for the last six amino acids of the coat gene, followed by the termination signal and an untranslated region. As part of the latter formed an overlap with the replicase ribosome binding site (Steitz, 1969), Nichols could conclude that the intercistronic region between the coat gene and the replicase gene was 36 nucleotides long.

We have mentioned already that the initiating AUG of the coat gene occurs on the top of a stable hairpin (Section 4.3.1; Steitz, 1969). Fragments were subsequently identified which included this hairpin and allowed investigators to extend the known sequence (Cory *et al.*, 1970; Adams *et al.*, 1972*a*). A region of 40 nucleotides before the initiating AUG of the coat gene was characterized; it contained three termination codons, a UAA and UGA in one phase and UAG in a second phase. Remaut and Fiers (1972) showed that the A protein gene of MS2 is terminated by a single UAG signal, because on infection of host cells which carry an amber suppressor gene with wild-type virus, a fourth virus-specific protein is produced. This polypeptide was shown to be formed by readthrough at the end of the A protein gene in cells containing an su_{am} allele and is indicated by A_s. A_s is about 30 amino acids longer than the normal A protein and is not incorporated in virus particles. By examination of the nucleotide sequence, it was predicted that the intercistronic region between the A protein gene and the coat gene would be 26 nucleotides long and that under conditions of suppression of UAG codons (amber), partial readthrough occurs, resulting in A_s protein which would be 27 amino acids longer and terminated by a UGA signal located already inside the coat gene, but in a different phase (i.e., the A_s protein gene and the coat gene overlap) (Remaut and Fiers, 1972). This prediction was fully proven when longer nucleotide sequences became available such that the reading frame of the A protein could be deduced (Contreras *et al.*, 1973). Further confirmation

came from amino acid sequencing data on the A protein (Vandekerckhove *et al.*, 1973; Vandekerckhove and van Montagu, 1977).

RNA fragments derived from the coat gene were the easiest to
identify, as the coat protein was the only virus-specific polypeptide for
which the amino acid sequence was known (Section 3.2). We have seen
in the introductory paragraph of this section that a fragment derived
from the R17 coat gene was the first to be sequenced and to allow a
direct comparison between the chemical structure of the genetic
information and the corresponding gene product (Adams *et al.*, 1969).
Soon other fragments derived from the coat gene were isolated and
characterized, in the case of R17 RNA (Jeppesen *et al.*, 1970, 1972), of
MS2 RNA (Min Jou *et al.*, 1971; Fiers *et al.*, 1971), and of f2 RNA
(Nichols and Robertson, 1971).

The amino acid sequences of the A protein and the viral replicase
polypeptide were not known, and therefore it was not so simple to
identify fragments derived from these genes. But the ribosome binding
regions including the information for the first few N-terminal amino
acids had been characterized (Section 4.3.1). Consequently, these
regions were extended by the isolation of fragments which formed an
overlap, e.g., for the A protein gene of R17 (Rensing *et al.*, 1973) and
for the MS2 replicase gene (Contreras *et al.*, 1972). Other fragments
were derived from internal regions of the genes and could not be exactly
positioned (Fiers *et al.*, 1971; Rensing and Schoenmakers, 1973; Rensing, 1973; Rensing *et al.*, 1973, 1974; Haegeman and Fiers, 1973). In
total, 23.9% of the R17 genome and 11.5% of the f2 genome has been
sequenced (reviewed by Min Jou and Fiers, 1976*b*). The comparison
between the structures of the group I phage RNAs will be discussed in
Section 5.7.2.

Applying a similar approach to the phage Qβ RNA, Hindley and
co-workers isolated and sequenced fragments derived from around the
ribosome binding sites of the coat and of the replicase gene (Porter and
Hindley, 1972; Porter *et al.*, 1974) (Fig. 7).

4.4.7. The Complete Structure of MS2 RNA

The overall structure of the viral RNA, as that of tRNA,
essentially consists of a series of hairpins linked by connecting segments. These basic units of secondary structure are then further folded
into a specific three-dimensional superstructure. Usually the top loops
of the hairpin as well as parts of the connecting segments are not or less

involved in secondary interactions and form the targets for single-strand-specific nucleases. Under normal conditions of partial digestion with ribonuclease T1 only the hairpins are preserved (Section 4.4.2). They may contain single-stranded tails, derived from the interconnecting segments, depending on whether or not exposed G residues are present. Also, cleavages may occur at G residues present in the top of a hairpin or in discontinuities of the stem. The products obtained from partial digestion are often complexes, held together by secondary interactions. Indeed, it was mentioned above that nearly all the secondary structure was still preserved at this stage (Fig. 8). In order to obtain pure molecules for nucleotide sequence analysis, the complexes have to be denatured and resolved in individual fragments. For fragments of chain length 70 and below, this resolution can be achieved by electrophoresis at pH 3.5 followed by homochromatography (Section 4.4.3). The fragments discussed in the preceding section had mainly been obtained by this approach. For the purification of longer fragments, however, the development of the two-dimensional polyacrylamide gel electrophoresis method (De Wachter and Fiers, 1972) has been absolutely essential. In this way, pure fragments of 125 nucleotides and longer have been obtained.

The next phase, then, consisted of the introduction of the so-called mild partial digestion conditions (Section 4.4.2). Under these conditions, usually not more than one cleavage occurs in the interconnecting segments, such that nearly all sequence information is still present on the separating, neutral gel [6% gel (De Wachter *et al.*, 1971)]. The resulting complexes are obviously larger and consist of one or more connected hairpins to which single-stranded tails are still attached. The versatility of the two-dimensional polyacrylamide gel electrophoresis method also allows resolution of these complexes into individual components. In this way larger fragments are obtained, sometimes exceeding 200 nucleotides in length.

Fragments derived from the MS2 coat gene could be identified and placed in the proper order, as the amino acid sequence of the protein was known. This allowed establishment of the first nucleotide sequence of a complete gene (Min Jou *et al.*, 1972). Overlapping segments, however, were seldom found, and it seems more as if the order in which the different susceptible G residues are cleaved is rather strict. Some sites (three in the case of the MS2 RNA coat gene) are so sensitive to hydrolysis by ribonuclease T1 that they are always split, even under the mildest digestion conditions. Hence all fragments that were characterized were subregions of four nonoverlapping primary fragments.

Their ordering and the knowledge that they are contiguous were based on the amino acid sequence data.

The approach so far, then, was still insufficient to derive the total nucleotide sequence of a viral RNA. By characterizing many hundreds of fragments it was possible to assign these to specific regions, corresponding to large primary fragments. The latter were recognized by the presence of one or more typical oligonucleotides which occur only once or a few times in the total sequence, such as (G)A-A-C-A-G. In this way, some 20–25 regions or RNA fragment families were characterized. For some of these, a very approximate location on the genome was known, e.g., when they contained an oligonucleotide which had previously been assigned to the 5' one-third or the 3' two-thirds part of the genome (Min Jou *et al.*, 1969; Jeppesen *et al.*, 1970).

An answer to this problem of overlaps, and the key to the elucidation of the total sequence of MS2 RNA, was the application of the enzyme ε-carboxymethyl-lysine-41-pancreatic ribonuclease A (CM-RNase). This derivative was first synthesized by Heinrikson (1965) and was shown by Goldstein (1967) to result in limited hydrolysis of 5 S RNA. As mentioned in Section 4.4.5, this enzyme cleaves almost exclusively between C-A and U-A (Contreras and Fiers, 1971), and is thus more restricted in its specificity than either RNase T1 or pancreatic RNase A. It has been enormously useful, both for solving the nucleotide sequence of longer T1 oligonucleotides (Section 4.4.4) and for ordering the oligonucleotides in RNA fragments (Section 4.4.5). Furthermore, it was established that the action of CM-RNase can be limited to single-stranded regions only. When MS2 RNA is digested at 15°C, no loss whatsoever in hypochromicity can be observed (cf. Fig. 8 for the analogous experiment with T1 RNase) (Ysebaert, 1975). Consequently, after partial digestion (20 min at a 1:600 w/w enzyme-to-substrate ratio) a series of products is obtained which still contain nearly all the secondary structure present in the original MS2 RNA molecule. These products, which correspond to the hairpins, can again by resolved first on a neutral 12% gel, resulting in a series of bands. The material present in each band usually consists of complexes, whose individual RNA fragments can be fractionated by two-dimensional gel electrophoresis. Also, by using milder digestion conditions (10 min at a 1:2000 w/w enzyme-to-substrate ratio) hairpins which often retain single-stranded tails from the connecting segments can be obtained. By systematically carrying out these fractionations, many hundreds of CM-RNase fragments have been isolated and characterized. Correlation of this information with the RNA fragment families derived from partial T1 RNase digestion provided all the necessary overlaps, and in this way the total nucleotide sequence of MS2 RNA was established (Fiers *et al.*, 1975, 1976; Vandenberghe *et al.*, 1975) (Fig. 5).

4.4.8.   Derivation of Secondary Structure Models

Several essential biological functions of the phage RNA must undoubtedly be explained on the basis of the three-dimensional folding of the molecule, e.g., control mechanisms regulating the expression of the A protein and of the replicase gene (Section 5.4), translational expression of the coat gene (Section 4.3.1), resistance against cytoplasmic mRNA-degrading enzymes, correct encapsidation, etc. Therefore, it seems proper that, starting from the primary nucleotide sequence, one should try to gain some insight into the secondary and perhaps even tertiary structure. The experiences with the simple tRNAs, however, present an indication that although a satisfactory secondary structure can be predicted (the cloverleaf), the real tertiary structure is much more intricate and at present for viral RNAs absolutely beyond the reach of theoretical prediction.

We have seen in Section 3.4 that under physiological conditions approximately $73\% \pm 5\%$ of the nucleotides in the viral RNA are involved in base-pair interactions, and this value may even be higher for the viral RNA inside the virions. Not only is this degree of secondary structure decidedly higher than what can be expected on a random basis, but moreover the structures are considerably more stable (Ricard and Salzer, 1975) (Section 3.4). Obviously, the whole approach of sequencing the viral RNA by partial digestion would be inconceivable were it not for the presence of a highly specific secondary structure, uniform over the whole population of molecules.

The derivation of the secondary structure models, as shown in Fig. 5, is partly based on experimental data and partly on theoretical considerations. It was mentioned in Section 4.4.2 and in the preceding section that under conditions of limited enzymatic digestion of MS2 RNA no loss of hypochromicity and hence no appreciable loss of secondary structure occur (Fig. 8). Partial digestion with T1 RNase is carried out at 0°C, which is 35°C below the temperature at which the first base-paired regions start to melt. Therefore, it is unlikely that much rearrangement can occur under these conditions, and we may assume that the secondary structure, still present in the complexes isolated by electrophoresis on a neutral polyacrylamide gel, corresponds to a large extent to aspects of the folding present in the original macromolecule.

There are numerous indications for an ordered structure in many of the isolated RNA fragments. On further digestion, for example, there may be more than a fiftyfold difference in susceptibility toward T1 RNase between a G residue in a stem of a hairpin and a G residue in a single-stranded tail. It is not unusual to find a hairpin in which the top loop is nicked, but the two strands remain together and behave as a single molecule until they are denatured in the first dimension of the two-dimensional separation method for the preparation of pure RNA fragments (Min Jou *et al.*, 1971; Contreras *et al.*, 1971). When the two strands are mixed, the hairpin readily re-forms. Occasionally, a fragment which corresponds to an uncleaved hairpin may, after denaturation and returning to neutral pH, not renature intramolecularly but form a dimer, another property typical of hairpin structures.

For the derivation of a secondary structure model, it is indicated to start from a fragment regularly found in the more severe type of partial T1 RNase digests. By scoring all segments of complementary base pairs, it is usually possible to write up one or more alternative models of secondary structure. The choice between these alternatives is then based on estimates of thermodynamic stability (see below). A hairpin which survives a partial T1 RNase digestion very often also survives, in a slightly different length, a partial CM-RNase digestion. Once the most stable segments have been identified, base-pairing schemes can be tried out for the remaining, weaker regions; these either form extensions of the hairpins or form structures on their own or may be involved in long-range interactions, which in this context means base pairing with a sequence from a quite different area in the phage RNA. The frequency with which a given RNA fragment occurs in a partial digest is actually a good measure of the susceptibility and hence the degree of exposition of particular sites in the superstructure. In the deduction of the MS2 RNA structure we found it useful to classify the cleavable sites in five categories (both for T1 RNase digests and for CM RNase digests): (1) positions which are always cleaved even under the mildest conditions used, (2) position which are usually cleaved and nearly always in the more severe type of partial digestion, (3) positions which are usually uncleaved in the milder digestion conditions but are split rather often in the more severe conditions, (4) positions which are usually not cleaved even under the more severe conditions, and (5) positions which were only very occasionally found to be cleaved. It may be noted that under the conditions used the majority of the sites remain completely resistant to enzymatic attack. A close scrutiny of the exact positions of these different types of cleavage sites in the secondary structure model reveals a remarkably good fit (this does not constitute completely independent information as the enzymatic susceptibility of the sites was often taken into account to derive the model). It is clear that the positions of type 1, where cleavage always occurs, are found only in single-stranded regions and most of them actually are located in the top loops of hairpins (Fiers *et al.*, 1975, 1976).

Ideally, one would like to predict the secondary structure purely on the basis of the primary nucleotide sequence information. The real conformation most likely corresponds to a state of minimum free energy. The free energy for a particular region can be seen as the algebraic sum of stabilizing and destabilizing features (Tinoco *et al.*, 1971; Delisi and Crothers, 1971). The stabilizing factors (negative free energy contribution) are of course the base-pair interactions, involving the H-bonding as well as the stacking effects. The destabilizing features (positive free energy contribution) are the hairpin loop, internal loops (nonmatching bases in the stem), and bulge loops (one or more looped-out nucleotides in one strand of the stem). Much effort has been spent on the study of the thermodynamic stability of various model compounds in order to arrive at the appropriate physicochemical values which could be used to predict the secondary structure of natural RNA (Fink and Crothers, 1972; Gralla and Crothers, 1973a; Uhlenbeck *et al.*, 1973; Borer *et al.* 1974). On the basis of such data, an improved system for estimating the stability of a given RNA structure was proposed (Tinoco *et al.*, 1973). In this revised method, the stabilizing contributions are based not on the nature of each base pair but rather on the nature of a stack of two base pairs. As mentioned above, consideration of the primary nucleotide sequence of a given region often allows the drawing of several variant models for the secondary structure, and the most stable one can then be chosen by calculating the estimated stability of each alternative. However, other evidence such as the position of the sites susceptible to single-strand specific nucleases should certainly also be taken into account, first because the stability estimates are far from perfect and second because other interactions, perhaps responsible for a tertiary structure, may stabilize one conformation rather than another.

The theoretical prediction of the stability of an RNA structure will certainly be refined in the future; for example, the zero contribution of G-U base pairs may be an underestimate, the nature (and the sequence) of the nucleotide(s) in bulges, internal hairpins, and hairpin loops may be important, the values for the destabilizing features need to be more accurately known, and so on. Obviously, it is desirable to develop a computer program that will predict the secondary structure on the basis of the primary nucleotide sequence. But it is not so simple to ensure that the program allows for the evaluation of all possible alternative conformations. Moreover, because of the uncertainties in the estimated stabilizing and especially destabilizing features, the conformation listed by the computer as of minimal free energy may in reality be less stable than the true conformation.

After a secondary structure model for a region of the viral RNA has been formulated, it is sometimes possible to support or disprove it by further experimentation. In the case of tRNA careful studies have shown that residues not involved in secondary or tertiary structure interactions can readily be modified by reagents such as methoxyamine, kethoxal, and carbodiimide (Rich and RajBhandary, 1976). This approach cannot be applied directly to phage RNA as the molecule is far too complex and hence the modified oligonucleotides cannot readily be identified. But these selective chemical modification reactions can be done, however, on isolated fragments and complexes which have retained or regained a secondary structure (Iserentant and Fiers, 1976). Also, complexes held together by secondary interactions can be taken apart, and the specificity of reassociation of the RNA fragments can be studied. *A posteriori* evidence for the secondary structure came also from comparative studies; it turned out that nucleotides involved in secondary structure interactions are less prone to mutational drift (Min Jou and Fiers, 1976*b*).

By the above procedures, the secondary structure model for MS2 RNA (Fig. 5) has been optimized. It should be considered as a best approximation, largely but not completely correct. Also, it is quite possible that for certain regions of the molecule alternative configurations may coexist (Min Jou *et al.*, 1972). Furthermore, such conformational rearrangements may even be intricately linked to the biological function, as is also believed to occur in tRNA (Rich and RajBhandary, 1976).

Attempts have been made to directly visualize aspects of the secondary structure by electron microscopy. The MS2 RNA was partially denatured in formamide before spreading and further sample preparation. A regular pattern of looplike structures could be observed and localized on the genome (Jacobson, 1976; Jacobson and Spahr, 1977). Unfortunately, these features are difficult to correlate with aspects of the secondary structure model shown in Fig. 5, and at present it is not clear why this is so. Edlind and Bassel (1977) used the same method to compare f2 RNA, Qβ RNA, and *Pseudomonas aeruginosa* PP7 RNA. For f2 RNA they obtained similar results as Jacobson, and moreover

they showed that these three almost unrelated phage RNAs all contain
near the center a loop of about 700 nucleotides. Possibly the loop is
formed by an interaction between a segment near the beginning of the
coat gene and a segment in the first part of the replicase gene
(nucleotides 1392–1408 and nucleotides 2127–2145; cf. Fig. 5) (also Fig.
3 in Fiers *et al.*, 1976). The former authors speculate that the central
loop may perhaps play a role in encapsidation.

4.5. Regions of Qβ RNA Sequenced by Partial Replication

An elegant procedure was worked out by Weissmann *et al.* (1973)
for sequencing terminal regions of Qβ RNA. When purified Qβ replicase is incubated with denatured double-stranded Qβ RNA (i.e., a mixture of plus and minus strands) in the presence of nucleotide precursors
but in the absence of host factors, the product synthesized is nearly
exclusively plus strand. It is possible to synchronize this reaction by
preincubation with GTP and ATP such that the enzyme pauses where it
has to insert the first pyrimidine nucleotide. Further elongation is then
allowed to proceed at 20°C for a limited time period by the addition of
UTP and CTP. This approach is straightforward, and moreover it
offers several other advantages: (1) As the product corresponds to a
limited region of the genome, the fingerprints are relatively simple. (2)
The product is synthesized *in vitro*, using each of the four NTPs in turn
in the form of the labeled [α-^{32}P]nucleoside triphosphate; therefore, the
possibility of relying on the nearest-neighbor effect considerably
facilitates the sequencing and the ordering of oligonucleotides (Bishop
et al., 1968). (3) By allowing the synchronized reaction to proceed for
increasing time periods, it is possible to order the main oligonucleotides
on the basis of their temporal appearance on the fingerprint. In this
way, the first 175 nucleotides of Qβ RNA were sequenced (Billeter *et
al.*, 1969) (Fig. 6), and this segment was subsequently extended to 330
(Weissmann *et al.*, 1973). Correlation with the sequence of the initiation region of the A2 protein gene allowed the conclusion that the first
Qβ gene starts at nucleotide 62–63 (Staples *et al.*, 1971). By using
longer periods of synthesis, it was possible to show that the coat protein
gene is located between the 1100th and the 1400th nucleotides from the
5′ terminus (Hindley *et al.*, 1970). This means that the gene order is
similar to that in the group I phages (Fig. 1).

The same approach has been used to sequence the last 160
nucleotides at the 3′ terminus (Goodman *et al.*, 1970; Weissmann *et al.*,
1973) (Fig. 6). In this case, Qβ RNA plus strands are used as a tem-

plate in the presence of host factors, such that the minus strand RNA is synchronously synthesized. The complement of this product corresponds of course to the 3′ end of the plus strand (except for the additional 3′-terminal A; Section 4.1.2).

In principle this approach of synchronized synthesis could be used to label selectively any region of the genome, by giving the labeled precursors only during a limited time interval. In reality, however, the synchronization cannot be maintained during prolonged incubation times. Nevertheless, procedures have been developed to label specifically some selected regions. For example, if Qβ plus-strand RNA with a ribosome bound to the coat gene initiator region is used as a template, the replicase can proceed with the synthesis of the minus strand only until it becomes blocked by this ribosome. By gently removing the latter without dissociation of the template–replicase–nascent minus-strand complex, and on addition of labeled NTPs, synthesis of a labeled region is obtained corresponding to the segment around and preceding the coat initiation codon (Kolakofsky *et al.*, 1973; Taniguchi and Weissmann, 1978).

As mentioned above, the synchronized synthesis approach offers several important advantages over the partial degradation procedures. However, no information is obtained on aspects related to the secondary structure.

4.6. Nucleotide Sequence of Small Qβ Replicase Template RNAs

Qβ replicase accepts not only full-size Qβ plus- or minus-strand RNA as a template for continuous propagation but also various types of smaller, specific RNA molecules (Eoyang and August, 1973). No host factors are required for the latter reaction. A first class of Qβ template molecules was generated by repeated transfers of Qβ RNA replication reaction mixtures, such that a selective pressure for shorter replication cycles was imposed (Mills *et al.*, 1967). After 74 transfers the RNA molecules (V-1 RNA) had decreased, presumably by successive deletions, to a size of 550 nucleotides. These "abridged" molecules were still related to Qβ RNA, as shown by hybridization (Mills *et al.*, 1968). Subsequently, molecules of the V-1 population were cloned, resulting in a homogeneous "strain" of molecules, V-2 RNA (Levisohn and Spiegelman, 1968). By imposing various types of selection pressure, other V-2-derived variants could be generated, e.g., synthesis in the presence of inhibitory agents such as tubercidin triphosphate (Levisohn and Spiegelman, 1969), ethidium bromide, or proflavin (Saffhill *et al.*, 1970).

A second class of small Qβ templates can be obtained by incubation of purified Qβ replicase in the absence of any template RNA. After a lag period of 2–20 min the enzymatic synthesis starts up and a "6 S"-type RNA is generated. It is not clear whether this is due to minute traces of 6 S-like RNAs derived from the infected cell which still contaminate the Qβ replicase preparation, or whether it is really due to *de novo* synthesis of polynucleotides and selection of the molecule which is most efficiently replicated (Sumper and Luce, 1975). One such variant, MDV-1 (for midivariant-1), was isolated and sequenced (Kacian *et al.*, 1972; Mills *et al.*, 1973). Each complementary strand is 218 nucleotides in length. Under optimal conditions of *in vitro* synthesis one molecule will autocatalytically give rise to 10^{12} copies in 20 min. MDV-1 has a considerably higher G-C content (70%) than Qβ RNA and each complementary strand has a rather strong secondary structure. One of the most interesting features of such small Qβ replicase templates is that they can be modified by selection pressure and that the resulting change in chemical structure can be correlated with a modification of its enzymological or physicochemical properties. For example, starting from MDV-1 RNA a mutant was selected whose propagation was less susceptible to ethidium bromide (Kramer *et al.*, 1974). This mutant MDV-1 RNA derivative turned out indeed to exhibit a lower affinity for binding the drug. Characterization by nucleotide sequence analysis revealed that the mutant was generated by three successive, independent mutations (three transitions).

Subsequently, it was found that some MDV-1 RNA preparations were contaminated by still a smaller Qβ template molecule, designated microvariant RNA (Mills *et al.*, 1975). It was isolated, propagated and characterized by complete sequence analysis. Microvariant RNA is only 114 nucleotides long, but its internal sequence does not reveal any relationship to that of MDV-1 RNA. Even more minute Qβ replicase template RNA molecules were characterized in the laboratory of Weissmann (Schaffner *et al.*, 1977). These closely related RNA species, nanovariant WS I, WS II, and WS III RNA, also appeared spontaneously on incubation of unprimed, purified Qβ replicase preparations. The nanovariant RNAs are only 91 nucleotides long and although they are 50 times shorter than Qβ RNA they are still efficiently bound to the Qβ replicase and propagated. The primary nucleotide sequence of the nanovariant RNA, microvariant RNA, and midivariant RNA has little in common, except that they all start with a series of G residues and end with a series of C residues. There is some relationship between the nucleotide sequence of midivariant RNA and the terminal regions of $Q\beta$ RNA. Although all these small template molecules must be bound by the replicase such that the 3' end comes in an appropriate position to initiate RNA synthesis, no similarity to the binding sites for replicase on the $Q\beta$ RNA (Section 4.3.5) can be detected. As discussed in Section 4.1.2, it is possible that initiation of RNA synthesis by phage-RNA-dependent RNA polymerase requires the stacking of several G nucleotides, which would explain why all templates start with a series of three or more G residues and end with three or more C residues. We also mentioned that the 3'-terminal A residue of all phage viral RNAs is not genetically encoded and may perhaps be added as part of a release mechanism to dissociate the newly synthesized RNA strand from the enzymatic replication complex. But even this feature is not constant: the nanovariant RNAs end indeed with . . . C-C-C-A_{OH} but the midivariant and the microvariant RNAs end with . . . C-C-C_{OH}.

4.7. 3'-Terminal Elongation, Reverse Transcription, and Cloning of Phage RNA

It is well known that nearly all eukaryotic messenger RNAs are polyadenylated at the 3' end. Possibly, this 3'-poly(A) tail is required to increase the half-life of the messenger in the eukaryotic cytoplasm (Huez *et al.*, 1975). The 3'-terminal poly(A) offers a convenient way to copy these mRNAs into cDNA by means of reverse transcriptase derived from avian oncornaviruses and using oligo(dT) as a primer. Considering the almost limitless possibilities of genetic engineering, it is only logical that efforts have been undertaken to bring the phage RNAs within the realm of this new technology.

Gilvarg *et al.* (1975) used terminal riboadenylate transferase isolated from calf thymus to polyadenylate $Q\beta$ RNA. Even short poly(A) tails led to complete loss of *in vitro* template activity for $Q\beta$ replicase (Devos *et al.*, 1976*b*; Gilvarg *et al.*, 1976). Remarkably, the 3'-polyadenylated $Q\beta$ RNA molecules retained full infectivity in a spheroplast system (Gilvarg *et al.*, 1975, 1976). As the progeny virions contain normal $Q\beta$ RNA, a correction system must be operative *in vivo*. Either the elongated $Q\beta$ RNA is trimmed back to normal size or (less likely in view of the *in vitro* replication data) the replication system skips the 3'-poly(A) tail and initiates the minus strand at the normal position.

An ATP:RNA adenyltransferase which is absolutely dependent on addition of an acceptor RNA has been purified from *E. coli* by Sippel (1973). Using this enzyme, Devos *et al.* (1976*a*) adenylated MS2 RNA without detectable internal nicking. The average length of the poly(A) tails could be controlled by the time of enzymatic reaction. Only about 50% of the MS2 RNA molecules acted as acceptors; presumably this was a conformation effect. On the other hand, more than 90% of the Qβ RNA molecules became polyadenylated under the same reaction conditions (Devos *et al.*, 1976*a,b*). At slightly higher pH and higher manganese-to-magnesium ratio, the same enzyme can also be used to transfer C residues to the 3' terminus of MS2 RNA (Devos *et al.*, 1977). This MS2 RNA-poly(C) can now be copied (but not propagated) by Qβ replicase.

MS2 RNA-poly(A) and Qβ RNA-poly(A) act as excellent templates for the synthesis of cDNA by means of reverse transcriptase from avian myeloblastosis virus and in the presence of oligo(dT) as a primer (Devos *et al.*, 1977). When one or more nucleoside triphosphates are used at low concentrations, discrete products are obtained, the sequence of which corresponds exactly to the complement of the nucleotide sequence of the 3'-terminal end of MS2 RNA or Qβ RNA as previously established.

At high NTP concentration and in the presence of pyrophosphate a full-length cDNA copy of MS2 RNA was obtained (Devos *et al.*, 1979). The cDNA can then be converted into duplex DNA and integrated into a bacterial plasmid. It was shown by restriction mapping and partial DNA sequence analysis that this DNA is a faithful and full-length copy, except for 14 nucleotides at the 5' end. Taniguchi *et al.* (1978) also polyadenylated the Qβ minus-strand RNA, and, by making cDNA copies from both plus and minus strands which could then be annealed, they were able to synthesize a full-length DNA copy of Qβ RNA. This duplex Qβ DNA was likewise introduced into an *E. coli* plasmid. Most remarkably, colonies of such transformed *E. coli* clones continuously release infectious Qβ virus. Presumably, the genetic information corresponding to the viral RNA is occasionally transcribed in the proper orientation and the longer RNA transcript may then be trimmed down to yield the normal Qβ RNA, because of the specific secondary and tertiary structure of the latter (alternative hypotheses are of course equally possible). The net result is that occasionally in the Qβ DNA-plasmid-containing bacteria such a process occurs, and once a normal size Qβ RNA molecule arises a regular lytic cycle rapidly ensues.

The availability of all the genetic information of these viral RNAs in the form of bacterial DNA plasmids offers many new avenues for further investigation.

5. BIOLOGICAL FUNCTIONS OF THE BACTERIOPHAGE GENOME

5.1. The Untranslated Regions

5.1.1. The 5′-Leader Sequence

The 5′-untranslated region is 129 nucleotides long in group I phages and 61–62 nucleotides in Qβ. In the leader sequence of the former group several potential AUG and GUG initiation codons are present, and the fact that these are not functional must be explained partly on the basis of additional requirements for interaction with the ribosome and partly by masking by secondary structure effects, as discussed in Section 4.3.1. Indeed, the first hairpin at the 5′ end of MS2–R17–f2 RNA is remarkably stable.

No information is available concerning the biological function of the 5′-leader sequence, and only some hypotheses can be formulated. It could be that its complement, i.e., the 3′-terminal region of the minus strand, requires a very well-defined three-dimensional conformation in order to allow initiation of plus-strand RNA synthesis. However, we note that the small Qβ variants can have widely different structures without impairment of their ability to be replicated (Section 4.6). Alternatively, a specific conformation of the leader sequence may be required for metabolic stability of the phage genome in the cytoplasm or for conferring on the whole macromolecule a proper tertiary structure such that it becomes encapsidated. A strong hint that the structure has a very important biological function comes from comparative studies of group I phage genomes (Robertson and Jeppesen, 1972; Min Jou and Fiers, 1976b). As far as these have been sequenced (Section 4.4.6), not a single mutation has been found in either the 5′-untranslated region or the 3′-untranslated region, while the variation in the translated regions is 4.2% for the comparison MS2-R17, 3.8% for MS2-f2, and 4.0% for R17-f2.

In more recent years it has become clear that not only animal and plant viral RNAs but also bacterial and eukaryotic messenger RNAs usually have long, untranslated, 5′-leader sequences. Whether the latter have a similar or a different *raison d'être* as in the phage RNAs is not known.

5.1.2. The 3'-Untranslated Sequence

The 3'-untranslated region in MS2 RNA is 174 nucleotides long. It has a tight secondary structure, and the model for this region is somewhat reminiscent of a tRNA cloverleaf (Fig. 5). Nevertheless, unlike several plant virus RNAs (Pinck *et al.*, 1970; Giegé *et al.*, 1978), it cannot be aminoacylated.

As has been discussed in the previous section for the 5'-terminal region of the phage minus strand, the 3'-terminal segment of the plus strand could also conceivably play an important role in the initiation process of RNA replication. Although only limited sequence information is available from the 3'-terminal region of the phages R17 and f2, it is so far identical to the MS2 RNA counterpart.

An ingenious and straightforward procedure was worked out by Weissmann and colleagues to probe the functional significance of the 3'-terminal region of Qβ RNA. We have mentioned already in Section 4.5 that in the absence of one or more nucleoside triphosphates the Qβ replication reaction becomes blocked at the empty site. By further addition of the mutagenic analogue N^4-hydroxy-CTP instead of CTP a mutation could be created at a well-defined position. In this way Qβ plus-strand RNA with an A instead of G residue at position 16 from the 3' terminus was obtained (Flavell *et al.*, 1974). This mutant could be replicated *in vitro* as well as wild type, but the *in vivo* infectivity was reduced to less than 5% (Sabo *et al.*, 1977). This indicated that the 3'-terminal region may have a more complex role *in vivo* than functioning as an initiator region for RNA-dependent RNA replication. Another mutant was prepared by a similar procedure (Domingo *et al.*, 1976). It had an A to G transition at position 40 from the 3' end. This mutant was viable, but its replication rate *in vivo* was only one-fourth of that of wild type, such that it became rapidly overgrown by wild-type revertants. This selective handicap may be due to a lesser affinity of the mutant RNA for the S1 protein, which is also a component of the Qβ replicase complex (Goelz and Steitz, 1977; cf. Section 4.3.2).

5.1.3. The Intercistronic Regions

The first intercistronic region in the group I phages is 26 nucleotides long and the second 36 nucleotides long. Not enough data are available to know whether these sequences are more or less conserved compared to the translated segments. We have seen in Section 4.3.1. that a naturally occurring mutation in the first intercistronic region is known. R17 RNA (Cambridge stock) has a G residue at ten nucleotides before the coat-initiating AUG, while MS2, f2, and R17 (Geneva stock) RNA have an A residue at this position. Although this mutation is expected to affect the interaction with the ribosome (Section 4.3.1), there is no evidence that it modulates the efficiency of translation of the coat gene.

A natural mutation is also known to occur in the second intercistronic region. It involves a U ↔ C transition at position 1732. This mutation affects the stability of the termination hairpin of the coat gene (Min Jou and Fiers, 1976b). Moreover, in phage R17 RNA, where position 1732 is a U residue, it is possible—at least in theory—that the intercistronic region could code for a hexapeptide (Nichols and Robertson, 1971; Robertson and Jeppesen, 1972). The latter statement cannot be made in the case of MS2 or f2 RNA, as here position 1732 is a C residue. It was proposed that this hexapeptide might play a role in restricting host RNA synthesis in the infected cell. However, such a peptide has never been found and there is no direct evidence to support this hypothesis.

It is perhaps remarkable that such extended intercistronic regions exist in the RNA phage genomes, while genes are often overlapping or contiguous in ϕX174 DNA and in some bacterial operons (Platt and Yanofsky, 1975; Sanger et al., 1977). Possibly, this may be related to the fact that in the latter systems transcriptional control mechanisms are operative, while all control functions for the differential and interdepent expression of the RNA phage genes have to be imprinted on the viral RNA structure itself (cf. Sections 4.3.1 and 5.4).

5.2. Viral Proteins

The amino acid sequence of the two structural proteins, the coat protein and the A protein, has been discussed in Sections 3.2 and 3.3 respectively (cf. Figs. 2 and 3). The amino acid sequence of the third MS2 gene product, the replicase subunit, is shown in Fig. 10. This polypeptide is 544 residues long, and, as previously only a few N-terminal residues had been directly determined (Lodish, 1968a; Osborn et al., 1970a), it was the first protein whose amino acid sequence was entirely established on the basis of the nucleotide sequence of its gene. The replicase subunit interacts with S1 and with Tu-Ts to form an

<u>AUG</u>·UCG·AAG·ACA·ACA·AAG·AAG·UUC·AAC·UCU·UUA·UGU·AUU·GAU·CUU·CCU·CGC·GAU·CUU·UCU·CUC
Ser Lys Thr Thr Lys Lys Phe Asn Ser Leu Cys Ile Asp Leu Pro Arg Asp Leu Ser Leu
20

1824
GAA·AUU·UAC·CAA·UCA·AUU·GCU·UCU·GUC·GCU·ACU·GGA·AGC·GGU·GAU·CCG·CAC·AGU·GAC·GAC
Glu Ile Tyr Gln Ser Ile Ala Ser Val Ala Thr Gly Ser Gly Asp Pro His Ser Asp Asp
40

1884
UUU·ACA·GCA·AUU·GCU·UAC·UUA·AGG·GAC·GAA·UUG·CUC·ACA·AAG·CAU·CCG·ACC·UUA·GGU·UCU
Phe Thr Ala Ile Ala Tyr Leu Arg Asp Glu Leu Leu Thr Lys His Pro Thr Leu Gly Ser
60

1944
GGU·AAU·GAC·GAG·GCG·ACC·CGU·CGU·ACC·UUA·GCU·AUC·GCU·AAG·CUA·CGG·GAG·GCG·AAU·GGU
Gly Asn Asp Glu Ala Thr Arg Arg Thr Leu Ala Ile Ala Lys Leu Arg Glu Ala Asn Gly
80

2004
GAU·CGC·GGU·CAG·AUA·AAU·AGA·GAA·GGU·UUC·UUA·CAU·GAC·AAA·UCC·UUG·UCA·UGG·GAU·CCG
Asp Arg Gly Gln Ile Asn Arg Glu Gly Phe Leu His Asp Lys Ser Leu Ser Trp Asp Pro
100

2064
GAU·GUU·UUA·CAA·ACC·AGC·AUC·CGU·AGC·CUU·AUU·GGC·AAC·CUC·CUC·UCU·GGC·UAC·CGA·UCG
Asp Val Leu Gln Thr Ser Ile Arg Ser Leu Ile Gly Asn Leu Leu Ser Gly Tyr Arg Ser
120

2124
UCG·UUG·UUU·GGG·CAA·UGC·ACG·UUC·UCC·AAC·GGU·GCU·CCU·AUG·GGG·CAC·AAG·UUG·CAG·GAU
Ser Leu Phe Gly Gln Cys Thr Phe Ser Asn Gly Ala Pro Met Gly His Lys Leu Gln Asp
110

2184
GCA·GCG·CCU·UAC·AAG·AAG·UUC·GCU·GAA·CAA·GCA·ACC·GUU·ACC·CCC·CGC·GCU·CUG·AGA·GCG
Ala Ala Pro Tyr Lys Lys Phe Ala Glu Gln Ala Thr Val Thr Pro Arg Ala Leu Arg Ala
160

2244
GCU·CUA·UUG·GUC·CGA·GAC·CAA·UGU·GCC·GCG·UGG·AUC·AGA·CAC·GCG·GUC·CGC·UAU·AAC·GAG
Ala Leu Leu Val Arg Asp Gln Cys Ala Ala Trp Ile Arg His Ala Val Arg Tyr Asn Glu
180

2304
UCA·UAU·GAA·UUU·AGG·CUC·GUU·GUA·GGG·AAC·GGA·GUG·UUU·ACA·GUU·CCG·AAG·AAU·AAU·AAA
Ser Tyr Glu Phe Arg Leu Val Val Gly Asn Gly Val Phe Thr Val Pro Lys Asn Asn Lys
200

2364
AUA·GAU·CGG·GCU·GCC·UGU·AAG·GAG·CCU·GAU·AUG·AAU·AUG·UAC·CUC·CAG·AAA·GGG·GUC·GGU
Ile Asp Arg Ala Ala Cys Lys Glu Pro Asp Met Asn Met Tyr Leu Gln Lys Gly Val Gly
220

2424
GCU·UUC·AUC·AGA·CGC·CGG·CUC·AAA·UCC·GUU·GGU·AUA·GAC·CUG·AAU·GAU·CAA·UCG·AUC·AAC
Ala Phe Ile Arg Arg Arg Leu Lys Ser Val Gly Ile Asp Leu Asn Asp Gln Ser Ile Asn
240

2484
CAG·CGU·CUG·GCU·CAG·CAG·GGC·AGC·GUA·GAU·GGU·UCG·CUU·GCG·ACG·AUA·GAC·UUA·UCG·UCU
Gln Arg Leu Ala Gln Gln Gly Ser Val Asp Gly Ser Leu Ala Thr Ile Asp Leu Ser Ser
260

2544
GCA·UCC·GAU·UCC·AUC·UCC·GAU·CGC·CUG·GUG·UGG·AGU·UUU·CUC·CCA·CCU·GAG·CUA·UAU·UCA
Ala Ser Asp Ser Ile Ser Asp Arg Leu Val Trp Ser Phe Leu Pro Pro Glu Leu Tyr Ser
280

2604
UAU·CUC·GAU·CGU·AUC·CGC·UCA·CAC·UAC·GGA·AUC·GUA·GAU·GGC·GAG·ACG·AUA·CGA·UGG·GAA
Tyr Leu Asp Arg Ile Arg Ser His Tyr Gly Ile Val Asp Gly Glu Thr Ile Arg Trp Glu
300

2664
CUA·UUU·UCC·ACA·AUG·GGA·AAU·GGG·UUC·ACA·UUU·GAG·CUA·GAG·UCC·AUG·AUA·UUC·UGG·GCA
Leu Phe Ser Thr Met Gly Asn Gly Phe Thr Phe Glu Leu Glu Ser Met Ile Phe Trp Ala
320

2724
AUA·GUC·AAA·GCG·ACC·CAA·AUC·CAU·UUU·GGU·AAC·GCC·GGA·ACC·AUA·GGC·AUC·UAC·GGG·GAC
Ile Val Lys Ala Thr Gln Ile His Phe Gly Asn Ala Gly Thr Ile Gly Ile Tyr Gly Asp
340

2784
GAU·AUU·AUA·UGU·CCC·AGU·GAG·AUU·GCA·CCC·CGU·GUG·CUA·GAG·GCA·CUU·GCC·UAC·UAC·GGU
Asp Ile Ile Cys Pro Ser Glu Ile Ala Pro Arg Val Leu Glu Ala Leu Ala Tyr Tyr Gly
360

2844
UUU·AAA·CCG·AAU·CUU·CGU·AAA·ACG·UUC·GUG·UCC·GGG·CUC·UUU·CGC·GAG·AGC·UGC·GGC·GCG
Phe Lys Pro Asn Leu Arg Lys Thr Phe Val' Ser Gly Leu Phe Arg Glu Ser Cys Gly Ala
380

2904
CAC·UUU·UAC·CGU·GGU·GUC·GAU·GUC·AAA·CCG·UUU·UAC·AUC·AAG·AAA·CCU·GUU·GAC·AAU·CUC
His Phe Tyr Arg Gly Val Asp Val Lys Pro Phe Tyr Ile Lys Lys Pro Val Asp Asn Leu
400

```
2964
   UUC·GCC·CUG·AUG·CUG·AUA·UUA·AAU·CGG·CUA·CGG·GGU·UGG·GGA·GUU·GUC·GGA·GGU·AUG·UCA
   Phe  Ala  Leu  Met  Leu  Ile  Leu  Asn  Arg  Leu  Arg  Gly  Trp  Gly  Val  Val  Gly  Gly  Met  Ser
                                                                                                    420

3024
   GAU·CCA·CGC·CUC·UAU·AAG·GUG·UGG·GUA·CGG·CUC·UCC·UCC·CAG·GUG·CCU·UCG·AUG·UUC·UUC
   Asp  Pro  Arg  Leu  Tyr  Lys  Val  Trp  Val  Arg  Leu  Ser  Ser  Gln  Val  Pro  Ser  Met  Phe  Phe
                                                                                                    440

3084
   GGU·GGG·ACG·GAC·CUC·GCU·GCC·GAC·UAC·UAC·GUA·GUC·AGC·CCG·CCU·ACG·GCA·GUC·UCG·GUA
   Gly  Gly  Thr  Asp  Leu  Ala  Ala  Asp  Tyr  Tyr  Val  Val  Ser  Pro  Pro  Thr  Ala  Val  Ser  Val
                                                                                                    460

3144
   UAC·ACC·AAG·ACU·CCG·UAC·GGG·CGG·CUG·CUC·GCG·GAU·ACC·CGU·ACC·UCG·GGU·UUC·CGU·CUU
   Tyr  Thr  Lys  Thr  Pro  Tyr  Gly  Arg  Leu  Leu  Ala  Asp  Thr  Arg  Thr  Ser  Gly  Phe  Arg  Leu
                                                                                                    480

3204
   GCU·CGU·AUC·GCU·CGA·GAA·CGC·AAG·UUC·UUC·AGC·GAA·AAG·CAC·GAC·AGU·GGU·CGC·UAC·AUA
   Ala  Arg  Ile  Ala  Arg  Glu  Arg  Lys  Phe  Phe  Ser  Glu  Lys  His  Asp  Ser  Gly  Arg  Tyr  Ile
                                                                                                    500

3264
   GCG·UGG·UUC·CAU·ACU·GGA·GGU·GAA·AUC·ACC·GAC·AGC·AUG·AAG·UCC·GCC·GGC·GUG·CGC·GUU
   Ala  Trp  Phe  His  Thr  Gly  Gly  Glu  Ile  Thr  Asp  Ser  Met  Lys  Ser  Ala  Gly  Val  Arg  Val
                                                                                                    520

3324
   AUA·CGC·ACU·UCG·GAG·UGG·CUA·ACG·CCG·GUU·CCC·ACA·UUC·CCU·CAG·GAG·UGU·GGG·CCA·GCG
   Ile  Arg  Thr  Ser  Glu  Trp  Leu  Thr  Pro  Val  Pro  Thr  Phe  Pro  Gln  Glu  Cys  Gly  Pro  Ala
                                                                                                    540

3384
   AGC·UCU·CCU·CGG·[UAG]
   Ser  Ser  Pro  Arg
                    544
```

Fig. 10. Replicase subunit gene of bacteriophage MS2. The total nucleotide sequence of the replicase subunit gene (numbering on the left) and the deduced amino acid sequence (numbering on the right) are shown. From Fiers *et al.* (1976).

enzymatically active complex (Section 4.3.5). At present the primary structure of the replicase subunit does not reveal any information on its biological properties, but it may form the basis for later studies on structure–function relationship and on possible evolutionary relatedness to other nucleic acid polymerases.

Some preliminary information on the chemical structure of the Qβ replicase polypeptide has been obtained such as tryptic fingerprints (Hindennach and Jockusch, 1974). Moreover, it could be synthesized in a cell-free system; the association with S1 and Tu-Ts did not occur right away, but an enzymatically active complex was formed by precipitation with ammonium sulfate (Happe and Jockusch, 1975).

5.3. Use of the Genetic Code

The principle of the genetic code was established in the early 1960s by genetic approaches (Crick *et al.*, 1961), and the potential triplet code was then deduced mainly by means of *in vitro* systems (Nirenberg *et al.*, 1966; Khorana *et al.*, 1966). Some information on the actual code words used *in vivo* became available by studies on mutant proteins, especially those resulting from shifts in reading frame (Okada *et al.*, 1970). But it was only with the advent of procedures to sequence the RNA phage genomes (Section 4.4.5) that extensive data became available on the actual occurrence of the different degenerate codons in natural messengers.

Forty-nine out of the 61 sense codons are used in the MS2 coat gene to code for 129 amino acids (Min Jou *et al.*, 1972) (Fig. 11). Although the sample is too small to permit definite conclusions, it seems that for some amino acids the choice between the different degenerate codons is nonrandom. Perhaps most noteworthy is that some codons are apparently avoided, like AUA for isoleucine (5% significance as tested by χ^2 analysis; the coat protein contains only eight isoleucine residues), UAU for tyrosine, AGU for serine, and ACA for threonine.

With the completion of the nucleotide sequence of the A protein gene (Fiers *et al.*, 1975), it became clear that in fact all 61 codons have been used to write up the genetic message of these phages. However,

		U		C		A		G		
U	Phe	1 3	Ser	3 2 2 2	Tyr	4	Cys	1 1	U C A G
	Leu	1			Ochre Amber	O O	Opal Trp	2	
C	Leu	2 2 2	Pro	2 1 2 1	His Gln	1 5	Arg	3 1	U C A G
A	Ile	4 4	Thr	4 4 1	Asn Lys	4 6 5 1	Ser Arg	4	U C A G
	Met	⊙ + 2							
G	Val	4 4 3 3	Ala	5 2 6 1	Asp Glu	1 3 2 3	Gly	3 3 2 1	U C A G

Fig. 11. Codons used in the MS2 coat protein gene. First letter of code word is indicated at the left, second letter on the top, and third letter at the right; e.g., the code word U-U-U is used once for phenylalanine and U-U-C is used three times. ⊙, Codon used for initiation.

	U	C	A	G	
U	Phe 19	Ser 15	Tyr (9)	Cys 6	U
	Phe 29	Ser 20	Tyr 32	Cys 6	C
	Leu 17	Ser 16	Ochre 1	Opal	A
	Leu (11)	Ser 22	Amber 2	Trp 23	G
C	Leu 15	Pro 17	His (6)	Arg 21	U
	Leu 26	Pro 10	His (9)	Arg 20	C
	Leu 15	Pro 9	Gln 17	Arg (10)	A
	Leu (9)	Pro 13	Gln 22	Arg (11)	G
A	Ile 12	Thr 19	Asn 17	Ser (8)	U
	Ile 25	Thr 21	Asn 28	Ser 16	C
	Ile (19)	Thr (13)	Lys 19	Arg (7)	A
	Met 2+18	Thr 14	Lys 26	Arg (6)	G
G	Val 21	Ala 26	Asp 28	Gly 37	U
	Val 21	Ala 21	Asp 22	Gly 16	C
	Val 16	Ala 21	Glu 16	Gly 12	A
	Val 1+18	Ala 23	Glu 28	Gly 16	G

Fig. 12. Codons used in the MS2 RNA genome. O, Not used in the coat gene. The numbers indicate the frequency with which each codon is used. The initiating methionine residues which are subsequently removed are indicated separately (the initiating methionine of the A protein is maintained). From Fiers et al. (1976).

the choice between the different degenerate codons for a given amino acid is often decidedly nonrandom. The codons used in the complete MS2 genome are summarized in Fig. 12, and on this basis statistically more meaningful conclusions can be drawn. For example, the codon GGU is decidedly preferred for glycine (0.1% significance), UAC is preferred for tyrosine (0.1% significance), and AUC is preferred over AUU for isoleucine (1% significance). The preference for arginine codons is CGPy > CGPu > AGPu (0.1% significance). Although it seems that flexible use is being made of the degeneracy of the genetic code, it remains nevertheless true that, for nearly any given third-letter position in the sequence, one nucleotide is clearly preferred over any other. Otherwise, the primary structure would simply not be constant and could never have been established. Although there is evidence for some fluctuation, this is actually very limited (Section 5.7).

On what basis then is the choice made between the different degenerate codons for a given amino acid? In some cases it may be a historical accident, like the choice between a UCX or an AGPy codon for serine; indeed, these are evolutionarily very distant and not interconvertible by a single mutation. In Sections 3.4 and 4.4.8 it was explained that the secondary (and presumably tertiary) structure is very specific and decidedly much higher than could be expected for a random polymer. This means that these conformational requirements impose some constraints on the nucleotide sequence. There is no reason to believe that this effect has actually influenced the amino acid sequence, but this cannot be ruled out, either. Alternatively, the secondary structure can be maximized by a proper choice of third letters, and by bringing complementary segments of a double helical region into proper register; there is more adaptability if the interchangeable third letters do not face each other in the double-stranded regions (Min Jou *et al.*, 1971). Some evidence supporting a choice of third letters on the basis of their base-pairing potentialities was originally obtained (at that time mostly regions with a strong hairpinlike secondary structure were studied). (Adams *et al.*, 1969; Fiers *et al.*, 1971; Min Jou *et al.*, 1971, 1972). When more nucleotide sequence data became available, however, this hypothesis could no longer be substantiated by statistically convincing data. It is likely that relatively few selected third letters are sufficient to bring the molecule from a random secondary structure (50–60% base pairing) to a level of a stable conformation as observed in the viral RNAs (73% ± 5% base pairing), and this low level of constraint may not be revealed by statistical analysis (Fiers *et al.*, 1976). Moreover, we have no way to assess the role of third letters in tertiary structure interactions.

But, as we have mentioned above, the choice between degenerate codons for some amino acids is decidedly nonrandom. Hence, at least in these instances, factors directly related to the translation process must play a predominant role. For some codons, like AUA for isoleucine and AGPu for arginine, the discriminant use may be related to a modulation control, as will be further discussed (Section 5.4.3). Fitch (1976) noted that among the pyrimidine-restricted codons (i.e., twofold degenerate codons of the type NNPy) in MS2 RNA, those ending in C are decidedly preferred over those ending in U. For fourfold degenerate codons there is a very clear preference for a pyrimidine in the third position; in fact, the ratio NNPy/NNPu for fourfold degenerate codons is very close to the ratio of twofold degenerate codons of the type NNPy over twofold degenerate codons of the type NNPu, but why this should be so is not clear.

Grosjean *et al.* (1978) introduced the concept of an optimum interaction energy between the codon and the anticodon. The interaction should be neither too strong nor too weak for optimal movement of the ribosome and minimal error frequency. There is conjectural evidence for such a view, e.g., when the third nucleotide in the anticodon of *E. coli* tRNA is an A or a U residue, then the adjacent nucleotide is invariably hypermodified, and it is believed that the latter residue significantly increases the stability of the codon-anticodon interaction (Grosjean *et al.*, 1976). Assuming such an optimal interaction energy, and considering that pyrimidines in the third position of all codons are read by a G residue (or the derived Q base), one would predict that for codons in which positions 1 and 2 are A or U, the third letter would preferentially be C, while for codons in which positions 1 and 2 are G or C, the third letter would rather be U (i.e., the wobbling G-U interaction would be less stabilizing than the nonwobbling G-C). In fact, this hypothesis is convincingly supported by the code word utilization in MS2 RNA (Fig. 12). Obviously, in codons of the type $_U^A\,_U^A$ Py, the latter residue is preferentially C, viz. for phenylalanine, tyrosine, isoleucine, and asparagine. Conversely, for codons of the type $_C^G\,_C^G$ Py, the latter is more often a U residue, viz. for proline, valine, and glycine (the CGPy codons for arginine are a different problem as they are recognized by a tRNA containing ICG in the anticodon). The hypothesis of optimalization of codon–anticodon interaction does not explain the preferential use in the case of codons ending with a purine residue, but most of these preferences are less pronounced. The use of synonymous codons is quite different in ϕX174 DNA (Sanger *et al.*, 1977); here a general and striking preference for U in the third position is observed. This may be due to other constraints, which for this system are more important than an optimalization of the translation efficiency, for example, asymmetrical synthesis of single-stranded DNA or packaging. The translation and replication efficiency of RNA phages seem indeed to be superior, considering their burst size of 5000–10,000 particles per cell, while a ϕX174-infected cell contains only about 200–400 virions (Sinsheimer, 1970).

The RNA phage system continues to reveal new facets of the mechanism of protein synthesis and the intricacies of the genetic code. Mitra *et al.* (1977) have observed that at least in an *in vitro* system programmed with MS2 RNA, each of three different isoaccepting tRNAs for valine is able to respond to all four valine codons. This means that under these conditions only two out of three codon letters are effectively read (Lagerkvist, 1978). The same presumably holds true for the glycine tRNAs.

For some classes of codons there is also evidence for context effects, i.e., that the choice of the third letter is influenced by the nature of the following codon. But these phenomena are at present too poorly understood to warrant discussion.

5.4. Regulatory Systems Controlling the Expression of the Viral Genes

5.4.1. Introduction

The expression of the three viral genes (four in the case of Qβ) is finely controlled, both in relative amount and in time. Considering the structure of the virion, the coat protein is needed and indeed synthesized in vastly larger amounts than the A protein. At later times of infection the enzyme responsible for viral RNA synthesis is present and properly functioning, and therefore it is logical that further synthesis of enzyme is turned off. These control mechanisms have been thoroughly discussed in previous reviews (Kozak and Nathans, 1972; Eoyang and August, 1974; Steitz, 1977), and therefore only the general aspects and their relationship to the viral RNA structure will be considered here.

5.4.2.   Intrinsic Efficiency of Ribosome Binding Sites

It is difficult to obtain unambiguous information on the intrinsic efficiency of initiation at the three viral genes, i.e., in the absence of secondary structure effects. Considering the many internal ribosome-binding-like regions which are nevertheless not functional (Section 4.3.1 and Table 11), it seems likely that even on the nascent strand local secondary structures are formed before the ribosomes have a chance to interact. Because of these conformation effects, the intrinsic initiation efficiency is difficult to measure directly. However, if the affinity of the ribosome for rebinding the isolated initiator region is used as an index for intrinsic gene initiation efficiency, then the relative order is clearly A protein > replicase > coat protein (Section 4.3.1). This relative order is compatible with the evidence suggesting that the A protein is exclusively synthesized on nascent chains, while the coat gene is largely if not completely started on mature viral RNA (see below). We have also mentioned before that initiation with an AUG codon or a GUG codon appears to be about equally efficient.

5.4.3.   Accessibility of the Ribosome Binding Sites

5.4.3a.   The Coat Protein Gene

When ribosomes are added to intact viral RNA, they bind only to the coat initiator region. We have mentioned in Section 4.3.1 that the three-dimensional structure may play a special role in promoting efficient initiation at this site. The coat gene is by far the most actively expressed (both *in vivo* and *in vitro*). This is not unexpected, as 180 coat molecules are required to encapsidate one viral RNA molecule.

There is good *in vivo* evidence that once the infection cycle is well under way (and synthesis of replicase is repressed) the completed viral RNA molecules serve only as messenger for coat protein production. Indeed, the polysome pattern in the infected cell shifts to lower size classes (Hotham-Iglewski and Franklin, 1967), and the smaller polysomes (trimers or less) synthesize only coat protein (Truden and Franklin, 1972).

5.4.3b.   The A Protein Gene

It has already been mentioned in Section 4.3.1 that the A protein initiation region (like the replicase region) is normally masked in the intact viral RNA molecule, and becomes accessible only after partial degradation. Under these conditions, unfortunately, the gene is badly damaged, and this at least partly explains why it is so difficult to obtain full-length A protein synthesis in *in vitro* translation systems. Only by the use of appropriate mutants could synthesis of A protein in an *in vitro* system unambiguously be demonstrated (Lodish and Robertson, 1969). That the masking is due to conformational constraints is further documented by the fact that formaldehyde treatment, incubation at higher temperature (this necessitates the use of *B. stearothermophilus* ribosomes), or the use of nascent strands all increase the relative initiation efficiency of the A protein gene (Lodish, 1975; Steitz, 1977). Therefore, the hypothesis was made that A protein is synthesized only on nascent strands, and that when the RNA chain grows longer a three-dimensional folding occurs which effectively shuts off further expression (Robertson and Lodish, 1970). Physiologically, this makes sense, as in fact only one A protein molecule is required per virion particle and therefore its synthesis should be limited. Actually, much more A protein is made than is needed, as the *in vivo* molar amount is about 10–15% of the coat protein (Nathans *et al.*, 1969; Vinuela *et al.*, 1967; Robertson and Lodish, 1970). When the secondary structure model for the A protein gene was worked out, it turned out that a segment, located at about two-thirds distance in the gene, remained single stranded after the normal hairpins had been identified, but could base-pair with the region just before the initiating GUG of the gene (Fig. 5). This model for autocontrol is not yet strongly supported by direct experimental data, but it nicely explains the aforementioned biological and biochemical observations. Also, the initiation region of the A2 protein gene in $Q\beta$ is inaccessible in the complete molecule, but it is still free in nascent Qβ RNA chains up to about 500 nucleotides in length (Staples *et al.*, 1971); these data then suggest a control system very similar to the model proposed for MS2.

5.4.3c. The Replicase Gene and the Polarity Effect

The initiator region of the replicase gene in the complete viral RNA molecule is also not freely accessible to ribosomes. In *in vitro* translation systems programmed with phage RNA the incorporation of histidine starts only after a certain lag period. As histidine is not present in the coat protein, its incorporation can be considered as a measure for replicase synthesis, and this identification can readily be confirmed by analysis of the products on polyacrylamide gels after denaturation with sodium dodecylsulfate. Characterization of the suppressor-sensitive mutants of the amber type (Section 5.6) (Horiuchi, 1975) revealed a class of mutants in the coat gene which gave only poor and delayed complementation (Gussin, 1966). These mutants were said to be polar: they were localized in one gene, the coat gene, and interfered with the expression of another gene, the replicase gene. These polar coat mutations were subsequently identified as being in position 6 of the coat gene, for R17, f2, and MS2 (Section 5.6). Amber mutations at position 50, 54, or 70 are not polar and do not interfere with the expression of the replicase gene. This means that translation of the coat gene is required for expression of the replicase gene. A plausible hypothesis for this polarity effect is that when ribosomes translate a region of the coat gene located between positions 6 and 50, they open up the secondary (and/or tertiary) structure such that the initiator region of the replicase gene becomes accessible for ribosomes. The secondary structure model of the coat gene, called the "flower model," provides an attractive basis for this control model (Min Jou *et al.*, 1972) (Fig. 5). When ribosomes translate the coat gene, they zipper open a base-paired region formed between nucleotides 1409–1433 and nucleotides 1738–1769. The former segment is localized indeed in the beginning of the coat gene (but distal from position 6), while the complementary segment encompasses the ribosome binding site of the replicase gene (Table 10). Unmasking of the latter segment thus allows expression of the latter gene.

It has long been unclear what the biological meaning of the polarity effect is. There is evidence that the effect is operative *in vivo* even in singly infected cells. When a polar mutant infects a nonpermissive cell, synthesis of replicase is retarded and the parental viral RNA fails to be converted into partially double-stranded structures (Roberts and Gussin, 1967). The polarity effect has also been observed in the case of the Qβ phage (Ball and Kaesberg, 1973). However, the situation is more complex, because coat protein mutants at increasing distance from the N terminus (positions 17, 37, and 86) showed a *gradual* diminution of the polar effect on the replicase gene. It should be recalled, in this respect, that there are about 600 nucleotides between the end of the Qβ coat gene and the beginning of the replicase gene (Fig. 1); therefore, the conformational effects may be more subtle, e.g., translation of the Qβ coat gene may result in progressive changes in the three-dimensional folding, such that the initiation region of the replicase gene becomes gradually more accessible to ribosomes.

The possible biological significance of the polar control will be discussed in Section 5.4.5b.

5.4.4. Possible Control of the Elongation Rate

In addition to the important controls which regulate the initiation frequency of the three viral genes, there may be a finer tuning by additional control mechanisms operating on the elongation rate. As stressed in Section 5.3, the virus-specific protein synthesis in infected cells is enormous, and therefore the process may have been optimized at different levels.

Once the degeneracy of the genetic code was recognized, it was soon realized that differential expression of genes could be achieved by selective use of the codon repertory (Ames and Hartman, 1963; Stent, 1964). This is called modulation control. In the case of the RNA phages one would expect that if codons exist which slow down the speed of translation, these would be avoided in the coat gene, as the product is needed in largest quantities. Inspection of the code word table for this gene reveals that a number of codons are indeed not used (Fig. 11). For many of these, this is only a coincidence or the consequence of the preferential use discussed in Section 5.3. Clearcut conclusions on the basis of statistical analyses cannot be obtained as the coat protein is only 129 amino acids long. Nevertheless, a χ^2 test shows that the absence of the AUA codon for isoleucine has less than a 5% chance to be not significant. Therefore, the possibility that AUA is a modulating triplet should be seriously considered. Strong support for this view comes from the fact that AUA is recognized by a specific isoaccepting tRNA which is present in minute amounts in *E. coli* (Caskey *et al.*, 1968; Harada and Nishimura, 1974). There is also some genetic evidence which points in the same direction; a silent mutation in the MS2 coat gene was shown to be due to a methionine → isoleucine interconversion. As transitions are much more frequent than transversions (Min Jou and Fiers, 1976*b*), one might expect that this mutation would correspond to an AUG → AUA change. Nucleotide sequence analysis of the mutant, however, revealed that the mutation was in fact AUG → AUU, which means that the argument for a modulating role for AUA was not invalidated (Min Jou *et al.*, 1976).

Also, the codons AGA and AGG for arginine are good candidates for a modulation function. They are not present in the coat gene, and they are recognized by a minor isoaccepting tRNA which represents only 2% of the arginine-specific tRNA (Caskey *et al.*, 1968; Anderson and Gilbert, 1969). We have mentioned in Section 5.3 that the constraints which govern the codon use in the phage φX174 genome may be quite different from those acting on the RNA phages. Nevertheless, we note that the codons which could possibly be implicated in modulation control are again conspicuously low, viz. AUA for isoleucine and AGA/AGG for arginine (Sanger *et al.*, 1977).

5.4.5. Translational Repression

5.4.5a. Translational Repression by Coat Protein

When techniques were worked out to specifically label and analyze the viral proteins it became clear that once the infection cycle was well under way and no more replicase enzyme was needed, its further synthesis was indeed shut off (Kozak and Nathans, 1972; Eoyang and August, 1974). This repression, however, did not occur when infection was started with a nonpolar coat mutant in a wild-type (nonsuppressor) host. Under the latter conditions considerable overproduction of the viral replicase protein is observed, and there is also more synthesis of virus-specific, double-stranded RNA, suggesting that the RNA replication becomes aberrant. Higher levels of enzyme activity were also detected in the cell extract (Lodish *et al.*, 1964). These observations led to the translational repressor hypothesis (Gussin, 1966). The coat protein would function as a repressor for the expression of the replicase gene. This hypothesis could soon be confirmed by *in vitro* protein synthesis systems programmed with phage RNA to which increasing amounts of coat protein were added (Sugiyama and Nakada, 1967, 1970; Ward *et al.*, 1968; Robertson *et al.*, 1968; Eggen and Nathans, 1969). We have seen in Section 4.3.6 that the region to which a single coat protein molecule binds has been well characterized. The protein interacts with a hairpin structure, which contains the initiating AUG of the replicase gene (Min Jou *et al.*, 1972; Gralla *et al.*, 1974), and thus prevents its further functioning. What is less clear, however, is how this single, specifically bound coat protein is again removed. Indeed, the infecting, parental RNA molecule must be free from such a repressor when it enters the cell. Perhaps encapsidation involves a rearrangement of the RNA conformation such that the repressor molecule is torn off.

The same control system applies to the phage Qβ. Amber mutants in the coat gene lead to overproduction of the replicase, and this over-producing system has been very useful for the preparation of purified Qβ replicase (Palmenberg and Kaesberg, 1973).

5.4.5b. Translational Repression by the Replicase

It was observed by Kolakofsky and Weissmann (1971) that a ribosome bound to Qβ RNA prevents further progression of the repli-case. Conversely, when replicase is present, binding of ribosomes to the viral RNA is drastically reduced. It was shown that replicase binds indeed around the coat gene initiation site (Section 4.3.5) (Weber *et al.*, 1972). Ribosomes translate of course the RNA in a 5′ to 3′ direction, while the replicase which synthesizes minus strands copies the plus strand in a 3′ to 5′ direction. Obviously, *in vivo* a dead-end situation has to be avoided in which a ribosome and a replicase-nascent minus-strand complex would mutually prevent further progression.

Therefore, the following model was proposed. The replicase binds to the coat region (the S site), whenever it has a chance (i.e., when unoccupied by a ribosome). Ribosomes in the process of translating the coat gene or the replicase gene continue their way, but no further initia-tions of the coat gene can take place. As we are dealing here with a completed viral RNA template, the A protein initiation region is already in the closed position (Section 5.4.3b). Once the ribosomes have cleared the first segment of the coat gene, the polarity effect comes into play. This means that the initiation region of the replicase now also becomes masked. Ribosomes which are still translating the replicase gene are allowed to finish their task, but after their release a template RNA molecule is left to which the replicase is already bound. Now the tertiary structure is such that the 3′ end comes at the proper orientation relative to the active site of the enzyme and viral RNA replication can start.

Many aspects of this model need further experimental support, and it is not known if it can also be applied to the group I phages. However, the scenario explains at least the *raison d'être* of the polarity effect and in general is very plausible and therefore attractive.

5.5. Termination Regions

Nichols (1970) was the first to have identified a termination region. He established the nucleotide sequence of an R17 RNA fragment part of which corresponded to the genetic information for the last six amino acids of the known coat protein. This coding information was followed by the double stop signal UAA UAG.

We have discussed in Sections 3.3 and 4.4.6 the biochemical evidence which led to the conclusion that the A protein gene is terminated by a single UAG codon, followed some 30 triplets further by another termination codon. Correlation of this information with the nucleotide sequence data allowed Contreras *et al.* (1973) to identify the terminating UAG codon at 26 nucleotides before the initiating AUG codon of the coat gene. This assignment was subsequently confirmed by the determination of the C-terminal sequence of the A protein (Vandekerckhove *et al.*, 1973; Vandekerckhove and van Montagu, 1977). The A protein gene of the phage R17 is also terminated by a UAG signal (Adams *et al.*, 1972a).

However, no information is available on the amino acid sequence of the viral replicase subunit. Vandenberghe *et al.* (1975) deduced the sequence of the last 361 nucleotides of MS2 RNA. Although the segment contains numerous termination codons, one open reading frame could be identified, which came to an end at a UAG codon located 174 nucleotides from the 3' end. If readthrough occurred (e.g., in an amber suppressor cell), a further seven amino acids would be added, and translation would then stop at a UAA codon. In fact, this is precisely what was observed by Atkins and Gesteland (1975). Replicase polypeptide synthesized under normal conditions had an appropriate molecular weight of 63,000, while under suppression conditions some of the product had an estimated size of 63,500, i.e., about five additional amino acids. Therefore, the above identification of the replicase termination codon is almost certainly correct. Atkins and Gesteland (1975) also noted that their *in vitro* system led to the synthesis of an additional replicase-related polypeptide with a molecular weight of 66,000. The origin of this product is not known.

The coat protein gene of the phage $Q\beta$ is terminated by a single UGA signal, and partial suppression (a UGA-stop is rather leaky) leads to the essential A1 (also called "IIb") protein (Section 3.3). The actual nucleotide sequence of this region is not yet known.

It is somewhat surprising that two out of three genes in MS2 end with the suppressible amber codon and not with the stronger UAA stop. Perhaps this is just a coincidence. It is remarkable to note on the secondary structure model of MS2 RNA (Fig. 5) that the termination codons of the three genes are all located near the top of a hairpin; even the second stop of the replicase gene is at a similar position. It would be of interest to known whether "termination loops" have a functional meaning. Release of ribosomes at the end of a message is rather complex and not yet understood in detail (Martin and Webster, 1975).

5.6. RNA Phage Mutants

Genetic approaches often provide the first tools to explore the molecular biology of biological systems. But genetic studies of RNA phages have been hampered by several drawbacks: (1) The spontaneous mutation rate and reversion rate are very high. It is difficult to maintain phage mutant stocks in which the number of wild-type revertants is less than 1%. (2) Recombination does not occur; hence only complementation analysis is possible and localization of mutations has to be done by chemical procedures. (3) Even complementation is an arduous task as only a minority of host cells become multiply infected. This is due to the scarcity of F^+ pili on the host cells [possibly one F^+ pilus allows only one phage to enter (Section 2.1)].

Only point mutations are known. Temperature-sensitive mutations can readily be isolated by the use of 34–35°C as permissive and 42°C as nonpermissive condition (at temperatures below 34°C the F^+ pilus receptor is poorly expressed) (Pfeiger et al., 1964; Zinder, 1965). The mutants could be assigned to two groups, presumably corresponding to the replicase and the coat gene. They have been very valuable for physiological studies, e.g., shifts from permissive to nonpermissive conditions, or vice versa.

Especially fruitful not only for our understanding of these RNA phage systems but also for revealing fundamental aspects of protein synthesis in general have been the suppressor-sensitive RNA phage mutants. Indeed, our current detailed knowledge of the biochemistry of suppression has largely been obtained by means of these RNA phage mutants.

Amber (UAG) mutants can readily be obtained either by treatment of the virions with nitrous acid or hydroxylamine or by phage growth in the presence of fluorouracil, and selection on appropriate bacterial strains. These mutants can be classified in different complementation groups, and further subgrouping is often possible on the basis of the response to different suppressor strains and, in the case of the coat gene, on whether or not the mutation is polar (Table 12). Each complementation group can then be correlated with a particular gene by analysis of the physiological defect in an su^- host (Table 12). The exact position of the mutation can be identified by analysis of the amino acid sequence of the mutant protein synthesized in a particular su^+ host and comparison with that of the wild-type protein. If only transitions are allowed, a UAG mutation could either arise from a CAG codon for glutamine or from UGG for tryptophan. All clearly identified amber mutations are of the former type.

Amber mutants in the A protein gene can be obtained with surprising ease. In fact 60–70% of the amber mutants are of this type (Tooze and Weber, 1967; Fiers *et al.*, 1969). Amber mutants in the A protein gene can even be suppressed by ochre-suppressing hosts (Table 12), which are known to have a low efficiency of suppression. Undoubtedly, this is due to the fact that *in vivo* much more A protein is synthesized relative to the small amount needed. The A protein mutants have not been characterized by detailed protein chemistry data, but Vandamme *et al.* (1972) could show that they fall in two groups. One group makes no detectable nonsense fragment *in vivo* (either it is very short or else it is hidden in the coat protein peak). The second group, however, produced in an su^- host a nonsense polypeptide which is 88% of full length. Correlation of this information with the amino acid sequence of the A protein (Fiers *et al.*, 1975) reveals indeed that the position of this mutation must correspond to the glutamine codon at nucleotide 1165–1167 (Fig. 3). There are 18 glutamine codons in the A protein gene (nine of which are coded by a CAG), and the fact that over one-third of the A protein mutants belong to this second group means that this position must correspond to a very pronounced mutational hot spot. Looking up this particular CAG codon in the secondary structure model (Fig. 5) reveals that it is indeed located in a single-stranded interior loop and is therefore, presumably, more accessible to the mutagenic agent (Fiers *et al.*, 1975).

Amber mutants in the coat gene could readily be localized as the protein chemistry is relatively easy. Combining the data for the phages f2, R17, and MS2, it is of interest to note that only mutations at positions 6, 50, 54, and 70 have been identified. For reasons not understood, mutation at position 6 has been observed only after HNO_2 or fluorouracil treatment, and not after hydroxylamine treatment. The following coat gene mutations have been identified: position 6 for f2, R17, and MS2; position 50 for R17 and MS2; position 54 for R17; and position 70 for f2 and MS2 (references are given in Footnote *b* to Table 12). As mentioned in Section 5.4.3c, only the mutants at position 6 are polar; all these mutations correspond to a CAG codon for glutamine. But, in addition, glutamine also occurs at positions 40 and 109, where mutations were never found. The latter position corresponds to a CAA codon, and, supposedly, mutation to an ochre codon would be lethal (the efficiency of suppression is too low for a protein needed in such large amounts). Identification of the CAG codons which can mutate (i.e., positions 6, 50, 54, and 70) in the secondary structure model of the coat gene (Min Jou *et al.*, 1972) (Fig. 5) reveals strikingly that each constitutes a discontinuity in the secondary structure, and therefore presumably becomes more prone to mutagenic attack. The CAG at position 40, where a mutation has never been found, is completely involved in a double-helical interaction.

Also, a series of UGA (opal) mutants have been isolated (van Montagu, 1968; Fiers *et al.*, 1969; Model *et al.*, 1969). The mutations were localized in either the A protein gene or the replicase gene. It may be noted here that *E. coli* K12 strains are rather leaky in their UGA-dependent termination, and in fact the phage Qβ has made use of this leakiness for translational control (Section 3.3). The leakiness of the su^- host can be reduced by an str^r mutation. The suppressor strain (*E. coli* CAJ 64) inserts tryptophan in the position corresponding to the UGA mutation (Chan *et al.*, 1971).

An interesting new class of mutants was called azures or reversed ambers (Horiuchi and Zinder, 1967; van Montagu, 1968; Fiers *et al.*, 1969). These grow normally on wild-type host strains but are restricted in amber suppressor strains. This restriction is proportional to the efficiency of the amber suppressing ability, and presumably an early event in the infection cycle is affected. A molecular explanation is not known, but it is tempting to correlate these observations with the fact that two out of three MS2 genes are terminated by a UAG codon. Perhaps a second mutation causes readthrough at the UAG termination to become a lethal event.

TABLE 12
Properties of Amber Mutants[a]

Mutation in cistron	Typical mutants[b]	Growth on[c]				Physiological effect in an *su*⁻ cell
		$su_I{}^+$	$su_{II}{}^+$	$su_{III}{}^+$	$su_{(UAA)}{}^{+d}$	
A protein	f2: *sus1*	+	+			Cell lyses with production of a normal burst of noninfectious, A–protein-defective particles; these are sensitive to ribonuclease, but if degradation is avoided the phage RNA can be isolated in an intact form, which is infectious in a spheroplast system
	R17: A3, A9, A30–A68	+	+	+	+	
	MS2: Class 1: 303, 900 (12 mutants)	+	+	+	+	MS2: Class 1: no nonsense polypeptide detected
	Class 2: 100, 302, 902 (7 mutants)	+	+	+	+	Class 2: synthesis of a nonsense polypeptide 88% of the normal length
	Qβ: 2, 203	+				Qβ: A1 protein mutants do not lyse host cells
Coat protein Polar Position 6	f2: *sus3*	+	–	–	–	Little effect on cellular growth rate; no phage antigen; no or poor complementation with replicase mutants (polar effect on replicase); decreased level of replicase activity
	R17: B2, B23–B29	+	±	–	–	
	MS2: 908	+	–	–	–	

Nonpolar						
Position 50	R17: B11, B22	+	±	±	−	Reduced cellular growth rate, but no lysis; normal complementation; enhanced level of virus-induced replicase activity and virus-specific double-stranded RNA
	MS2: 623	+	−	±	−	
	111	+	±	±	−	
	904	+	−	−	−	
Position 54	R17: B17–21	+	±	−	−	
Position 70	f2: sus11	+	−	−	−	
	MS2: Mu9	+	±	±	−	
	601	+	−	−	−	
Unidentified	Qβ: 11, 12	+	−	−	−	
Replicase	f2: sus10	+	±	+		No viral RNA synthesis; no effect on growth of host cell; no phage antigen
	R17: C13	+	+	+	−	
		C8, C14, C15, C16	±	+	+	
	MS2: 607	+	+	+		
	Qβ: 12, 01	+	+	+		

[a] From Fiers (1974).

[b] References: f2 mutants: Zinder and Cooper (1964), Lodish and Zinder (1966). R17 mutants: Gussin (1966), Tooze and Weber (1967). MS2 mutants: Vinuela et al. (1968). Over 100 mutants were isolated and characterized by M. van Montagu (personal communication) and partially described in van Montagu et al. (1967), Fiers et al. (1969), van de Kerckhove et al. (1971), Vandamme et al. (1972). Qβ mutants: Horiuchi and Matsuhashi (1970), Horiuchi et al. (1971).

[c] Very often, efficiency of plating (e.o.p.) and not actual growth was tested; ± means either very small plaques or decreased e.o.p.

[d] Ochre suppressor strains suppress both UAA and UAG, but at very low efficiency (1–5%).

Mutants can also be immunologically or physically selected. These presumably correspond to alterations in the surface properties of the virion particle, and hence allow probing of which regions are oriented toward the solvent. The first class is anti-MS2 serum-resistant mutants (van Assche *et al.*, 1972), and the second class has been selected on the basis of altered electrophoretic mobility (van Assche and van Montagu, 1974). Still another class of mutants was selected by being conditionally lethal on wild-type strains but viable on *E. coli* strains which were ribonuclease I deficient. All three classes have been characterized at the level of the coat protein sequence (Section 3.2).

A new area in genetics has begun with the development of procedures to obtain a mutation at a preselected site (Flavell *et al.*, 1974). Such mutations have been obtained in the ribosome binding region of the Qβ coat gene (Section 4.3.1) and the untranslated 3'-terminal segment of Qβ RNA (Section 5.1.2).

5.7. General Properties of the Viral Nucleotide Sequence

5.7.1. Intrinsic Properties

It has long been known that the bacteriophage RNA genomes have a very high spontaneous mutation rate. For example, each stock of bacteriophage Qβ contains an appreciable proportion of temperature-sensitive mutants (Valentine *et al.*, 1969). Conversely, the high reversion rate of any type of mutant is one of the reasons why genetic studies with these phages are rather difficult. The spontaneous generation of new variants can of course create serious problems for nucleotide sequence analysis. Nevertheless, in the laboratory of the author the stock of MS2 which has been used over the years has remained quite constant. But, on several occasions, a preparation turned out to contain a (silent) mutation; an example is given by Min Jou *et al.* (1972). All such changes which have been analyzed turned out to be transition mutations. Nevertheless, when MS2 RNA was converted into DNA and a single molecule was cloned, no discrepancies with the published RNA sequence were observed [almost 20% has been rechecked by this approach (Devos *et al.*, 1979)]. Other examples of apparently neutral point mutations have been reported for R17 RNA (Cory *et al.*, 1970; Bernardi and Spahr, 1972); these changes do of course affect the stability of the hairpins in which they occur (Min Jou and Fiers, 1976*b*).

The nucleotide heterogeneity of a Qβ phage stock has been studied in more detail by Domingo *et al.* (1978). They estimate that each molecule deviates from the ideal standard sequence in one or two positions. These authors propose that the phage stock is in a dynamic equilibrium, with mutants arising continuously at each replication round. However, the standard wild-type sequence has a selective advantage, such that a near-constant genotype is maintained. If this interpretation is correct, it would mean that nearly each nucleotide (including all the third letters of the degenerate codons) has a defined biological or structural role, such that selection pressure toward reversion to wild type is imposed.

One can also ask whether the primary nucleotide sequence may still reveal clues as to its possible evolutionary origin. An important mechanism that has been used by nature to increase the coding potential of the genetic material is by gene duplication, and some evidence for duplication of segments of the viral RNA has been obtained. The first indication came from an analysis of the pancreatic ribonuclease products (Section 4.2.1); some of the polypurine tracts seemed related to each other (Min Jou and Fiers, 1969; Thirion and Kaesberg, 1970). Cory *et al.* (1970) pointed out that the segment from nucleotides 44 to 55 in R17 RNA might have been duplicated to give the segment 56–67, which contains eight out of 12 identical residues. This region is homologous to a sequence in Qβ RNA (following section), and here one can propose a similar repeat, viz. nucleotides 101–112 repeated in nucleotides 113–124, containing nine out of 12 identical residues. Another example is a segment of 25 nucleotides located in the last part of the A protein gene which is repeated somewhat further; in this case one base change and three one-nucleotide deletions or insertions are required to make the segments identical (Rensing, 1973). Still another example of a repeat can be found in the region preceding the Qβ coat gene; a segment of 33 nucleotides is apparently duplicated, with a conservation of 21 residues (Porter and Hindley, 1972). More such cases can be found by inspection of the MS2 RNA sequence. Although the above examples of duplications seem convincing, a careful evaluation is clearly needed in order to assess the degree of statistical significance.

One of the first intriguing features which was revealed by analysis of the primary structure of the viral RNA genomes concerned the rhythmic distribution of purine tract frequencies (Fiers *et al.*, 1965). Total digestion of MS2 RNA with pancreatic ribonuclease results in products of the form $(Pu)_{n-1} Py$, which can be separated according to the chain length n (Section 4.2.1). When the frequencies (i.e., quantitative amounts) of these products were compared to those expected for a random sequence of the same base composition, it was found that the deviations from randomness showed a rhythmic pattern: the deviations for odd values of n were positive and those for even numbers were negative. This means that a relative excess was observed for $(Pu)_2Py$, $(Pu)_4Py$, and $(Pu)_6Py$. A similar property could be demonstrated for the RNAs derived from R17 (Sinha *et al.*, 1965*a*), M12 (Sinha *et al.*, 1965*b*), and $\mu2$ (Matthews, 1968). A more detailed analysis has shown that this property not only is almost certainly significant (at the level of about 1%) but also occurs in several sequenced bacteriophage λ mRNAs and in the $Q\beta$ coat initiation region (Elton and Fiers, 1976). Various explanations have been offered for this strange observation (Fiers *et al.*, 1965; Fiers, 1966; Elton and Fiers, 1976). Possibly it is a remnant of a pattern present in an original stretch of nucleotides from which the viral RNAs have evolved by repeated duplications; possibly it stems from an earlier evolutionary period when the defined tertiary structure was not yet achieved and a rhythmic distribution gave a higher percentage of base pairing to a randomly folded chain; possibly it is related to a subtle influence exerted on the RNA polymerase by the nearest and the second-nearest residue on the incorporation of the following nucleotide. These, however, are only speculations, and the phenomenon has not really been explained in a satisfactory way.

5.7.2. Comparative Studies of Viral RNAs

The group I phages are closely related to each other as evidenced by immunological data and by the amino acid sequence of their coat protein (Sections 2.1 and 3.2). This relationship was soon confirmed and expressed in quantitative terms when actual nucleotide sequence information of the viral RNAs became available (De Wachter *et al.*, 1971*b*; Min Jou *et al.*, 1971; Fiers *et al.*, 1971; Nichols and Robertson, 1971; Ling, 1971; Adams *et al.*, 1972*a,b*; Robertson and Jeppesen, 1972). Later on, more sequences of viral RNA segments were elucidated (the complete sequence of MS2 RNA; nearly one-quarter of R17 RNA) and a compilation of all the analyses was made by Min Jou and Fiers (1976*b*). There is no evidence that any of the phages MS2, R17, and f2 differ from each other by more than a number of point mutations (i.e., there is no evidence for insertions or deletions). These three prototype phages seem to be independently derived from a common ancestor. As we have mentioned in Section 5.1, no mutation has so far been found in the terminal untranslated regions. This seems to suggest a very important biological role for these parts of the molecule. The overall variability amounts to 3.9% for the comparison MS2-R17, 3.4%

for MS2-f2, and 3.7% for R17-f2 (as the variability is zero for the untranslated terminal regions, the values are slightly higher when only the translated regions are considered; cf. Section 5.1.1). Of the 26 nucleotide changes observed between MS2 and R17, only four lead to an amino acid change, the other 22 being neutral. This means that there is a strong selection pressure to maintain the specific amino acid sequence of the different proteins. Moreover, the amino acid changes which do survive are of a conservative nature (Thr ↔ Ala; Arg ↔ Lys; Ser ↔ Asn). As discussed by Min Jou and Fiers (1976b), the ratio of silent mutations to those which affect the amino acid sequence is in the same range for RNA bacteriophages and for hemoglobins.

Of the mutations which could be unambiguously compared, 31 (86%) are transitions and only five (14%) are transversions. C ↔ U transitions are slightly more frequent than G ↔ A interchanges, but the difference is not statistically significant. The prevalence of transitions over transversions can readily be explained by G-U wobble pairing during replication (during either plus-strand or minus-strand synthesis).

By comparing the number of mutations in single-stranded regions to those in double-stranded stems, it could be deduced that the latter were 2.5 times less frequent than expected on a random basis. This clear effect implies of course that the structure shown in Fig. 5 must be largely correct. Moreover, the result also indicates that this secondary (and tertiary) structure must have an important biological role, so that it tends to be maintained in evolution.

Bacteriophage Qβ shows almost no immunological cross-reactivity with the group I phages (Section 2.1). Also, no homology could be detected by competition hybridization (Weissmann and Ochoa, 1967). Nevertheless, various evidence suggests a common ancestry. Not only is the organization of the genome similar (Fig. 1), but the coat proteins also show a certain degree of relatedness (Fig. 2). Moreover, nucleotide sequence analysis has revealed several examples of presumptive homology. The region from positions 5 to 22 in R17 (or MS2) RNA contains 17 nucleotides also present in a corresponding Qβ RNA segment (Adams and Cory, 1970). Somewhat farther in the 5'-initial segment, there is a region from positions 44 to 71 (in R17-MS2), for which 20 out of 28 nucleotides are identical in a corresponding segment of Qβ RNA. Remarkably, this segment is part of the untranslated region in R17 RNA but is located inside the A2 cistron in Qβ RNA, suggesting that the site of initiation for the latter gene has been fixed only after the phage ancestors diverged. Another example of homology is found around the ribosome binding region of the replicase gene (Porter *et al.*,

1974); 22 out of 33 nucleotides are identical in MS2 RNA and in Qβ RNA. Also, nine out of the first 17 amino acids in the replicase subunits are identical. At the 3' end 16 out of 24 nucleotides (and one deletion) are again identical (Cory *et al.*, 1970). Obviously, this degree of relatedness should be expressed in statistically meaningful estimates. This has to some extent already been done for the ribosome binding regions (Köhler and Rohloff, 1974). Undoubtedly, more sequence information on the phage Qβ genome will soon be forthcoming, and this will allow a detailed and quantitative comparison.

6. CONCLUDING REMARKS

In the introduction (Section 1) we have already stressed the important role played by the RNA phages as a tool to understand the fundamental biology not just of RNA viruses in general but even more of the prokaryotic host cell. Our present knowledge of protein synthesis, both from a mechanistic and from an information-processing point of view, stems mainly from the use of phage viral RNAs as readily available, well-characterized messengers. Fundamental aspects of translation, such as initiation, termination, suppression, modulation, and translational repression, have been clarified by means of these RNA genomes. The elucidation of the complete structure of bacteriophage MS2 RNA allowed investigators for the first time to relate all the biological functions of an organism (if a virus is regarded as such) to the information content of its genome. Nevertheless, although the number of publications dealing with RNA phages has decreased considerably in recent years, important lacunae in our knowledge still remain—for example, what is the mechanism of cell lysis, why is the viral RNA apparently stable toward the messenger-RNA-degrading enzyme systems, what is the detailed three-dimensional structure of the viral RNA, what conformational rearrangements accompany the diverse biological functions of the RNA, what is the detailed mechanism of RNA replication and what determines the asymmetry of plus- and minus-strand synthesis, what is the nature of the defect in some odd phage mutants, and so on. It is to be hoped that these questions will be further explored and ultimately solved.

ACKNOWLEDGMENTS

The research in the author's laboratory was mainly supported by the FKFO of Belgium. I thank M. Billeter, J. A. Steitz, M. van

Montagu and C. Weissmann for helpful comments and permission to quote unpublished results.

7. LITERATURE

7.1. Reviews

Bradley, D. E., 1967, Ultrastructure of bacteriophages and bacteriocins, *Bacteriol. Rev.* **31**:230.

Eoyang, L., and August, J. T., 1974, Reproduction of RNA bacteriophages, in: *Comprehensive Virology*, Vol. 2 (H. Fraenkel-Conrat and R. R. Wagner, eds.), p. 1, Penum Press, New York.

Fiers, W., 1974, RNA bacteriophages, in: *Handbook of Genetics*, Vol. 1 (R. C. King, ed.), p. 271, Plenum Press, New York.

Hindley, J., 1973, Structure and strategy in phage RNA, in: *Progress in Biophysics and Molecular Biology*, Vol. 26 (J. A. V. Butler and D. Noble, eds.), p. 269, Pergamon Press, Oxford.

Hohn, T., and Hohn, B., 1970, Structure and assembly of simple RNA bacteriophages, *Adv. Virus Res.* **16**:43,

Kozak, M., and Nathans, D., 1972, Translation of the genome of a ribonucleic acid bacteriophage, *Bacteriol. Rev.* **36**:109.

Lodish, H. F., 1968, The replication of RNA-containing bacteriophages, in: *Progress in Biophysics and Molecular Biology* (J. A. V. Butler and D. Noble, eds.), p. 285, Pergamon Press, Oxford.

Lodish, H. F., 1976, Translational control of protein synthesis, *Annu. Rev. Biochem.* **45**:39.

Stavis, R. L., and August, J. T., 1970, The biochemistry of RNA bacteriophage replication, *Annu. Rev. Biochem.* **45**:527.

Steitz, J. A., 1979, Genetic signals and nucleotide sequences in messenger RNA, in: *Biological Regulation and Development*, Vol. 1: *Gene Expression* (R. Goldberger, ed.), p. 349, Plenum Press, New York.

Valentine, R. C., Ward, R., and Strand, M., 1969, The replication cycle of RNA bacteriophages, *Adv. Virus Res.* **15**:1.

Weissmann, C., 1974, The making of a phage, *FEBS Lett.* **40**:S10.

Weissmann, C., and Ochoa, S., 1967, Replication of phage RNA, *Progr. Nucleic Acid Res. Mol. Biol.* **6**:353.

Weissmann, C., Billeter, M. A., Goodman, H. M., Hindley, J., and Weber, H., 1973, Structure and function of phage RNA, *Annu. Rev. Biochem.* **42**:303.

Zinder, N. D., 1965, RNA phages, *Annu. Rev. Microbiol.* **19**:455.

Zinder, N. D. (ed.), 1975, *RNA Phages*, Cold Spring Harbor Laboratory, Cold Spring Harbor, N.Y.

7.2. Specific References

Achtman, M., Willetts, N., and Clark, A. J., 1971, Beginning a genetic analysis of conjugational transfer determined by the F factor in *Escherichia coli* by isolation and characterization of transfer-deficient mutants, *J. Bacteriol.* **106**:529.

Adams, J. M., and Cory, S., 1970, Untranslated nucleotide sequence at the 5'-end of R17 bacteriophage RNA, *Nature (London)* **227**:570.

Adams, J. M., Jeppesen, P. G. N., Sanger, F., and Barrell, B. F., 1969, Nucleotide sequence from the coat protein cistron of R17 bacteriophage RNA, *Nature (London)* **223**:1009.

Adams, J. M., Cory, S., and Spahr, P. F., 1972*a*, Nucleotide sequences of fragments of R17 bacteriophage RNA from the region immediately preceding the coat protein cistron, *Eur. J. Biochem.* **29**:469.

Adams, J. M., Spahr, P. F., and Cory, S., 1972*b*, Nucleotide sequence from the 5' end to the first cistron of R17 bacteriophage ribonucleic acid, *Biochemistry* **11**:976.

Ames, B. N., and Hartman, P. E., 1963, The histidine operon, *Cold Spring Harbor Symp.* **28**:349.

Ammann, J., Delius, H., and Hofschneider, P. H., 1964, Isolation and properties of an intact phage-specific replicative form of RNA phage M12, *J. Mol. Biol.* **10**:557.

Anderson, W. F., and Gilbert, J. M., 1969, Translational control of in vitro hemoglobin synthesis, *Cold Spring Harbor Symp.* **34**:585.

Argetsinger, J., 1968, A slowly sedimenting, infective form of bacteriophage R17, *J. Mol. Biol.* **33**:947.

Argetsinger, J. E., and Gussin, G. N., 1966, Intact ribonucleic acid from defective particles of bacteriophage R17, *J. Mol. Biol.* **21**:421.

Argetsinger-Steitz, J., 1968*a*, Identification of the A protein as a structural component of bacteriophage R17, *J. Mol. Biol.* **33**:923.

Argetsinger-Steitz, J., 1968*b*, Isolation of the A protein from bacteriophage R17, *J. Mol. Biol.* **33**:937.

Argetsinger-Steitz, J., Wahba, A. J., Langhrea, M., and Moore, P. B., 1977, Differential requirements for polypeptide chain initiation complex formation at the three bacteriophage R17 initiator regions, *Nucleic Acids Res.* **4**:1.

Atkins, J. F., and Gesteland, R. F., 1975, The synthetase gene of the RNA phages R17, MS2 and f2 has a single UAG terminator codon, *Mol. Gen. Genet.* **139**:19.

August, J. T., Banerjee, A. K., Eoyang, L., Franze de Fernandez, T., Hori, K., Kuo, C. H., Rensing, U., and Shapiro, L., 1968, Synthesis of bacteriophage $Q\beta$ RNA, *Cold Spring Harbor Symp. Quant. Biol.* **33**:73.

Aviv, H., Bovine, J., Loyd, B., and Leder, P., 1972, Translation of bacteriophage $Q\beta$ messenger RNA in a murine Krebs 2 ascites tumor cell-free system, *Science* **178**:1293.

Ball, L. A., and Kaesberg, P., 1973, A polarity gradient in the expression of the replicase gene of RNA bacteriophage $Q\beta$, *J. Mol. Biol.* **74**:547.

Bamford, O. H., Palva, E. T., and Lounatmaa, K., 1976, Ultrastructure and life cycle of the lipid-containing bacteriophage $\phi6$, *J. Gen. Virol.* **32**:249.

Banerjee, A. K., Kuo, C. H., and August, J. T., 1969*a*, Replication of RNA viruses. VIII. Direction of chain growth in the $Q\beta$ RNA polymerase reaction, *J. Mol. Biol.* **40**:445.

Banerjee, A. K., Rensing, U., and August, J. T., 1969*b*, Replication of RNA viruses. X. Replication of a natural 6 S RNA by the $Q\beta$ RNA polymerase, *J. Mol. Biol.* **45**:181.

Bassel, B. A., Jr., and Spiegelman, S., 1967, Specific cleavage of $Q\beta$ RNA and identification of the fragment carrying the 3'-OH terminus, *Proc. Natl. Acad. Sci. USA* **58**:1155.

Bastin, M., Dasgupta, R., Hall, T. C., and Kaesberg, P., 1976, Similarity in structure and function of the 3'-terminal region of the four brome mosaic viral RNA's, *J. Mol. Biol.* **103**:737.

Bendis, I., and Shapiro, L., 1970, Properties of *Caulobacter* ribonucleic acid bacteriophage φCb5, *J. Virol.* **6**:847.

Benike, C., McClements, W., and Davis, J. W., 1975, The molecular size of the RNA genome of *Pseudomonas aeruginosa* bacteriophage PP7, *Virology* **66**:625.

Bernardi, A., and Spahr, P.-F., 1972, Nucleotide sequence at the binding site for coat protein on RNA of bacteriophage R17, *Proc. Natl. Acad. Sci. USA* **69**:3033.

Billeter, M. A., Libonati, M., Vinuela, E., and Weissmann, C., 1966, Replication of viral RNA. X. Turnover of virus-specific double-stranded RNA during replication of phage MS2 in *Escherichia coli*, *J. Biol. Chem.* **241**:4750.

Billeter, M. A., Dahlberg, J. E., Goodman, H. M., Hindley, J., and Weissmann, C., 1969, Sequence of the first 175 nucleotides from the 5'-terminus of Qβ RNA synthesized *in vitro*, *Nature (London)* **224**:1083.

Billeter, M., Parsons, J. T., and Coffin, J. M., 1974, The nucleotide sequence complexity of avian tumor virus RNA, *Proc. Natl. Acad. Sci. USA* **71**:3560.

Bishop, D. H. L., and Bradley, D. E., 1965, Determination of base ratios of six ribonucleic acid bacteriophages specific to *Escherichia coli*, *Biochem. J.* **95**:82.

Bishop, D. H. L., Claybrook, J. R., Pace, N .R., and Spiegelman, S., 1967, An analysis by gel electrophoresis of Qβ-RNA complexes formed during the latent period of an *in vitro* synthesis, *Proc. Natl. Acad. Sci. USA* **57**:1474.

Bishop, D. H. L., Mills, D. R., and Spiegelman, S., 1968, The sequence at the 5'-terminus of a self-replicating variant of viral Qβ ribonucleic acid, *Biochemistry* **7**:3744.

Blumenthal, T., Landers, T. A., and Weber, K., 1972, Bacteriophage Qβ replicase contains the protein biosynthesis elongation factors EFTu and EFTs, *Proc. Natl. Acad. Sci. USA* **69**:1313.

Boedtker, H., 1960, Configurational properties of tobacco mosaic virus ribonucleic acid, *J. Mol. Biol.* **2**:171.

Boedtker, H., 1967, The reaction of ribonucleic acid with formaldehyde. I. Optical absorbance studies, *Biochemistry* **6**:2718.

Boedtker, H., 1968, Dependence of the sedimentation coefficient on molecular weight of RNA after reaction with formaldehyde, *J. Mol. Biol.* **35**:61.

Boedtker, H., 1971, Conformation independent molecular weight determination of RNA by gel electrophoresis, *Biochim. Biophys. Acta* **240**:448.

Borer, P. N., Dengler, B., and Tinoco, I., Jr., 1974, Stability of Ribonucleic acid double-stranded helices, *J. Mol. Biol.* **86**:843.

Borst, P., and Weissmann, C., 1965, Replication of viral RNA. VIII. Studies on the enzymatic mechanism of replication of MS2 RNA, *Proc. Natl. Acad. Sci. USA* **54**:982.

Bosch, L. (ed.), 1972, *The Mechanism of Protein Synthesis and Its Regulation*, North-Holland, Amsterdam.

Bradley, D. E., 1964, Some preliminary observations on filamentous and RNA bacteriophages, *J. Ultrastruct. Res.* **10**:385.

Bradley, D. E., 1966, The structure and infective process of a *Pseudomonas aeruginosa* bacteriophage containing ribonucleic acid, *J. Gen. Microbiol.* **45**:83.

Braun, R., and Behrens, K., 1969, A ribonuclease from *Physarum:* Biochemical properties and synthesis in the mitotic cycle, *Biochim. Biophys. Acta* **195**:87.

Briand, J. P., Richards, K. E., Witz, J., and Hirth, L., 1976, Structure of the amino-acid accepting 3′-end of high-molecular weight eggplant mosaic virus RNA, *Proc. Natl. Acad. Sci. USA* **73**:737.

Briand, J. P., Jonard, G., Guilley, H., Richards, K., and Hirth, L., 1977, Nucleotide sequence (*n* = 159) of the amino acid accepting 3′-OH extremity of turnip yellow mosaic virus RNA and the last portion of its coat protein cistron, *Eur. J. Biochem.* **72**:453.

Brinton, C. C., Jr., 1971, The properties of sex pili, the viral nature of "conjugal" genetic transfer systems, and some possible approaches to the control of bacterial drug resistance, *Critical Rev. Microbiol.* **1**:105.

Brinton, C. C., Gemski, P., and Carnahan, J., 1964, A new type of bacterial pilus genetically controlled by the fertility factor of *E. coli* K12 and its role in chromosome transfer, *Proc. Natl. Acad. Sci. USA* **52**:776.

Brownlee, G. G., 1972, Determination of sequences in RNA, in: *Laboratory Techniques in Biochemistry and Molecular Biology*, Vol. 3, Part 1 (T. S. Work and E. Work, eds.), pp. 1–266, North-Holland, Amsterdam.

Brownlee, G. G., and Sanger, F., 1969, Chromatography of ^{32}P-labelled oligonucleotides on thin layers of DEAE-cellulose, *Eur. J. Biochem.* **11**:395.

Brownlee, G. G., Sanger, F., and Barrell, B. G., 1968, The sequence of 5 S ribosomal ribonucleic acid, *J. Mol. Biol.* **34**:379.

Camerini-Otero, R. D., Franklin, R. M., and Day, L. A., 1974, Molecular weights, dispersion of refractive index increments, and dimensions from transmittance spectrophotometry: Bacteriophages R17, T7 and PM2, and TMV, *Biochemistry* **13**:3763.

Capecchi, M. R., and Webster, R. E., 1975, Bacteriophage RNA as template for *in vitro* protein synthesis, in: *RNA Phages* (N. D. Zinder, ed.), p. 279, Cold Spring Harbor Laboratory, Cold Spring Harbor, N.Y.

Capecchi, M. R., Hughes, S. H., and Wahl, G. M., 1975, Yeast supersuppressors are altered tRNAs capable of translating a nonsense codon *in vitro*, *Cell* **6**:269.

Carmichael, G. C., Weber, K., Niveleau, A., and Wahba, A. J., 1975, The host factor required for RNA phage Qβ RNA replication *in vitro*, *J. Biol. Chem.* **250**:3607.

Caskey, C. T., Beaudet, A., and Nirenberg, M., 1968, RNA codons and protein synthesis. 15. Dissimilar responses of mammalian and bacterial transfer RNA fractions to messenger RNA codons, *J. Mol. Biol.* **37**:99.

Chan, T.-S., Webster, R. E., and Zinder, N. D., 1971, Suppression of UGA codon by a tryptophan tRNA, *J. Mol. Biol.* **56**:101.

Clark, B. F. C., and Marcker, K. A., 1966, The role of *N*-formyl-methionyl-tRNA in protein biosynthesis, *J. Mol. Biol.* **17**:394.

Contreras, R., and Fiers, W., 1971, A new method for partial digestion useful for sequence analysis of polynucleotides, *FEBS Lett.* **16**:281.

Contreras, R., and Fiers, W., 1975, A method for the isolation of cytidylate series from ribonuclease T_1-oligonucleotides, *Anal. Biochem.* **67**:319.

Contreras, R., Vandenberghe, A., Min Jou, W., De Wachter, R., and Fiers, W., 1971, Studies on the bacteriophage MS2 nucleotide sequence of a 3′-terminal fragment (*n* = 104), *FEBS Lett.* **18**:141.

Contreras, R., Vandenberghe, A., Volckaert, G., Min Jou, W., and Fiers, W., 1972, Studies on the bacteriophage MS2. XIX. Some nucleotide sequences from the RNA polymerase gene, *FEBS Lett.* **24**:339.

Contreras, R., Ysebaert, M., Min Jou, W., and Fiers, W., 1973, Bacteriophage MS2

RNA: Nucleotide sequence of the end of the A protein gene and the intercistronic region, *Nature (London) New Biol.* **241**:99.

Cory, S., Spahr, P. F., and Adams, J. M., 1970, Untranslated nucleotide sequence in R17 bacteriophage RNA, *Cold Spring Harbor Symp. Quant. Biol.* **35**:1.

Cory, S., Adams, J. M., Spahr, P.-F., and Rensing, U., 1972, Sequence of 51 nucleotides at the 3'-end of R17 bacteriophage RNA, *J. Mol. Biol.* **63**:41.

Crick, F. H. C., Leslie Barnett, F. R. S., Brenner, S., and Watts-Tobin, R. J., 1961, General nature of the genetic code for proteins, *Nature (London)* **192**:1227.

Crothers, D. M., Cole, P. E., Hilbers, C. W., and Schulman, R. G., 1974, The molecular mechanism of thermal unfolding of *Escherichia coli* formylmethionine transfer RNA, *J. Mol. Biol.* **87**:63.

Crowther, R. A., Amos, L. A., and Finch, J. T., 1975, Three-dimensional image reconstructions of bacteriophages R17 and f2, *J. Mol. Biol.* **98**:631.

Curtiss, L. K., and Krueger, R. G., 1974, Localization of coliphage MS2 A-protein, *J. Virol.* **14**:503.

Czernilofsky, A. P., Kurland, C. G., and Stoffler, G., 1975, 30 S ribosomal proteins associated with the 3'-terminus of 16 S RNA, *FEBS Lett.* **58**:281.

Dahlberg, A. E., and Dahlberg, J. E., 1975, Binding of ribosomal protein S1 of *Escherichia coli* to the 3' end of 16 S rRNA, *Proc. Natl. Acad. Sci. USA* **72**:2940.

Dahlberg, J. E., 1968, Terminal sequence of bacteriophage RNAs, *Nature (London)* **220**:548.

Datta, N., Hedges, R. W., Shaw, E. J., Sykes, R. B., and Richmond, M. H., 1971, Properties of an R factor from *Pseudomonas aeruginosa*, *J. Bacteriol.* **108**:1244.

Davies, J. W., and Kaesberg, P., 1973, Translation of virus mRNA: Synthesis of bacteriophage Qβ proteins in a cell-free extract from wheat embryo, *J. Virol.* **12**:1434.

Davis, J. E., and Benike, C., 1974, Translation of virus mRNA: Synthesis of bacteriophage PP7 proteins in cell-free extracts from *Pseudomonas aeruginosa*, *Virology* **61**:450.

Davis, J. E., Strauss, J. H., and Sinsheimer, R. L., 1961, Bacteriophage MS2: Another RNA phage, *Science* **134**:1427.

Delisi, C., and Crothers, D. M., 1971, Prediction of RNA secondary structure, *Proc. Natl. Acad. Sci. USA* **68**:2682.

Devos, R., Gillis, E., and Fiers, W., 1976a, The enzymic addition of poly(A) to the 3'-end of RNA using bacteriophage MS2 RNA as a model system, *Eur. J. Biochem.* **62**:401.

Devos, R., van Emmelo, J., Seurinck-Opsomer, C., Gillis, E., and Fiers, W., 1976b, Addition by ATP:RNA adenyltransferase from *Escherichia coli* of 3'-linked oligo(A) to bacteriophage Qβ RNA and its effect on RNA replication, *Biochim. Biophys. Acta* **447**:319.

Devos, R., van Emmelo, J., Celen, P., Gillis, E., and Fiers, W., 1977, Synthesis of discrete reverse transcripts of in vitro polyadenylated bacteriophage RNA by AMV-dependent DNA polymerase, *Eur. J. Biochem.* **79**:419.

Devos, R., van Emmelo, J., Contreras, R., and Fiers, W., 1979, Construction and characterization of a plasmid containing a nearly full-size copy of bacteriophage MS2 RNA, *J. Mol. Biol.* **128**:595.

De Wachter, R., and Fiers, W., 1967, Studies on the bacteriophage MS2. IV. The 3'-OH terminal undecanucleotide sequence of the viral RNA chain, *J. Mol. Biol.* **30**:507.

De Wachter, R., and Fiers, W., 1969, Sequences at the 5′-terminus of bacteriophage Qβ RNA, *Nature (London)* **221**:233.

De Wachter, R., and Fiers, W., 1970, The 5′-terminal nucleotide sequence of bacteriophage MS2 RNA, *Cold Spring Harbor Symp. Quant. Biol.* **35**:11.

De Wachter, R., and Fiers, W., 1971, Fractionation of RNA by electrophoresis on polyacrylamide gel slabs, in: *Methods in Enzymology*, Vol. 21 (L. Grossman and K. Moldave, eds.), p. 167, Academic Press, New York.

De Wachter, R., and Fiers, W., 1972, Preparative two-dimensional polyacrylamide gel electrophoresis of ^{32}P-labeled RNA, *Anal. Biochem.* **49**:184.

De Wachter, R., Verhassel, J. P., and Fiers, W., 1968a, The 5′-terminal end group of the RNA of the bacteriophage MS2, *Biochim. Biophys. Acta* **157**:195.

De Wachter, R., Verhassel, J. P., and Fiers, W., 1968b, Studies on the bacteriophage MS2. V. The 5′-terminal tetranucleotide sequence of the viral RNA chain, *FEBS Lett.* **1**:93.

De Wachter, R., Merregaert, J., Vandenberghe, A., Contreras, R., and Fiers, W., 1971a, Studies on the bacteriophage MS2: The untranslated 5′-terminal nucleotide sequence preceding the first cistron, *Eur. J. Biochem.* **22**:400.

De Wachter, R., Vandenberghe, A., Merregaert, J., Contreras, R., and Fiers, W., 1971b, The leader sequence from the 5′-terminus to the A-protein initiation codon in MS2 virus RNA, *Proc. Natl. Acad. Sci. USA* **68**:585.

Dhaese, P., Vandekerckhove, J., Vingerhoed, J. P., and van Montagu, M., 1977, Studies on PRR1, an RNA bacteriophage with broad host range, *Arch. Intern. Physiol. Biochim.* **85**:168.

Dhillon, E. K. S., and Dhillon, T. S., 1974, Synthesis of indicator strains and density of ribonucleic acid-containing coliphages in sewage, *Appl. Microbiol.* **27**:840.

Domingo, E., Flavell, R. A., and Weissmann, C., 1976, *In vitro* site-directed mutagenesis: Generation and properties of an infectious extracistronic mutant of bacteriophage Qβ, *Gene* **1**:3.

Domingo, E., Sabo, D., Taniguchi, T., and Weissmann, C., 1978, Nucleotide sequence heterogeneity of an RNA phage population, *Cell* **13**:735.

DuBow, M. S., and Blumenthal, T., 1975, Host factor for coliphage Qβ RNA replication is present in *Pseudomonas putida*, *Mol. Gen. Genet.* **141**:113.

Dunker, A. K., and Paranchych, W., 1975, On the structure of R17 phage, *Virology* **67**:297.

Edlind, T. D., and Bass, A. R., 1977, Secondary structure of RNA from bacteriophage f2, Qβ and PP7, *J. Virol.* **24**:135.

Eggen, K., and Nathans, D., 1969, Regulation of protein synthesis directed by coliphage MS2 RNA. II. *In vitro* repression by phage coat protein, *J. Mol. Biol.* **39**:293.

Elton, R. A., and Fiers, W., 1976, Rhythmic variations in purine run frequencies in bacteriophage RNA, *J. Theor. Biol.* **63**:49.

Engelhardt, D. L., and Zinder, N. D., 1964, Host-dependent mutants of the bacteriophage f2. III. Infective RNA, *Virology* **23**:582.

Engelhardt, D. L., Robertson, H. D., and Zinder, N. D., 1968, *In vitro* translation of multistranded RNA from *Escherichia coli* infected by bacteriophage f2, *Proc. Natl. Acad. Sci. USA* **59**:972.

Enger, M. D., and Kaesberg, P., 1965, Comparative studies of the coat proteins of R17 and M12 bacteriophages, *J. Mol. Biol.* **13**:260.

Enger, M. D., Stubbs, E. A., Mitra, S., and Kaesberg, P., 1963, Biophysical characteristics of the RNA-containing bacterial virus R17, *Biochemistry* **49**:857.

Eoyang, L., and August, J. T., 1971, Qβ RNA polymerase from phage Qβ-infected *E.
coli*, in: *Procedures in Nucleic Acid Research*, Vol. 2 (G. L. Cantoni and D. R.
Davies, eds.), p. 829, Harper and Row, New York.

Eoyang, L., and August, J. T., 1974, Reproduction of RNA bacteriophages, in:
Comprehensive Virology, Vol. 2 (H. Fraenkel-Conrat and R. R. Wagner, eds.), p.
1, Plenum Press, New York.

Erikson, R. L., and Franklin, R. M., 1966, Symposium on replication of viral nucleic
acids. I. Information and properties of a replicative intermediate in the biosynthesis of viral ribonucleic acid, *Bacteriol. Rev.* **30**:267.

Feary, T. W., Fisher, E., Jr., and Fisher, T. N., 1963, A small RNA-containing *Pseudomonas aeruginosa* bacteriophage, *Biochem. Biophys. Res. Commun.* **10**:359.

Feary, T. W., Fisher, E., Jr., and Fisher, T. N., 1964, Isolation and preliminary characteristics of three bacteriophages associated with a lysogenic strain of *Pseudomonas
aeruginosa*, *J. Bacteriol.* **87**:196.

Fedoroff, N., 1975, Replicase of the phage f2, in: *RNA Phages* (N. D. Zinder, ed.), p.
235, Cold Spring Harbor Laboratory, Cold Spring Harbor, N.Y.

Fedoroff, N. V., and Zinder, N. D., 1971, Structure of the poly(G) polymerase
component of the bacteriophage f2 replicase, *Proc. Natl. Acad. Sci. USA* **68**:1838.

Fenwick, M. L., Erikson, R. L., and Franklin, R. M., 1964, Replication of the RNA of
bacteriophage R17, *Science* **146**:527.

Fiers, W., 1966, The rhythmic genetic code of RNA-bacteriophages, *Nature (London)*
212:822.

Fiers, W., 1967, Studies on the bacteriophage MS2. III. Sedimentation heterogenity of
viral RNA preparations, *Virology* **33**:413.

Fiers, W., 1974, RNA-bacteriophages, in: *Handbook of Genetics* (R. C. King, ed.), p.
271, Plenum Press, New York.

Fiers, W., 1975, Chemical structure and biological activity of bacteriophage MS2-
RNA, in: *RNA Phages* (N. D. Zinder, ed.), p. 353, Cold Spring Harbor Laboratory, Cold Spring Harbor, N.Y.

Fiers, W., Lepoutre, L., and Vandendriessche, L., 1965, Studies on the bacteriophage
MS2. I. Distribution of purine sequences in the viral RNA and in yeast RNA, *J.
Mol. Biol.* **13**:432.

Fiers, W., De Wachter, R., Min Jou, W., and van Styvendaele, B., 1968, The structure
of bacteriophage RNA, in: *First Congress of Virology, Helsinki 1968* (J. L. Melnick, ed.), p. 30, Karger, Basel.

Fiers, W., van Montagu, M., De Wachter, R., Haegeman, G., Min Jou, W., Messens,
E., Remaut, E., Vandenberghe, A., and van Styvendaele, B., 1969, Studies on the
primary structure and the replication mechanism of bacteriophage RNA, *Cold
Spring Harbor Symp. Quant. Biol.* **34**:697.

Fiers, W., Contreras, R., De Wachter, R., Haegeman, G., Merregaert, J., Min Jou,
W., and Vandenberghe, A., 1971, Recent progress in the sequence determination of
bacteriophage MS2-RNA, *Biochimie* **53**:495.

Fiers, W., Contreras, R., Duerinck, F., Haegeman, G., Merregaert, J., Min Jou, W.,
Raeymaekers, A., Volckaert, G., Ysebaert, M., van de Kerckhove, J., Nolf, F.,
and van Montagu, M., 1975, A-protein gene of bacteriophage MS2, *Nature
(London)* **256**:273.

Fiers, W., Contreras, R., Duerinck, F., Haegeman, G., Iserentant, D., Merregaert, J., Min Jou, W., Molemans, F., Raeymaekers, A., Vandenberghe, A., Volckaert, G., and Ysebaert, M., 1976, Complete nucleotide sequence of bacteriophage MS2-RNA: Primary and secondary structure of the replicase gene, *Nature (London)* **260**:500.

Fink, T. R., and Crothers, D. M., 1972, Free energy of imperfect nucleic acid helices. I. The bulge effect, *J. Mol. Biol.* **66**:1.

Fisby, D. P., Newton, C., Carey, N. H., Fellner, P., Newman, J. F. E., Harris, T. J. R., and Brown, F., 1976, Oligonucleotide mapping of picornavirus RNAs by two-dimensional electrophoresis, *Virology* **71**:379.

Fishbach, F. A., Harrison, P. M., and Anderegg, J. W., 1965, An X-ray scattering study of the bacterial virus R17, *J. Mol. Biol.* **13**:638.

Fitch, W. M., 1976, Is there selection against wobble in codon-anticodon pairing? *Science* **194**:1173.

Flavell, R. A., Sabo, D. L., Bandle, E. F., and Weissmann, C., 1974, Site-directed mutagenesis: Generation of an extracistronic mutation in bacteriophage Qβ RNA, *J. Mol. Biol.* **89**:255.

Fraenkel-Conrat, H., 1954, Reaction of nucleic acid with formaldehyde, *Biochim. Biophys. Acta* **15**:307.

Fraenkel-Conrat, H., 1957, Degradation of tobacco mosaic virus with acetic acid, *Virology* **4**:1.

Francke, B., and Hofschneider, P.H., 1966, Infectious nucleic acids of *E. coli* bacteriophages. IX. Sedimentation constants and strand integrity of infectious M12 phage replicative-form RNA, *Proc. Natl. Acad. Sci. USA* **56**:1883.

Franklin, R. M., 1966, Purification and properties of the replicative intermediate of the RNA bacteriophage R17, *Proc. Natl. Acad. Sci. USA* **55**:1504.

Franklin, R. M., 1967, Replication of bacteriophage ribonucleic acid: Some physical properties of single-stranded, double-stranded, and branched viral ribonucleic acid, *J. Virol.* **1**:64.

Fukuma, I., and Cohen, S. S., 1975, Polyamines in bacteriophage R17 and its RNA, *J. Virol.* **16**:222.

Garwes, D., Sillero, A., and Ochoa, S., 1969, Virus-specific proteins in *E. coli* infected with phage Qβ, *Biochim. Biophys. Acta* **186**:166.

Gesteland, R. F., 1966, Isolation and characterization of ribonuclease I mutants of *Escherichia coli*, *J. Mol. Biol.* **16**:67.

Gesteland, R. F., and Boedtker, H., 1964, Some physical properties of bacteriophage R17 and its ribonucleic acid, *J. Mol. Biol.* **8**:496.

Gesteland, R. F., Wolfner, M., Grisafi, P., Fink, G., Botstein, D., and Ruth, J. R., 1976, Yeast suppressors of UAA and UAG nonsense codons work efficiently in vitro via tRNA, *Cell* **7**:381.

Ghosh, H. P., Soll, D., and Khorana, H. G., 1967, Studies on polynucleotides. LXVII. Initiation of protein synthesis in vitro as studied by using ribopolynucleotides with repeating nucleotide sequences as messenger, *J. Mol. Biol.* **25**:275.

Giegé, R., Briand, J. P., Mengual, R., Ebel, J. P., and Hirth, L., 1978, Valylation of the two RNA components of turnip yellow mosaic virus and specificity of the tRNA amino-acylation reaction, *Eur. J. Biochem.* **84**:251.

Gilvarg, C., Bollum, F. J., and Weissmann, C., 1975, The *in vitro* addition of a poly-adenylate sequence to the 3' end of phage Qβ RNA and the biological activity of the product, *Proc. Natl. Acad. Sci. USA* **72**:428.

Glitz, D. G., and Eichler, D., 1971, Nucleotides at the 5'-linked ends of bromegrass mosaic virus RNA and its fragments, *Biochim. Biophys. Acta* **238**:224.

Goelz, S., and Steitz, J. A., 1977, *Escherichia coli* ribosomal subunit S1 recognizes two sites in bacteriophage Qβ RNA, *J. Biol. Chem.* **252**:5177.

Goldberg, M. L., and Steitz, J. A., 1974, Cistron specificity of 30 S ribosomes heterologously reconstituted with components from *Escherichia coli* and *Bacillus stearothermophilus*, *Biochemistry* **13**:2123.

Goldstein, J., 1967, Digestion of ribonucleic acid by an alkylated ribonuclease, *J. Mol. Biol.* **25**:123.

Goodman, H. M., Billeter, M. A., Hindley, J., and Weissmann, C., 1970, The nucleotide sequence at the 5'-terminus of the Qβ RNA minus strand, *Proc. Natl. Acad. Sci. USA* **67**:921.

Gould, H., 1966, The specific cleavage of ribonucleic acid from reticulocyte ribosomal subunits, *Biochemistry* **5**:1103.

Gralla, J., and Crothers, D. M., 1973*a*, Free energy of imperfect nucleic acid helices. II. Small hairpin loops, *J. Mol. Biol.* **73**:497.

Gralla, J., and Crothers, D. M., 1973*b*, Free energy of imperfect nucleic acid helices. III. Small internal loops resulting from mismatches, *J. Mol. Biol.* **78**:301.

Gralla, J., and Delisi, C., 1974, mRNA is expected to form stable secondary structures, *Nature (London)* **248**:330.

Gralla, J., Steitz, J. A., and Crothers, D. M., 1974, Direct physical evidence for secondary structure in an isolated fragment of R17 Bacteriophage RNA, *Nature (London)* **248**:204.

Granboulan, N., and Franklin, R. M., 1966, Electron microscopy of viral RNA, replicative form and replicative intermediate of the bacteriophage R17, *J. Mol. Biol.* **22**:173.

Granboulan, N., and Franklin, R. M., 1968, Replication of bacteriophage ribonucleic acid: Analysis of the ultrastructure of the replicative form and the replicative intermediate of bacteriophage R17, *J. Virol.* **2**:129.

Griffin, B. E., 1971, Separation of ^{32}P-labeled ribonucleic acid components. The use of polyethylenimine-cellulose (TLC) as a second dimension in separating oligoribonucleotides of 4.5 S and 5 S from *E. coli*, *FEBS Lett.* **15**:165.

Groner, Y., Pollack, Y., Berissi, H., and Revel, M., 1972, Cistron specific translation control protein in *Escherichia coli*, *Nature (London) New Biol.* **239**:16.

Grosjean, H., Soll, D. G., and Crothers, D. M., 1976, Studies of the complex between transfer RNAs with complementary anticodons. I. Origins of enhanced affinity between complementary triplets, *J. Mol. Biol.* **103**:499.

Grosjean, H., Sankoff, D., Min Jou, W., Fiers, W., and Cedergren, R. J., 1978, Bacteriophage MS2 RNA: A correlation between the stability of the codon–anticodon interaction and the choice of code words, *J. Mol. Evol.* **12**:113.

Gross, H. J., Duerinck, F. R., and Fiers, W., 1970, The tRNA pyrophosphorylase activity of *Escherichia coli:* A study on substrate specificity, *Eur. J. Biochem.* **17**:116.

Gupta, S. L., Chen, J., Schaefer, L., Lengyel, P., and Weissmann, S. M., 1970, Nucleotide sequence of a ribosome attachment site of bacteriophage f2 RNA, *Biochem. Biophys. Res. Commun.* **39**:883.

Gussin, G. N., 1966, Three complementation groups in bacteriophage R17, *J. Mol. Biol.* **21**:435.

Haegeman, G. and Fiers, W., 1973, Studies on the bacteriophage MS2: An internal nucleotide fragment resembling some ribosomal binding sites, *Eur. J. Biochem.* **36**:135.

Haegeman, G., Min Jou, W., and Fiers, W., 1971, Studies on the bacteriophage MS2. IX. The heptanucleotide sequences present in the pancreatic ribonuclease digest of viral RNA, *J. Mol. Biol.* **57**:597.

Happe, M., and Jockush, H., 1975, Phage Qβ replicase: Cell-free synthesis of the phage-specific subunit and its assembly with host subunits to form active enzyme, *Eur. J. Biochem.* **58**:359.

Harada, F., and Nishimura, S., 1974, Purification and characterization of AUA specific isoleucine transfer ribonucleic acid from *Escherichia coli* B, *Biochemistry* **13**:300.

Haruna, I., and Spiegelman, S., 1965a, Specific template requirements of RNA replicases, *Proc. Natl. Acad. Sci. USA* **54**:579.

Haruna, I., and Spiegelman, S., 1965b, Recognition of size and sequence by an RNA replicase, *Proc. Natl. Acad. Sci. USA* **54**:1189.

Haruna, I., Nozu, K., Ohtaka, Y., and Spiegelman, S., 1963, An RNA "replicase" induced by and selective for a viral RNA: Isolation and properties, *Proc. Natl. Acad. Sci. USA* **50**:905.

Haruna, I., Nishihara, T., and Watanabe, I., 1967, Template activity of various phage RNA for replicases of Qβ and VK phages, *Proc. Jpn. Acad.* **46**:375.

Haruna, I., Itoh, Y. H., Yamane, K., Miyake, T., Shiba, T., and Watanabe, I., 1971, Isolation and properties of RNA replicases induced by SP and FI phages, *Proc. Natl. Acad. Sci. USA* **68**:1778.

Haselkorn, R., 1962, Studies on infectious RNA from turnip yellow mosaic virus, *J. Mol. Biol.* **4**:357.

Heinrikson, R. L., 1966, On the alkylation of amino acid residues at the active site of ribonuclease, *J. Biol. Chem.* **241**:1393.

Heisenberg, M., 1966, Formation of defective bacteriophage particles by fr amber mutants, *J. Mol. Biol.* **17**:136.

Held, W. A., Gette, W. R., and Nomura, M., 1974, Role of 16 S ribosomal ribonucleic acid and the 30 S ribosomal protein S12 in the initiation of natural messenger ribonucleic acid translation, *Biochemistry* **13**:2115.

Hilbers, C. W., and Schulman, R. G., 1974, Assignment of the hydrogen bonded proton resonances in (*Escherichia coli*) tRNA^{GLU} by sequential melting, *Proc. Natl. Acad. Sci. USA* **71**:3239.

Hindennach, I., and Jockush, H., 1974, Peptide mapping of Qβ proteins using cell-free synthesis, *Virology* **60**:327.

Hindley, J., and Staples, D. H., 1969, Sequence of a ribosome binding site in bacteriophage Qβ-RNA, *Nature (London)* **224**:964.

Hindley, J., Staples, D. H., Billeter, M. A., and Weissmann, C., 1970, Location of the coat cistron on the RNA of phage Qβ, *Proc. Natl. Acad. Sci. USA* **67**:1180.

Hirata, A. A., Hung, P. P., Overby, L. R., and McIntire, F. C., 1972, Antibody response to bacteriophage Qβ and its structural components in rabbits, *Immunochemistry* **9**:555.

Ho, N. W. Y., and Gilham, P. T., 1967, The reversible chemical modification of uracil, thymine, and guanine nucleotides and the modification of the action of ribonuclease on ribonucleic acid, *Biochemistry* **6**:3632.

Hofschneider, P. H., 1963, Untersuchungen über "kleine" *E. coli* K12 Bakteriophagen, *Z. Naturforsch.* **18b**:203.

Hofstetter, H., Monstein, H. J., and Weissmann, C., 1974, The readthrough protein A1 is essential for the formation of viable Qβ particles, *Biochim. Biophys. Acta* **374**:238.

Hohn, T., 1967, Formation of defective bacteriophage particles by fr amber mutants, *Eur. J. Biochem.* **2**:152.

Holley, R. W., Apgar, J., Everett, G. A., Madison, J. T., Marquisee, M., Merrill, S. H., Penswick, J. R., and Zamir, A., 1965, Structure of a ribonucleic acid, *Science* **147**:1462.

Horiuchi, K., 1975, Genetic studies of RNA phages, in: *RNA Phages* (N. D. Zinder, ed.), p. 29, Cold Spring Harbor Laboratory, Cold Spring Harbor, N.Y.

Horiuchi, K., and Adelberg, E. A., 1965, Growth of male-specific bacteriophage in *Proteus mirabilis* harboring F-genomes derived from *Escherichia coli*, *J. Bacteriol.* **89**:1231.

Horiuchi, K., and Matsuhashi, S., 1970, Three cistrons in bacteriophage Qβ, *Virology* **42**:49.

Horiuchi, K., and Zinder, N. D., 1967, Azure mutants: A type of host-dependent mutant of the bacteriophage f2, *Science* **156**:1618.

Horiuchi, K., Webster, R. E., and Matsuhashi, S., 1971, Gene products of bacteriophage Qβ, *Virology* **45**:429.

Hotham-Iglewski, B., and Franklin, R. M., 1967, Replication of bacteriophage ribonucleic acid: Alterations in polyribosome patterns and association of double-stranded RNA with polyribosomes in *Escherichia coli* infected with bacteriophage R17, *Proc. Natl. Acad. Sci. USA* **58**:743.

Hotham-Iglewski, B., Phillips, L. A., and Franklin, R. M., 1968, Viral RNA transcription–translation complex in *Escherichia coli* infected with bacteriophage R17, *Nature (London)* **219**:700.

Huez, G., Marbaix, G., Hubert, E., Cleuter, Y., Leclercq, M., Chantrenne, H., Devos, R., Soreq, H., Nudel, U., and Littauer, U. Z., 1975, Readenylation of poly-adenylate-free globin messenger RNA restores its stability *in vivo*, *Eur. J. Biochem.* **59**:589.

Inouye, H., Pollack, Y., and Petre, J., 1974, Physical and functional homology between ribosomal protein S1 and interference factor i, *Eur. J. Biochem.* **45**:109.

Isenberg, H., Cotter, R. I., and Gratzer, W. B., 1971, Secondary structure and interaction of RNA and protein in a bacteriophage, *Biochim. Biophys. Acta* **232**:184.

Iserentant, D., and Fiers, W., 1976, Modification of some hairpin loops of the MS2 genome with the methoxyamine reagent, *Arch. Intern. Physiol. Biochim.* **84**:165.

Isono, K., and Isono, S., 1976, Lack of ribosomal protein S1 in *Bacillus stearothermophilus*, *Proc. Natl. Acad. Sci. USA* **73**:767.

Isono, S., and Isono, K., 1975, Role of ribosomal protein S1 in protein synthesis: Effects of its addition to *Bacillus stearothermophilus* cell-free system, *Eur. J. Biochem.* **56**:15.

Jacobson, A. B., 1976, Studies on secondary structure of single-stranded RNA from bacteriophage MS2 by electron microscopy, *Proc. Natl. Acad. Sci. USA* **73**:307.

Jacobson, A. B., and Spahr, P. F., 1977, Studies on the secondary structure of single-stranded RNA from the bacteriophage MS2. II. Analysis of the RNase IV cleavage products, *J. Mol. Biol.* **115**:279.

Jacrot, B., Chauvin, C., and Witz, J., 1977, Comparative neutron small-angle scattering study of small spherical RNA viruses, *Nature (London)* **266**:417.

Jay, E., Bambara, R., Padmanabhan, R., and Wu, R., 1974, DNA sequence analysis:

A general, simple and rapid method for sequencing large oligoribonucleotide fragments by mapping, *Nucleic Acids Res.* **1**:331.

Jeppesen, P. G. N., 1971, The nucleotide sequences of some large ribonuclease T1 products from bacteriophage R17 ribonucleic acid, *Biochem. J.* **124**:357.

Jeppesen, P. G. N., Nichols, J. L., Sanger, F., and Barrell, B. G., 1970a, Nucleotide sequences from bacteriophage R17 RNA, *Cold Spring Harbor Symp. Quant. Biol.* **35**:13.

Jeppesen, P. G. N., Steitz, J. A., Gesteland, R. F., and Spahr, P. F., 1970b, Gene order in the bacteriophage R17 RNA: 5'-A protein–coat protein–synthetase-3', *Nature (London)* **226**:230.

Jeppesen, P. G. N., Barrell, B. F., Sanger, F., and Coulson, A. R., 1972, Nucleotide sequences of two fragments from the coat protein cistrons of bacteriophage R17 ribonucleic acid, *Biochem. J.* **128**:993.

Johnson, B., and Szekely, M., 1977, Specific binding site of *E. coli* initiation factor 3 (IF3) at a 3'-terminal region of MS2 RNA, *Nature (London)* **267**:550.

Kacian, D. L., Mills, D. R., and Spiegelman, S., 1971, The mechanism of Qβ replication: Sequence at the 5'-terminus of a 6 S RNA template, *Biochim. Biophys. Acta* **238**:212.

Kacian, D. L., Mills, D. R., Kramer, F. E., and Spiegelman, S., 1972, A replicating RNA molecule suitable for a detailed analysis of extracellular evolution and replication, *Proc. Natl. Acad. Sci. USA* **69**:3038.

Kamen, R., 1969, Infectivity of bacteriophage R17 RNA after sequential removal of 3'-terminal nucleotides, *Nature (London)* **221**:321.

Kamen, R., 1970, Characterization of the subunits of Qβ replicase, *Nature (London)* **228**:527.

Kamen, R., Kondo, M., Romer, W., and Weissmann, C., 1972, Reconstitution of Qβ replicase lacking subunit α with protein-synthesis-interference factor i, *Eur. J. Biochem.* **31**:44.

Kamen, R. I., Monstein, H. J., and Weissmann, C., 1974, The host factor requirement of Qβ RNA replicase, *Biochim. Biophys. Acta* **366**:292.

Kelley, J. J., Frist, R. H., and Kaesberg, P., 1971, Chromatography of ribonuclease T1 digests of RNA on DEAE-cellulose and DEAE-Sephadex, *Anal. Biochem.* **44**:328.

Kelly, R. B., Gould, J. L., and Sinsheimer, R. L., 1965, The replication of bacteriophage MS2. IV. RNA components specifically associated with infection, *J. Mol. Biol.* **11**:562.

Khorana, H. G., Buchi, H., Ghosh, H., Gupta, N., Jacob, T. M., Kossel, H., Morgan, R., Narang, S. A., Ohtsuka, E., and Wells, R. D., 1966, Polynucleotide synthesis and the genetic code, *Cold Spring Harbor Symp. Quant. Biol.* **31**:39.

Kitano, T., 1966a, Male specific bacteriophage in *Shigella flexneri*. I. Formation of male *Shigella flexneri* by F' mediated transfer with *Escherichia coli*, *Jpn. J. Med. Sci. Biol.* **19**:65.

Kitano, T., 1966b, Male specific bacteriophage in *Shigella flexneri*. II. Growth characteristics of phage in F'⁺ *Shigella*, *Jpn. J. Med. Sci. Biol.* **19**:171.

Knolle, P., and Hohn, T., 1975, Morphogenesis of RNA phages, in: *RNA Phages* (N. D. Zinder, ed.), p. 147, Cold Spring Harbor Laboratory, Cold Spring Harbor, N.Y.

Köhler, E., and Rohloff, H., 1974, Homologies in nucleotide sequences of RNA-phages Qβ and R17, *Z. Naturforsch.* **29c**:433.

Kolakofsky, D., and Weissmann, C., 1971, Possible mechanism for transition of viral RNA from polysome to replication complex, *Nature* (*London*) *New Biol.* **231**:42.

Kolakofsky, D., Billeter, M. A., Weber, H., Weissmann, C., 1973, Resynchronization of RNA synthesis by coliphage Qβ replicase at an internal site of the RNA template, *J. Mol. Biol.* **76**:271.

Kondo, M., Gallerani, R., and Weissmann, C., 1970, Subunit structure of Qβ replicase, *Nature* (*London*) **228**:525.

Konigsberg, W., Maita, T., Katze, J., and Weber, K., 1970, Amino acid sequence of the Qβ coat protein, *Nature* (*London*) **227**:271.

Konings, R. N. H., Ward, R., Francke, B., and Hofschneider, P. H., 1970, Gene order of RNA bacteriophage M12, *Nature* (*London*) **226**:604.

Kozak, M., and Nathans, D., 1971, Fate of maturation protein during infection by coliphage MS2, *Nature* (*London*) *New Biol.* **234**:209.

Kozak, M., and Nathans, D., 1972, Translation of the genome of a ribonucleic acid bacteriophage, *Bacteriol. Rev.* **36**:109.

Krahn, P. M., O'Callaghan, R. J., and Paranchych, W., 1972, Stages in phage R17 infection. VI. Injection of A protein and RNA into the host cell, *Virology* **47**:628.

Kramer, F. R., Mills, D. R., Cole, P. E., Nishihara, T., and Spiegelman, S., 1974, Evolution *in vitro:* Sequence and phenotype of a mutant RNA resistant to ethidium bromide, *J. Mol. Biol.* **89**:719.

Krueger, R. G., 1965, The effect of streptomycin on antibody synthesis *in vitro*, *Proc. Natl. Acad. Sci. USA* **54**:144.

Krueger, R. G., 1969, Serological relatedness of the ribonucleic acid-containing coliphages, *J. Virol.* **4**:567.

Lagerkvist, U., 1978, "Two out of three": An alternative method for codon reading, *Proc. Natl. Acad. Sci. USA* **75**:1759.

Langbeheim, M., Arnon, R., and Sela, M., 1976, Antiviral effect on MS2 coliphage obtained with a synthetic antigen, *Proc. Natl. Acad. Sci. USA* **73**:4636.

Lee, Y. F., and Wimmer, E., 1976, "Fingerprinting" high molecular weight RNA by two-dimensional gel electrophoresis: Application to poliovirus RNA, *Nucleic Acids Res.* **3**:1647.

Leffler, S., and Szer, W., 1973, Messenger selection by bacterial ribosomes, *Proc. Natl. Acad. Sci. USA* **70**:2364.

Leffler, S., and Szer, W., 1974, Purification and properties of initiation factor IF-3 from *Caulobacter crescentus*, *J. Biol. Chem.* **249**:1458.

Leffler, S., Hierowski, M., Poindexter, J. S., and Szer, W., 1971, Large scale isolation of the *Caulobacter* bacteriophage ϕCb5 and its RNA genome, *FEBS Lett.* **19**:112.

Leipold, B., and Hofschneider, P. H., 1975, Isolation of an infectious RNA–A-protein complex from the bacteriophage M12, *FEBS Lett.* **55**:50.

Levisohn, R., and Spiegelman, S., 1968, The cloning of a self-replicating RNA molecule, *Proc. Natl. Acad. Sci. USA* **60**:866.

Levisohn, R., and Spiegelman, S., 1969, Further extracellular Darwinian experiments with replicating RNA molecules: Diverse variants isolated under different selective conditions, *Proc. Natl. Acad. Sci. USA* **63**:805.

Lin, L., and Schmidt, J., 1972, Adsorption of a ribonucleic acid bacteriophage of *Pseudomonas aeruginosa*, *Arch. Mikrobiol.* **83**:120.

Lin, J.-Y., Tsung, C. M., and Fraenkel-Conrat, H., 1967, The coat protein of the RNA bacteriophage MS2, *J. Mol. Biol.* **24**:1.

Ling, V., 1971, Sequence at the 5'-end of bacteriophage f2 RNA, *Biochem. Biophys. Res. Commun.* **42**:82.

Ling, V., 1972, Fractionation and sequences of the large pyrimidine oligonucleotides from bacteriophage fd DNA, *J. Mol. Biol.* **64**:81.

Litvak, S., Tarrago, A., Tarrago-Litvak, L., and Allende, J. E., 1973, Elongation factor–viral genome interaction dependent on the aminoacylation of TYMV and TMV RNAs, *Nature (London) New Biol.* **241**:88.

Lodish, H. F., 1968a, Bacteriophage f2 RNA: Control of translation and gene order, *Nature (London)* **220**:345.

Lodish, H. F., 1968b, Polar effects of an amber mutation in f2 bacteriophage, *J. Mol. Biol.* **32**:47.

Lodish, H. F., 1969, Species specificity of polypeptide chain initiation, *Nature (London)* **224**:867.

Lodish, H. F., 1970a, Specificity in bacterial protein synthesis: Role of initiation factor and ribosomal subunits, *Nature (London)* **226**:705.

Lodish, H. F., 1970b, Secondary structure of bacteriophage f2 ribonucleic acid and the initiation of *in vitro* protein biosynthesis, *J. Mol. Biol.* **50**:689.

Lodish, H. F., 1975, Regulation of *in vitro* protein synthesis by bacteriophage RNA by RNA tertiary structure in: *RNA Phages* (N. D. Zinder, ed.), p. 301, Cold Spring Harbor Laboratory, Cold Spring Harbor, N.Y.

Lodish, H. F., 1976, Translational control of protein synthesis, *Annu. Rev. Biochem.* **45**:39.

Lodish, H. F., and Robertson, H. D., 1969, Cell-free synthesis of bacteriophage f2 maturation protein, *J. Mol. Biol.* **45**:9.

Lodish, H. F., and Zinder, N. D., 1966, Mutants of the bacteriophage f2. VIII. Control mechanisms for phage-specific syntheses, *J. Mol. Biol.* **19**:333.

Lodish, H. F., Cooper, S., and Zinder, N. D., 1964, Host-dependent mutants of the bacteriophage f2. IV. On the biosynthesis of a viral RNA polymerase, *Virology* **24**:60.

Lodish, H. F., Horiuchi, K., and Zinder, N. D., 1965, Mutants of bacteriophage f2, V. On the production of non-infectious phage particles, *Virology* **27**:139.

Loeb, T., and Zinder, N. D., 1961, A bacteriophage containing RNA, *Proc. Natl. Acad. Sci. USA* **47**:282.

Lucas-Lenard, J., and Lipmann, F., 1971, Protein biosynthesis, *Annu. Rev. Biochem.* **40**:409.

Maita, T., and Konigsberg, W., 1971, The amino acid sequence of the Qβ coat protein, *J. Biol. Chem.* **246**:5003.

Marvin, D. A., and Hoffmann-Berling, H., 1963, A fibrous DNA phage (fd) and a spherical RNA phage (fr) specific for male strains of *E. coli*, *Z. Naturforsch.* **186**:884.

Martin, J., and Webster, R. E., 1975, The *in vitro* translation of a terminating signal by a single *Escherichia coli* ribosome: The fate of the subunits, *J. Biol. Chem.* **250**:8132.

Matthews, H. R., 1968, The distribution of purine nucleotides in μ2 viral ribonucleic acid, *J. Gen. Virol.* **3**:403.

Matthews, K., and Cole, R. D., 1972a, Shell formation by capsid protein of f2 bacteriophage, *J. Mol. Biol.* **65**:1.

Matthews, K., and Cole, R. D., 1972b, Interaction of lysozyme with f2 bacteriophage, *J. Mol. Biol.* **68**:173.

McPhie, P., Hounsell, J., and Gratzer, W. B., 1966, The specific cleavage of yeast ribosomal ribonucleic acid with nucleases, *Biochemistry* **6**:988.

Merregaert, J., 1976, Struktuur van de amino-terminus van het A-eiwitgen en van een polynukleotidefragment uit het replikase-gebied van de RNA Bateriofaag MS2, Ph.D. dissertation, University of Ghent, Belgium.

Messens, E., and van Montagu, M., 1968, The synthesis of nucleoside 2'(3')-phosphate 5'-triphosphates, *FEBS Lett.* **1**:326.

Meyer, F., Weber, H., Vollenweider, H. J., and Weissmann, C., 1975, The binding sites of Qβ RNA, *Experientia* **31**:143.

Mills, D. R., Peterson, R. L., and Spiegelman, S., 1967, An extracellular Darwinian experiment with a self-duplicating nucleic acid molecule, *Proc. Natl. Acad. Sci. USA* **58**:217.

Mills, D. R., Bishop, D. H. L., and Spiegelman, S., 1968, The mechanism and direction of RNA synthesis templated by free minus strands of a "little" variant of Qβ RNA, *Proc. Natl. Acad. Sci. USA* **60**:713.

Mills, D. R., Kramer, F. R., and Spiegelman, S., 1973, Complete nucleotide sequence of a replicating RNA molecule, *Science* **180**:916.

Mills, D. R., Kramer, F. R., Dobkin, C., Nishihara, T., and Spiegelman, S. 1975, Nucleotide sequence of microvariant RNA: Another small replicating molecule, *Proc. Natl. Acad. Sci. USA* **72**:4252.

Min Jou, W., and Fiers, W., 1969, Studies on the bacteriophage MS2. VII. Structure determination of the longer polypurine sequences present in the pancreatic ribonuclease digest of the viral RNA, *J. Mol. Biol.* **40**:187.

Min Jou, W., and Fiers, W., 1970, The 3'-terminal nucleotide sequence (n = 16) of bacteriophage MS2 RNA, *FEBS Lett.* **9**:222.

Min Jou, W., and Fiers, W., 1976a, Sequence determination of Gp-rich oligonucleotides by means of the kethoxal modification, *FEBS Lett.* **66**:77.

Min Jou, W., and Fiers, W., 1976b, Studies on the bacteriophage MS2. XXXIII. Comparison of the nucleotide sequence in related bacteriophage RNAs, *J. Mol. Biol.* **106**:1047.

Min Jou, W., Fiers, W., Goodman, H., and Spahr, P., 1969, Allocation of polypurine tracts to two fragments of bacteriophage MS2 RNA, *J. Mol. Biol.* **42**:143.

Min Jou, W., Haegeman, G., and Fiers, W., 1971, Studies on the bacteriophage MS2: Nucleotide fragments from the coat protein cistron, *FEBS Lett.* **13**:105.

Min Jou, W., Haegeman, G., Ysebaert, M., and Fiers, W., 1972, Nucleotide sequence of the gene coding for the bacteriophage MS2 coat protein, *Nature (London)* **237**:82.

Min Jou, W., van Montagu, M., and Fiers, W., 1976, On the possible modulating role of the isoleucine AUA-codon in bacteriophage MS2 RNA, *Biochem. Biophys. Res. Commun.* **73**:1083.

Mitra, S., Enger, M. D., and Kaesberg, P., 1963, Physical and chemical properties of RNA from the bacterial virus R17, *Proc. Natl. Acad. Sci. USA* **50**:68.

Mitra, S. K., Lustig, F., Akesson, B., and Lagerkvist, U., 1977, Codon–anticodon recognition in the valine codon family, *J. Biol. Chem.* **252**:471.

Miyake, T., Shiba, T., and Watanabe, I., 1967, Grouping of RNA phages by a millipore filtration method, *Jpn. J. Microbiol.* **11**:203.

Miyake, T., Shiba, T., Sakurai, T., and Watanabe, I., 1969, Isolation and properties of two new RNA phages SP and FI, *Jpn. J. Microbiol.* **13**:375.

Miyake, T., Haruna, I., Shiba, T., Itoh, H., Yamane, K., and Watanabe, I., 1971,

Grouping of RNA phages based on the template specificity of their RNA replicases, *Proc. Natl. Acad. Sci. USA* **68**:2022.

Modak, M. J., and Notani, G. W., 1969, Properties of RNA containing bacteriophage f4, *Experientia* **25**:1027.

Model, P., Webster, R. E., and Zinder, N. D., 1969, The UGA codon in vitro: Chain termination and suppression, *J. Mol. Biol.* **43**:177.

Moore, C. M., Farron, F., Bohnert, D., and Weissmann, C., 1971, Possible origin of a minor virus specific protein (A1) in Qβ particles, *Nature (London) New Biol.* **234**:204.

Morrison, T. G., and Lodish, H. F., 1973, Translation of bacteriophage Qβ RNA by cytoplasmic extracts of mammalian cells, *Proc. Natl. Acad. Sci. USA* **70**:315.

Morrison, T. G., and Lodish, H. F., 1974, Recognition of protein synthesis initiation signals on bacteriophage ribonucleic acid by mammalian ribosomes, *J. Biol. Chem.* **249**:5860.

Musso, R. E., de Crombrugghe, B., Pastan, I., Sklar, J., Yot, P., and Weissman, S., 1971, The 5'-terminal nucleotide sequence of galactose messenger ribonucleic acid of *Escherichia coli*, *Proc. Natl. Acad. Sci. USA* **71**:4940.

Nathans, D., Oeschger, M. P., Eggen, K., and Shimura, Y., 1966, Bacteriophage-specific proteins in *E. coli* infected with an RNA bacteriophage, *Proc. Natl. Acad. Sci. USA* **56**:1844.

Nathans, D., Oeschger, M. P., Polmar, S. K., and Eggen, K., 1969, Regulation of protein synthesis by coliphage MS2 RNA. I. Phage protein and RNA synthesis in cells infected with suppressible mutants, *J. Mol. Biol.* **39**:279.

Nichols, J. L., 1970, Nucleotide sequence from the polypeptide chain termination region of the coat protein cistron in bacteriophage R17 RNA, *Nature (London)* **225**:147.

Nichols, J. L., and Robertson, H. D., 1971, Sequences of RNA fragments from the bacteriophage f2 coat protein cistron which differ from their R17 counterparts, *Biochim. Biophys. Acta* **228**:676.

Nirenberg, M., Caskey, T., Marshall, R., Brimacombe, R., Kellogg, D., Doctor, B., Hatfield, D., Levin, J., Rottman, F., Pestka, S., Wilcox, M., and Anderson, F., 1966, The RNA code and protein synthesis, *Cold Spring Harbor Symp. Quant. Biol.* **31**:11.

Nishihara, T., and Watanabe, I., 1969, Discrete buoyant density distribution among RNA phages, *Virology* **39**:360.

Nishihara, T., Haruna, I., and Watanabe, I., 1969, Comparison of coat proteins from three groups of RNA phages, *Virology* **37**:153.

Nishihara, T. Nozu, Y., and Okada, Y., 1970, Amino acid sequence of the coat protein of the RNA phage ZR, *J. Biochem. Jpn.* **67**:403.

Ocada, Y., Amagase, S., and Tsugita, A., 1970, Frameshift mutation in the lysozyme gene of bacteriophage T4: Demonstration of the insertion of five bases, and a summary of *in vivo* codons and lysozyme activities, *J. Mol. Biol.* **54**:219.

Olsen, R. H., and Shipley, P., 1973, Host range and properties of the *Pseudomonas aeruginosa* R factor R1822, *J. Bacteriol.* **113**:772.

Olsen, R. H., and Thomas, D. D., 1973, Characteristics and purification of PRP1, an RNA phage specific for the broad host range *Pseudomonas* R1822 drug resistance plasmid, *J. Virol.* **12**:1560.

Oriel, P. J., and Koenig, J. A., 1968, The optical rotary dispersion of MS2 bacteriophage, *Arch. Biochem. Biophys.* **127**:274.

Osborn, M., Weber, K., and Lodish, H. F., 1970a, Amino terminal peptides of RNA phage proteins synthesized in the cell free system, *Biochem. Biophys. Res. Commun.* **91**:748.

Osborn, M., Weiner, A. M., and Weber, K., 1970b, Large scale purification of A-protein from bacteriophage R17, *Eur. J. Biochem.* **17**:63.

Overby, L. R., Barlow, G. H., Doi, R. H., Jacob, H., and Spiegelman, S., 1966a, Comparison of two serologically distinct ribonucleic acid bacteriophages. II. Properties of the nucleic acids and coat proteins, *J. Bacteriol.* **92**:739.

Overby, L. R., Barlow, G. H., Doi, R. H., Jacob, H., and Spiegelman, S., 1966b, Comparison of two serologically distinct ribonucleic acid bacteriophages. I. Properties of the viral particles, *J. Bacteriol.* **91**:442.

Palmenberg, A., and Kaesberg, P., 1973, Amber mutant of bacteriophage Qβ capable of causing overproduction of Qβ replicase, *J. Virol.* **11**:603.

Paranchych, W., 1975, Attachment, ejection and penetration stages of the RNA phage infectious process, in: *RNA Phages* (N. D. Zinder, ed.), p. 85, Cold Spring Harbor Laboratory, Cold Spring Harbor, N.Y.

Paranchych, W., and Graham, A. F., 1962, Isolation and properties of an RNA-containing bacteriophage, *J. Cell. Comp. Physiol.* **60**:199.

Paranchych, W., Krahn, P. M., and Bradley, R. D., 1970, Stages in phage R17 infection, *Virology* **41**:465.

Pfeifer, D., Davis, J. E., and Sinsheimer, R. L., 1964, The replication of bacteriophage MS2. III. Asymmetric complementation between temperature-sensitive mutants, *J. Mol. Biol.* **10**:412.

Pilly, D., Niemeye, A., Schmidt, M., and Bargetzi, J. P., 1978, Enzymes for RNA sequence analysis, *J. Biol. Chem.* **253**:437.

Pinck, M., Yot, P., Chapeville, F., and Duranton, H. M., 1970, Enzymatic binding of valine to the 3'-end of TYMV-RNA, *Nature (London)* **226**:954.

Pinder, J. C., Staynov, D. Z., and Gratzer, W. B., 1974, Electrophoresis of RNA in formamide, *Biochemistry* **13**:5373.

Platt, T., and Yanofsky, C., 1975, An intercistronic region and ribosome-binding site in bacterial messenger RNA, *Proc. Natl. Acad. Sci. USA* **72**:2399.

Porter, A. G., and Hindley, J., 1973, The binding of Qβ initiated fragments to *E. coli* ribosomes, *FEBS Lett.* **33**:339.

Porter, A. G., Hindley, J., and Billeter, M. A., 1974, A sequence of 83 nucleotides containing the replicase cistron ribosome binding site of phage Qβ RNA, *Eur. J. Biochem.* **41**:413.

Radloff, R. J., and Kaesberg, P., 1973, Electrophoretic and other properties of bacteriophage Qβ: The effect of a variable number of read-through proteins, *J. Virol.* **11**:116.

RajBhandary, U. L., 1968, Studies on polynucleotides. LXXVII. The labeling of end groups in polynucleotide chains: The selective modification of diol end groups in ribonucleic acids, *J. Biol. Chem.* **243**:556.

Randerath, K., Randerath, E., Chia, L. S. Y., Gupta, R. C., and Sivarajan, M., 1974, Sequence analysis of nonradioactive RNA fragments by periodate–phosphatase digestion and chemical tritium labeling: Characterization of large oligonucleotides and oligonucleotides containing modified nucleosides, *Nucleic Acids Res.* **1**:1121.

Rappaport, I., 1970, An analysis of the inactivation of MS2 bacteriophage with antiserum, *J. Gen. Virol.* **6**:25.

Reich, E., 1974, Tumor-associated fibrinolysis, in: *Control of Proliferation in Animal*

Cells (B. Clarkson and R. Baserga, eds.), p. 351, Cold Spring Harbor Laboratory, Cold Spring Harbor, N.Y.

Remaut, E., and Fiers, W., 1972, Studies on the bacteriophage MS2. XVI. The termination signal of the A-protein cistron, *J. Mol. Biol.* **71**:243.

Rensing, U. F. E., 1973, A sequence of seventy-three nucleotides from the coliphage R17 genome, *Biochem. J.* **131**:593.

Rensing, U., and August, J. T., 1969, The 3'-terminus and the replication of phage RNA, *Nature (London)* **224**:853.

Rensing, U. F. E., and Coulson, A., 1973, Nucleotide sequences of similar size from the coliphage R17 genome, *Biochem. J.* **131**:605.

Rensing, U. F. E., and Schoenmakers, J. G. G., 1973, A sequence of 50 nucleotides from coliphage R17 RNA, *Eur. J. Biochem.* **33**:8.

Rensing, U. F. E., Coulson, A., and Schoenmakers, J. G. G., 1974, A sequence of 54 nucleotides from the A-protein cistron of coliphage R17 RNA. *Eur. J. Biochem.* **41**:431.

Ricard, B., and Salzer, W., 1975, Secondary structure formed by random RNA sequences, *Biochem. Biophys. Res. Commun.* **63**:548.

Rice, R. H., and Horst, J., 1972, Isoelectric focussing of viruses in polyacrylamide gels, *Virology* **49**:602.

Rich, A., and RajBhandary, U. L., 1976, Transfer RNA: Molecular structure, sequence and properties, *Annu. Rev. Biochem.* **45**:805.

Roblin, R., 1968, The 5'-terminus of bacteriophage R17 RNA: pppGp . . ., *J. Mol. Biol.* **31**:51.

Roberts, J. W., and Gussin, G. N., 1967, Polarity in an amber mutant of bacteriophage R17, *J. Mol. Biol.* **30**:565.

Robertson, H. D., and Jeppesen, P. G. N., 1972, Extent of variation in three related bacteriophage RNA molecules, *J. Mol. Biol.* **68**:417.

Robertson, H. D., and Lodish, H. F., 1970, Messenger characteristics of nascent bacteriophage RNA, *Proc. Natl. Acad. Sci. USA* **67**:710.

Robertson, H. D., and Zinder, N. D., 1968, Identification of the terminus of nascent f2 bacteriophage RNA, *Nature (London)* **220**:69.

Robertson, H. D., and Zinder, N. D., 1969, Purification and properties of nascent f2 phage ribonucleic acid, *J. Biol. Chem.* **244**:5790.

Robertson, H. D., Webster, R. E., and Zinder, N. D., 1968, Bacteriophage coat protein as repressor, *Nature (London)* **218**:533.

Robinson, W. E., Frist, R. H., and Kaesberg, P., 1969, Genetic coding: Oligonucleotide coding for the first six amino acid residues of the coat protein of R17 bacteriophage, *Science* **166**:1291.

Rohrmann, G. F., and Krueger, R. G., 1970, Precipitation and neutralization of bacteriophage MS2 by rabbit antibodies, *J. Immunol.* **104**:353.

Sabo, D. L., Domingo, E., Bandle, E. F., Flavell, R. A., and Weissmann, C., 1977, A guanosine to adenosine transition in the 3' terminal extracistronic region of bacteriophage Qβ RNA leading to loss of infectivity, *J. Mol. Biol.* **112**:235.

Saffhill, R., Schneider-Bernloehr, H., and Orgel, L. E., 1970, In vitro selection of bacteriophage Qβ ribonucleic acid variants resistant to ethidium bromide, *J. Mol. Biol.* **51**:531.

Sakurai, T., Miyake, T., Shiba, T., and Watanabe, I., 1968, Isolation of a possible fourth group of RNA phages, *Jpn. J. Microbiol.* **12**:544.

Samuelson, G., and Kaesberg, P., 1970, An artificial top component of R17 bacteriophage, *J. Mol. Biol.* **47**:87.

Sanger, F., and Brownlee, G. G., 1967, A two-dimensional fractionation method for radioactive nucleotides, in: *Methods in Enzymology*, Vol. 12A (L. Grossman and K. Moldave, eds.), p. 361, Academic Press, New York.

Sanger, F., Brownlee, G. G., and Barrell, B. G., 1965, A two-dimensional fractionation procedure for radioactive nucleotides, *J. Mol. Biol.* **13**:373.

Sanger, F., Air, G. M., Barrell, B. G., Brown, N. L., Coulson, A. R., Fiddes, J. C., Hutchison, C. A., III, Slocombe, P. M., and Smith, M., 1977, Nucleotide sequence of bacteriophage ϕX174 DNA, *Nature (London)* **265**:687.

Schaffner, W., Ruegg, K. J., and Weissmann, C., 1977, Nanovariant RNAs: Nucleotide sequence and interaction with bacteriophage Qβ replicase, *J. Mol. Biol.* **117**:877.

Schmidt, J. M., 1966, Observations on the adsorption of *Caulobacter* bacteriophages containing ribonucleic acid, *J. Gen. Microbiol.* **45**:347.

Schmidt, J. M., and Stanier, R. Y., 1965, Isolation and characterization of bacteriophage active against stalked bacteria, *J. Gen. Microbiol.* **39**:95.

Schreier, M. H., Staehelin, T., Gesteland, R. F., and Spahr, P. F., 1973, Translation of bacteriophage R17 and Qβ RNA in a mammalian cell-free system, *J. Mol. Biol.* **75**:575.

Schubert, D., and Franck, H., 1970, The use of 2-chloroethanol for reversible depolymerization of the protein shell of bacteriophage fr, *Z. Naturforsch.* **25b**:711.

Scott, D. W., 1965, Serological cross reactions among the RNA-containing coliphages, *Virology* **26**:85.

Semancik, J. S., Vidaver, A. K., and van Etten, J. L., 1973, Characterization of a segmented double-helical RNA from bacteriophage ϕ6, *J. Mol. Biol.* **78**:617.

Senear, A. W., and Steitz, J. A., 1976, Site-specific interaction of Qβ host factor and ribosomal protein S1 with Qβ and R17 bacteriophage RNAs, *J. Biol. Chem.* **251**:1902.

Shapiro, L., and Agabian-Keshishian, N., 1970, Specific assay for differentiation in the stalked bacterium *Caulobacter crescentus*, *Proc. Natl. Acad. Sci. USA* **67**:200.

Shapiro, L., and Bendis, I., 1975, RNA phages of bacteria other than *E. coli*, in: *RNA Phages* (N. D. Zinder, ed.), p. 397, Cold Spring Harbor Laboratory, Cold Spring Harbor, N.Y.

Shapiro, L., Agabian-Keshishian, N., and Bendis, I., 1971, Bacterial differentiation, *Science* **173**:884.

Shiba, R., 1975, Reconstitution of an infectious complex in RNA phages, *Proc. Mol. Biol. Meeting Jpn.*, p. 4.

Shiba, T., and Miyake, T., 1975, New type of infectious complex of *E. coli* RNA phage, *Nature (London)* **254**:157.

Shine, J., and Dalgarno, L., 1974, The 3'-terminal sequence of *Escherichia coli* 16 S ribosomal RNA: Complementarity to nonsense triplets and ribosome binding sites, *Proc. Nat. Acad. Sci. USA* **71**:1342.

Shine, J., and Dalgarno, L., 1975a, Terminal sequence analysis of bacterial ribosomal RNA: Correlation between the 3'-terminal-polypyrimidine sequence of 16 S RNA and translational specificity of the ribosome, *Eur. J. Biochem.* **57**:221.

Shine, J., and Dalgarno, L., 1975b, Determinant of cistron specificity in bacterial ribosomes, *Nature (London)* **254**:34.

Silberklang, M., Prochiantz, A., Haenni, A. L., and RajBhandary, U. L., 1977, Studies on the sequence of the 3'-terminal region of turnip yellow mosaic virus RNA, *Eur. J. Biochem.* **72**:465.

Silverman, P. M., Mobach, H. W., and Valentine, R. C., 1967, Sex hair (F pili) mutants of *E. coli, Biochem. Biophys. Res. Commun.* **27**:412.

Sinha, N. K., Enger, M. D., and Kaesberg, P., 1965*a*, Comparison of the pancreatic ribonuclease digestion products of R17 viral RNA and M12 viral RNA, *J. Mol. Biol.* **12**:299.

Sinha, N. K., Fujimura, R. K., and Kaesberg, P., 1965*b*, Ribonuclease digestion of R17 viral RNA, *J. Mol. Biol.* **11**:84.

Sinsheimer, R. L., 1970, The life cycle of a single-stranded DNA virus (ϕX174), in: *The Harvey Lectures*, Series 64, p. 69, Academic Press, New York.

Slegers, H., and Fiers, W., 1972*a*, Bacteriophage MS2 RNA and *Escherichia coli* 23 S ribosomal RNA have a similar conformation after reaction with formaldehyde at low pH, *FEBS Lett.* **21**:127.

Slegers, H., and Fiers, W., 1972*b*, Studies on the bacteriophage MS2. XXII. Conformation of MS2 RNA in acid medium, *Biopolymers* **12**:2007.

Slegers, H., and Fiers, W., 1972*c*, Studies on the bacteriophage MS2. XXIII. Fixation of the MS2 RNA acid structure by formaldehyde, *Biopolymers* **12**:2023.

Slegers, H., Clauwaert, J., and Fiers, W., 1973, Studies on the bacteriophage MS2. XXIV. Hydrodynamic properties of the native and acid MS2 RNA structures, *Biopolymers* **12**:2033.

Southern, E. M., 1974, An improved method for transferring nucleotides from electrophoresis strips to thin layers of ion-exchange cellulose, *Anal. Biochem.* **62**:317.

Southern, E. M., and Mitchell, A. R., 1971, Chromatography of nucleic acid digests on thin layers of cellulose impregnated with polyethyleneimine, *Biochem. J.* **123**:613.

Spahr, P. F., and Gesteland, R. F., 1968, Specific cleavage of bacteriophage R17 RNA by an endonuclease isolated from *E. coli* MRE-600, *Proc. Natl. Acad. Sci. USA* **59**:876.

Spahr, P. F., Farber, M., and Gesteland, R. F., 1969, Binding site on R17 RNA for coat protein, *Nature (London)* **222**:455.

Spahr, G., Mirault, M.-E., Imaizumi, T., and Scherrer, K., 1976, Molecular-weight determination of animal-cell RNA by electrophoresis in formamide under fully denaturing conditions on exponential polyacrylamide gels, *Eur. J. Biochem.* **62**:313.

Sprague, K. U., and Steitz, J. A., 1975, The 3'-terminal oligonucleotide of *E. coli* 16 S ribosomal RNA: The sequence in both wild-type and RNase III⁻ cells is complementary to the polypurine tracts common to mRNA initiator regions, *Nucleic Acids Res.* **2**:787.

Sprague, K. U., Steitz, J. A., Grenley, R. M., and Stocking, C. E., 1977, 3'-Terminal sequence of 16 S rRNA do not explain translational specificity differences between *E. coli* and *B. stearothermophilus* ribosomes, *Nature (London)* **267**:462.

Staehelin, M., 1959, Deactivation of virus nucleic acid with glyoxal derivatives, *Biochim. Biophys. Acta* **31**:448.

Stanley, W. B., Jr., Salas, M., Wahba, A. J., and Ochoa, S., 1966, Translation of the genetic message: Factors involved in the initiation of protein synthesis, *Proc. Natl. Acad. Sci. USA* **56**:290.

Staples, D. H., and Hindley, J., 1971, Ribosome binding site of Qβ RNA polymerase cistron, *Nature (London) New Biol.* **234**:211.

Staples, D. H., Hindley, J., Billeter, M. A., and Weissmann, C., 1971, Localization of Qβ maturation cistron ribosome binding site, *Nature (London) New Biol.* **234**:202.

Steege, D. A., 1977, 5′-terminal nucleotide sequence of *Escherichia coli* lactose repressor mRNA: Features of translational initiation and reinitiation sites, *Proc. Natl. Acad. Sci. USA* **74**:4163.

Steinschneider, A., and Fraenkel-Conrat, H., 1966, Studies of nucleotide sequences in tobacco mosaic virus ribonucleic acid. IV. Use of aniline in stepwise degradation, *Biochemistry* **5**:2735.

Steitz, J. A., 1969, Polypeptide chain initiation: Nucleotide sequences of the three ribosomal binding sites in bacteriophage R17 RNA, *Nature (London)* **224**:957.

Steitz, J. A., 1972, Oligonucleotide sequences of replicase initiation site in Qβ RNA, *Nature (London) New Biol.* **236**:71.

Steitz, J. A., 1973a, Specific recognition of non-initiated regions in RNA bacteriophage messengers by ribosomes of *Bacillus stearothermophilus*, *J. Mol. Biol.* **73**:1.

Steitz, J. A., 1973b, Discriminatory ribosome rebinding of isolated regions of protein synthesis initiation from the ribonucleic acid of bacteriophage R17, *Proc. Natl. Acad. Sci. USA* **70**:2605.

Steitz, J. A., 1974, Specific recognition of the isolated R17 replicase initiator region by R17 coat protein, *Nature (London)* **248**:223.

Steitz, J. A., 1979, Genetic signals and nucleotide sequences in messenger RNA, in: *Biological Regulation and Development*, Vol. 1: *Gene Expression* (R. Goldberger, ed.), p. 349, Plenum Press, New York.

Steitz, J. A., and Jakes, K., 1975, How ribosomes select initiator regions in mRNA: Base pair formation between the 3′ terminus of 16 S rRNA and the mRNA during initiation of protein synthesis in *Escherichia coli*, *Proc. Natl. Acad. Sci. USA* **72**:4734.

Steitz, J. A., and Steege, D. A., 1977, Characterization of two mRNA·rRNA complexes implicated in the initiation of protein biosynthesis, *J. Mol. Biol.* **114**:545.

Steitz, J. A., Sprague, K. U., Steege, D. A., Yuan, R. C., Laughrea, M., Moore, P. B., and Wahba, A. J., 1977, RNA-RNA and protein-RNA interactions during the initiation of protein synthesis. In: *Symposium on Nucleic Acid–Protein Recognition* (R. Vogel, ed.), p. 491, Academic, New York.

Stent, G. S., 1964, The operon: On its third anniversary, *Science* **144**:816.

Stoll, E., Wilson, K. J., Reiser, J., and Weissmann, C., 1977a, Revised amino acid sequence of Qβ coat protein between positions 1 and 60, *J. Biol. Chem.* **252**:990.

Stoll, E., Wilson, J., and Weissmann, C., 1977b, The revised amino-acid sequence of Qβ coat protein, *Experientia* **32**:813.

Strauss, J. H., Jr., and Sinsheimer, R. L., 1963, Purification and properties of bacteriophage MS2 and of its ribonucleic acid, *J. Mol. Biol.* **7**:43.

Strauss, J. H., Jr., and Sinsheimer, R. L., 1967, Characterization of an infectivity assay for the ribonucleic acid of bacteriophage MS2, *J. Virol.* **1**:711.

Strauss, J. H., and Sinsheimer, R. L., 1968, Initial kinetics of degradation of MS2 ribonucleic acid by ribonuclease, heat, and·alkali and the presence of configurational restraints in the ribonucleic acid, *J. Mol. Biol.* **34**:453.

Strauss, J. H., Jr., Kelly, R. B., and Sinsheimer, R. L., 1968, Denaturation of RNA with dimethyl sulfoxide, *Biopolymers* **6**:793.

Stubbs, G., Warren, S., and Holmes, K., 1977, Structure of RNA and RNA binding site in tobacco mosaic virus from 4-Å map calculated from X-ray fibre diagrams, *Nature (London)* **267**:216.

Sugiyama, T., 1965, 5'-Linked end group of RNA from bacteriophage MS2, *J. Mol. Biol.* **11**:856.

Sugiyama, T., 1971, Interaction of MS2 coat protein with MS2 RNA, *Recent Progr. Microbiol.* **10**:296.

Sugiyama, T., and Nakada, D., 1967, Control of translation of MS2 RNA cistrons by MS2 coat protein, *Proc. Natl. Acad. Sci. USA* **57**:1744.

Sugiyama, T., and Nakada, D., 1968, Translational control of bacteriophage MS2 RNA cistrons by MS2 coat protein: Polyacrylamide gel electrophoresis analysis of proteins synthesized in vitro, *J. Mol. Biol.* **31**:431.

Sugiyama, T., Hebert, R. R., and Hartman, K. A., 1967, Ribonucleoprotein complexes formed between bacteriophage MS2 RNA and MS2 protein *in vitro*, *J. Mol. Biol.* **25**:455.

Sumper, M., and Luce, R., 1975, Evidence for de novo production of self-replicating and environmentally adapted RNA structures by bacteriophage Qβ replicase, *Proc. Natl. Acad. Sci. USA* **72**:162.

Szekely, M., and Sanger, F., 1969, Use of polynucleotide kinase in fingerprinting non-radioactive nucleic acids, *J. Mol. Biol.* **43**:607.

Szer, W., Hermoso, J. M., and Leffler, S., 1975, Ribosomal protein S1 and polypeptide chain initiation in bacteria, *Proc. Natl. Acad. Sci. USA* **72**:2325.

Takanami, M., 1966, The 5'-terminus of *E. coli* ribosomal RNA and f2 bacteriophage RNA, *Cold Spring Harbor Symp. Quant. Biol.* **31**:611.

Takanami, M., Yan, Y., and Jukes, T. H., 1965, Studies on the site of ribosomal binding of f2 bacteriophage RNA, *J. Mol. Biol.* **12**:761.

Taniguchi, T., and Weissmann, C., 1978, Site-directed mutations in the initiator region of the bacteriophage Qβ coat cistron and their effect on ribosome binding, *J. Mol. Biol.* **118**:533.

Taniguchi, T., Palmieri, M., and Weissmann, C., 1978, Qβ DNA-containing hybrid plasmids giving rise to Qβ phage formation in the bacterial host, *Nature (London)* **274**:223.

Thirion, J.-P., and Kaesberg, P., 1968a, The pyrimidine catalogs of M12 and R17 ribonucleic acids, *J. Mol. Biol.* **33**:379.

Thirion, J.-P., and Kaesberg, P., 1968b, Sequence determination of oligonucleotides obtained from pancreatic ribonuclease digests of M12 and R17 RNAs, *Biochim. Biophys. Acta* **161**:247.

Thirion, J.-P., and Kaesberg, P., 1970, Base sequence of polypurine regions of the RNAs of bacteriophages R17 and M12, *J. Mol. Biol.* **47**:193.

Thomas, C. J., Jr., and Hartman, K. A., 1973, Raman studies of nucleic acids. VIII. Estimation of RNA secondary structure from Raman scattering by phosphate-group vibrations, *Biochim. Biophys. Acta* **312**:311.

Thomas, C. J., Jr., Prescott, B., McDonald-Ordzie, P. E., and Hartman, K. A., 1976, Studies of virus structure by laser-Raman spectroscopy, *J. Mol. Biol.* **102**:103.

Tinoco, I., Jr., Uhlenbeck, O. C., and Levine, M. D., 1971, Estimation of secondary structure in ribonucleic acids, *Nature (London)* **230**:362.

Tinoco, I., Jr., Borer, P. N., Dengler, B., Levine, M. D., Uhlenbeck, O. C., Crothers, D. M., and Gralla, J., 1973, Improved estimation of secondary structure in ribonucleic acids, *Nature (London) New Biol.* **246**:40.

Tooze, J., and Weber, K., 1967, Isolation and characterization of amber mutants of bacteriophage R17, *J. Mol. Biol.* **28**:311.

Truden, J. L., and Franklin, R. M., 1972, Polysomal localization of R17 bacteriophage-specific protein synthesis, *J. Virol.* **9**:75.

Turchinsky, M. F., Musova, K. S., and Budowsky, E. I., 1974, Conversion of non-covalent interactions in nucleoproteins into covalent bonds: Bisulfide-induced formation of polynucleotide-protein crosslinks in MS2 bacteriophage virions, *FEBS Lett.* **38**:304.

Uhlenbeck, O. C., Borer, P. N., Dengler, B., and Tinoco, I., Jr., 1973, Stability of RNA hairpin loops: A_6-C_m-U_6, *J. Mol. Biol.* **73**:483.

Van Assche, W., and van Montagu, M., 1974, Isolation of acidic coat mutants of the RNA bacteriophage MS2 by use of polyacrylamide gel electrophoresis, *Arch. Intern Physiol. Biochim.* **82**:778.

Van Assche, W., Vandekerckhove, J., Gielen, J., and van Montagu, M., 1972, Anti-serum-resistant mutants of the RNA bacteriophage MS2, *Arch. Intern. Physiol. Biochim.* **80**:410.

Van Assche, W., Vandekerckhove, J., and van Montagu, M., 1974, Mutation sites in the coat-protein gene of bacteriophage MS2, *Arch. Intern. Physiol. Biochim.* **82**:1020.

Vandamme, E., Remaut, E., van Montagu, M., and Fiers, W., 1972, Studies on the bacteriophage MS2. XVII. Suppressor-sensitive mutants of the A-protein cistron, *Mol. Gen. Genet.* **117**:219.

Vandekerckhove, J., 1972, Bepaling van de aminozuursekwenties van wild-type- en mutant manteleiwit bij de bacteriofaag MS2, Ph.D. dissertation, University of Ghent, Belgium.

Vandekerckhove, J. S., and van Montagu, M., 1977, Sequence of the A-protein of coliphage MS2, *J. Biol. Chem.* **252**:7773.

Vandekerckhove, J., Gielen, J., Lenaerts, A., van Assche, W., and van Montagu, M., 1971, Difference between the nitrous acid-induced and the hydroxylamine-induced amber mutants in the RNA bacteriophage MS2. *Arch. Intern. Physiol. Biochim.* **79**:636.

Vandekerckhove, J. S., Nolf, F., and van Montagu, M., 1973, The amino acid sequence at the carboxyl terminus of the maturation protein of bacteriophage MS2, *Nature (London) New Biol.* **241**:102.

Vandekerckhove, J., van Assche, W., Vingerhoed, J.-P., and van Montagu, M., 1975, Approaches to the determination of the protein configuration in particles of bacteriophage MS2, *Abstr. 3rd Int. Congr. Virol.*, Madrid.

Vandenberghe, A., van Styvendaele, B., and Fiers, W., 1969, Studies on the bacteriophage MS2. VI. The nucleoside 5'-triphosphate end groups of the replicative intermediate and the replicative form, *Eur. J. Biochem.* **7**:174.

Vandenberghe, A., Min Jou, W., and Fiers, W., 1975, 3'-Terminal nucleotide sequence ($n = 361$) of bacteriophage MS2 RNA, *Proc. Natl. Acad. Sci. USA* **72**:2559.

van Dieijen, G., van Knippenberg, P., and van Duin, J., 1976, The specific role of ribosomal protein S1 in the recognition of native phage RNA, *Eur. J. Biochem.* **64**:511.

van Dieijen, G., van Knippenberg, P. H., van Duin, J., Koekman, B., and Pouwels, P. H., 1977, The effect of the ribosomal protein S1 from *Escherichia coli* on the synthesis *in vitro* of bacterial-, DNA phage- and RNA phage proteins, *Mol. Gen. Genet.* **153**:75.

van Duin, J., Kurland, C. G., Dondon, J., and Grunberg-Manago, M., 1975, Near neighbors of IF3 bound to 30 S ribosomal subunits, *FEBS Lett.* **59**:287.

van Etten, J. L., Vidaver, A. K., Koski, R. K., and Burnett, J. P., 1974, Base composition and hybridization studies of the three double-stranded RNA segments of bacteriophage $\phi6$, *J. Virol.* **13**:1254.

van Montagu, M., 1968, Studies with amber and UGA mutants of the RNA phage MS2, *Arch. Intern. Physiol. Biochim.* **76**:393.

van Montagu, M., Leurs, C., Brachet, P., and Thomas, R., 1967, A set of amber mutants of bacteriophages λ and MS2 suitable for the identification of suppressors, *Mutat. Res.* **4**:698.

Vasquez, C., Granboulan, N., and Franklin, R. M., 1966, Structure of the ribonucleic acid bacteriophage R17, *J. Bacteriol.* **92**:1779.

Verbraeken, E., and Fiers, W., 1972a, Studies on the bacteriophage MS2. XX. Expansion of the virion in low salt, *Virology* **50**:690.

Verbraeken, E., and Fiers, W., 1972b, Further evidence on the role of the A-protein in bacteriophage MS2 particles, *FEBS Lett.* **28**:89.

Vidaver, A. K., Koski, R. K., and van Etten, J. L., 1973, Bacteriophage φ6: A lipid-containing virus of *Pseudomonas phaseolicola*, *J. Virol.* **11**:799.

Vinuela, E., Algranati, I. D., and Ochoa, S., 1967, Synthesis of virus-specific proteins in *Escherichia coli* infected with the RNA bacteriophage MS2, *Eur. J. Biochem.* **1**:3.

Vinuela, E., Algraniti, I. D., Feix, G., Garwes, D., Weissmann, C., and Ochoa, S., 1968, Virus-specific proteins in *Escherichia coli* infected with some amber mutants of phage MS2, *Biochim. Biophys. Acta* **155**:558.

Volckaert, G., and Fiers, W., 1973, Studies on the bacteriophage MS2: G-U-G as the initiation codon of the A-protein cistron, *FEBS Lett.* **35**:91.

Volckaert, G., and Fiers, W., 1974, A simple and highly sensitive method for sequence determination of ^{32}P-labeled oligonucleotides, *Anal. Biochem.* **62**:573.

Volckaert, G., and Fiers, W., 1977, Micro thin-layer techniques for rapid sequence analysis of ^{32}P-labeled RNA: Double digestion and pancreatic ribonuclease analysis, *Anal. Biochem.* **83**:228.

Volckaert, G., Min Jou, W., and Fiers, W., 1976, Analysis of ^{32}P-labeled bacteriophage MS2-RNA by a mini-fingerprinting procedure, *Anal. Biochem.* **72**:433.

Vollenweider, H. J., Koller, T. H., Weber, H., and Weissmann, C., 1976, Physical mapping of Qβ RNA, *J. Mol. Biol.* **101**:367.

Wahba, A. J., Miller, M. J., Niveleau, A., Landers, T. A., Carmichael, G., Weber, K., Hawley, D. A., and Slobin, L. J., 1974, Subunit I of Qβ replicase and 30 S ribosomal protein S1 of *Escherichia coli*, *J. Biol. Chem.* **249**:3314.

Walz, A., Pirrotta, U., and Ineichen, K., 1976, λ Repressor regulates the switch between P_R and P_{RM} promoters, *Nature (London)* **262**:665.

Ward, R., Strand, M., and Valentine, R. C., 1968, Translational repression of f2 protein synthesis, *Biochem. Biophys. Res. Commun.* **30**:310.

Watanabe, H., and Watanabe, M., 1970, Comparative biology of five RNA phages, R23, f2, Qβ, R34, and R40, *Can. J. Microbiol.* **16**:859.

Watanabe, I., Miyake, T., Sakurai, T., Shiba, T., and Ohno, T., 1967a, Isolation and grouping of RNA phages, *Proc. Jpn. Acad.* **43**:204.

Watanabe, I., Nishihara, T., Kaneko, H., Sakurai, T., and Osawa, S., 1967b, Group characteristics of RNA phages, *Proc. Jpn. Acad.* **43**:210.

Watanabe, M., and August, J. T., 1968, Identification of guanosine triphosphate on the 5'-terminus of RNA from bacteriophage Qβ and R23, *Biochemistry* **59**:513.

Watanabe, M., Watanabe, H., and August, J. T., 1968, Replication of RNA bacteriophage R23. I. Quantitative aspects of phage RNA and protein synthesis, *J. Mol. Biol.* **33**:1.

Weber, K., 1967, Amino acid sequence studies on the tryptic peptides of the coat protein of the bacteriophage R17, *Biochemistry* **6**:3144.

Weber, H., 1976, The binding site for coat protein on bacteriophage Qβ RNA, *Biochim. Biophys. Acta* **418**:175.

Weber, K., and Konigsberg, W., 1967, Amino acid sequence of the f2 coat protein, *J. Biol. Chem.* **242**:3563.

Weber, K., and Konigsberg, W., 1975, Proteins of the RNA phage, in: *RNA Phages* (N. D. Zinder, ed.), p. 51, Cold Spring Harbor Laboratory, Cold Spring Harbor, N.Y.

Weber, H., and Weissmann, C., 1970, The 3'-termini of bacteriophage Qβ plus and minus strands, *J. Mol. Biol.* **51**:215.

Weber, H., Billeter, M. A., Kahane, S., Weissmann, C., Hindley, J., and Porter, A., 1972, Molecular basis for repressor activity of Qβ replicase, *Nature (London)* **237**:166.

Weber, H., Kamen, R., Meyer, F., and Weissmann, C., 1974, Interactions between Qβ replicase and Qβ RNA, *Experientia* **30**:711.

Weiner, A. M., and Weber, K., 1971, Natural read-through at the UGA termination signal of Qβ coat protein cistron, *Nature (London) New Biol.* **234**:206.

Weiner, A. M., and Weber, K., 1973, A signal UGA codon functions as a natural termination signal in the coliphage Qβ coat protein cistron, *J. Mol. Biol.* **80**:837.

Weiner, A. M., Platt, T., and Weber, K., 1972, Amino terminal sequence analysis of protein purified on a nanomole scale by gel electrophoresis, *J. Biol. Chem.* **247**:3242.

Weissmann, C., and Ochoa, S., 1967, Replication of phage RNA, *Progr. Nucl. Acid. Res. Mol. Biol.* **6**:353.

Weissmann, C., Billeter, M. A., Goodman, H. M., Hindley, J., and Weber, H., 1973, Structure and function of phage RNA, *Annu. Rev. Biochem.* **42**:303.

Weith, H. L., and Gilham, P. T., 1967, Structural analysis of polynucleotides by sequential base elimination: The sequence of the terminal decanucleotide fragment of the ribonucleic acid from bacteriophage f2, *J. Am. Chem. Soc.* **89**:5473.

Weith, H. L., and Gilham, P. T., 1969, Polynucleotide sequence analysis by sequential base elimination: 3'-Terminus of phage Qβ RNA, *Science* **166**:1004.

Weppelman, R. M., and Brinton, C. C., Jr., 1971, The infection of *Pseudomonas aeruginosa* by RNA pilus phage PP7: The adsorption organelle and the relationship between phage sensitivity and the division cycle, *Virology* **44**:1.

Wittman-Liebold, B., and Wittman, H. G., 1967, Coat proteins of strains of two RNA viruses: Comparison of their amino acid sequences, *Mol. Gen. Genet.* **100**:358.

Wong, K., Morgan, A. R., and Paranchych, W., 1974, Controlled cleavage of phage R17 RNA within the virion by treatment with ascorbate and copper (II), *Can. J. Biochem.* **52**:950.

Wong, K. L., Wong, Y. P., and Kearns, D. R., 1975, Investigation of the thermal unfolding of secondary and tertiary structure in *E. coli* tRNA^{fMET} by high-resolution NMR, *Biopolymer* **14**:749.

Ysebaert, M., 1975, Nukleotidesekwentiebepaling van een intercistronisch gebied en van segmenten uit de drie genen, leidend tot de volledige struktuuropheldering van bakteriofaag MS2 RNA, Ph.D. dissertation, University of Ghent, Belgium.

Zinder, N. D., 1965, RNA phages, *Annu. Rev. Biochem.* **33**:455.

Zinder, N. D. (ed.), 1975, *RNA Phages*, Cold Spring Harbor Laboratory, Cold Spring Harbor, N.Y.

Zinder, N. D., and Cooper, S., 1964, Host-dependent mutants of the bacteriophage f2.
    I. Isolation and preliminary classification, *Virology* **23**:152.
Zipper, P., and Folkhard, W., 1975, A small-angle X-ray scattering investigation on the
    structure of the RNA from bacteriophage MS2, *FEBS Lett.* **56**:283.
Zipper, P., Kratky, O., Herrmann, R., and Hohn, T., 1971, An X-ray small angle study
    of the bacteriophage fr and R17, *Eur. J. Biochem.* **18**:1.

CHAPTER 4

DNA Sequencing of Viral Genomes

Gillian M. Air

Department of Microbiology
The John Curtin School of Medical Research
Australian National University
Canberra, A.C.T.
Australia

1. INTRODUCTION

In his book *Biochemistry* Lehninger (1970) illustrated the complexity of the genetic material by devoting a full page to closely spaced arrays of A, G, C, and T letters, calling this "an imaginary base sequence for the chromosome of bacteriophage ϕX174" and pointing out that this is one of the smallest DNA genomes known. There has been a remarkable revolution in DNA sequencing technology since that page was composed. Not only has the real nucleotide sequence of ϕX174 been published (Sanger *et al.*, 1977a), but also DNA sequences of bacteriophages G4 (Godson *et al.*, 1978) and fd (Schaller *et al.*, 1978) and an animal virus, SV40 (Reddy *et al.*, 1978a; Fiers *et al.*, 1978) are completed, or nearly so, and a remarkable array of DNA sequences from various sources is fast accumulating.

The two techniques which made sequencing of whole genomes a relatively short-term project are those of Sanger and Coulson (1975) and Maxam and Gilbert (1977). Both methods depend on the fact that single-stranded DNA fragments will run on polyacrylamide gel electrophoresis strictly according to size. Hence if, in a set of different-length fragments from a fixed end point, the terminal (or terminal plus one) nucleotide of each product is identified, then the sequence of neucleotides can be read from the position of each product on the gel. The method of sorting the various size classes of oligonucleotides according to the sequence is entirely different in the two techniques. Sanger and Coulson (1975) use a staggered primed synthesis of DNA, incorporating an $[\alpha\text{-}^{32}P]$deoxyribonucleoside triphosphate, while Maxam and Gilbert (1977) use partial chemical degradation after labeling one end of the oligonucleotide with ^{32}P. Both methods have been greatly facilitated by the increasing catalogue of sequence-specific endonucleases, the restriction enzymes (Roberts, 1976). Using one or more restriction enzymes, practically any region of DNA can be broken down into fragments of 100–200 nucleotide pairs, which is the ideal length for either of the rapid sequence methods.

1.1. The Sanger and Coulson Sequencing Method

Otherwise known as the "plus and minus" technique, the Sanger and Coulson (1975) method involves two stages of DNA synthesis. Starting with a single-stranded DNA template, a complementary sequence is annealed as primer. The primer can be a synthetic oligonucleotide or, usually easier to obtain, a double-stranded restriction fragment of which only the strand complementary to the template will anneal. The four deoxynucleoside triphosphates, one of which is $\alpha\text{-}^{32}P$ labeled, and *Escherichia coli* DNA polymerase I are added. DNA synthesis is random, and to ensure a mixture of lengths of the synthesized products aliquots are taken at various times and the synthesis is terminated. All these aliquots are recombined, when ideally every possible length of product from one to, say, 200 residues is present. If the primer is a long fragment, it is removed with the appropriate restriction enzyme and the remaining products are resolved by polyacrylamide gel electrophoresis in urea. Each band on the gel is related to the next slowest by addition of one nucleotide. Two methods are used to identify this nucleotide for each size of synthesized DNA. In theory, either the "minus" or the "plus" system alone is sufficient, but in practice neither works perfectly all the time and both are used to obtain the sequence.

1.1.1. The Minus System

The synthesized mixture of oligonucleotides is divided into eight aliquots: four for the minus reaction and four for the plus reactions. In the minus system the oligonucleotides are elongated with DNA polymerase and three nucleoside triphosphates. The fourth triphosphate is missing; hence in each of the four reaction mixtures, missing dATP, dGTP, dCTP, and dTTP, respectively, synthesis continues to the point where it stops because the nucleoside triphosphate specified by the template is missing. The "−A" mix, for instance, which started with every possible length of product, now contains only those lengths where the next nucleotide would be an A. The "−G" mix contains a different set of lengths of oligonucleotides, where the next residue would be a G, and so for the −C and −T mixes. The result is that every possible length of product is now in one mix or another, and when the four mixes are run side by side on a polyacrylamide gel after cleaving off the restriction fragment primer and dissociating the template by heating in formamide, the sequence of nucleotides can be read off an autoradiograph of the gel by noting in which mix each band (size) occurs, starting with the smallest fragments at the bottom of the gel.

1.1.2.   The Plus System

To the second four aliquots of the original elongation mix are added dATP, dGTP, dCTP, or dTTP, and DNA polymerase from phage T4-infected *E. coli* (T4 polymerase). This enzyme degrades double-stranded DNA from the 3′ end, but if a single nucleoside triphosphate is present the exonuclease action effectively stops, since the nucleotide is polymerized in faster than it is exonucleased out (Englund, 1971, 1972). Hence the "+A" mix will contain only those products where A is the 3′ nucleotide: the pattern of bands should be the same as in the −A reaction, but one nucleotide longer. The sequence can therefore be read from an autoradiograph of the polyacrylamide gel with all four plus reactions run side by side. In practice, the four minus reactions and the four plus reactions are run on the same gel so that use can be made of the one-nucleotide relationship between a "−N" and a "+N" product.

1.1.3.   Interpretation of the Sequence

Ideally, either the minus or the plus system should give the complete nucleotide sequence of 100–200 residues, but certain problems can occur. The most important is that where there is a "run" of a particular nucleotide only one product is usually seen, which is the shortest in the minus reaction and the longest in the plus reaction. Measuring the distance between these products indicates the number of nucleotides not seen, but where the run is of four nucleotides or more, and especially toward the top of the gel, it is difficult to be sure of the length of the run. Sometimes bands are missing completely, and occasionally artifact bands appear. These missing and extra bands are usually not consistent in different incorporations, and repeating the experiment will often remove any ambiguities. Persistent problems can occur where there is secondary structure in the DNA template (Fiddes, 1976). Priming from another site or using the complementary single strand as template helps to confirm the sequence. Modifications have been made to the original procedure (Air *et al.*, 1976*b*; Brown and Smith, 1977*b*), but it is wise to check the sequence obtained by some other method, such as depurination analysis of both strands of a short restriction fragment (Fiddes, 1976; Brown and Smith, 1977*b*), or in coding regions the sequence can be compared to a known amino acid sequence (Air *et al.*, 1975, 1976*a*,*b*; Barrell *et al.*, 1976).

The four gels shown in Fig. 1 plus one other give a continuous sequence of 352 nucleotides from gene G of ϕX174 (Air *et al.*, 1976*b*). Each experiment was repeated several times to check that the results were consistent, but since the entire sequencing procedure is completed in 24 hr the time and effort involved are remarkably small for such a large amount of information.

1.2. The Maxam and Gilbert Sequencing Method

The chemical method of sequencing can be applied to either single- or double-stranded DNA fragments. The fragment is labeled at one end: at the 3' end using terminal transferase (Roychoudhury *et al.*, 1976) and [α-^{32}P]-ATP or at the 5' end using polynucleotide kinase (Richardson, 1971; van de Sande *et al.*, 1973; Lillehaug and Kleppe, 1975) and [γ-^{32}P]-ATP. In general, the latter reaction is more satisfactory for the sequence work, since [γ-^{32}P]-ATP can be obtained at over 10 times the specific activity of [α-^{32}P]-ATP. The complementary strands of the fragment are separated by electrophoresis after denaturation, or else the fragment is cleaved by another restriction enzyme into two unequal fragments which are separated as the double-stranded structures, each having the ^{32}P end-label on only one strand.

The DNA is then partially degraded by reagents which first damage then excise a base from its sugar. This sugar is very susceptible to alkali or amine cleavage of both 3' and 5' phosphates. Although there are no reagents of absolute base specificity for cleavage, the purine and pyrimidine reagents will, under appropriate conditions, preferably attack adenine or guanine, or cytosine or thymine, respectively. Since the ^{32}P label is at only one end of the DNA fragment, partial cleavage will generate a series of products which can be seen on the autoradiograph of an acrylamide gel only when that end is intact. In other words, a specific set of lengths is obtained for cleavage at a specific nucleotide, and the sequence is read off the autoradiograph as in the Sanger and Coulson (1975) method.

1.2.1. Purine Cleavage

Dimethylsulfate methylates guanine at the N-7 position and adenine at the N-3 (Lawley and Brookes, 1963). The methylation weakens the glycosidic bond, which breaks on heating and alkali then cleaves the sugar–phosphate bonds. Since guanine methylates fivefold faster than adenine, the reaction mixture when run on the acrylamide gel shows dark bands where a guanine has reacted and light bands where there was an adenine in the sequence. The difference in intensities is not always so marked as expected; hence in another reaction mix the methylated DNA is treated with dilute acid. The glycosidic bond of methylated adenine is less stable than that of methylated guanine, and the adenines are preferentially released, giving darker bands than those of guanines. Comparison of the two sets of conditions enables the sequence to be read.

1.2.2. Pyrimidine Cleavage

Hydrazine is used to cleave thymine and cytosine (Cashmore and Petersen, 1969); then treatment with piperidine displaces the products

---

→

Fig. 1. Four autoradiographs of sequences from gene G of ϕX174 determined by the Sanger and Coulson (1975) method. A: The sequence obtained by priming with fragments *Hha*2. The nucleotide numbered "1" is 57 residues from the priming site and the sequence is read to 145 nucleotides from the site. B: The sequence primed by fragment *Hinf*4. The first nucleotide shown is 31 from the priming site. Although the sequence extends for 91 nucleotides, there are several artifact bands, while other bands were missing. This experiment was repeated several times to obtain the sequence shown, which was confirmed by the amino acid sequence. C: The sequence primed by fragment *Hap*5. The gel shown is the long electrophoretic run, in which the first nucleotide indicated is 107 from the priming site. The short electrophoresis run (not shown) overlapped the data obtained from gel B. D: The sequence primed by fragment *Hinf*8. The continuous sequence obtained from five polyacrylamide gel electrophoreses is 352 nucleotides long. From Air *et al.* (1976*b*), with permission.

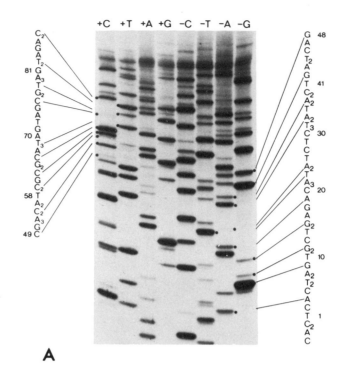

A

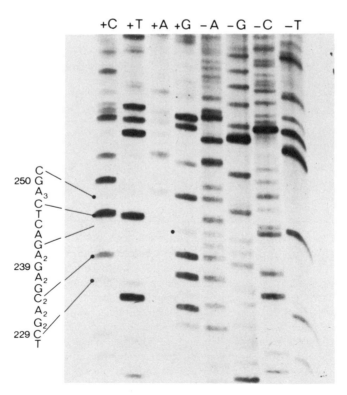

C

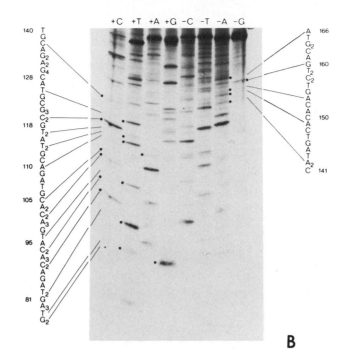

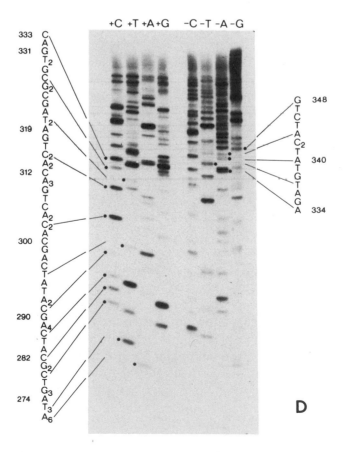

of hydrazinolysis from the sugars and catalyzes cleavage of the phosphate bonds. The reaction is much the same for thymine and cytosine, but in 2 M NaCl the reaction of thymine is suppressed and bands are obtained only from cytosine. The complete sequence can therefore be read from four slots on the gel: G > A; A > G; C + T; C.

One distinct advantage of this method is that every band in a run can usually be seen; hence there is less doubt about the length of the sequence. The chemical method is also less sensitive to any secondary structure in the DNA, which can lead to problems in interpreting results from the enzymatic method of Sanger and Coulson. Sometimes the distinction between G and A is not clear enough to be confident of the sequence (Scherer *et al.*, 1977; Efstratiadis *et al.*, 1977), or the resolution of a run of bands is poor (Bennett *et al.*, 1978), and alternative methods (including sequencing the complementary strand) are required to confirm the sequence.

Figure 2 shows two autoradiographs of Maxam–Gilbert gels of a sequence from the VP2-VP3 gene of SV40. The sequences run in both directions from an *AluI* restriction site and total 112 nucleotides. Longer electrophoresis of the same reaction mixes extended the sequence obtained to 179 nucleotides (Contreras *et al.*, 1977*a*).

1.3.   Chain-Termination Sequencing Method

Sanger *et al.* (1977*b*) have developed a DNA sequencing method which is considerably simpler than either the plus-minus or the Maxam–Gilbert technique. This method relies on primed synthesis of DNA, incorporating a [^{32}P]-dNTP, but also including an abnormal nucleoside triphosphate which is incorporated but which terminates DNA synthesis. The terminators which have been used are 2′,3′-dideoxy-(thymidine, cytidine, adenosine, and guanosine) triphosphates. The four arabinoside triphosphates can also be used when *E. coli* DNA polymerase I is the synthesizing enzyme and low temperature is used. Mammalian DNA polymerases and the *E. coli* enzyme at 37°C, such as during removal of the primer by a restriction enzyme, may not terminate at the arabinotide, so the dideoxy derivatives are probably more reliable. The proportion of dideoxy or arabinoside to normal triphosphate is such that only partial incorporation of the terminator occurs.

The sample of template single-stranded DNA with annealed primer is therefore divided into four, and each aliquot is incubated with the four deoxyribonucleoside triphosphates (one of which is α-^{32}P labeled),

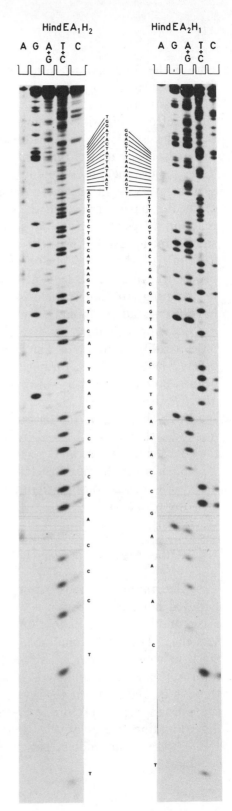

Fig. 2. Two autoradiographs of the Maxam and Gilbert (1977) method to obtain a sequence from the VP2-VP3 gene of SV40 (Contreras *et al.*, 1977*a*). The sequences run in both directions from an *Alu*I site. *Hind*EA$_2$H$_1$ is the coding strand sequence commencing with the T of the *Alu* recognition sequence AGCT. *Hind*EA$_1$H$_2$ is the complementary strand sequence commencing with the T of the restriction site sequence. The sequences read total 112 nucleotides. Longer electrophoresis runs of the same mixtures enabled another 29 nucleotides to be added to the sequence from *Hind*EA$_1$H$_2$ and 38 to that from *Hind*EA$_2$H$_1$, so that the continuous sequence of 179 nucleotides was obtained from four polyacrylamide gels.

one of the four chain-terminating inhibitors, and DNA polymerase I (Klenow fragment). After the incubation a "cold" chase is given to avoid any termination due to the limiting concentration of the ^{32}P-labeled nucleoside triphosphate. Elongation of individual DNA molecules is therefore stopped whenever an inhibitor molecule is incorporated. This happens randomly, so when the mix containing dideoxy-TTP, for instance, is run on a polyacrylamide gel, a radioactive band is seen at every position where there is a T since a certain proportion of molecules have terminated there. The pattern of bands from the four reaction mixes then gives the sequence as in the plus-minus method. A significant advantage over the plus-minus method is that every band in a "run" of the same nucleotide appears, as in the Maxam–Gilbert procedure. In general, sequences from 15 to about 200 nucleotides from the priming site can be determined in one experiment, and sequences have been read to about 300 nucleotides (Sanger *et al.*, 1977*b*). There are occasional artifact bands, not so many as on plus-minus gels, and more readily eliminated. The most serious problem is compression of bands where the DNA forms stable base-paired loops. This has largely been overcome by the use of much thinner polyacrylamide gels (Sanger and Coulson, 1978). Sanger *et al.* (1977*b*) still consider that the sequence obtained by the terminator method, as well as the other rapid methods, should be checked by some other method or by priming on the complementary strand.

Barnes (1978) has developed a method similar in principle, but incorporating randomly a ribonucleotide instead of the terminator, then cleaving with alkali.

1.4. Other Methods of Sequencing DNA

The rapid methods can potentially give sequences of several hundred nucleotides within a week, but problems and ambiguities can arise, and it is advisable to obtain data by other methods to confirm the sequence. The provisional sequence read from gels provides a framework in which the particular methods which will give the most useful information can be planned. If small oligonucleotides are sequenced there is no requirement for several sets since the gel sequence provides the overlapping. Therefore, even though the older methods of sequence determination are relatively time consuming, the proverbial "roll of DEAE paper and endless patience" are not required to confirm a gel sequence.

Methods of sequencing DNA have been comprehensively reviewed by Murray and Old (1974), Salser (1974), and Wu *et al.* (1976). There is therefore no need to go into too much detail in this chapter, but the more commonly used methods can be outlined. The enzymes and chemicals used to cleave DNA are shown in Table 1.

1.4.1. Transcription into RNA

One of the major difficulties in early DNA sequence work was the lack of single-base-specific enzymes. Therefore, the DNA is often transcribed into RNA where the standard RNA sequencing techniques can be applied to digestion products of T1, U2, and pancreatic ribonucleases (Barrell, 1971). Transcription has been extensively used in the SV40 sequence work (see Section 3.1.).

1.4.2. Direct Sequencing of DNA

The depurination reaction of Burton and Petersen (1960) is still a useful and simple tool. Brown and Smith (1977*b*) were able to confirm a long sequence from ϕX174 by depurinating both strands of small restriction fragments (preferably <100 nucleotides) using in turn ^{32}P-labeled dATP or dGTP to identify the purine at the 3' end of each pyrimidine tract. By determining the composition of each product, the 3' purine, and the relative amounts of each isostich, the sequence they had obtained by the Sanger and Coulson (1975) method was shown to be correct.

Small restriction enzyme fragments or products of digestion with, say, endonuclease IV can be sequenced by partial spleen or venom phosphodiesterase digestion. These are exonucleases acting at a 5'-hydroxyl and 3'-hydroxyl group, respectively. If necessary, a 5' or 3' phosphate can be removed with bacterial alkaline phosphatase. The method used by Ling (1972*a,b*) to sequence pyrimidine tracts up to 20 nucleotides in length was partial exonuclease digestion with separation of the products by electrophoresis at pH 3.5 on cellulose acetate and homochromatography on DEAE-cellulose thin layers in the second dimension (Brownlee and Sanger, 1969). Since the T and C nucleotides have different mobilities on electrophoresis, and homochromatography separates according to size, a trail of spots is obtained up the chromatography plate representing every possible product of the exonu-

TABLE 1
Methods of Cleaving DNA^a

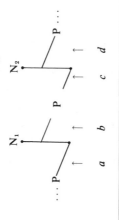

Procedure	Substrate	Type of reaction	Specificity of cleavage	Predominant reaction products (5'→3')
Snake venom phosphodiesterase	RNA, ssDNA	Exonuclease	At b where N_2 is the 3' terminus and carries a 3'—OH group	pN
Spleen phosphodiesterase	RNA, ssDNA	Exonuclease	At c where N_1 is the 5' terminus and carries a 5'—OH group	Np
Alkaline phosphatase (bacteria)	RNA, DNA	Phosphatase	At a where N_1 is the 5' terminus; at d where N_2 is the 3' terminus	P_i and oligonucleotide with 3'—OH and 5'—OH groups
Exonuclease III (E. coli)	dsDNA	Exonuclease and phosphatase	At b (and d) where N_2 is the 3' terminus and carries 3'—OH (or -P)	pN
λ Exonuclease	dsDNA	Exonuclease	At b where N_1 is the 5' terminus and carries a 5'-P	pN

Enzyme	Substrate	Type	Specificity	Products
Micrococcal nuclease	DNA, RNA	Endonuclease	At c where N_1 and N_2 are any nucleotides	Np, $NpNp$
Endonuclease IV (T4-infected $E.\ coli$)	ssDNA	Endonuclease	At b where N_1N_2 is TC	$pC \cdots T$
Deoxyribonuclease I (pancreas)	DNA	Endonuclease	At b where N_1 and N_2 are any nucleotides	Nucleotides and small oligonucleotides $pN \cdots N$, pN
Deoxyribonuclease II (spleen)	DNA	Endonuclease	At c where N_1 and N_2 are any nucleotides	Nucleotides and small oligonucleotides $N \cdots Np$, Np
Restriction enzymes	dsDNA[b]	Endonuclease	At b where N_1 and N_2 are part of the appropriate recognition sequence	$pN \cdots N$
Formic acid plus diphenylamine	DNA	Depurination	At c where N_1N_2 is PyPu; at b where N_1N_2 is PuPu	Pyrimidine tracts $pPy \cdots Pyp$
Hydrazine followed by alkaline hydrolysis	DNA	Depyrimidination	At c where N_1N_2 is PuPy; at b where N_1N_2 is PyPu	Purine tracts $pPu \cdots Pup$
Dimethylsulfate followed by alkaline hydrolysis	DNA	Depurination	At c where N_1N_2 is PyPu; at b where N_1N_2 is PuPy	$pPy \cdots Pyp$
Ribonuclease T1	RNA[c]	Endonuclease	At c where N_1 is G	$Np \cdots Gp$
Ribonuclease T2	RNA[c]	Endonuclease	At c where N_1 is usually A, sometimes G	$Np \cdots Ap$
Ribonuclease U2	RNA[c]	Endonuclease	At c where N_1 is a purine	$Np \cdots Pup$
Pancreatic ribonuclease	RNA[c]	Endonuclease	At c where N_1 is a pyrimidine	$Np \cdots Pyp$
Alkali	RNA[c]	Esterolysis	At c where N_1 is any nucleotide	Mixture of 2' and 3' nucleotides

[a] For details of individual enzymes, see Boyer (1971); restriction enzymes are reviewed by Roberts (1976).
[b] Some restriction enzymes may also cleave ssDNA.
[c] Or ribosubstituted DNA.

clease. From the relationship of each spot to the one before, Ling (1972*b*) could identify whether the difference was due to loss of a C or a T, and hence deduce the sequence. Ziff *et al.* (1973), Galibert *et al.* (1974), and Sedat *et al.* (1976) extended this method to identify all four nucleotides and determined sequences from DNA, labeled with ^{32}P *in vivo*, digested with endonuclease IV. Other laboratories have used this method extensively, often with 5′ end-labeling and venom phosphodiesterase (Ysebaert *et al.*, 1976; Subramanian *et al.*, 1977*a*). An example of a sequence determined by partial exonuclease digestion is shown in Fig. 3. In this case pancreatic DNAse has been added to extend the exonuclease data (Van de Voorde *et al.*, 1976).

1.4.3. Primed Synthesis—Ribonucleoside Substitution

Labeling of a DNA strand with ^{32}P *in vitro* is much more efficient than the *in vivo* incorporation of ^{32}P, and since the label can be restricted to one nucleoside triphosphate, nearest-neighbor analysis can give useful information. The α-^{32}P incorporated is at the 5′ site, and as most enzyme digestions or chemical degradations cleave the 5′ phosphate bond, the input ^{32}P becomes the 3′ phosphate of the next nucleotide. As previously mentioned, there is a lack of known deoxyribonucleases of single-base specificity, whereas several ribonucleases do have this property. Sanger *et al.* (1973) used the observations of Berg *et al.* (1963) and Salser *et al.* (1972) that, in the presence of manganese ion instead of magnesium, *E. coli* DNA polymerase I will insert ribonucleotides into the synthesized sequence. Therefore, if three deoxyribonucleoside triphosphates and one ribonucleoside triphosphate are present, e.g., rCTP, every C in the synthesized oligonucleotide is susceptible to alkali or pancreatic ribonuclease cleavage. By substituting different ribotriphosphates a set of overlapping oligonucleotides can be obtained and sequenced. Van de Voorde *et al.* (1974) used the opposite approach, inserting one deoxynucleotide into an RNA transcript. If dCTP is used, for instance, pancreatic ribonuclease will cleave only at U residues.

These are the major methods used at present to obtain extensive DNA sequence data or to confirm sequences obtained by the Sanger and Coulson (1975) or Maxam and Gilbert (1977) techniques. Individual variations have been introduced, which are noted in later sections of this chapter as DNA sequence information available for each virus is discussed.

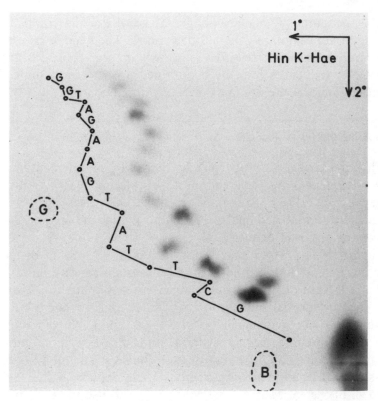

Fig. 3.   A sequence of 14 nucleotides obtained by partial venom phosphodiesterase and DNase I digestion of an end-labeled fragment of SV40. Although longer sequences have been obtained with this method, the reading becomes less reliable with longer products. The first dimension is electrophoresis at pH 3.5 on cellulose acetate, and the second dimension is homochromatography on a DEAE-cellulose thin layer. B and G mark the positions of xylene cyanol and orange G dye markers. From Van de Voorde *et al.* (1976), with permission.

2. DNA SEQUENCES FROM BACTERIOPHAGE GENOMES

2.1. The Bacteriophage λ

Bacteriophage λ has been intensively studied for some years. It grows easily; therefore, the phage, its DNA, and some of its gene products are readily detected and isolated. Much is known about the genetic and physical map, and interest has been focused particularly on the control processes which determine a temperate or lysogenic mode of replication. Details of λ knowledge up to 1970–1971 are given in Hershey (1971). Since that time considerable effort has gone into sequencing the regions of DNA of most interest.

The genome of bacteriophage λ is a double-stranded DNA molecule of approximately 49,000 base pairs. The genetic map of some of the more significant features is shown in Fig. 4. The areas from which DNA sequences have been obtained are the ends, the origin of replication, and the site of major transcriptional control.

2.1.1. The Cohesive Ends

The circularization of λ DNA by means of complementary single-stranded sequences at each end of the molecule was established by Hershey *et al.* (1963). By filling in these ends using *E. coli* DNA polymerase I and labeled nucleoside triphosphates the sequence of these cohesive regions was deduced (Wu and Kaiser, 1968; Wu, 1970; Wu and Taylor, 1971). The repair reactions could be limited by omitting one or more nucleoside triphosphates. The products were digested with pancreatic DNase or micrococcal nuclease, fractionated by two-dimensional electrophoresis and chromatography, and further analyzed by digestion with spleen exonuclease or snake venom phosphodiesterase. By labeling the repair products with ^{3}H and ^{32}P, the terminal nucleotide could be identified, and eventually the sequences of the 12-nucleotide single-stranded complementary regions were deduced. The sequences are shown in Fig. 5. Murray and Murray (1973) used 5'-terminal label-

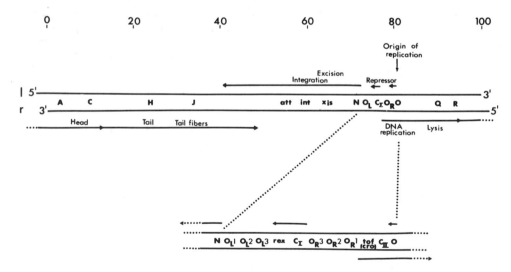

Fig. 4.   Map of the λ genome. The major leftward (O_L) and rightward (O_R) operators are shown, and horizontal arrows indicate the leftward and rightward mRNA species. Some of the major gene functions are indicated. The 5' cohesive ends are exaggerated in this diagram. Adapted from Szybalski *et al.* (1969), Murray and Old (1974), and Ptashne *et al.* (1976).

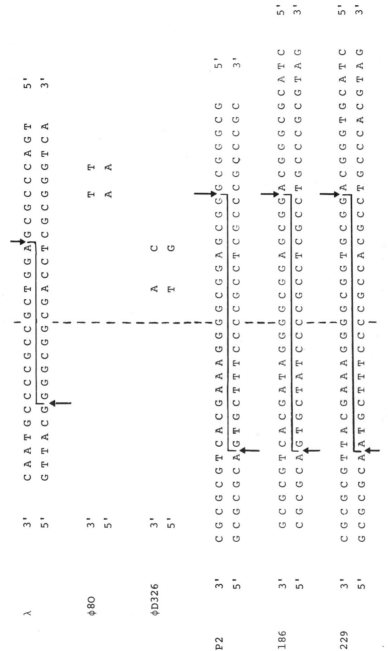

Fig. 5. Cohesive end sequences of temperate coliphages. Arrows indicate the sites of cleavage by the *ter* enzyme(s). The sequences of φ80 and φD326 are the same as λ except for the two differences shown in each. The dashed line indicates the axis of twofold rotational symmetry. Adapted from Murray *et al.* (1975, 1977) and Wu *et al.* (1976).

ing and limited digestion with pancreatic DNase followed by venom phosphodiesterase treatment to show that the cohesive end sequences are identical in other lambdoid phages—82, 21, 424, and ϕ80—but Murray *et al.* (1975) have shown that two bases differ in the DNA of lambdoid phage ϕD326. The 3'-terminal sequences of λ DNA were determined using the exonuclease-repair reaction of T4 DNA polymerase (Weigel *et al.*, 1973), and partial data for this region were obtained using the *E. coli* DNA polymerase I repair reaction (Brezinski and Wang, 1973). Jay *et al.* (1974) extended the 3' sequences in λ DNA to 10 at the left-hand end and 7 at the right-hand end. These sequences are included in Fig. 5. Bambara and Wu (1975) have sequenced the 3' terminus of ϕ80 DNA, and the two base changes found are indicated in Fig. 5.

2.1.2. The Origin of Replication

Replication of λ DNA is bidirectional (Schnös and Inman, 1970), starting from a well-defined region of the physical and genetic map (Fig. 4). The λ replicator has now been precisely located by genetic analysis (Furth *et al.*, 1977) and by nucleotide sequence analysis of *ori*⁻ mutants (Denniston-Thompson *et al.*, 1977). The essential region is at least 26 nucleotide pairs long and lies within the coding sequence of the structural gene O. The *ori*⁻ mutants were chosen to retain O function, and in the *ori*⁻ deletion mutants sequenced, all are deleted by multiples of three nucleotides so there is no frameshift in the O protein. The sequence of the *ori* region shows unusual features such as an unbroken tract of 18 pyrimidines on the r strand and many runs of four or five identical nucleotides. In the region sequenced there is no extended symmetrical structure which would provide a model for bidirectional initiation of replication. The role of RNA synthesis in λ DNA replication is also not understood. It was suggested that a small RNA molecule (*oop*), encoded near the replication origin, primes DNA replication (Hayes and Szybalski, 1973), but all the *ori*⁻ mutations lie at least 450 nucleotide pairs to the right of the *oop* RNA initiation (which is leftward).

2.1.3. The λ Operators

Lysogeny or virulence when λ infects *E. coli* is determined by a complex control system. The essential event in establishing the lysogenic state is production of a phage-coded repressor molecule which binds to the major promoters for leftward and rightward transcription of the genome. The operators can be isolated as protected fragments by binding repressor to the DNA and digesting with pancreatic DNase. Where repressor is bound, the DNA is resistant to nuclease attack and fragments of 35–100 nucleotide pairs have been isolated (Maniatis and Ptashne, 1973*a*). Using mutants defective in one or other of the promoters, the leftward and rightward promoters could be isolated separately. From the sizes of the protected regions at varying concentrations of repressor, it was apparent that each operator contains three repressor binding sites, one repressor molecule protecting about 30 nucleotide pairs from nuclease digestion. (For a review, see Ptashne *et al.*, 1976.) Sequence analysis of the λ operators made use of restriction enzymes which cut the DNA in the operator regions. The original sequence determination, that of the major leftward operator, was carried out by Maniatis *et al.* (1974). The methods used were those adapted for DNA sequencing from the well-established RNA sequencing technology (Sanger *et al.*, 1973). The protected DNA fragments were degraded with endonucleases to yield oligonucleotides of lengths up to about 30 residues. The sequence of these was established by partial digestion with spleen and venom phosphodiesterases. By these methods many sequence data were collected (Maniatis *et al.*, 1974, 1975; Pirrotta, 1975). More recently the sequences of the three right and three left operators have been completed using the Maxam–Gilbert (1977) method (Humayun *et al.*, 1977*a*). The combined results are shown in Fig. 6. As indicated, the leftward operators are concerned with an mRNA which contains at the 5′ end the genetic information for the structural polypeptide of the N gene. Dahlberg and Blattner (1975) sequenced 149 nucleotides of this RNA and obtained incomplete data into the operator region by transcribing an RNA molecule from the complementary strand. These "upstream" data fit the sequence obtained by Maniatis *et al.* (1974). In the mRNA sequence Dahlberg and Blattner (1975) looked for possible initiation codons for the N gene product. The first such codon is GUG at position 90, since AUG and GUG codons occurring farther toward the 5′ end of the mRNA are followed shortly by termination codons. As yet there are no further genetic or amino acid data for the N gene product which would confirm or dimiss this GUG as an initiation codon.

Each of the left and right λ operators spans some 80 base pairs and contains three repressor binding sites. These are designated O_L1, O_L2, O_L3 and O_R1, O_R2, O_R3. Each is 17 base pairs long and shows

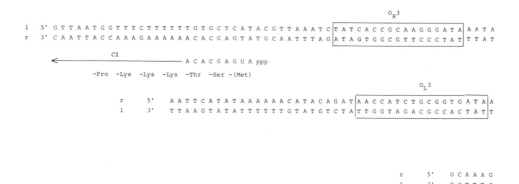

Fig. 6. Nucleotide sequences of the λ operators. Note that the orientation of the O_L and P_O sequences is reversed from that on the map in Fig. 4. The RNA start sequences for the CI. *tof*, N, and "*oop*" RNA are indicated, with the N-terminal amino acid sequence of the cI (repressor) protein. The 17 base-pair repressor binding sites in the O_L

considerable similarity to the others. There is an axis of partial rotational symmetry through the ninth base pair of each, and they are separated from each other by A·T-rich sequences. The strongest repressor binding sites are O_L1 and O_R1 (Maniatis and Ptashne, 1973*a,b*). Humayun *et al.* (1977*b*) reported somewhat different results of repressor binding experiments from those of Maniatis *et al.* (1973) for reasons which are not clear, but further characterization of the region may clarify the mechanism of repressor binding to these sites.

The topology of repressor binding has been investigated using the protection from methylation of G nucleotides as was worked out for the *lac* repressor binding site (Gilbert *et al.*, 1976). The results imply that the repressor is bound in the major groove of the helix (Humayun *et al.*, 1977*b*). The situation is therefore somewhat different from that for *lac*, where nucleotides are protected from methylation in both the major and minor grooves (Gilbert *et al.*, 1976).

The promoters associated with the λ operators have also been investigated. The standard protection experiment, in which a fragment of DNA is not sensitive to nuclease attack when RNA polymerase is bound, yielded a fragment of about 45 base pairs (Walz and Pirrotta, 1975). As found with similar RNA polymerase-protected fragments from other phages (Schaller *et al.*, 1975; Pribnow, 1975*b*), the protected λ fragments will not rebind the polymerase after the complex is dissociated. Two promoter mutations have been sequenced from λ (Meyer *et al.*, 1975; Kleid *et al.*, 1976), and both lie outside the polymerase-protected sequence. Ptashne *et al.* (1976) report that, using

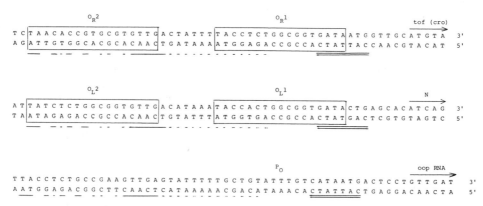

and O_R sequences are boxed, and nucleotides which are identical (———) or partially homologous (AT vs. GC; ---) in the three promoter regions are indicated by underlining. Data from Humayun *et al.* (1977a) and Scherer *et al.* (1977).

λ exonuclease and S1 nuclease in a protection experiment with the rightward promotor, the protected fragment is about 65 nucleotide pairs in length, and includes the promotor mutation site. This longer fragment does rebind the polymerase if dissociated after nuclease treatment. One interesting phenomenon is that O_R3 contains RNA polymerase recognition sites for transcription in both directions. To the right is made the mRNA of the *tof* gene, while to the left, on the complementary strand, is the mRNA for the *cI* (repressor) gene (Ptashne *et al.*, 1976).

There are in fact two promoters for transcription of the *cI* gene (Ptashne *et al.*, 1976). In the initial stages of lysogeny, transcription is from a promoter about 1000 bases to the right of the *cI* gene (P_{RE}, or promoter for repressor establishment = P_O). RNA from this promoter has a long leader sequence, and just before the AUG initiating codon for repressor synthesis is a sequence of six nucleotides which are complementary to the 3′ end of the 16 S ribosomal RNA and may be concerned with ribosome binding (Shine and Dalgarno, 1974; Steitz and Jakes, 1975). Later in infection, the *cI* gene is transcribed from a much closer promoter (P_{RM} or promoter for repressor maintenance) as shown in Fig. 6. The 5′-terminal nucleotide of RNA transcribed from this promoter is the A of the AUG which initiates *cI* protein (repressor) synthesis (Humayun *et al.*, 1977a). In other words, this mRNA does not have any leader sequence which could include a ribosome binding site. This mRNA also contains the genetic information for the *rex* gene (see Fig. 4). Humayun (1977) has determined a sequence of 57 nucleotide pairs which includes the codons for the known C-terminal amino acid sequence of the *cI* protein. A few nucleotides after the termination codon for *cI* (repressor) protein is a sequence with very high complementarity to the 3′ end of 16 S ribosomal RNA, and Humayun (1977) suggests this as the ribosome binding site for the *rex* gene, which would initiate at a following GUG codon. In this way, the mRNA from the P_{RM} promoter would be translated into the *rex* protein with high efficiency, but since there is no ribosome binding sequence for the *cI* protein the repressor would be made in very small amounts. This low production of repressor is required to maintain lysogeny. At the onset of lysogeny much more repressor is required, and this is translated from the P_{RE} promoter mRNA where there is a long leader sequence that does contain a "ribosome binding" sequence (Ptashne *et al.*, 1976; Humayun, 1977). Since the mechanisms involved in ribosome binding and translational control are not clear, these ideas are still speculative, but the nucleotide sequence determined through this region is a basis for further experimentation.

The first structural gene from the rightward operators of λ is *tof* (or *cro*). Using the chemical sequencing method of Maxam and Gilbert (1977), the nucleotide sequence of the *cro* gene has been determined by Roberts *et al.* (1977). The amino acid sequence of the *cro* protein has been determined by Hsiang *et al.* (1977) and agrees precisely with that predicted by the DNA sequence from the initiating ATG (which in the mRNA has been sequenced in a ribosome binding site by Steege, 1977) to the terminating TAA.

The same sequence has been determined by Schwarz *et al.* (1978); this sequence is then continued through the *cII* structural gene; the "*oop*" RNA sequence, and into the *O* gene; a total of just over 1000 nucleotide pairs. The sequence of the promoter preceding initiation of the 4 S *oop* RNA primer has been determined by Scherer *et al.* (1977) using the Maxam and Gilbert (1977) method. Their sequence determination extends into the 4 S RNA which was sequenced by Dahlberg and Blattner (1973) but differs at three positions. Part of the sequence has also been reported by Kleid *et al.* (1976), and the overlapping region agrees with the sequence of Scherer *et al.* (1977). The promoter sequence shows some similarities to the other λ promoters.

2.1.4. The Attachment Sites

A key process in lysogeny is integration of the circularized phage genome into the host chromosome by reciprocal exchange between a specific site in the phage DNA molecule and a specific site in the *E. coli* chromosome, the *att* sites. The product of the phage gene *int*, mapping to the right of *att*, is required for both integration and excision; in addition, excision requires the product of the *xis* gene mapping to the right of *int* (see Fig. 4).

Genetic work by Shulman and Gottesman (1973) suggested a common sequence in the bacterial and phage *att* sites, although such a common core could not be seen by electron microscope heteroduplex analysis, indicating that it is short. Landy and Ross (1977) have sequenced the two phage and two bacterial *att* sites using the Maxam and Gilbert (1977) procedure and found a common sequence 15 nucleotide pairs in length. The sequences determined total about 1000 nucleotide pairs, and there are several interesting features such as inverted repeats, a seven-base-pair palindrome, and a strong homology with the IS1 insertion sequence.

Davies *et al.* (1977) have also sequenced the *att* site of λ, using the Sanger and Coulson (1975) method with some use of the Maxam and Gilbert (1977) procedure. They determined 320 nucleotide pairs, including the *att* site and a possible C-terminal sequence of the *int* protein. There are three nucleotide differences in this sequence compared to that of Landy and Ross (1977), all being A in the l strand instead of the Ts found by Landy and Ross (1977).

Further work on the sequence analysis and studies on interaction with the *int* and *xis* gene products should help to determine the molecular mechanism of the integration–excision process of lysogeny.

2.2. Bacteriophages P2, 299, and 186

Phage P2 and its relatives are a group of temperate coliphages which resemble bacteriophage λ in that the genome is a linear, duplex molecule of DNA with 5′ cohesive ends, but differ in that the cohesive ends are longer and there is no significant homology detected between the nucleotide sequences (see Murray and Old, 1974). Murray *et al.* (1977) have determined the 3′-terminal sequences from DNA of phages P2, 299, and 186. When added to the sequences previously determined of the 5′ cohesive ends (Murray and Murray, 1973; Padmanabhan *et al.*, 1974), sequences of 33 base pairs are known for each of the three bacteriophages. In the fully base-paired situation (i.e., circularized) the sequences are not identical but all contain an axis of twofold symmetry through the central nucleotide pair. The terminal sequences of P2, 299, and 186 are included in Fig. 5. The symmetrical elements of these sequences may be involved in their recognition by the phage-coded enzyme(s) by which the double-stranded circular molecule is cleaved to generate the single-stranded cohesive ends (Murray *et al.*, 1977).

2.3. Bacteriophage T7

The genome of bacteriophage T7 is a linear, double-stranded DNA of about 40,000 nucleotide pairs. This genome contains terminally redundant sequences of about 260 nucleotide pairs (Ritchey *et al.*, 1967), and a model of DNA replication has been proposed which involves these repetitious ends in cleaving concatemeric DNA. The cleavage mechanism results in 5′ single-stranded complementary segments of about 260 nucleotides at each end of the DNA. These cohesive ends can be filled in by a DNA polymerase to give the terminally redundant sequences (Watson, 1972). Some sequence data were obtained for the 5′ and 3′ ends of the r and l strands (Weiss and Richardson, 1976; Englund, 1972; Price *et al.*, 1973). Loewen (1975) extended the 5′-terminal sequences by labeling whole T7 DNA with $[\gamma\text{-}^{32}P]$-ATP and polynucleotide kinase (Richardson, 1972) and partially digesting the fragments with pancreatic deoxyribonuclease. The resulting oligonucleotides were separated by electrophoresis and homochromatography, and the sequence was completed with the use of snake venom phosphodiesterase.

The sequences of 18 nucleotides at the 5′ end of the l strand and 15 nucleotides at the 5′ end of the r strand have been determined (Loewen, 1975). There is a certain amount of homology in the sequences to the 3′ side of the nick in each strand that may be concerned with recognition of the sequence by the endonuclease(s) which act on the concatemer, and further sequence work may clarify whether there are one or two endonucleases involved (Watson, 1972; Loewen, 1975).

Other regions of T7 DNA have been obtained by sequencing the *in vitro* RNA transcript. Arrand and Hindley (1973) sequenced a fragment of RNA which was protected from nuclease digestion by ribosome binding. Robertson *et al.* (1977) and Rosenberg and Kramer (1977) have sequenced regions around the sites of ribonuclease III cleavage by which the long, polycistronic early messenger RNA is processed into monocistronic messengers. They find that the cleavage site sequence is usually (but not exclusively)

$$5'\quad \text{U-U-U-A-U}_{\text{OH}}\ _p\text{G-A-U}\quad 3'$$

Considerable stable hairpin looping around the cleavage site is possible in at least two cases (Robertson *et al.*, 1977; Rosenberg and Kramer, 1977), but as pointed out by Robertson *et al.* (1977) this may not be particularly significant since a similar structure can be drawn in the phage R17 sequence where there is no ribonuclease III cleavage.

One major promoter sequence in T7 has been obtained by Pribnow (1975). A promoter specific for the T7 RNA polymerase has been sequenced by Oakley and Coleman (1977).

2.4. Bacteriophage ϕX174

The circular, single-stranded DNA of bacteriophage ϕX174 was the first DNA genome to be sequenced in full. Although some regions are subject to confirmation, Sanger *et al.* (1977a) have published a DNA sequence of 5375 nucleotides. As would be expected, knowledge of the DNA sequence does not mean that everything about ϕX174 is understood. However, the sequence enables accurate and precise location of the known features, such as the gene boundaries, the transcription starts and stops, and the replication origin, even though the control mechanisms operating are far from clear.

The methods used in the ϕX174 sequence work form a history of the development of DNA sequencing technology. The major part of the sequence was determined using the rapid "plus-minus" method of Sanger and Coulson (1975), but the older techniques were used to confirm the extensive data obtained. Since the plus and minus method gives 100 or more nucleotides at a time, there was no need for overlapping sequences when checking the gel sequences with small oligonucleotides.

The first nucleotide sequences established from ϕX174 were pyrimidine tracts. When products from the Burton and Petersen (1960) depurinations were fractionated in two dimensions, the longer products could be obtained sufficiently pure for sequence analysis by partial spleen and venom phosphodiesterases (Ling, 1971, 1972a,b; Harbers *et al.*, 1976). The corresponding depyrimidination reaction has not been so successful, although Chadwell (1974) improved the procedure and sequenced all the longer purine tracts in ϕX174 DNA.

Since the viral strand DNA of ϕX174 has the same polarity as the messenger RNA, it will bind ribosomes in a pseudoinitiation complex and thus a region of DNA is protected from endonuclease digestion. Such a protected 50-residue fragment was sequenced by Robertson *et al.* (1973) and Barrell *et al.* (1975). The sequence they obtained contained an ATG triplet and the amino acid sequence predicted if this was a protein initiation codon proved to be the N-terminal sequence of the coat protein specified by gene G (Air and Bridgen, 1973).

The major problem in DNA sequence determination at this stage was a lack of base-specific enzymes to generate fragments of a suitable length for sequencing. The rapid increase in the number of known restriction enzymes (Roberts, 1976) has now almost eliminated the difficulty, but Ziff *et al.* (1973) were able to obtain reasonable-sized fragments (50–200 nucleotides long) by partial digestion with endonuclease IV. Under the conditions they used, in which secondary structure would be maximized, they obtained a series of overlapping fragments from one area of the genome, representing about 10% of the whole. Further sequence analysis of the fragments (Galibert *et al.*, 1974; Sedat *et al.*, 1976) showed that they contained the coding sequence for the N-terminal part of the major capsid protein (gene F), the amino acid sequence of which was known (Air, 1976).

These methods of direct DNA sequencing all relied on DNA which was labeled with ^{32}P *in vivo*. Such labeling is not very efficient, and the short half-life of the isotope means that by the end of a series of procedures to sequence the fragment of DNA the results can often not be seen.

In vitro labeling offers two major advantages over the *in vivo* experiments. First, the label is introduced with high efficiency and can be restricted to a particular region of interest. Second, since the precursors used are nucleoside triphosphates, the ^{32}P label can be restricted to each of the four in turn; thus the radioisotope is being used as part of the sequence determination as well as a means of seeing amounts too small to detect chemically. One approach is to transcribe the DNA into RNA using purified RNA polymerase and [α-^{32}P] nucleoside triphosphates. The RNA can be sequenced by the well-established RNA sequencing methods (Barrell, 1971). Blackburn (1975, 1976) transcribed whole single-stranded ϕX174 DNA and some mapped endonuclease IV and restriction enzyme fragments. The results, combined with those from direct DNA sequencing (Galibert *et al.*, 1974; Sedat *et al.*, 1976; Ziff *et al.*, 1973), protein sequences (Air, 1976), and the plus-minus method (Sanger and Coulson, 1975), gave a continuous sequence of 281 nucleotides from the N-terminal region of gene F (Air *et al.*, 1976*a*).

DNA sequencing techniques using primed synthesis with DNA polymerase and α-^{32}P-labeled deoxyribonucleoside triphosphates were also developed (Sanger *et al.*, 1973). Incorporation of a ribonucleoside triphosphate, e.g., CTP, instead of the deoxyribonucleoside triphosphate facilitated the sequence determination—the synthesized strand could then be cleaved at the ribonucleotide by either alkali or the base-specific ribonucleases. With a synthetic decanucleotide primer the known sequence of the ribosome-protected region at the beginning of the gene G was extended back toward gene F (Donelson *et al.*, 1975).

Transcription of restriction fragments and results from the plus-minus method and amino acid sequencing gave a continuous sequence of 195 nucleotides from the N-terminal region of gene G (Air *et al.*, 1975).

The known sequences at this stage totaled just over 500 nucleotides, which had been obtained over some years. The development of the plus-minus method (described in Section 1), together with the rapidly increasing numbers of available restriction enzymes, made the next 4000 nucleotides comparatively easy, even if some regions do still need further confirmation.

Restriction enzyme maps of ϕX174 have been constructed in many laboratories. The enzymes and maps used in the sequence work were *Hind*II, *Hae*III, and *Hpa*I+II (Lee and Sinsheimer, 1974); *Hin*HI and *Hap*II (Hayashi and Hayashi, 1974); *Alu*I (Vereijken *et al.*, 1975); *Pst*I (Brown and Smith, 1976); *Hha*I, *Alu*I, *Hae*II, and *Hap*II (Jeppesen *et al.*, 1976); *Mbo*II (N. L. Brown, C. A. Hutchison III, and M. Smith, unpublished results); *Taq*I (Sato *et al.*, 1977); *Hha*I and *Hinf*I (Baas *et al.*, 1976*a*); and *Hph*I (Hutchison, unpublished results). In some cases the published maps can be corrected now that the whole sequence is known (Sanger *et al.*, 1977*a*). In the DNA sequence determination, fragments of double-stranded DNA obtained by digestion with these enzymes were used as primers on either the viral or complementary single strand. Ideally, overlapping sequences were obtained from several primers and on both strands. Where the restriction sites were too far apart for this multiple confirmation of the sequence, other methods such as depurination analysis and ribosubstitution were used. In one region, between genes F and G, the plus-minus method did not give good results, apparently because of the secondary structure (Fiddes, 1976), but, even so, the sequence which was obtained could be used to predict which alternative techniques would be useful, and to provide the overlaps between short oligonucleotides sequenced independently.

2.4.1. The Genetic Map of ϕX174 DNA

Interpretation of the ϕX174 DNA sequence reported by Sanger *et al.* (1977*a*) was greatly facilitated by the detailed studies on the genetics of the bacteriophage. The genetic map which was constructed by Benbow *et al.* (1971, 1972, 1974) showed nine genes, in the order on the circular map A-B-C-D-E-(J)-F-G-H. Gene J was identified with a small basic protein in the virion, but the genetic evidence was weak. Gene F coded for the capsid protein of the phage, genes G and H for the virion "spike" components, E for the lysis function, and A, B, C, and D were all involved in DNA replication, viral DNA synthesis, and morphogenesis. The molecular weights of the proteins coded by these genes were determined in several laboratories by polyacrylamide gel electrophoresis in sodium dodecylsulfate (SDS) (Burgess and Denhardt, 1969; Benbow *et al.*, 1972; and see Barrell *et al.*, 1976; Denhardt, 1975). While the values obtained for the coat proteins and for gene D protein were fairly consistent, the molecular weight estimates for the products of genes A, B, C, and E varied widely, partly because they are made in lower amounts and therefore are difficult to identify *in vivo* or *in vitro* (reviewed by Denhardt, 1975, 1977). The extent of each of the genes was related to the restriction maps by the marker-rescue method (Hutchison and Edgell, 1971) by Weisbeek *et al.* (1976), Borrias *et al.* (1976), and Weisbeek *et al.* (1977). It was therefore known in which regions of the DNA sequence the various genes were located, and the boundaries of genes D, J, F, G, and H were clearly identified by correlating the DNA sequence with the known protein amino acid sequences via the genetic code (Air *et al.*, 1975, 1976*a,b*; Barrell *et al.*, 1976; Fiddes, 1976; Sanger *et al.*, 1977*a*). The other genes have been located, albeit without direct proof of which initiation codon is used, by sequencing termination mutants (amber or ochre) in each gene to determine the reading frame and, where several mutants were available, to check that the nucleotide sequence was the correct length—i.e., that the reading frame did not change from one end of the gene to the other (Barrell *et al.*, 1976; Slocombe, 1977; Brown and Smith 1977*a,b*; Smith *et al.*, 1977; Sanger *et al.*, 1977*a*). Once the reading frame of the nucleotide sequence is established, the protein sequence can be read off in triplet codons until a termination codon is reached. This will presumably define the C terminus of the protein. In the absence of protein sequence data, the N terminus of the protein is not so easily identified. An initiation codon, ATG or GTG, is required to the 5′ side (upstream) of the mutation which has been sequenced and downstream from any termination codon in that reading frame. Sometimes there is a choice, and the ϕX174 initiation codons were selected on the basis of the sequence preceding the initiating codon having some degree of complementarity to the 3′ end of 16 S ribosomal RNA (Shine and Dalgarno, 1974). In the case of gene B the sequence of a ribosome-protected fragment of RNA (Ravetch *et al.*, 1977) lent support to this reasoning (Brown and Smith, 1977*a*,*b*).

The result is that a revised genetic map of ϕX174 can be drawn, accurate to the nucleotide level, and it is shown in Fig. 7. Nucleotide sequence and protein sequence work showed that the small basic protein of the virion tentatively assigned to gene J by Benbow *et al.* (1972) was indeed coded by the phage, and in the position on the genetic map as given by Benbow *et al.* (1972), even though the mutation by which gene J was defined was subsequently mapped as a double mutant in genes A and E (Weisbeek *et al.*, 1976, 1977; Smith *et al.*, 1977).

A more surprising feature of the map is the positions of genes D and E (Barrell *et al.*, 1976) and A and B (Brown and Smith, 1977*a*; Smith *et al.*, 1977). Since alignment of protein and nucleotide sequences showed the gene order D-J-F, Barrell *et al.* (1976) located mutants in gene E, which genetic mapping had placed between genes D and J–F,

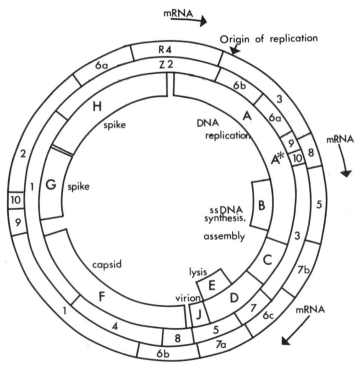

Fig. 7.   Genetic and physical map of ϕX174. The outermost circle shows the *Hind*II map (R), the middle circle the *Hae*III map (Z), and the inner circles the gene products with the functions of each. A* results from an internal initiation within gene A. The mRNA initiation sites are indicated by arrows. Adapted from Barrell *et al.* (1976) and Sanger *et al.* (1977*a*).

by rescue of the mutation (Hutchison and Edgell, 1971). Spheroplasts are infected with mutant single-stranded DNA to which are annealed purified restriction fragments from wild-type double-stranded DNA. Where the fragment anneals around the site of mutation, wild-type progeny phage particles are produced. The gene E mutants tested by this method all mapped in fragment *Hae*III,7. Since the complete D amino acid sequence was known, and had been correlated to the nucleotide sequence, and this sequence included the whole of fragment *Hae*III,7, gene E is located with gene D. The two genes are genetically entirely distinct, and the most plausible explanation was that gene E was translated in a different reading frame to gene D, from the same nucleotide sequence. This was confirmed by sequencing several gene E mutants (Barrell *et al.*, 1976) and a wild-type revertant of one of them. Figure 8 shows part of the plus and minus (Sanger and Coulson, 1975) gel where a gene E mutant is compared to a revertant. A single nucleotide difference is clearly seen. Viral strand DNA was used as the template, so the sequences shown are the complementary strand. The viral strand sequences are therefore

revertant   5'-G-T-G-G-G-A-T-A-3'
am3   5'-G-T-A-G-G-A-T-A-3'

The amber codon sequence TAG is changed to TGG in the revertant, which is the same as the wild-type sequence, and defines the reading frame for the gene-E-coded protein. This reading frame is displaced one nucleotide to the right of that used to code for the gene D protein. Figure 9 shows the nucleotide sequence through this region and the amino acid sequences of the two proteins. The gene E protein sequence extends to the first termination codon in this reading frame, which is close to the gene D protein termination. There is no direct evidence to show which initiation codon is used, but consideration of possible ribosome-binding by complementarity to the 3' end of 16 S ribosomal RNA (Shine and Dalgarno, 1974; Steitz and Jakes, 1975) favors the ATG indicated in Fig. 9. The only other possibility is the preceding GTG (Barrell *et al.*, 1976). In either case, the entire coding sequence of the gene E protein lies within the sequence coding for the gene D protein. Also shown in Fig. 9 is the sequence coding for the N-terminal part of the gene J protein (gene J being now defined as coding for the small basic virion protein). The initiation ATG for gene J overlaps the D terminating TAA by one nucleotide.

This remarkable compression of the ϕX174 genetic map is repeated in genes A and B. The estimated molecular weights of the gene

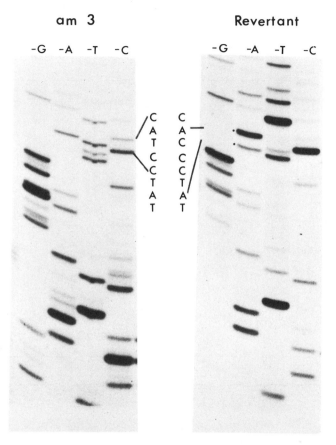

Fig. 8. Nucleotide sequences obtained by the Sanger and Coulson (1975) method comparing ϕX174 *am3* and a wild-type revertant. The autoradiographs of polyacrylamide gels show sequences within fragment *Hae*III,7, in which the *am3* mutation was located by the marker-rescue technique (see Barrell *et al.*, 1976). The sequences shown are of the complementary strand; the viral (coding strand) sequences are therefore

am3	5′	GT<u>A</u>GGATA
revertant	5′	GT<u>GG</u>GATA

From Air and Hutchison (unpublished results).

A and B proteins were rather too large for the space available if they were separately coded. Precise genetic mapping onto restriction fragments had given unexpected results, in that gene A mutants were mapped on both sides of gene B mutants (Borrias *et al.*, 1976). Ravetch *et al.* (1977a) isolated a ribosome-protected fragment of RNA from within the gene A coding sequence, and the overlap was established by showing that the initiation sequence predicted from it was in the same reading frame as a gene B amber mutant, yet displaced by one

D

         G-A-G-T-C-C-G-A-T-G-C-T-G-T-C-A-A-C-A-C-A-C-T-A-A-T-A-G-G-T-A-A-G-A-A-A-T-C-[A-T-G]-
         Hinf 16a↑16b   D start
                   ↑ mRNA start

D   Ser - Gln - Val - Thr - Glu - Gln - Ser - Val - Arg - Phe - Gln - Thr - Ala - Ser - Ile - Lys - Leu - Ile -
     A-G-T-C-A-A-G-T-T-A-C-T-G-A-A-C-A-A-A-G-T-T-C-G-T-T-T-C-C-A-A-A-C-C-G-C-T-T-C-T-A-T-T-A-A-G-C-T-T-A-T-T-
Hinf 16b↑1   10   20   30   Hae III 3↑7   40   Alu 6↑1 50   60

D   Gln - Ala - Ser - Ala - Val - Leu - Asp - Leu - Thr - Glu - Asp - Asp - Phe - Leu - Thr - Ser - Asn - Lys -
     C-A-G-G-C-T-T-C-T-G-C-C-G-T-T-T-T-G-G-A-T-T-T-A-A-C-C-G-A-A-G-A-T-G-A-T-T-T-C-G-A-T-T-T-C-T-G-A-C-G-A-G-T-A-A-C-A-A-A-A-
         70   80   Mbo II   Taq 4↑5 1↑7   110   120
                                      E (Met)>Val-
                                      E start

D   Val - Trp - Ile - Ala - Thr - Asp - Arg - Ser - Arg - Ala - Arg - Arg - Cys - Val - Glu - Ala - Cys - Val - Tyr - Gly -
     G-T-T-T-G-G-A-T-T-G-C-T-A-C-T-G-A-C-C-G-C-T-C-T-C-G-T-G-C-T-C-G-T-C-G-C-T-G-C-G-T-T-G-A-G-G-C-T-T-G-C-G-T-T-T-A-T-G-G-T-
        130   140   150   160   170
                                          [A-T-G]-G-T- E start

                                      Leu
    Ter   Ter   ↑
     ↑   ↑
E   Arg - Trp - Thr - Leu - Trp - Asp - Thr - Leu - Ala - Phe - Leu - Leu - Leu - Ser - Leu - Leu - Pro - Ser -
     G-T-T-T-G-G-A-C-T-T-T-G-A-C-A-C-C-C-T-C-G-T-C-C-G-T-C-G-C-C-G-C-T-T-C-C-T-G-C-T-C-C-T-G-T-T-C-C-T-G-C-C-T-C-C-G-C-T-T-C-
                             210

D   Thr - Leu - Asp - Phe - Val - Gly - Tyr - Pro - Arg - Phe - Glu - Phe - Ile - Ala - Ala - Val -
     A-C-G-C-T-G-G-A-C-T-T-T-G-T-G-G-G-A-T-A-C-C-C-T-C-G-C-T-T-T-C-G-A-G-T-T-T-A-T-T-G-C-T-G-C-C-G-T-C-
     ↓   ↓   ↓   ↓ 230
     A am27, amN11   A am3, am34   A am3   T dE3, dE5

```
E   Leu - Leu - Ile - Met - Phe - Ile - Pro - Ser - Thr - Phe - Lys - Arg - Pro - Val - Ser - Ser - Trp - Lys - Ala - Leu -

D   Ile - Ala - Tyr - Tyr - Val - His - Pro - Val - Asn - Ile - Gln - Thr - Ala - Cys - Leu - Ile - Met - Glu - Gly - Ala -

    A-T-G-C-T-T-A-T-T-A-T-G-T-T-C-A-T-C-C-C-G-T-C-A-A-C-A-T-T-C-A-A-A-C-G-G-C-C-T-G-T-C-T-C-A-T-C-A-T-G-G-A-A-G-G-C-G-C-T-
                250              Hind 6c↑7a        270       Hae III 7↑5                              Hha 4↑13


E   Asn - Leu - Arg - Lys - Thr - Leu - Leu - Met - Ala - Ser - Ser - Val - Arg - Leu - Lys - Pro - Leu - Asn - Cys - Ser -

D   Glu - Phe - Thr - Glu - Asn - Ile - Ile - Glu - Arg - Pro - Val - Lys - Ala - Ala - Glu - Leu - Phe -

    G-A-A-T-T-T-A-C-G-G-A-A-A-A-C-A-T-T-A-T-T-A-A-T-G-G-C-G-T-C-G-A-G-C-G-T-C-C-G-G-T-T-A-A-A-G-C-C-G-C-T-G-A-A-T-T-G-T-T-C-
              310              Taq 5↑3    320    Hap 1↑3  340                     350                      360


E   Arg - Leu - Pro - Cys - Val - Tyr - Ala - Gln - Glu - Thr - Leu - Thr - Phe - Leu - Leu - Thr - Gln - Lys - Lys - Thr -

D   Ala - Phe - Thr - Leu - Arg - Val - Arg - Ala - Gly - Asn - Thr - Asp - Val - Leu - Thr - Asp - Ala - Glu - Glu - Asn -

    G-C-G-T-T-T-A-C-C-T-T-G-C-G-T-G-T-A-C-G-C-G-C-A-G-G-A-A-A-C-A-C-T-G-A-C-G-T-T-A-C-T-G-A-T-C-G-C-G-A-A-G-A-A-A-A-C-
              370          Hha 13↑11           390                     400          Mbo II 410               420


E   Cys - Val - Lys - Asn - Tyr - Val - Arg - Lys - Glu          J      Ser - Lys - Gly - Lys - Lys - Arg - Ser -

D   Val - Arg - Gln - Lys - Leu - Arg - Ala - Glu - Gly - Val - Met            J

    G-T-G-C-G-T-C-A-A-A-A-A-T-T-A-C-G-T-G-C-G-G-A-A-G-G-A-G-T-G-A-[T-G-A]-[T-A]-T-G-T-C-T-A-A-A-G-G-T-A-A-A-A-A-A-C-G-T-T-C-T-G
     7↑3                   430               440           E stop  D stop   J start            470                      480
```

Fig. 9. Nucleotide sequence through genes D and E of φX174. The amino acid sequences of the D and J proteins have been determined. That of the E protein was inferred from the DNA sequence and the *am3* mutation as described in the text. From Barrell *et al.* (1976), with permission.

nucleotide from the reading frame assigned to gene A (Brown and Smith, 1977a,b). Nucleotide sequence determinations of other A and B mutants confirmed these reading frames (Smith *et al.*, 1977) and showed that the B protein terminates 28 codons before termination of the A protein, i.e., that gene B is totally contained within gene A. Further genetic mapping of many mutants in genes A and B by Weisbeek *et al.* (1977) suggested that gene B originated within gene A and terminated close to and possibly before the gene A termination.

The A termination codon overlaps by four nucleotides the most probable initiating codon for gene C in the sequence A-$\overline{\text{T-G-A}}$ (Sanger *et al.*, 1977a) since the sequence of a gene C ochre termination mutant has set the reading frame for the C protein (B. G. Barrell, unpublished results). Although the sequence was not finally confirmed, the termination codon TGA for gene C overlaps the gene D initation codon in the same relationship as the gene A–gene C overlap, the sequence being again A-T-G-A. (Sanger *et al.*, 1977a; B. G. Barrell, unpublished results).

The coat protein genes of ϕX174 are spaced in a comparatively expansive fashion. Between genes J and F there is an intergenic space of 39 nucleotides, and between genes G and H are 11 nucleotides. Between genes F and G is a sequence of 111 nucleotides which contains terminators in all three phases and so cannot be translated (Fiddes, 1976). The sequence contains a prominent region of hyphenated 2-fold molecular symmetry, the central portion of which has a sequence of 17 A·T base pairs, flanked by regions very rich in G·C base pairs. A hairpin loop can be drawn in the viral strand sequence which corresponds in pyrimidine tracts to the major nuclease-resistant (double-stranded) product from whole viral strand isolated by Bartok *et al.* (1975). The length of this untranslated region in the economical ϕX174 genome and the peculiarities in the sequence suggest that there is some particular function, although none has been mapped here (Fiddes, 1976). The secondary structure of the single strand is reminiscent of the origin of replication sequences in SV40 (Subramanian *et al.*, 1977), but in ϕX174 the origin of viral strand synthesis has been located by several techniques inside the gene A coding region (see Fig. 7), while synthesis of the complementary strand is initiated at many sites (see Denhardt, 1975, 1977). In the SV40 genome there are long tracts of continuous A·T base pairs before the sites of initiation of early and late messenger RNA, but no promoters have been located in this part of the ϕX174 genome. Fiddes (1976) suggested that one possible function is the binding site for the H protein, which is the "pilot protein" during infection (Jazwinski *et al.*, 1975a,b,c).

2.4.2.   Transcription of ϕX174

Attempts to characterise and map the messenger RNA molecules in ϕX174 *in vitro* (Smith and Sinsheimer, 1976; Grohmann *et al.*, 1975; Axelrod, 1976) and *in vivo* (Hayashi *et al.*, 1976) showed a much more complex pattern than is obtained, for instance, in the filamentous single-stranded phages (see Section 2.6). Three *in vitro* mRNA classes have been characterized by sequence analysis of the 5' ends (Smith and Sinsheimer, 1976; Grohmann *et al.*, 1975; Axelrod, 1976), and these 5' sequences have been located in the sequence of the ϕX174 genome (Sanger *et al.*, 1977a) at the map positions for *in vivo* mRNA starts (Hayashi *et al.*, 1976). Two of them correspond to RNA polymerase binding sites mapped by Chen *et al.* (1973). The characteristic promoter sequence (T-A-T-Pu-A-T-Pu: Pribnow, 1975) is not perfect in any of the ϕX174 sequences, but elements of it are present in all cases. The features essential to a promoter site are still unclear (Okomoto *et al.*, 1977).

There appear to be many transcription termination sites in ϕX174, some *rho* dependent, others *rho* independent (Axelrod, 1976; Hayashi *et al.*, 1976). The results from several laboratories all indicated that there is one major termination site, which is *rho* independent, but its map position varied dramatically. Smith and Sinsheimer (1976) placed it in the gene C region, while Axelrod (1976) and Hayashi *et al.* (1976) placed it before gene A. The differences probably arise from the fact that the map positions could be determined for the 5' ends directly, but the 3' ends were mapped by estimating the length of the RNA by gel electrophoresis, a notoriously dubious procedure. Taking the majority estimate of the principal termination site, Sanger *et al.* (1977a) found the sequence T-T-T-T-T-T-A just before the gene A coding region, which is similar to the 3' ends of many mRNA molecules and may act as a termination signal (Bertrand *et al.*, 1975; Lee *et al.*, 1976; Sogin *et al.*, 1976; Rosenberg *et al.*, 1976; Sugimoto *et al.*, 1977). Just before this T_6A sequence is a region of possible base pairing which may also be significant in termination (Rosenberg *et al.*, 1976; Sugimoto *et al.*, 1977). In ϕX174 there was a complication in this interpretation since the proposed termination site was 20 nucleotides to the 3' side of the mRNA initiation site, and Sanger *et al.* (1977a) have suggested that the hairpin loop is indeed involved in termination. Since the newly initiated mRNA is too short to form such a double-stranded region the polymerase will read through the terminator, while RNA initiated at other sites will form the hairpin and terminate.

It will be interesting to find out which messenger RNA molecules are involved in synthesizing which proteins. In the filamentous bacteriophages some proteins appear to be expressed from any mRNA carrying the coding information (see Section 2.6), but the presence of overlapping genes in ϕX174 suggests that other control mechanisms may operate to determine which of the overlapping genes is translated. In the A-B region gene B has a separate promoter; thus the mRNA initiated here does not contain the initiating codon for gene A, or for the protein resulting from initiation within gene A in the same reading frame, A* (Denhardt, 1975; Brown and Smith, 1977a). In the D-E overlapping region there is apparently no such separate promoter for gene E (Barrell *et al.*, 1976).

2.4.3. The Origin of Replication in ϕX174

The origin of viral strand synthesis has been located in gene A at a precise point (Baas *et al.*, 1976b). This origin has also been characterized by location of gaps in replicating double-stranded molecules. Eisenberg *et al.* (1975) investigated such gaps by filling them in with labeled nucleotides and by depurination analysis of the labeled material. They identified, in particular, the product C_6T. Sanger *et al.* (1977a) find the sequence C-T-C-C-C-C-C in this region, but the surrounding sequence does not show the spectacular symmetry and base pairing observed in SV40 (Subramanian *et al.*, 1977b) or fd (Gray *et al.*, 1978) origins. There is an A·T-rich region, surrounded by two G·C-rich regions, which may have some significance, but ϕX174 replication may prove to be somewhat different from that of fd. Not very much is known about the synthesis of the complementary strand. Initiation apparently occurs at many sites around the genome, in contrast to the single site in fd which is the same as for viral strand synthesis (Tabak *et al.*, 1974; Denhardt, 1977).

The exact position of the gene A protein induced nick is six nucleotides downstream of the CTC_5 sequence (Langeveld *et al.*, 1978).

2.4.4. Translation of ϕX174 proteins

The proteins coded by ϕX174 genes A, B, C, D, E, F, G, H, and J were almost all identified by polyacrylamide gel electrophoresis in sodium dodecylsulfate, but for some gene products the identification was not entirely clear, and for the gene B protein, in particular, the band was clear enough on the gels but the molecular weight estimates varied considerably depending on the gel system used (see Denhardt, 1975). Once the proteins are identified in the nucleotide sequence, not only can a precise length be assigned but so can the entire amino acid sequence. The nucleotide sequence determination is faster and probably more reliable than protein sequencing (Air *et al.*, 1976*b*) even when the proteins are relatively easy to obtain in sufficient amounts. Of the ϕX174-coded proteins, the coat proteins (genes F, G, H, and J) and one intracellular protein, made in extremely high amounts (gene D), have been purified for amino acid sequence work. The J protein was sequenced by Freymeyer *et al.* (1977). Complete amino acid sequences were determined for the G and D proteins (Air *et al.*, 1975, 1976*b*; Barrell *et al.*, 1976), and most of the F protein sequence is known (Air, 1976; Air *et al.*, 1978). Some peptides of the H protein have been sequenced, including the N-terminal and C-terminal regions (Sanger *et al.*, 1977*a*; Air, unpublished results). In every protein the N- and C-terminal sequences matched the initiation and termination predicted from the nucleotide sequence, so none of these proteins is made as a longer precursor. This is one property which cannot be seen in the DNA sequence, and it should be emphasized that the sequence of amino acids read from the nucleotide sequence may be longer than the *in vivo* protein. With this proviso, the amino acid sequences of all the ϕX174 proteins are known.

In assigning initiation codons to genes where no amino acid sequence was available, the Shine and Dalgarno (1974) proposal that the sequence before the initiation codon has some complementarity to the 3' end of 16 S ribosomal RNA (Sanger *et al.*, 1977*a*; Barrell *et al.*, 1976) was taken into account. There is indeed some complementarity in all known ϕX174 initiation sequences, but there is no obvious relationship between the extent of possible base pairing and the amount of protein synthesis (Sanger *et al.*, 1977*a*) or whether the site is protected by ribosomes *in vitro* (Ravetch *et al.*, 1977*a*).

In the earliest correlations between nucleotide sequences and amino acid sequences, a marked pattern in the use of codons was observed. There was a particular preference for T at the variable third position in degenerate codons (Air *et al.*, 1975, 1976*a,b*). This trend has been continued as more data became available (Sanger *et al.*, 1977*a*). ϕX174 is rich in T, but the significance of this finding is not known at this stage. The filamentous phages fd, f1, and M13 have a very similar overall base composition to ϕX174, and it will be interesting when the sequence data from these phages is analyzed to see if the third T phenomenon occurs in these phages. On the other hand, phage G4

(ϕX174-like) has a base composition almost complementary to that of ϕX174.

The ϕX174 DNA sequence has now been confirmed and completed (Sanger *et al.*, 1978) using the chain-termination method (Sanger *et al.*, 1977*b*).

2.5.   Bacteriophage G4

G4 is an isometric phage similar to ϕX174. It has a single-stranded DNA genome approximately 5550 nucleotides long, which codes for the same series of nine proteins as ϕX174 (Godson, 1974).

G4 has a single unique origin of synthesis of the viral DNA strand which is located within the A gene, as in ϕX174. However, unlike ϕX174, G4 also has a single unique origin of synthesis of complementary strand DNA, which maps approximately 100° away on the circular genome. Fiddes *et al.* (1978) have determined the nucleotide sequence around both of these replication origins. They found that the viral strand origin, within gene A, shows considerable homology with the ϕX174 origin. The complementary strand origin was located in the untranslated region between genes F and G. Although such an untranslated intergenic region exists in ϕX174 (Fiddes, 1976), there is no sequence homology with the G4 sequence in the same region. The G4 origin sequence does, however, show extensive sequence homology with the bacteriophage λ origin of DNA replication (Denniston-Thompson *et al.*, 1977).

A complete nucleotide sequence has been obtained for the G4 DNA (Godson *et al.*, 1978). Despite a 40% base sequence difference in the genome, the proteins are similar to those of ϕX174, including the overlapping genes B within A, and E within D. In addition, a gene "K," which was not detected genetically, could be postulated from the DNA sequence in both G4 and ϕX174, overlapping genes A and C. This protein has now been detected and partially sequenced from G4 (Shaw *et al.*, 1978).

2.6.   Bacteriophage S13

Bacteriophage S13 is almost identical to ϕX174 in size and in physical and biological characteristics. At least eight of the nine ϕX174 genes have been demonstrated in S13, and their order on the genetic map is the same (Yeng *et al.*, 1970; Baker and Tessman, 1967; Benbow *et al.*, 1971). Restriction endonuclease analyses indicate extensive sequence homology (Grosveld *et al.*, 1976; Godson, 1976; Hayashi and Hayashi, 1974).

Furthermore, Tessman *et al.* (1976) made a detailed study of the proteins produced by the two phages. They found that the proteins coded by genes A (and the internal initiation product A*) C, F, and G of S13 comigrate on SDS-acrylamide gel electrophoresis with corresponding ϕX174 proteins, while the gene products of D and H are slightly altered in mobility in S13. Since the migration of the ϕX174 D protein is anomalous (Barrell *et al.*, 1976), the difference in migration of the S13 protein may well not involve a size difference. The gene B protein has a markedly greater mobility in S13 compared to ϕX174, and Tessman *et al.* (1976) concluded that the gene B protein of S13 is considerably smaller than that of ϕX174. The longer pyrimidine oligonucleotides of S13 were isolated and sequenced by Harbers *et al.* (1976), and most were identical with those from ϕX174.

Grosveld and Spencer (1977) have sequenced 190 nucleotides of S13 DNA in gene A, just before the gene B out-of-phase initiation. There are three nucleotide differences from the ϕX174 sequence (Brown and Smith, 1977b; Sanger *et al.*, 1977a), two of which would not alter the A protein sequence. The third would result in a threonine in ϕX174 becoming a serine in S13. The methods used by Grosveld and Spencer (1977) were digestion of separated single strands of restriction fragments with endonuclease IV and sequencing by partial spleen or venom phosphodiesterases after *in vitro* labeling of the 3' end with terminal transferase (Roychoudhury *et al.*, 1976) or the 5' end with polynucleotide kinase (Richardson, 1965; Delaney and Spencer, 1976). The preparation of T4 endonuclease IV (Sadowski and Bakyta, 1972) was modified by Grosveld and Spencer (1977) to ensure there was no contaminating 3' endonuclease activity. Kaptein and Spencer (1978) used similar techniques to investigate the priming potential of the longer pyrimidine tracts.

2.7. Bacteriophages f1, fd, M13, and ZJ-2

The F-specific filamentous coliphages f1, fd, ZJ-2, and M13 are so similar in properties that they can be discussed together. Van den Hondel and Schoenmakers (1976) have shown that there are several differences in the restriction enzyme maps and therefore in nucleotide sequence, but no significant functional or genetic differences have been observed.

The genome of these phages consists of a covalently closed single-stranded DNA molecule. There has been some confusion over the length (see Denhardt, 1975), but sequence work and physicochemical studies both now indicate a length close to 6400 nucleotides (Van den Hondel and Schoenmakers, 1976; Day and Berkowitz, 1977). The filamentous phages have been recently reviewed in some detail (Denhardt, 1975).

A provisional DNA sequence for the fd genome is available (Schaller and Takanami, 1978; Beck *et al.*, 1978).

The genetic map, containing eight genes (I to VIII), was constructed for bacteriophage f1 by Lyons and Zinder (1972), and the only alteration in the map since then is the transposition of genes V and VII (Vovis *et al.*, 1975). The gene order is the same in M13 (Van den Hondel *et al.*, 1975). Restriction maps of the genomes of f1, fd, M13, and ZJ-2 have been determined for several enzymes (Tabak *et al.*, 1974; Horiuchi *et al.*, 1975; Seeburg and Schaller, 1975; Takanami *et al.*, 1975; Van den Hondel and Schoenmakers, 1975, 1976; Van den Hondel *et al.*, 1976; Vovis *et al.*, 1975). The boundaries of the genes could then be located more precisely, mostly by the use of *in vitro* transcription–translation systems to determine the size of polypeptide coded by each gene, and in which restriction fragments the genes are located (Model and Zinder, 1974; Konings, 1973; Konings *et al.*, 1975; Van den Hondel *et al.*, 1975).

The genetic map of M13 is shown in Fig. 10, the maps of f1 and fd being almost identical at this level. In between genes IV and II is a long (approximately 450 nucleotides) intergenic region (Vovis *et al.*, 1975; Van den Hondel *et al.*, 1976) which contains the origins of both viral and complementary strand DNA synthesis (Horiuchi and Zinder, 1976; Suggs and Ray, 1977; Van den Hondel *et al.*, 1976). The gene products, with their estimated molecular weights, are indicated in Fig. 10. Complete amino acid sequences have been determined for two of these gene products. The gene V protein, which binds strongly to newly synthesized viral DNA until exchanged for coat protein in the cell membrane, was sequenced by Cuypers *et al.* (1974) from M13 and by Nakashima *et al.* (1974) from fd. The major coat protein, coded by gene VIII, was originally sequenced by Asbeck *et al.* (1969). When DNA sequencing suggested there was an error in the amino acid sequence (Sanger *et al.*, 1973), Nakashima and Konigsberg (1974) found that the fd coat protein contains an extra amino acid, making the total length 50 amino acids instead of the 49 reported by Asbeck *et al.* (1969). The ZJ-2 coat protein is also 50 amino acids long, with a single

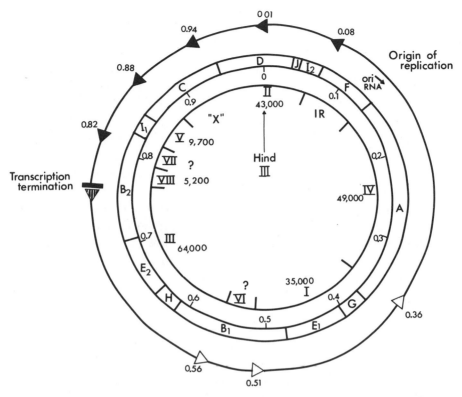

Fig. 10.   Genetic and physical map of bacteriophage M13. There are slight differences in the restriction maps of fd and f1. The outermost circle shows the promoters: ▶ indicates G and ▷ indicates A as the initiating nucleotide of the mRNA. ▷ is unknown. The solid bar is the central transcription terminator. The middle circles show the *Hap*I restriction map (fragments A, B_1, B_2, etc.), and the innermost circle indicates genes (I–VIII) with the approximate molecular weights of the gene products. IR indicates the intergenic region, which does not code for protein. Protein "X" apparently results from an internal initiation within gene II. Adapted from Edens *et al*. (1976) and Schaller *et al*. (1976).

amino acid difference (Snell and Offord, 1972). The N-terminal sequence of the gene III protein, which is present in one copy per virion at one end of the phage particle, has been determined by Goldsmith and Konigsberg (1977).

2.7.1.   Transcription of f1, fd, and M13

The direction of transcription of the filamentous phage genome was first indicated by the finding that mutations in gene III were polar to genes VI and VIII (Lyons and Zinder, 1972). This orientation was confirmed by sizes of amber fragments produced by the various genes affected (Model and Zinder, 1974), and is indicated in Fig. 10. Chan *et al.* (1975) showed that most, if not all, f1 mRNA has the same polarity as the viral DNA, and Jacob and Hofschneider (1969) could not find any RNA complementary to the viral strand DNA in M13 infected cells.

Promoters have been located by mapping RNA polymerase-protected double-stranded DNA fragments onto the restriction map (Seeburg and Schaller, 1975), by mapping the RNA transcripts (Okamoto *et al.*, 1975; Edens *et al.*, 1976) or by determining which proteins are synthesized from the mapped transcripts *in vitro* (Chan *et al.*, 1975; Edens *et al.*, 1976). These results all agreed that transcription is initiated at several sites around the genome (at least eight) and terminates at a single unique site (Sugiura *et al.*, 1969; Edens *et al.*, 1975), which is *rho* independent (Takanami *et al.*, 1971). These sites are shown on the genetic map in Fig. 10. Takanami *et al.* (1970) investigated the 5'-terminal sequences of several fd mRNAs made *in vitro*, and numerous sequence data have been obtained for some transcripts using RNA sequencing techniques by Sugimoto *et al.* (1975*a,b*, 1977). In addition, Takanami's group have used nonspecific transcription of restriction fragments to obtain the sequence of the DNA preceding the major mRNA starts, i.e., the promoters, at map positions G0.94 (Sugimoto *et al.*, 1975*a,b*) and G0.98 (Takanami *et al.*, 1976; Sugimoto *et al.*, 1977). Schaller *et al.* (1975) have also sequenced the G0.94 promoter. This promoter is located within the gene II coding region preceding the initiation of the "X" protein translation (Edens *et al.*, 1976). Beck *et al.* (1978) have sequenced the promoter preceding gene II. Much effort has been put into trying to elucidate what features make a "promoter," but so far the mechanisms of polymerase binding and initiation of RNA synthesis are far from clear. Seeburg *et al.* (1977) have shown that there is no correlation between tightness of polymerase binding and speed of dissociation. Although there is no sequence common to all promoters, parts of the "T-A-T-Pu-A-T-Pu" sequence noted by Pribnow (1975*b*) and Schaller *et al.* (1975) are conserved in all phage promoters and may be significant. Since the piece of DNA which is protected by RNA polymerase, about 40 nucleotides in length, will not rebind to polymerase after dissociation (Schaller *et al.*, 1975; Maurer *et al.*, 1974), there must be some other requirement for polymerase binding. Okamoto *et al.* (1977) have used an *Hha*I site five base pairs upstream from the T-A-T-A-A-T sequence (15 base pairs upstream from the RNA initiation site) to join the promoter sequence to DNA fragments derived from other regions of the genome. Any of the fragments tested restored promoter function, and Okamoto *et al.* (1977) concluded that the requirement was for a contiguous DNA region rather than for a specific sequence.

The six promoters mapped by Seeburg and Schaller (1975) agree in map position with six of the eight found by Edens *et al.* (1976). Okamoto *et al.* (1975) detected three of these, plus another A-start messenger at map position 0.46. As shown in Fig. 10 there are clearly promoters preceding genes VI, I, IV, II, V, and VIII. In addition there is a promoter within gene I (Okamoto *et al.*, 1975) and there are two promoters within gene II (Edens *et al.*, 1976). One of these may precede the X protein, which appears to result from an internal initiation within gene II (Konings *et al.*, 1975). No promoter was found preceding gene III. The suggestions were made that the mRNA for this protein is obtained either by incomplete termination at the central terminator (Seeburg and Schaller, 1975; Edens *et al.*, 1976) or from a promoter which requires special conditions to be observed in *in vitro* systems. (Chan *et al.*, 1975; Seeburg and Schaller, 1975). Attempts to characterize transcripts made *in vivo* have led to confusing results (Jacob *et al.*, 1973).

Sugimoto *et al.* (1977) sequenced the whole of the RNA transcript from the G0.82 promoter preceding gene VIII to the central terminator. The 3' end of this transcript is therefore assumed to be the same in the longer RNA molecules made from all the other promoters. The 3' end terminates with a run of eight U residues, similar to the poly(U) sequences seen at the 3' ends of several RNA species (Bertrand *et al.*, 1975; Lee *et al.*, 1976; Sogin *et al.*, 1976; Rosenberg *et al.*, 1976). There is also a region of possible base pairing just before the 3' terminus, which is probably stable since this region can be isolated as a ribonuclease-T1-resistant core. The whole sequence is shown in Fig. 11.

2.7.2.   Translation of fd, f1, and M13

The DNA of the filamentous phages codes for at least eight proteins (Lyons and Zinder, 1972). Five of these gene products were identified *in vivo* (Henry and Pratt, 1969; Webster and Cashman, 1973; Lin and Pratt, 1974). Using *in vitro* systems for coupled transcription and translation of phage DNA, Model and Zinder (1974) working with f1 and Konings *et al.* (1975) working with M13 reported the same

```
                              20              40              60              80
ppp GGGGUCAAAGAUGAGUGUUUUAGUGUAUUCUUUCGCCUCUUUCGUUUUAGGUGGUGCCUUCGUAGUGGCAUUACGUAUU-

                    100             120             140
UUACCCGUUUAAUGGAAACUUCCUC AUG AAA AAG UCU UUA GUC CUC AAA GCC UCC GUA GCC GUU GCU ACC CUC GUU-
                          Met Lys Ser Leu Val Leu Lys Ala Ser Val Ala Thr Leu Val
                          ────────────────────────────────────────────────────────
                          Ribosome binding site
                          ── Coat protein ──→

     160             180             200             220
CCG AUG CUG UCU UUC GCU GCU GAG GGU GAC GAU CCC GCA AAA GCG GCC UUU GAC UCC CUG CAA GCC UCA GCG-
Pro Met Leu Ser Phe Ala Ala Glu Gly Asp Asp Pro Ala Lys Ala Ala Phe Asp Ser Leu Gln Ala Ser Ala

     240             260             280             300
ACC GAA UAU AUC GGU UAU GCG UGG GCG AUG GUU GUC AUU GUC GGC GCA ACU AUC GGU AUC AAG CUG UUU-
Thr Glu Tyr Ile Gly Tyr Ala Trp Ala Met Val Val Val Ile Val Gly Ala Thr Ile Gly Ile Lys Leu Phe
                                                               Ala in ZJ-2

              320             340
AAG AAA UUC ACC UCG AAA GCA AGC UGAUAAACCGAUACAAUUA    UUUUUU OH
Lys Lys Phe Thr Ser Lys Ala Ser                    A . U
                                                   A . U
                                                   G . C
                                                   G . C    360
                                                   C . G
                                                   U . A
                                                   C . G
                                                   C . G
                                                     U   U
                                                      U U
```

Fig. 11.   Nucleotide sequence of the mRNA initiated at the G0.82 promoter of fd and the amino acid sequence of the gene VIII precursor protein for which it codes. The region of secondary structure near the 3' terminus may be involved in termination. Adapted from Sugimoto *et al.* (1977).

results. The products of genes I, II, III, IV, V, and VIII could be clearly identified, and their molecular weights determined in various SDS-polyacrylamide gel electrophoresis systems. The molecular weight of the gene VIII product (the major coat protein) *in vitro* is somewhat larger than that of the protein isolated from phage particles (Konings *et al.*, 1975). This was predicted by Pieczenik *et al.* (1974), who isolated and sequenced a fragment of f1 mRNA which was protected against nuclease digestion by ribosomes. The fragment was from the smallest transcript, which codes only for the gene VIII product; hence the ribosomes would be expected to protect the initiation region for the coat protein. The amino acid sequence which could be read from the RNA sequence in the protected fragment did not correspond to the known N-terminal amino acid sequence of the coat protein (Asbeck *et al.*, 1969), and Pieczenik *et al.* (1974) postulated the existence of an N-terminal precursor sequence which was cleaved off before the coat protein was incorporated into the virion. Konings *et al.* (1975) estimated that the difference in length was about 20 amino acids, and Model *et al.* (personal communication) have obtained fragmentary amino acid sequence data from the *in vitro* gene VIII product which agrees with the initiation sequence of Pieczenik *et al.* (1974). The uncertainty in the precursor length has been resolved by Sugimoto *et al.* (1977), who have sequenced the whole of the small messenger RNA which codes for the gene VIII protein. There is a sequence of 23 amino acids from the initiation codon identified by Pieczenik *et al.* (1974) to the N-terminal amino acid of the virion coat protein. This sequence is shown in Fig. 11. One interesting feature is that since the coat protein of ZJ-2 differs from fd and f1 by substitution of alanine for threonine at position 36 (Snell and Offord, 1972), a single base mutation causing this substitution would create an *Alu*I site in ZJ-2 which is not present in fd. The next *Alu*I site in both phages is 14 base pairs away. Hence ZJ-2 would have an extra 14-long *Alu*I fragment, with a corresponding shortening of the adjacent fragment (fragment D of Van den Hondel *et al.*, 1976).

In the comparative studies of Van den Hondel and Schoenmakers (1976) no differences were observed in the *Alu*I maps of f1, fd, M13, and ZJ-2 in the gene VIII region. In their Fig. 5 the smallest fragments do not appear, but fragment D of ZJ-2 is distinctly faster than that of fd, f1, and M13, as would be expected if it were 14 base pairs shorter.

The complete amino acid sequence of the gene V (DNA binding) protein is also known (Cuypers *et al.*, 1974; Nakashima *et al.*, 1974). One of the ribosome-protected RNA sequences obtained by Pieczenik *et al.* (1974) predicted an N-terminal amino acid sequence which matches the gene V protein sequence; hence there is no processing at the N terminus of this protein. The molecular weights of the f1 and M13 *in vitro* products are the same as the *in vivo* proteins (Model and Zinder, 1974; Konings *et al.*, 1975).

The products of genes I (involved in morphogenesis) and III (the minor virion component) have been identified without ambiguities (Model and Zinder, 1974; Konings *et al.*, 1975), although the gene III protein *in vitro* has a higher molecular weight than the *in vivo* product, indicating the synthesis of a longer precursor (Konings *et al.*, 1975). Both investigating groups had trouble with multiple products from gene IV, interpreting their results as arising from premature termination. Both groups also found an extra protein from the gene II region (protein X), which has now been identified as a product of gene II and not an extra gene. It probably arises by initiation of translation in a separate mRNA which has its promoter within gene II (Edens *et al.*, 1976; Van den Hondel *et al.*, 1976). So far, no products synthesized *in vivo* or *in vitro* have been identified with gene VI or VII, even though there are amber mutants in both these genes, implying that they must be translated (Model and Zinder, 1974; Konings *et al.*, 1975; Chan *et al.*, 1975). Their amino acid sequences can be inferred from the DNA sequence (Schaller and Takanami, 1978).

Regulation of the amounts of each protein synthesized appears to be at least partly at the transcriptional level. The phenomenon of several promoters but only one major terminator provides a simple mechanism for this, since the proteins required in greatest amounts (gene products V and VIII) are close to the central terminator and therefore are coded by all the different lengths of mRNA molecules. For most genes, the amount of protein synthesized is related to the number of copies present (Chan *et al.*, 1975; Edens *et al.*, 1975; Seeburg and Schaller, 1975). In the case of gene VII, however, this can hardly be the case since, although placed between the two most noticeable gene products, the protein cannot be detected.

2.7.3. The Origin of Replication

The synthesis of double stranded DNA from the infecting single-stranded viral DNA and its subsequent replication have been extensively reviewed by Denhardt (1975) and Ray (1977). To summarize very briefly, synthesis of the first complementary strand is initiated from an RNA primer (Wickner *et al.*, 1972; Geider and Kornberg, 1974) at a specific site on the genome which has been mapped (1) by localizing the specific gap in double-stranded DNA left by excision of the primer

RNA (Griffith and Kornberg, 1974; Suggs and Ray, 1977; Tabak *et al.*, 1974), (2) by pulse-labeling replicating DNA as was used by Danna and Nathans (1972) to locate the origin of replication of SV40 DNA (Horiuchi and Zinder, 1976; Van den Hondel *et al.*, 1976; Suggs and Ray, 1977), and (3) by localizing a specific piece of DNA which is protected from nuclease digestion when complexed with RNA polymerase and DNA unwinding protein (Geider and Kornberg, 1974; Sigal *et al.*, 1972; Schaller *et al.*, 1976). The results all indicate that both strands of DNA are initiated in the same region, at 0.05–0.10 map unit (see Fig. 10). Gray *et al.* (1978) have sequenced the protected *ori* DNA fragment by the Maxam and Gilbert (1977) method applied to both strands and further confirmed by depurination analysis or the Sanger and Coulson (1975) method. The sequence is shown in Fig. 12. It contains extended palindromic sequences which result in stable hairpin loops in the single-stranded DNA, and long runs of pyrimidine nucleotides. These features are similar to those found in the replication origin sequences of plasmid *col*E1 (Tomizawa *et al.*, 1977) and SV40 (Subramanian *et al.*, 1977*b*), suggesting that such structures destabilize the double helix and therefore activate replication. Since the fd origin sequenced by Gray *et al.* (1978) does not correspond to any of the promoters previously detected, some such special mechanisms for RNA polymerase binding must be operating. The origin of replication in f1 also contains extensive potential secondary structure (Ravetch *et al.*, 1977*b*).

2.7.4. Other DNA Sequences from f1

The amino acid sequence of the fd coat protein as originally published (Asbeck *et al.*, 1969) contained the sequence Trp-Met-Val-. Since the codons specifying Trp and Met are not degenerate, the nucleotide sequence U-G-G-A-T-G-G-T would be expected at this site. Sanger *et al.* (1973) synthesized the octanucleotide complementary to the coding sequence and used it as a primer to determine an adjacent sequence of 50 nucleotides in f1 DNA. Since the sequence they obtained did not code for the coat protein, Sanger *et al.* (1973) suggested that the Trp-Met sequence was wrong, especially since the ZJ-2 sequence in this region was known to be Trp-Ala-Met (Snell and Offord, 1972). The extra Ala residue was confirmed in fd by Nakashima and Konigsberg (1974). However, the result is that a clear sequence of 50 nucleotides obtained from the synthetic primer is known, which must come from

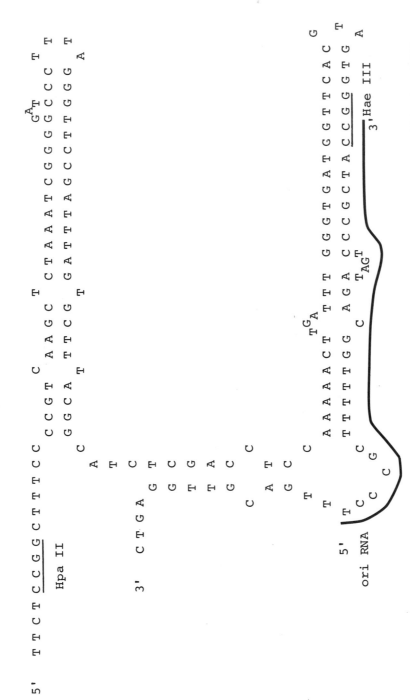

Fig. 12. Secondary structure of fd viral DNA at the origin of replication. The sequence of the *ori* RNA which primes DNA synthesis is indicated by the bold line. Adapted from Gray *et al.* (1978).

some other part of the f1 genome. The DNA sequence of Schaller and Takanami (1978) shows these nucleotides at the very end of gene II.

Of the sequences of ribosome-protected RNA fragments from f1 obtained by Pieczenik *et al.* (1974), two could be identified as the initiation regions for the gene V protein and the precursor gene VIII (coat) protein. The third sequence, of 14 nucleotides, remained unidentified until the complete fd DNA sequence was obtained. It is the initiation sequence for gene IV (Schaller and Takanami, 1978).

3. DNA SEQUENCES FROM ANIMAL VIRUSES

3.1. Simian Virus 40

Simian vacuolating virus 40 (SV40) is a small mammalian virus with oncogenic properties. Oncogenic viruses have come under intensive study over the past few years in an effort to understand the control mechanisms involved (for reviews, see Tooze, 1973; Tooze and Sambrook, 1974; Eckhard, 1974). SV40 is one of the smallest of such viruses, which has two important consequences. First, since its genetic capacity is so limited (about 5200 nucleotide pairs), it is dependent on host cell proteins for most of the processes involved in replication of its DNA, transcription and processing of viral message, and synthesis of viral proteins. Therefore, a detailed study of these mechanisms in the virus should reflect how such functions operate in the host cell. Second, the small size of SV40 means that it is feasible to obtain precise molecular information. The nucleotide sequence of the entire genome has recently been completed (Reddy *et al.*, 1978a; Fiers *et al.*, 1978).

Much of the sequence of SV40 obtained in Weissman's laboratory was from RNA transcripts using the basic RNA sequencing methods (Barrell, 1971). The RNA was labeled *in vivo* (Zain *et al.*, 1973) or *in vitro* using *E. coli* RNA polymerase (Subramanian *et al.*, 1977a). The *in vivo* RNA was annealed to DNA restriction fragments immobilized on nitrocellulose filters, eluted, and digested with enzymes such as pancreatic, T1, or U2 ribonucleases; the protected fragment purified by electrophoresis and homochromatography (Brownlee and Sanger, 1969) and sequenced by spleen and venom phosphodiesterases. A detailed description of these methods as applied to SV40 is given by Marotta *et al.* (1974).

As the number of known restriction enzymes increased, and small (~100 bp) fragments of DNA could be isolated, these were sequenced directly. The ends were labeled with $[\gamma\text{-}^{32}P]$-ATP and polynucleotide kinase (Maniatis *et al.*, 1975), and the 3'-terminal sequence was determined using limited venom phosphodiesterase (Galibert *et al.*, 1974). More recently these end-labeled fragments have been sequenced by the Maxam and Gilbert (1977) method. Most of the SV40 sequences obtained in Weissman's laboratory have been checked by two of these approaches, or by sequencing both strands of the DNA.

The methods used by Fiers and his collaborators are basically the same. They have used *in vitro* RNA transcripts labeled internally with one or another [^{32}P]nucleoside triphosphate (Volckaert *et al.*, 1976, 1977). The transcripts were digested with pancreatic, T1, or U2 ribonuclease and sequenced by standard methods (Barrell, 1971). Some sequences were obtained by substituting a deoxyribonucleoside triphosphate for the normal precursor. For example, if dG is incorporated, ribonuclease U2 will cleave only at the A residues. Similarly, if dU is incorporated, pancreatic ribonuclease will be specific for C residues (Van de Voorde *et al.*, 1974). DNA fragments have been sequenced directly by 5'-end labeling and partial venom phosphodiesterase digestion, or by the partial chemical degradation of Maxam and Gilbert (1977) (Ysebaert *et al.*, 1976; Contreras *et al.*, 1977; Van Heuverswyn *et al.*, 1977; Volckaert *et al.*, 1977; Van de Voorde *et al.*, 1976).

3.1.1. The Genetic and Physical Maps of SV40

The genome of SV40 is a double-stranded, covalently closed circular DNA of molecular weight about 3.4×10^6 or approximately 5200 base pairs. Physical maps were first compiled by Danna and Nathans (1971) and Danna *et al.* (1973). Since then most new restriction enzymes have been tested on SV40 DNA, and an extensive catalogue of sites is now available (for a review, see Roberts, 1976). These have been invaluable in locating genetic sites and in the nucleotide sequence analysis. The marker-rescue technique (Edgell *et al.*, 1972; Hutchison and Edgell, 1971) in which individual wild-type restriction fragments annealed to mutant single-strand circles are used to infect cells and thus ascertain which restriction fragment "rescues" the mutation to produce wild-type progeny has been adapted for SV40. Lai and Nathans (1974) mapped a number of temperature-sensitive mutants, both early and late, in this way. Restriction fragments have also been used to map the origin of replication of the SV40 genome. Replication was found to be bidirectional from a precise region of the genome and to terminate at a specific site on the opposite side of the DNA (Nathans and Danna, 1972; Danna and Nathans, 1972). The early and late messenger RNA molecules have also been mapped (Khoury *et al.*, 1974; Sambrook *et al.*, 1972, 1973; Dhar *et al.*, 1974, 1977*b*; May *et al.*, 1977). The major early and late mRNAs are both initiated near the origin of replication in opposite directions and terminate near the DNA replication terminus.

The SV40 gene products which are clearly identified are the three structural proteins VPI (MW 43,000), VP2 (MW 38,000), and VP3 (MW 27,000) and an early protein (A protein) of molecular weight 85,000. VP1, VP2, and VP3 are all transcribed from late mRNA, VP3 apparently being part of the VP2 amino acid sequence (Crawford, 1973).

The genetic and physical map of SV40 is summarized in Fig. 13.

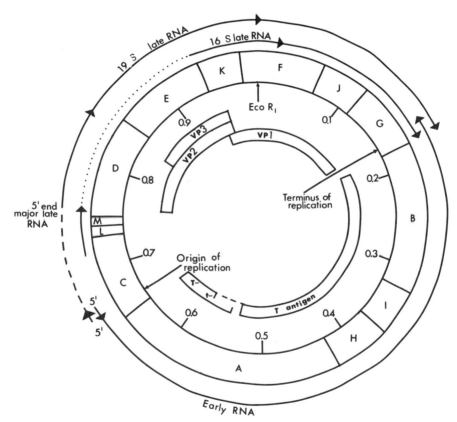

Fig. 13.   Genetic and physical map of SV40. The outer lines indicate the 5′ and 3′ ends of the major early and late species of RNA. The dashed line indicates a minor late RNA, and the dotted line indicates where the 5′ end of 16 S late RNA is joined to RNA sequences coded by a different region of the genome. The middle circle shows the *Hin*dII + III restriction map, while the gene products are innermost. The map was compiled from numerous sources cited in the text.

More detailed information is given by the nucleotide sequence of the DNA.

3.1.2. The Origin of Replication and Initiation of Transcription

As shown in Fig. 13, the 5' ends of early and late mRNA are complementary in nucleotide sequence since they are transcribed from opposite strands of the same DNA duplex sequence. This overlapping region also contains the origin of DNA replication (Danna and Nathans, 1972). The nucleotide sequence through this region has been determined (Subramanian *et al.*, 1977*a,b,c,d*; Dhar *et al.*, 1977*a,b*) and is shown in Fig. 14. Although the exact nucleotides which initiate DNA synthesis are unknown, the region shows an amazing degree of symmetry and repeating sequences, including a tandem repeat of 21 nucleotides and another of 55 nucleotides (Subramanian *et al.*, 1977*b,d*). Within the sequence of 60 nucleotides the hexanucleotide sequence G-G-G-C-G-G occurs six times (Subramanian *et al.*, 1977*b*), and just before the VP2-initiating ATG triplet is a nearly perfect tandem repeat (19 out of 20 nucleotides are identical) (Dhar *et al.*, 1977*a*). These sequences may play a similar role to the noncoding reiterated sequences in most eukaryotic cell DNA (Lewin, 1975), but as yet such function is unknown.

Transcription of both early and late mRNAs begins in the same region, but since the mRNA isolated *in vivo* may have undergone processing the 5' ends may not reflect a transcription initiation event (Dhar *et al.*, 1977*a*). However, the DNA preceding the sequence complementary to the 5' ends of cytoplasmic RNAs is characteristic—before the 5' end of early RNA is a sequence of 17 consecutive A·T pairs (Subramanian *et al.*, 1977*b*), while preceding the 5' end of late RNA is a sequence of 14 consecutive A·T pairs. Before the 5' end of "restart" late RNA (see Fig. 13) there is a sequence where 19 of 23 base pairs are A·T. These A·T-rich regions could be part of the promoters which initiate transcription or be a recognition sequence for processing enzymes (Dhar *et al.*, 1977*a*).

Dhar *et al.* (1974*a*) located the 3' ends [before the poly(A)] of the early and late transcripts by hybridization of *in vivo* transcripts to restriction fragments. Both early and late RNAs terminate very close to the *Hin*dB-G junction, and very close to the site where DNA synthesis terminates, within *Hin*dG (Danna and Nathans, 1972). May *et al.* (1977) have obtained the same result using electron microscopy. The 3' end [before the poly(A)] of the early mRNA contains at least 50 nucleotides after the last possible protein termination codon (Dhar *et al.*, 1974*b*). The 3' end of the late messenger RNA, at the *Hind*B-G junction, is approximately 70 nucleotides from the termination codon which ends the major coat protein (Celma *et al.*, 1977; Dhar *et al.*, 1974*a*).

3.1.3. The Early Region of SV40

Studies on the expression of the early region *in vivo* and *in vitro* have detected only one virus-specific protein, the A protein (see Rundell *et al.*, 1977; Anderson *et al.*, 1977). This A protein has been identified with the virus-specific T antigen which appears in infected cells (Rundell *et al.*, 1977). Other virus-specific antigens, the U antigen in the nucleus and the TSTA (tumor-specific transplantation antigen) on the cell surface, are also expressions of the early region of the SV40 genome, but there is no evidence that they are virus coded. One reason for assuming that they are not was that the molecular weight of the A protein (T antigen) estimated by electrophoresis on SDS-polyacrylamide gels was greater than 85,000. Since the early mRNA contains fewer than 2600 nucleotides, it seemed to contain only the T-antigen-coding sequence. Dhar *et al.* (1977*a*) found that the nucleotide sequence of the first 300 or so nucleotides of early RNA has termination codons (UGA, UAA, or UAG) in the three possible translation phases. Since all three termination codons have been found to operate in eukaryotic cells (Forget *et al.*, 1975; Efstratiadis *et al.*, 1977; Browne *et al.*, 1977; Proudfoot, 1977), the T antigen seemed not to be initiated before 0.595 map unit (Fig. 13). Thimmappaya and Weissman (1977) have sequenced another region of 70 base pairs about 0.545 map unit, and again there are terminators in all three reading frames. The 3' end of early mRNA is located near map position 0.160 (Khoury *et al.*, 1975; Dhar *et al.*, 1974*a,b*). Sequences obtained by Dhar *et al.*

Fig. 14.   Sequence around the origin of replication of SV40. A: The nucleotide sequence of the *Eco*RII-G fragment, containing parts of *Hind*C and *Hind*A (see Fig. 13). The "early" and "late" mRNA starts are indicated. Sequences possessing 2-fold rotational axes of symmetry appear within boxes drawn with solid lines; the rotational axes are shown as dashed lines within the boxes. True palindromes appear in the boxes drawn with dashed lines. Repeating sequences are shown within boxes drawn with alternate dashes and dots. The 17-long A·T-containing sequence which is flanked by G·C-rich sequences is shown in the box drawn with dotted lines. AUG triplets marked by arrows are possible protein initiation codons. B: Possible secondary structure in the *Eco*RII-G nucleotide sequence. From Subramanian *et al.* (1977*b*), with permission.

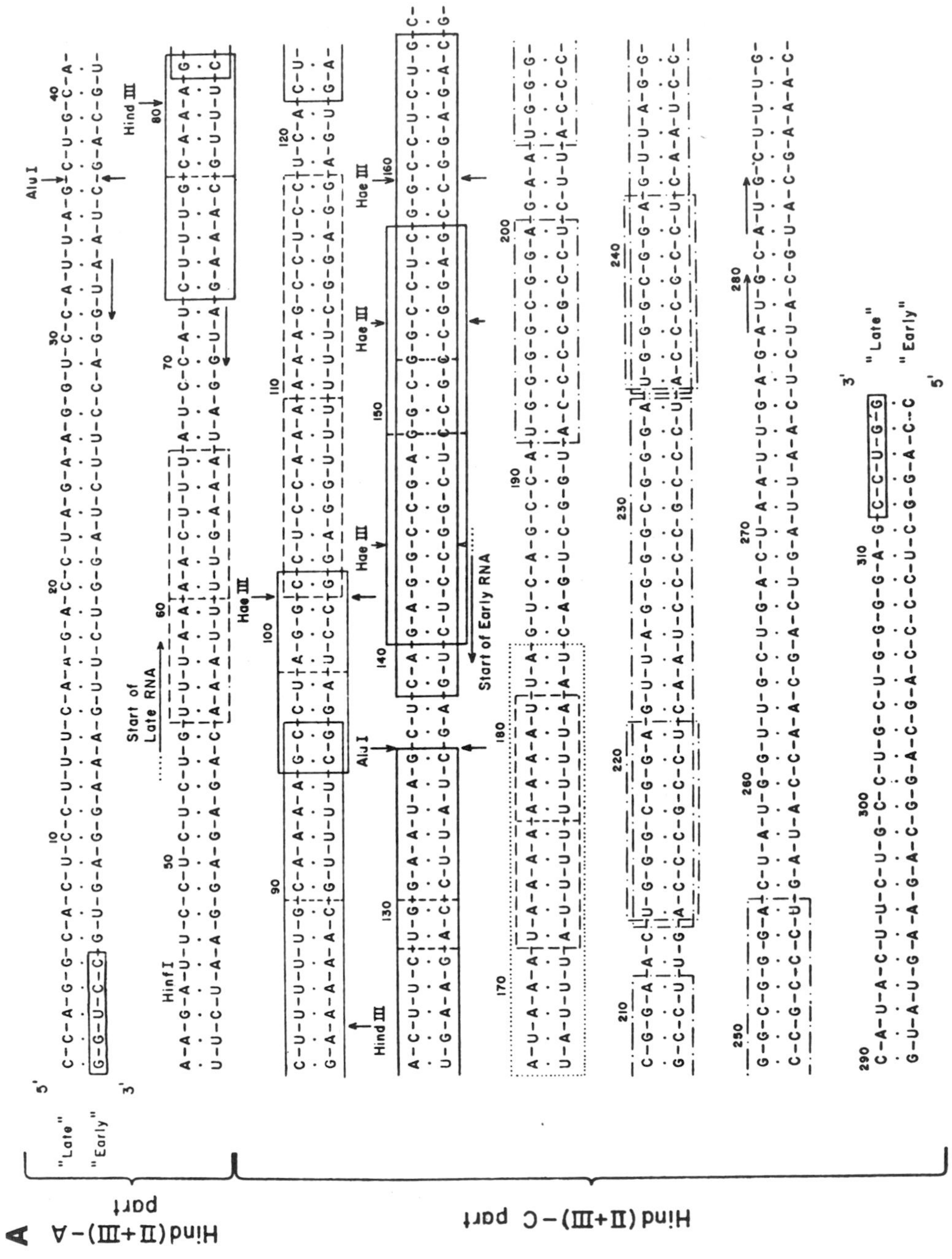
A
Hind(II+III)-A part
Hind(II+III)-C part
"Late"
"Early"
Start of Late RNA
Start of Early RNA
Hinf I
Hind III
Hae III
Alu I

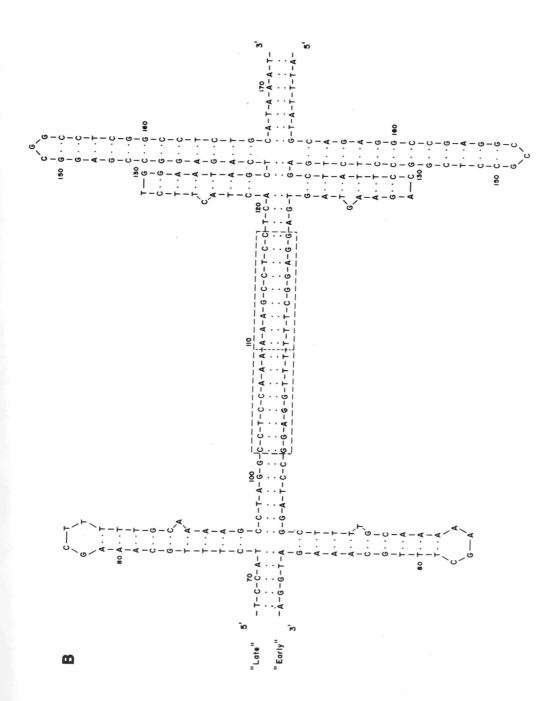

(1974*a,b*) at about 0.175 map unit contain termination codons in all three phases; hence the molecular weight of the T antigen could not be more than 70,000. There has been one reported molecular weight of this value (Del Villano and Defendi, 1973), but other estimates are much higher (Prives *et al.*, 1977; Tegtmeyer *et al.*, 1977), although the SDS gel mobility has been reported as varying with the gel system used (Rundell *et al.*, 1977). Volckaert *et al.* (1977) have sequenced the *Hin*dH (Fig. 13) fragment and found terminators in two reading frames. The third is therefore assigned to code for part of the T-antigen amino acid sequence.

The question is then: what is the function of the 25% (approximately 650 nucleotides) of the early mRNA which is apparently not translated into T antigen? There are results that suggest that host range mutants and temperature-sensitive early mutants might complement each other (Fluck *et al.*, 1976), and in the related polyoma virus some host range mutants have mapped in the 5′-terminal region of the early region while the early temperature-sensitive mutants in both polyoma and SV40 map beyond 0.545 map unit (Lai and Nathans, 1975; Feunteun *et al.*, 1976; Miller and Fried, 1976). Deletion mutants between 0.59 and 0.54 map unit do not affect the T antigen (A protein) (Shenk *et al.*, 1976). On the other hand, TSTA and U antigen, but not T antigen, are expressed during infection with the adeno-SV40 hybrid which contains only the segment of the early region of the SV40 genome spanning *Hin*d fragments H, I, and B (Lebowitz *et al.*, 1974) or is lacking early sequence from 0.54 to 0.67 (Lewis, 1977).

The anomalies in the early region coding capacity of SV40 have been recently resolved by the discovery that the "splicing" phenomenon, where the final (translated) messenger RNA contains segments from different regions of the genome (Celma *et al.*, 1977; Berget *et al.*, 1977; Klessig, 1977; Chow *et al.*, 1977*a,b*), is not restricted to noncoding sequences. In the β-globin and ovalbumin genes, for instance, there are relatively long (>500 nucleotide pairs) sequences which interrupt the coding sequences found in the messenger RNA (Tilghman *et al.*, 1978; Weinstock *et al.*, 1978).

When isolated from productively infected or transformed cells, two major forms of T antigen are detected. These are referred to as "large T" and "small t" and have apparent molecular weights of 90,000–100,000 and 15,000–20,000, respectively. Peptide mapping has shown that they have amino acid sequences in common (Prives *et al.*, 1977) and their N termini are identical (Paucha *et al.*, 1978) at 0.65 map unit (Fig. 13).

In the DNA sequence of SV40 (Fiers *et al.*, 1978; Reddy *et al.*, 1978*b*) the initiation codon for t and T is followed by 174 codons before a termination codon, and this appears to code for the t amino acid sequence (Volckaert *et al.*, 1978). The model proposed for large T synthesis is that it is initiated at the same codon as small t but is coded by two noncontiguous segments. One is from 0.65 to almost 0.59, and a second from 0.53 to 0.17 (Crawford *et al.*, 1978). Thus the region around 0.545 which contains termination codons in all three region frames is exluded from the T coding sequence. Mutants with deletions between 0.54 and 0.59 produce normal-sized T antigen, while small t is reduced in size (Sleigh *et al.*, 1978). Further protein sequencing work, or nucleic acid sequence determination of the mature mRNA, will be required to precisely locate the boundaries of the intervening DNA which does not code for protein.

3.1.4. The Late Region of SV40

Transcription of one species of late RNA is initiated at about 0.65 map unit (Fig. 13). As previously discussed, the 5' end overlaps the 5' end of early RNA which is transcribed from the complementary strand. The genes expressed from late RNA are the structural proteins VP1, VP2, and VP3. The molecular weights of these proteins (Salzman and Khoury, 1974; Rozenblatt *et al.*, 1976; Crawford, 1973) indicate that they would require most of the late RNA sequence (approximately 2000 nucleotides) for coding, but peptide data have shown that VP2 and VP3 contain common amino acid sequences (Crawford, 1973).

The nucleotide sequence reported by Dhar *et al.* (1977*a*) extending from 0.595 to 0.790 (Fig. 13) contains the 5'-terminal sequence of late RNA, although there is a major species of late RNA initiated at 0.775. The sequence of RNA from 0.65 to 0.75 contains terminators in all three reading frames (Dhar *et al.*, 1977*a*). Dhar *et al.* (1978) have extended this sequence through the 5' end of the late restart RNA (at 0.775) to 0.83. The first possible initiation codon for the structural protein VP2 is 40 nucleotides from the *Hin*dM-D junction within *Hin*dD. The sequence preceding this codon has some strange features in addition to the reiterated sequences discussed above (Dhar *et al.*, 1977*a,b*; Subramanian *et al.*, 1977*b*). Large amounts of RNA are present in infected cells complementary to part of *Hin*dC, while RNA transcribed from a short segment prior to the initiation codon could not be detected. Parts of this region (*Hin*dL and M, and part of *Hin*dC) have also been sequenced in Fiers's laboratory (Ysebaert *et al.*, 1976; Van Heuverswyn *et al.*, 1977) and part of *Hin*dM by Tu *et al.* (1976).

Reddy *et al.* (1977*b*) have completed the coding sequences for VP2 and VP3, most of which has also been determined by Fiers *et al.* (1975)

and Contreras *et al.* (1977*a*). Although there exist as yet no protein sequence data for VP2 and VP3, the reading frame which extends for 340 codons before the next terminator must contain the VP2 coding sequence. The initiation codon is not so easy to identify. The protein cannot be initiated before the codon chosen by Reddy *et al.* (1977*b*) since there is a termination codon in this reading frame to the 3′ side of the next AUG triplet. The 5′ end of large, late mRNA is located by electron microscopy (May *et al.*, 1977) and sequence analysis (Dhar *et al.*, 1977*a*) very cose to the *Hind*C-D junction, and the proposed VP2 protein initiation codon is close to the 5′ end of this mRNA. The next AUG codon is 107 codons downstream from the VP2 initiation codon, and this is proposed as the initiator for VP3, giving a protein of 229 amino acids in the same reading frame as VP2. More direct confirmation of these initiation sites is required, but the data on the amino acid composition of VP3 (Greenway and LeVine, 1973) agree to some extent with those obtained from the nucleotide sequence. There is, however, an alarming discrepancy between the composition and sequence in the glycine content of VP3.

The initiation codon for the major structural protein VP1 has been localized near the *Hind*E-K junction since the 16 S mRNA, which directs synthesis of VP1, is initiated here (May *et al.*, 1977). The termination region is within *Hind*G (Dhar *et al.*, 1974*a*). Since the N-terminal amino acid sequence has been determined (Lazarides *et al.*, 1974), the codons specifying the sequence can be located in the DNA sequence (Celma *et al.*, 1977; Contreras *et al.*, 1977*a*). This sequence in fact occurs before the termination codon for the VP2 and VP3 proteins, but in a different reading frame. This is the first demonstration that the phenomenon of overlapping genes found in ϕX174 (Barrell *et al.*, 1976; Smith *et al.*, 1977) occurs also in an animal virus. In the SV40 case there are 114 nucleotides translated in two different reading frames. The VP1 sequence extends for 361 codons before the first termination codon is reached (Pan *et al.*, 1977). This would predict a molecular weight of the protein of about 40,000, in reasonable agreement with the observed value of 43,000. The amino acid composition obtained from the DNA sequence is also in good agreement with analysis of the protein (Greenway and LeVine 1973). Parts of the VP1 coding sequence had been determined previously by Contreras *et al.* (1977*b*) and by Van de Voorde *et al.* (1976).

A section of the sequences of VP1, VP2, and VP3 is shown in Fig. 15. The DNA sequence extending beyond the C-terminal amino acids of VP1 has also been established (Zain *et al.*, 1978), thus overlapping

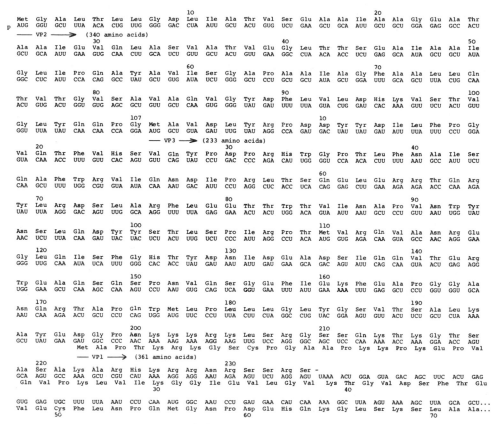

Fig. 15. Nucleotide sequence which codes for the structural proteins VP2, VP3, and part of VP1 of SV40. The sequence is shown from the initiating AUG codon of VP2, the amino acid sequence of which is inferred from the DNA sequence. VP3 arises from an internal initiation within VP2 as shown. VP1 initiates before the ends of VP2 and VP3, but in a different reading frame. The sequence is from Reddy *et al.* (1978*a*). Contreras *et al.* (1977*a*) have reported the sequence from amino acid 45 of VP3 to the C terminus of VP3 and demonstrated the same overlapping of the initiation of VP1. Preceding this, however, there are two nucleotide differences from the sequence obtained by Reddy *et al.* (1978*a*). These are in codons 110 (GUG) and 113 (CGA).

the early sequences described above and completing the nucleotide sequence of the SV40 genome. Since the mRNA for VP1 extends to the *Hin*dG-B junction (Dhar *et al.*, 1974*b*), there are about 70 untranslated nucleotides between the termination codon and the poly(A) tract at the 3' end of the messenger. However, oligonucleotide analysis of the 16 S mRNA which codes for VP1 showed extra sequences not present in the DNA sequence from this region (Aloni *et al.*, 1977; Celma *et al.*, 1977;

Haegeman and Fiers, 1978). Since the total SV40 sequence is known, these extra sequences could be searched for. They are located within part of *Hin*dC and in the small fragments *Hin*dL and M (Fig. 13) but not extending into *Hin*dD. The 200-nucleotide sequence is covalently attached to the 16 S RNA coding for VP1, 1000 nucleotides away. This "agnogene" sequence contains an ATG codon followed by 59 sense codons before the first terminator, but it is not known if a small polypeptide is produced (Celma *et al.*, 1977). This phenomenon is also found in transcription of adenovirus late genes (Berget *et al.*, 1977; Klessig, 1977; Chow *et al.*, 1977a,b) (see Section 3.3).

3.2. Polyoma Virus

Polyoma is a small oncogenic virus, very similar in genetic and physical characteristics to SV40. Both viruses contain a circular, double-stranded DNA molecule of about 5000 base pairs, which replicates bidirectionally from a single unique site on the genome and terminates at a site almost directly opposite on the circular map. Polyoma produces early and late messenger RNA, each involving about 50% of the genome. The 5' ends of the early and late transcripts both map very close to the origin of DNA replication, and the 3' ends map very close to the DNA replication termination site (Kamen *et al.*, 1974; Griffin *et al.*, 1974), precisely as found in SV40 (Dhar *et al.*, 1974a; Khoury *et al.*, 1974; Danna and Nathans, 1972). However, there appears to be very little nucleotide sequence homology, as examined by hybridization (Ferguson and Davis, 1975) or restriction enzyme mapping (see Roberts, 1976).

The nucleotide sequence of a fragment of polyoma DNA which contains the origin of DNA replication (Miller and Fried, 1976) has been determined by Soeda *et al.* (1977). They used two methods for the sequence analysis. Most of the information was obtained from the Maxam and Gilbert (1977) method, with 5' regions of the sequences being confirmed by partial digestion of 5' end-labeled fragments by pancreatic deoxyribonuclease I. The resulting olignucleotides were separated by electrophoresis on cellulose acetate at pH 3.5 followed by homochromatography in the second dimension on PEI plates as described by Volckaert *et al.* (1976).

A sequence of 74 nucleotide pairs was obtained, which contains a possible region of base pairing as shown in Fig. 16. The sequence does not show significant homology to the origin of replication of SV40, but there is an A·T-rich true palindromic sequence flanked by G·C-rich

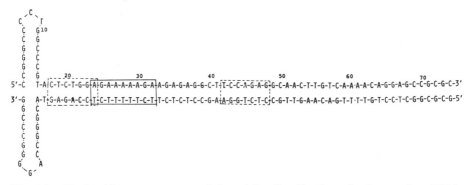

Fig. 16.   Nucleotide sequence around the origin of replication of polyoma virus DNA. The sequence contains a G·C-rich stretch with a 2-fold axis of symmetry and therefore possible secondary structure as shown. There is an A·T-rich stretch with true palindromic sequences (boxed with solid lines) and two inverted repeats (boxed with dashed lines). The top line is the "late" strand, the lower line the "early" strand of polyoma DNA. From Soeda *et al.* (1977), with permission.

hairpin loops, reminiscent of the region preceding the early messenger RNA start in SV40 (Subramanian *et al.*, 1977*b*).

3.3.   Adenoviruses

The genome of human adenoviruses is a linear duplex DNA of molecular weight around 23×10^6 representing approximately 35,000 nucleotide pairs (Green *et al.*, 1970). More than 80 distinct adenovirus serotypes have been isolated from human and animal sources (Wilner, 1969), but molecular studies have been concentrated on three human serotypes—adenoviruses 2, 5, and 12. Filter hybridization and heteroduplex mapping indicate 85–90% homology between genomes of Ad2 and Ad5, while these have less than 25% homology to the Ad12 genome (for reviews, see Green *et al.*, 1970; Philipson *et al.*, 1975; Ginsberg and Young, 1977).

When adenovirus infects permissive cells it can undergo productive infection. In nonpermissive cells the virus may bring about cell transformation. In productive infection the viral DNA rapidly enters the nucleus and transcription of early genes begins. At the onset of viral DNA replication, transcription of the late genes is initiated (Green *et al.*, 1970). In transformed cells the viral DNA is integrated into the host genome (Green, 1970). Infectious virus particles cannot be found in or induced from the transformed cells, but expression of some viral genes can be demonstrated, in particular transcription into specific mRNA molecules (Green *et al.*, 1970). Transformed cells contain two specific antigens, the T antigen and a transplantation antigen (TSTA), but so far these have not been conclusively shown to be encoded by the adenovirus genome. The relationship between transformation and tumor induction by adenoviruses has been reviewed by Philipson *et al.* (1975). *In vitro* transformation can be brought about by infecting cells with DNA fragments, specifically from the left-hand end of the genome (Graham *et al.*, 1974). Gallimore *et al.* (1974) showed that different cell lines of transformed cells contain in common the left-hand 14% of the genome, along with sequences from other parts of the DNA which vary between the cell lines. No cell line has been found with a complete adenovirus genome, which accounts for the inability to obtain infectious virus from transformed cells by physical or chemical treatments (Weber, 1974). *In situ* hybridization studies have not located adenovirus DNA on specific chromosomes (McDougall *et al.*, 1972; Loni and Green, 1973). Although there is particular interest in the processes involved in transformation and tumorigenesis, at the molecular level it is more practical to study situations on productive infection, and a certain amount is now known about transcription, translation, and replication of these viruses.

3.3.1. Adenovirus 2

Ad2 restriction maps have been prepared for the enzymes *Eco*RI (Mulder *et al.*, 1974); *Hpa*I (Mulder *et al.*, 1974); *Bam*I, *Hin*dIII, and *Sma*I (quoted in Sambrook *et al.*, 1975); and *Bal*I (quoted in Klessig, 1977). For nomenclature and details of these restriction enzymes, see Roberts (1976).

Transcripts of Ad2 synthesized during the early and late phases have been located on the restriction maps. The results have been reviewed by Philipson (1977), Flint (1977), Philipson *et al.* (1975), Chow *et al.* (1977*a*) and Ginsberg and Young (1977).

In the period before onset of viral DNA replication, most of both strands of the viral genome appear to be expressed in RNA isolated from the nucleus, but in cytoplasmic RNA only four short regions of the genome are represented (Philipson, 1977). These have been mapped on restriction fragments by hybridization in an aqueous polymer two-phase system (Philipson, 1977) and by electron microscopy (Chow *et al.*, 1977*a*). The resulting composite transcription map is shown in Fig. 17. The two strands of adenovirus-2 DNA are designated either "r" and "l" (indicating the strands from which rightward and leftward mRNA synthesis originates) or "h" and "l" [indicating heavy and light bouyant density in CsCl when complexed with poly(UG)], as indicated in Fig. 17. The four early cytoplasmic RNA species are located as shown, two transcribed from the r (l) strand, originating at 1.3–11.1 and 78.6–86.2 map units, and two from the l (h) strand at map units 62.4–67.9 and 91.5–96.8 (Chow *et al.*, 1977*a*). By *in vitro* translation of these mRNAs some of the polypeptides coded by them have been identified on SDS-polyacrylamdie gel electrophoresis (Anderson *et al.*, 1974; Walter and Maizel, 1974; Oberg *et al.*, 1975; Lewis *et al.*, 1976), and these are indicated in Fig. 17. The major early protein with an assigned function is the DNA binding protein (Fig. 17) which is involved in initiation and elongation in DNA synthesis (Van de Vliet *et al.*, 1977).

The late proteins are somewhat easier to characterize since almost all are structural components of the virion. One exception is a 100,000 MW protein found in messenger ribonucleoprotein particles in infected cells (Lindberg and Sundquist, 1974). The late RNA has been characterized in the nucleus (Weber *et al.*, 1977; Goldberg *et al.*, 1977) as a rightward-transcribing unit extending from 20 to 100 map units, close to 25,000 nucleotides in length, initiated at a specific site. Post-transcriptional cleavage would then give rise to the cytoplasmic mRNAs. The proteins coded by these mRNAs have been mapped (Eron *et al.*, 1974*a*,*b*; Lewis *et al.*, 1975), and the major ones are included in Fig. 17.

As the transcription maps were refined, some rather strange facts emerged. The information available at present indicates that many late

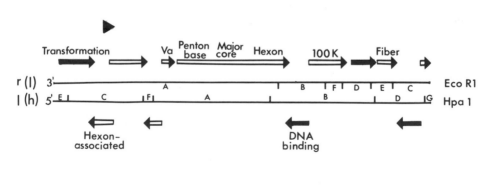

Fig. 17.   Map of the adenovirus 2 genome. Arrows indicate major species of RNA: →, early mRNA; ⇒, late mRNA. Some of the major functions coded by these mRNAs are indicated. ▶ represents the start of large, late, nuclear RNA. The restriction maps for *Eco*RI and *Hpa*I are shown. Adapted from Philipson *et al.* (1975) and Flint (1977).

mRNAs have sequences from several, well-separated parts of the genome. By hybridizing the mRNA which codes for the hexon protein of the adenovirus coat, Berget *et al.* (1977) demonstrated that it contained sequences from four separate regions of DNA, which was nicely visualized when the hexon mRNA was hybridized to the long *Eco*RI fragment A which extends from the left-hand side of the genome to about the end of the hexon gene. Three loops of unhybridized DNA could be seen. The only interpretation of this pattern is that the hexon mRNA consists of four distinct sequences. At the 5' end are a small number of nucleotides complementary to 16.8 map units on the r strand. Next come approximately 80 nucleotides from 19.8 map units, then 110 nucleotides from 26.9, and finally the region coding for the hexon polypeptide between 51.7 and 61.2 map units.

Independently, several approaches to transcription mapping in the Cold Spring Harbor Laboratory led to the same conclusions. Gelinas and Roberts (1977) found that many, and possibly all, late mRNAs contain an identical sequence at the 5' end, the capped structure being $7mG^{5'}ppp^{5'}A^mC^mU(C_4,U_3)G$. When fiber or 100K mRNA (see Fig. 17) was hybridized to DNA fragments, this oligonucleotide was very susceptible to ribonuclease T1 digestion (Klessig, 1977). This suggested that the 5' end of the mRNAs was not coded by the DNA sequence adjacent to the protein-coding region of these genes. The capped structures are protected from RNase action when the mRNAs are hybridized to a fragment mapping between 14.7 and 17, while the rest of the noncoding leader sequence hybridizes between 25.5 and 27.9. Chow *et al.* (1977*a,b*) found in electron microscope studies that the 5' ends of fiber and 100K mRNAs are complementary to sequences near positions 17, 20, and 27. This leader sequence is therefore common to at least the hexon, fiber, and 100K gene mRNAs and may contain some control function. The site of complementarity of the 5'-terminal oligonucleotide maps at the same position as the initiation site of the very long transcripts isolated from the nucleus (Weber *et al.*, 1977; Goldberg *et al.*, 1977). Since the large nuclear RNAs are polyadenylated at the 3' end (Darnell *et al.*, 1973) and capped at the 5' end (Shatkin, 1976), the model proposed by Klessig (1977) is that this single large RNA can be looped out and pieces ligated together to make up the various species of late mRNA. With the common leader sequence these late genes could then be under coordinate control.

One nucleotide sequence determination in the internal regions of the adenovirus genome is the "VA RNA." This low-molecular-weight RNA accumulates in infected cells both early and late in infection. It is 156 nucleotides in length, and the sequence was determined by Ohe and

Weissman (1970). There were several points of heterogeneity in the molecule. The sequence can be drawn into extensively base-paired structures, and there is a region somewhat homologous to several tRNA sequences. This RNA maps at 30 map units (Fig. 17) (Mathews, 1975), adjacent to another small RNA which is present only early in infection, but as yet there is still no evidence as to the function of either species.

Zain and Roberts (1978) have sequenced one of the recombination sites in the adeno-SV40 hybrid virus Ad2$^+$ND$_1$ and in Ad2 using the Maxam and Gilbert (1977) method. The corresponding sequence in SV40 is known (Dhar et al., 1974b; Reddy et al., 1978b; Fiers et al., 1978). In the hybrid about 850 nucleotide pairs of SV40 DNA from map position 0.11 are integrated in Ad2 from 86 map units. The sequence of the hybrid is identical to that of the respective parent virus on each side of the recombination site, but there are no sequence homologies with the other parent which would explain why integration occurs at that particular locus.

3.3.2. Replication of Adenovirus 2

Adenovirus DNA on denaturation and renaturation at low concentrations yields single-stranded circles (Garon et al., 1972; Wolfson and Dressler, 1972). Both strands are able to circularize, and they are opened by exonuclease III, which acts on a 3' end if it is part of a duplex DNA molecule. The most reasonable interpretation of these observations is that the single-strand circles are held by a "panhandle" structure, i.e., that the ends of adenovirus DNA form an inverted terminal repetition. The 3' nucleotide sequences were determined by Steenbergh et al. (1975). The method used was that of Englund (1971, 1972), which is based on the repair (exonuclease plus polymerase) activity of T4 DNA polymerase. Incubation of a linear duplex DNA with T4 polymerase in the presence of a single deoxyribonucleoside triphosphate results in exonucleolytic activity from the 3' end until the mononucleotide released is replacable with the dNTP which is present. Then it is essentially replaced faster than it is removed, and exonuclease activity stops at that point. By using each of the four dNTPs in turn, Steenbergh et al. (1972) found that the 3' sequence at both ends of the genome was pGpApTpG (3'), confirming the existence of a certain degree of terminal repetition. The length of the inverted terminal repeat was estimated by restriction enzyme analysis to be 100–140 nucleotide pairs (Roberts et al., 1974) and by exonuclease III inhibition of single-strand circle formation to be not more than 110 nucleotides (Robinson and Bellett, 1975). The sequences of the ends have now been extended by Arrand and Roberts (1977) using the Maxam–Gilbert (1977) method on material labeled at the 3' end with $[\alpha\text{-}^{32}P]$-dGTP and T4 polymerase. The sequence is shown in Fig. 18. The ends are identical for 102 nucleotide pairs, then show a marked divergence. This terminal sequence is not palindromic. Covalently attached to the 5' end of each strand is a protein (Rekosh et al., 1977; Carusi, 1977). This protein has been proposed to function in DNA replication (Rekosh et al., 1977), which is initiated at each 5' end of the genome (Horwitz, 1976; Weingartner et al., 1976).

The mechanism of replication of adenovirus DNA is not obvious (Watson, 1972; Bellett and Younghusband, 1972). Wu et al. (1977) observed some type of secondary structure at the ends of Ad2 DNA in the electron microscope, which has been interpreted as a hairpin structure that could initiate DNA synthesis, but as pointed out by Stillman et al. (1977) the available evidence does not support hairpin-priming in adenovirus DNA replication.

3.3.3. Adenovirus 5

Although detailed transcription maps are known for Ad2 DNA, the genetics of Ad5 is much more advanced through the use of mutants (Williams et al., 1974; Ginsberg and Young, 1977), two of which represent early functions required for viral DNA synthesis (Russell et al., 1974). Flint et al. (1976) have drawn up early and late mRNA maps by hybridization to restriction fragments. The maps are very similar to those of Ad2 (Fig. 17).

Replication of Ad5 also follows closely that of Ad2. Sussenbach and Kuijk (1977) have shown that termination of replication is at the ends of the genome, in accord with a displacement synthesis model, and Sussenbach et al. (1976) have reported that initiation occurs at both ends of the genome. A protein is covalently attached to the 5' end of Ad5 DNA with similar properties to that of Ad2 (Rekosh et al., 1977). The four terminal nucleotides at the ends of the DNA are identical (Steenbergh et al., 1975).

3.3.4. Adenovirus 12

Transcription maps of Ad12 have been prepared for nuclear and cytoplasmic RNAs from productively infected cells and in transformed

Protein
|
5' C A T C A T C A T A A T A T A C C T T A T T T T G G A T T G A A G C C A A T A T G A T A A A T G A G G
3' T A G T A G T A T T A T A T G G A A T A A A A C C T A A C T T C G G T T A T T A C T T A T T A C T C C
                                                                            MnlI

5' G G G T G G A G T T T G T G A C G T G G C G C G G G G G C G T G G G A A C G G G G C G G G T G A C G T A G
3' C C C A C C C T C A A A C A C T G C A C C G C G C C C C C G C A C C C C T T G C C C C G C C A C T G C A T C
                                  HhaI   HphI

Right
5' G T T T T A G G G C G G A G T A A C T T G C A T G T A T T G G G
3' C A A A A T C C C G C C T C A T T G A A C G T A C A T A A C C C

Left
5' T A G T G T G G C G G A A G T G T G A T G T G T T G C A A G T G T G G C G G A A C A C A T G T A A G C G C C C G G – 3'
3' A T C A C A C C G C C T T C A C A C T A C A C A A C G T T C A C A C C G G C G C C T T G T G T A C A T T C G C G G C C – 5'
                                                                                    HpaII
                                                                                    HhaI
                                                                                    HaeII

Fig. 18. Nucleotide sequence of the ends of adenovirus-2 DNA. The sequences of the left and right ends are identical for 102 nucleotides as shown. A protein is covalently attached to the 5' C at both ends (Arrand and Roberts, personal communication). The ends of adenovirus-5 have also been determined by Steenbergh, Maat, Van Ormondt, and Sussenbach (personal communication). The first 102 nucleotides are identical to the sequence shown here except for insertion of ^A_T between residues 8 and 9.

cells. The maps have many features in common with the Ad2 and Ad5 maps, but the genetics has not yet been worked out at a detailed level (Ortin *et al.*, 1977).

Initiation and termination sites of Ad12 DNA replication are located at the ends of the genome, and DNA synthesis proceeds bidirectionally (Ariga and Shimojo, 1977).

3.4. Adeno-Associated Virus

Adeno-associated virus (AAV) is a parvovirus, replication of which requires helper adenovirus. Individual AAV virions contain a linear single-stranded DNA of molecular weight 1.4×10^6 (about 4400 nucleotides), and the complementary DNA strands are encapsidated in different particles (Berns and Adler, 1972; Berns, 1974).

Straus *et al.* (1976) have isolated replicative intermediates of AAV DNA which are consistent with a "self-priming" mode of replication, in which both 3' ends can form base-paired hairpin loops. The resulting double-stranded region can then act as the primer to synthesize the complementary strand. This model implies that the ends of AAV are symmetrical. Fife *et al.* (1977) have demonstrated that both ends of AAV DNA contain regions which will rapidly re-form double-stranded structures after denaturation, which suggests that the terminal sequences are symmetrical. The duplex structures involve up to 4% of the DNA. The nucleotide sequence of each 5' end is heterogeneous, the major sequences obtained being

T-T-G-G-C-C-A   (35%)

T-G-G-C-C-A   (50%)

G-G-C-C-A   (Minor component)

Data from the 3' ends show the same heterogeneity, suggesting that the multiple 5'-end sequences are not generated by contaminating exonucleases (Fife *et al.*, 1977). Further sequence work should distinguish between the various models of AAV DNA replication which have been proposed from the limited data available.

4. GENERAL CONCLUSIONS

Two points became very clear during the preparation of this chapter. One was that a vast number of nucleotide sequence data have accumulated very rapidly since the development of the new technologies (Sanger and Coulson, 1975; Maxam and Gilbert, 1977). The second is that sequence analysis does not solve all problems. Promoter sequences are still mysterious; although in *E. coli* the seven-nucleotide sequence (T-A-T-Pu-A-T-Pu) described by Pribnow (1975*b*) appears to have some significance, in some *E. coli* promoters only four of the seven nucleotides are present. At this low degree of homology it is difficult to be sure of the alignment to compare sequences, but no more than two nucleotides can be conserved in all promoters, suggesting that other factors are involved. There have been several attempts to locate significant features of the sequence of a promoter "upstream" from the T-A-T-Pu-A-T-Pu, but the lack of significant homology and the experiments of Okamoto *et al.* (1977) on the effect of attaching a "foreign" piece of DNA (Section 2.6) exclude such a simple mechanism for RNA polymerase recognition.

The same problem applies to ribosome recognition sites. The complementarity between the 3' end of the *E. coli* 16 S ribosomal RNA and the mRNA sequence preceding an initiator codon noted by Shine and Dalgarno (1974) is present, but its extent is quite varied (e.g., Sanger *et al.*, 1977*a*) and initiation codons cannot be identified with confidence in the absence of more data. The situation is further complicated by the λ mRNA, which has no sequence preceding the initiating AUG (Section 2.1).

Origins of replication are also quite varied in nucleotide sequence, although this may be less surprising in view of the different mechanisms involved. The SV40 origin (Section 3.1) has very extensive symmetry, repeated sequences, and potential secondary structure. The f1 origin (Section 2.6) has some potential secondary structure and a pyrimidine-rich sequence. The λ origin (Section 2.1) is characterized mainly by runs of identical nucleotides or very asymmetrical distribution of pyrimidines and purines, with some repeats and inverted repeats. The ϕX174 origin (Section 2.4) shows no particular features except a pyrimidine sequence CTC_5.

It is therefore obvious that sequence analysis alone is not enough to work out mechanisms and control of replication, transcription, and translation. In conjunction with other studies it is, however, an invaluable aid to interpreting results of genetic analysis, binding studies, kinetics, and all the other biological experiments. The methods of nucleotide sequence analysis are now routine and do not require particular training or expensive equipment, and it is to be hoped that the literature from now on can contain more data and less speculation in the case of problems such as adenovirus replication (Section 3.3).

ACKNOWLEDGMENTS

I am indebted to the many colleagues who supplied unpublished material, which has added immensely to the content of this chapter. I am very much aware that as the rapid methods for sequencing DNA are becoming widespread the sequences described here may seem trifling compared to those that may be available by the time this volume is published. However, it is clear that some of the older DNA sequencing methods will continue to be useful in particular situations and for confirming rapid data, and I have described the available data on the replication, transcription, and translation of each genome. The resulting genetic maps can be refined as more sequence information becomes available.

I am grateful to my colleagues here in Canberra, particularly Drs. G. W. Both and B. W. Stillman, for their comments and critical reading of the manuscript.

5. REFERENCES

Air, G. M., 1976, Amino acid sequences from the gene F (capsid) protein of bacteriophage φX174, *J. Mol. Biol.* **107**:433.

Air, G., and Bridgen, J., 1973, Correlation between a coat protein amino-terminal sequence and a ribosome-binding DNA sequence from φX174, *Nature (London) New Biol.* **241**:40.

Air, G. M., Blackburn, E. H., Sanger, F., and Coulson, A. R., 1975, The nucleotide and amino acid sequences of the 5′ (N) terminal region of gene G of bacteriophage φX174, *J. Mol. Biol.* **96**:703.

Air, G. M., Blackburn, E. H., Coulson, A. R., Galibert, F., Sanger, F., Sedat, J. W., and Ziff, E. B., 1976a, Gene F of bacteriophage φX174: Correlation of nucleotide sequences from the DNA and amino acid sequences from the gene product, *J. Mol. Biol.* **107**:445.

Air, G. M., Sanger, F., and Coulson, A. R., 1976b, Nucleotide and amino acid sequences of gene G of φX174, *J. Mol. Biol.* **108**:519.

Air, G. M., Coulson, A. R., Fiddes, J. C., Friedmann, T., Hutchison, C. A., III, Sanger, F., Slocombe, P. M., and Smith, A. J. H., 1978, Nucleotide sequence of the F protein coding region of bacteriophage φX174 and amino acid sequence of its product, *J. Mol. Biol.* **125**:247.

Aloni, Y., Dhar, R., Laub, O., Horowitz, M., and Khoury, G., 1977, Novel mechanism for RNA maturation: The leader sequences of Simian virus 40 mRNA are not transcribed adjacent to the coding sequences, *Proc. Natl. Acad. Sci. USA* **74**:3686.

Anderson, C. W., Lewis, J. B., Atkins, J. F., and Gesteland, R. F., 1974, Cell-free synthesis of adenovirus-2 specific proteins programmed by fractionated mRNA: A comparison of polypeptide product size and messenger RNA lengths, *Proc. Natl. Acad. Sci. U.S.A.* **71**:2756.

Anderson, J. L., Chang, C., Mora, P., and Martin, R. B., 1977, Expression and thermal stability of simian virus 40 tumor-specific transplantation antigen and tumore antigen in wild type- and *ts A* mutant-transformed cells, *J. Virol.* **21**:459.

Ariga, H., and Shimojo, H., 1977, Initiation and termination sites of adenovirus 12 DNA replication, *Virology* **78**:415.

Arrand, J., and Hindley, J., 1973, Nucleotide sequence of a ribosome binding site on RNA synthesized in vitro from coliphage T7, *Nature (London) New Biol.* **244**:10.

Asbeck, F., Bayreuther, K., Kohler, H., von Wettstein, G., and Braunitzer, G., 1969, Die Konstitution des Hull Proteins des Phages fd, *Hoppe Seylers Z. Physiol. Chem.* **350**:1047.

Axelrod, N., 1976, Transcription of bacteriophage φX174 in vitro: Selective initiation with oligonucleotides, *J. Mol. Biol.* **108**:753.

Baas, P. D., van Heusden, G. P. H., Vereijken, J. M., Weisbeek, P. J., and Jansz, H. S., 1976a, Cleavage map of bacteriophage φX174 RF DNA by restriction enzymes, *Nucleic Acids Res.* **3**:1947.

Baas, P. D., Jansz, H. S., and Sinsheimer, R. L., 1976b, Bacteriophage φX174 DNA synthesis in a replication-deficient host: Determination of the origin of φX DNA replication, *J. Mol. Biol.* **102**:633.

Baker, R., and Tessman, I., 1967, The circular genetic map of phage S13, *Proc. Natl. Acad. Sci. USA* **58**:1438.

Bambara, R., and Wu, R., 1975, DNA sequence analysis: Terminal sequences of bacteriophage φ80, *J. Biol. Chem.* **250**:4607.

Barnes, W. M., 1978, DNA sequencing by partial ribosubstitution, *J. Mol. Biol.* **119**:83.

Barrell, B. G., 1971, Fractionation and sequence analysis of radioactive nucleotides, in: *Procedures in Nucleic Acids Research*, Vol. 2 (G. L. Cantoni and D. R. Davies, eds.), pp. 751–779, Harper and Row, New York.

Barrell, B. G., Weith, H. L., Donelson, J. E., and Robertson, H. D., 1975, Sequence analysis of the ribosome-protected bacteriophage φX174 DNA fragment containing the gene G initiation site, *J. Mol. Biol.* **92**:377.

Barrell, B. G., Air, G. M., and Hutchison, C. A., III, 1976, Overlapping genes in bacteriophage φX174, *Nature (London)* **264**:34.

Bartok, K., Harbers, B., and Denhardt, D. T., 1975, Isolation and characterization of self-complementary sequences from φX174 viral DNA, *J. Mol. Biol.* **99**:93.

Beck, E., Sommer, R., Auerswald, E. A., Kurz, C., Zink, B., Osterburg, G., Schaller, H., Sugimoto, K., Sugisaki, H., Okamoto, T., and Takanami, M., 1978, Nucleotide sequence of bacteriophage fd DNA, *Nucleic Acids Res.* **5**:4495.

Bellett, A. J. D., and Younghusband, H. B., 1972, Replication of the DNA of chick embryo lethal orphan virus, *J. Mol. Biol.* **72**:691.

Benbow, R. M., Hutchison, C. A., III, Fabricant, J. D., and Sinsheimer, R. L., 1971, Genetic map of bacteriophage φX174, *J. Virol.* **7**:549.

Benbow, R. M., Mayol, R. F., Picchi, J. C., and Sinsheimer, R. L., 1972, Direction of translation and size of bacteriophage φX174 cistrons, *J. Virol.* **10**:99.

Benbow, R. M., Zuccarelli, A. J., Davis, G. C., and Sinsheimer, R. L., 1974, Genetic recombination in bacteriophage φX174, *J. Virol.* **13**:898.

Bennett, G. N., Schweingruber, M. E., Brown, K. D., Squires, C., and Yanofsky, C., 1978, Nucleotide sequence of the promoter-operator region of the tryptophan operon of *Escherichia coli*, *J. Mol. Biol.* **121**:113.

Berg, P., Fancher, H., and Chamberlin, M., 1963, The synthesis of mixed polynu-
cleotides containing ribo- and deoxyribonucleotides by purified preparations of
DNA polymerase from *Escherichia coli*, in: *Symposium on Informational
Macromolecules* (H. Vogel, V. Bryson, and J. O. Lampen, eds.). pp. 467–483,
Academic Press, New York.

Berget, S. M., Moore, C., and Sharp, P. A., 1977, Spliced segments at the 5' terminus
of adenovirus 3 late mRNA, *Proc. Natl. Acad. Sci. USA* **74**:3171.

Bernardi, G., 1966, Spleen acid ribonuclease, in: *Procedures in Nucleic Acid Research*,
Vol. 1 (G. L. Cantoni and D. R. Davies, eds.), pp. 37–45, Harper and Row, New
York.

Berns, K. I., 1974, Molecular biology of the adeno-associated viruses, *Current Topics
Microbiol. Immunol.* **65**:1.

Berns, K. I., and Adler, S., 1972, Separation of two types of adeno-associated virus
particles containing complementary polynucleotide chains, *J. Virol.* **9**:394.

Bertrand, K., Korn, L., Lee, F., Platt, T., Squires, C. L., Squires, C., and Yanofsky,
C., 1975, New features of the regulation of the tryptophan operon, *Science* **189**:22.

Blackburn, E. H., 1975, Transcription by *Escherichia coli* RNA polymerase of a single-
stranded fragment of bacteriophage φX174 DNA 48 residues in length, *J. Mol.
Biol.* **93**:367.

Blackburn, E. H., 1976, Transcription and sequence analysis of a fragment of bacteriophage φX174 DNA, *J. Mol. Biol.* **107**:417.

Borrias, W. E., Weisbeek, P. J., and Van Arkel, G. A., 1976, An intracistronic region
of gene A of bacteriophage φX174 not involved in progency RF DNA synthesis,
Nature (London) **261**:245.

Boyer, P. D. (ed.), 1971, *The Enzymes IV*, 3rd ed., Academic Press, New York.

Brezinski, D., and Wang, J. C., 1973, The 3' terminal nucleotide sequences of λ DNA,
Biochem. Biophys. Res. Commun. **50**:398.

Brown, N. L., and Smith, M., 1976, The mapping and sequence determination of the
single site in φX174 am 3 replicative form DNA cleaved by restriction endonuclease *Pst* 1, *FEBS Lett.* **65**:284.

Brown, N. L., and Smith, M., 1977a, DNA sequence of a region of the φX174 genome
coding for a ribosome binding site, *Nature (London)* **265**:695.

Brown, N. L., and Smith, M., 1977b, The sequence of a region of bacteriophage φX174
DNA coding for parts of genes *A* and *B*, *J. Mol. Biol.* **116**:1.

Browne, J. K., Paddock, G. V., Liu, A., Clarke, P., Heindell, H. C., and Salser, W.,
1977, Nucleotide sequences from the rabbit beta globin gene inserted into *Escherichia coli* plasmids, *Science* **195**:389.

Brownlee, G. G., and Sanger, F., 1969, Chromatography of ^{32}P-labelled oligonucleotides on thin layers of DEAE cellulose, *Eur. J. Biochem.* **11**:395.

Burgess, A. B., and Denhardt, D. T., 1969, Studies on φX174 proteins. I. Phage-
specific proteins synthesized after infection of *Escherichia coli*, *J. Mol. Biol.*
44:377.

Burton, K., and Petersen, G. B., 1960, The frequencies of certain sequences of
nucleotides in deoxyribonucleic acid, *Biochem. J.* **75**:17.

Carusi, E. A., 1977, Evidence for blocked 5' termini in human adenovirus DNA,
Virology **76**:380.

Cashmore, A. R., and Petersen, G. B., 1969, The degradation of DNA by hydrazine: A
critical study of the suitability of the reaction for the quantitative determination of
purine nucleotide sequences, *Biochim. Biophys. Acta* **174**:591.

Celma, M. L., Dhar, R., Pan, J., and Weissman, S. M., 1977, Comparison of the nucleotide sequence of the messenger RNA for the structural protein of SV40 with the DNA sequence encoding the amino acids of the protein, *Nucleic Acids Res.* **4**:2549.

Chadwell, H. A., 1974, Ph.D. Thesis, University of Cambridge.

Chan, T. S., Model, P., and Zinder, N. D., 1975, In vitro protein synthesis directed by separated transcripts of bacteriophage f1 DNA, *J. Mol. Biol.* **99**:369.

Chen, C. Y., Hutchison, C. A., III, and Edgell, M. H., 1973, Isolation and genetic localization of three φX174 promoter regions, *Nature (London) New Biol.* **243**:233.

Chow, L. T., Roberts, J. M., Lewis, J. B., and Broker, T. R., 1977*a*, A map of cytoplasmic RNA transcripts from lytic adenovirus type 2, determined by electron microscopy of RNA:DNA hybrids, *Cell* **11**:819.

Chow, L. T., Gelinas, R. E., Broker, T. R., and Roberts, R. J., 1977*b*, An amazing sequence arrangement at the 5′ ends of adenovirus-2 messenger RNA, *Cell* **12**:1.

Contreras, R., Rogiers, R., Van de Voorde, A., and Fiers, W., 1977*a*, Overlapping of the VP2-VP3 gene and the VP1 gene in the SV40 genome, *Cell* **12**:529.

Contreras, R., Volckaert, G., Thys, F., Van de Voorde, A., and Fiers, W., 1977*b*, Nucleotide sequence of the restriction fragment *Hind* F-EcoR$_I$ 2 of SV40 DNA, *Nucleic Acids Res.* **4**:1001.

Crawford, L. V., 1973, Proteins of polyoma virus and SV40, *Br. Med. Bull.* **39**:253.

Crawford, L. V., Cole, C. N., Smith, A. E., Pancha, E., Tegtmeyer, P., Rundell, K., and Berg, P, 1978, Organization and expression of early genes of simian virus 40, *Proc. Natl. Acad. Sci. USA* **75**:117.

Cunningham, L., Catlin, B. W., and de Garilhe, M. P., 1956, Deoxyribonuclease of *Micrococcus pyrogenes*, *J. Am. Chem. Soc.* **78**:4642.

Cuypers, T., Van der Ouderaa, F. J., and de Jong, W. W., 1974, The amino acid sequence of gene 5 protein of bacteriophage M13, *Biochem. Biophys. Res. Commun.* **59**:557.

Dahlberg, J. E., and Blattner, F. R., 1973, In vitro transcription products of lambda DNA: Nucleotide sequences and regulatory sites, in: *Virus Research* (C. F. Fox and W. S. Robinson, eds.), pp. 533–543, Academic Press, New York.

Dahlberg, J. E., and Blattner, F. R., 1975, Sequence of the promoter–operator proximal region of the major leftward RNA of bacteriophage lambda, *Nucleic Acids Res.* **2**:1441.

Danna, K. J., and Nathans, D., 1971, Specific cleavage of simian virus 40 DNA by restriction endonuclease of *Hemophilus influenzae*, *Proc. Natl. Acad. Sci. USA* **68**:2913.

Danna, K. J., and Nathans, D., 1972, Bidirectional replication of simian virus 40 DNA, *Proc. Natl. Acad. Sci. USA* **69**:3097.

Danna, K. J., Sack, G. H., and Nathans, D., 1973, Studies of simian virus 40 DNA. VII. A cleavage map of the SV40 genome, *J. Mol. Biol.* **78**:363.

Darnell, J. E., Jr., Jelinek, W. R., and Molloy, G. R., 1973, Biogenesis of mRNA: Genetic regulation in mammalian cells, *Science* **181**:1215.

Davies, R. W., Schreier, P. H., and Büchel, D. E., 1977, Nucleotide sequence of the attachment site of coliphage lambda, *Nature (London)* **270**:757.

Day, L. A., and Berkowitz, S. A., 1977, The number of nucleotides and the density and refractive index increments of fd DNA, *J. Mol. Biol.* **116**:603.

Delaney, A. D., and Spencer, J. H., 1976, Nucleotide clusters in deoxyribonucleic acids.

XIII. Sequence analysis of the longer unique pyrimidine oligonucleotides of bacteriophage S13 SNA by a method using unlabeled starting oligonucleotides, *Biochim. Biophys. Acta* **435**:269.

Del Villano, B. C., and Defendi, V., 1973, Characterization of the SV40 T antigen, *Virology* **51**:34.

Denhardt, D. T., 1975, The single-stranded DNA phages, *CRC Critical Rev. Microbiol.* **4**:161.

Denhardt, D. T., 1977, The isometric single-stranded DNA phages, in: *Comprehensive Virology*, Vol. 7 (H. Fraenkel-Conrat and R. R. Wagner, eds.) pp. 1–104, Plenum, New York.

Denniston-Thompson, K., Moore, D. D., Kruger, K. E., Furth, M. E. and Blattner, F. R., 1977, Physical structure of the replication origin of bacteriophage lambda, *Science* **198**:1051.

Dhar, R., Subramanian, K., Zain, B. S., Pan, J., and Weissman, S. M., 1974*a*, Nucleotide sequence about the 3' terminus of SV40 DNA transcripts and the region where DNA synthesis is initiated, *Cold Spring Harbor Symp. Quant. Biol.* **39**:153.

Dhar, R., Zain, B. S., Weissman, S. M., Pan, J., and Subramanian, K. N., 1974*b*, Nucleotide sequences of RNA transcribed in infected cells and by *Escherichia coli* RNA polymerase from a segment of simian virus 40 DNA, *Proc. Natl. Acad. Sci. USA* **71**:371.

Dhar, R., Subramanian, K. N., Pan, J., and Weissman, S. M., 1977*a*, Structure of a large segment of the genome of simian virus 40 that does not encode known proteins, *Proc. Natl. Acad. Sci. USA* **74**:827.

Dhar, R., Subramanian, K. N., Pan, J., and Weissman, S. M., 1977*b*, Nucleotide sequence of a fragment of SV40 DNA that contains the origin of DNA replication and specifies the 5' ends of "early" and "late" viral RNA. IV. Localization of the SV40 DNA complementary to the 5' ends of viral mRNA, *J. Biol. Chem.* **252**:368.

Dhar, R., Reddy, V. B., and Weissman, S. M., 1978, Nucleotide sequence of the DNA encoding the 5' terminal sequences of SV40 late RNA, *J. Biol. Chem.* **253**:612.

Donelson, J. E., Barrell, B. G., Weith, H. L., Kössell, H., and Schott, H., 1975, The use of primed synthesis by DNA polymerase 1 to study an intercistronic sequence of ϕX174, *Eur. J. Biochem.* **58**:383.

Eckhart, W., 1974, Genetics of DNA tumor viruses, *Annu. Rev. Genet.* **8**:301.

Edens, L., Konings, R. N. H., and Schoenmakers, J. G. G., 1975, Physical mapping of the central terminator for transcription of the bacteriophage M13 genome, *Nucleic Acids Res.* **2**:1811.

Edens, L., Van Wezenbeek, P., Konings, R. N. H., and Schoenmakers, J. G. G., 1976, Mapping of promoter sites on the genome of bacteriophage M13, *Eur. J. Biochem.* **70**:577.

Edgell, M. H., Hutchison, C. A., and Sclair, M., 1972, Specific endonuclease R fragments of bacteriophage ϕX174 deoxyribonucleic acid, *J. Virol.* **9**:574.

Efstratiadis, A., Kafatos, F., and Maniatis, T., 1977, The primary structure of rabbit β-globin mRNA as determined from cloned DNA, *Cell* **10**:571.

Eisenberg, S., Harbers, B., Hurs, C., and Denhardt, D. T., 1975, The mechanism of replication of ϕX174 DNA. XII. Non-random location of gaps in nascent ϕX174 RF II DNA, *J. Mol. Biol.* **99**:107.

Englund, P. T., 1971, Analysis of nucleotide sequences at 3' termini of duplex DNA with the use of T4 DNA polymerase, *J. Biol. Chem.* **246**:3269.

Englund, P. T., 1972, The 3′ terminal nucleotide sequences of T7 DNA, *J. Mol. Biol.* **66**:209.

Ensinger, M. J., and Ginsberg, H. S., 1972, Selection and preliminary characterization of temperature-sensitive mutants of type 5 adenovirus, *J. Virol.* **10**:328.

Eron, L., Callahan, R., and Westphal, H., 1974a, Cell-free synthesis of adenovirus coat proteins, *J. Biol. Chem.* **249**:6331.

Eron, L., Westphal, H., and Callahan, R., 1974b, In vitro synthesis of adenovirus core proteins, *J. Virol.* **14**:375.

Ferguson, J., and Davis, R. W., 1975, An electron microscopic method for studying and mapping the region of weak sequence homology between simian virus 40 and polyoma DNAs, *J. Mol. Biol.* **94**:135.

Feunteun, J., Sompayrac, L., Fluck, M., and Benjamin, T., 1976, Localization of gene functions in polyoma virus DNA, *Proc. Natl. Acad. Sci. USA* **73**:4169.

Fiddes, J. C., 1976, Nucleotide sequence of the intercistronic region between genes G and F in bacteriophage φX174 DNA, *J. Mol. Biol.* **107**:1.

Fiddes, J. C., Barrell, B. G., and Godson, G. N., 1978, Nucleotide sequences of the separate origins of synthesis of bacteriophage G4 viral and complementary DNA strands, *Proc. Natl. Acad. Sci. USA* **75**:1081.

Fiers, W., Contreras, R., Haegeman, G., Rogiers, R., Van de Voorde, A., Van Heuverswyn, H., Van Herreweghe, J., Volkaert, G., and Ysebaert, M., 1978, Complete nucleotide sequence of SV40, *Nature (London)* **273**:113.

Fiers, W. Rogiers, S., Soeda, E., Van de Voorde, A., Van Heuverswyn, H., Van Herreweghe, J., Volckaert, G., and Yang, R., 1975, Nucleotide sequence analysis of SV40 DNA, *Proc. 10th FEBS Meet., Paris*, pp. 17–33.

Fife, K. H., Berns, K. I., and Murray, K., 1977, Structure and nucleotide sequences of the terminal regions of adeno-associated virus DNA, *Virology* **78**:475.

Flint, J., 1977, The topography and transcription of the adenovirus genome, *Cell* **10**:153.

Flint, S. J., Berget, S. M., and Sharp, P. A., 1976, Adenovirus transcription. III. Mapping of viral RNA sequences in cells productively infected by adenovirus type 5, *Virology* **72**:443.

Fluck, M., Staneloni, R., Feunteun, J., Sompayrac, L., and Benjamin, T., 1976, Relationships between non-transforming mutants of polyoma virus, in: *Abstracts of the Tumor Virus Meeting* (W. Eckhardt, ed.), Cold Spring Harbor Laboratory, Cold Spring Harbor, N.Y.

Forget, B., Marotta, C. A., Weissman, S. M., Cohen-Solal, M., 1975, Nucleotide sequences of the 3′-terminal untranslated region of messenger RNA for human beta globin chain, *Proc. Natl. Acad. Sci. USA* **72**:3614.

Freymeyer, D. K., Shank, P. R., Edgell, M. H., Hutchison, C. A., III, and Vanaman, T. C., 1977, Amino acid sequence of the small core protein from bacteriophage φX174, *Biochemistry* **16**:4550.

Furth, M. E., Blattner, F. R., McLeester, C., and Dave, W. F., 1977, Genetic structure of the replication origin of bacteriophage lambda, *Science* **198**:1046.

Galibert, F., Sedat, J., and Ziff, E., 1974, Direct determination of DNA nucleotide sequences: Structure of a fragment of bacteriophage φX174 DNA, *J. Mol. Biol.* **87**:377.

Gallimore, P. H., Sharp, P. A., and Sambrook, J., 1974, Viral DNA in transformed cells. II. A study of the sequences of adenovirus 2 DNA in nine lines of transformed rat cells using specific fragments of the viral genome, *J. Mol. Biol.* **89**:49.

Garon, C. F., Berry, K. N., and Rose J. A., 1972, A unique form of terminal redundancy in adenovirus DNA molecules, *Proc. Nat. Acad. Sci. USA* **69**:2391.

Geider, K., and Kornberg, A., 1974, Conversion of the M13 viral single strand to the double-stranded replicative form by purified proteins, *J. Biol. Chem.* **249**:3999.

Gelinas, R. E., and Roberts, R. J., 1977, One predominant 5'-undecanucleotide in adenovirus 2 late messenger RNA, *Cell* **11**:533.

Gilbert, W., Maxam, A., and Mirzabekov, A., 1976, Contacts between the *lac* repressor and DNA revealed by methylation. in: *Control of Ribosome Synthesis* (N. Kjeldgaard and O. Maaløe, eds.), The Alfred Benzon Symposium IX, pp. 139–148, Munksgaard, Copenhagen.

Ginsberg, H. S., and Young, C. S. H., 1977, Genetics of adenoviruses, in: *Comprehensive Virology*, Vol. 9 (H. Fraenkel-Conrat and R. R. Wagner, eds.), pp. 27–88, Plenum, New York.

Godson, G. N., 1974, Evolution of φX174. Isolation of four new φX-like phages and comparison with φX174, *Virology* **58**:272.

Godson, G. N., 1976, Evolution of φX174. III. Restriction map of S13 and its alignment with that of φX174, *Virology* **75**:263.

Godson, G. N., Barrell, B. G., and Fiddes, J. C., 1978, Nucleotide sequence of bacteriophage G4 DNA, *Nature (London)* **276**:236.

Goldberg, S., Weber, J., and Darnell, J. E., Jr., 1977, The definition of a large viral transcription unit late in Ad 2 infection of HeLa cells: Mapping by effects of ultraviolet irradiation, *Cell* **10**:617.

Goldsmith, M. E., and Konigsberg, W. H., 1977, Adsorption protein of the bacteriophage fd: Isolation, molecular properties, and location in the virus, *Biochemistry* **16**:2686.

Graham, F. L., Abrahams, P. J., Warnaar, S. O., Mulder, C., de Vries, F. A. J., Fiers, W., and Van der Eb, A. J., 1974, Studies on in vitro transformation with viral DNA and DNA fragments, *Cold Spring Harbor Symp. Quant. Biol.* **39**:637.

Gray, C. P., Sommer, R., Polke, C., Beck, E., and Schaller, H., 1978, Structure of the origin of DNA replication of bacteriophage fd, *Proc. Natl. Acad. Sci. USA* **75**:50.

Green, M., 1970, Oncogenic viruses, *Annu. Rev. Biochem.* **39**:701.

Green, M., Parsons, J. T., Piña, M., Fujinaga, K., Caffier, H., and Landgraf-Leurs, I., 1970, Transcription of adenovirus genes in productively-infected and in transformed cells, *Cold Spring Harbor Symp. Quant. Biol.* **35**:803.

Greenway, P. J., and Le Vine, D., 1973, Amino acid compositions of simian virus 40 structural proteins, *Biochem. Biophys. Res. Commun.* **52**:1221.

Griffin, B. E., and Fried, M., 1976, Structural mapping of the DNA of an oncogenic virus (polyoma viral DNA), in: *Methods in Cancer Research*, Vol. 12 (H. Busch, ed.), pp. 49–86, Academic Press, New York.

Griffin, B., Fried, M., and Cowie, A., 1974, Polyoma DNA: A physical map, *Proc. Natl. Acad. Sci. USA* **71**:2077.

Griffith, J., and Kornberg, A., 1974, Mini M13 bacteriophage: Circular fragments of M13 DNA are replicated and packaged during normal infections, *Virology* **59**:139.

Grohmann, K., Smith, L. H., and Sinsheimer, R. L., 1975, A new method for isolation and sequence determination of 5' terminal regions of bacteriophage φX174 in vitro mRNAs, *Biochemistry* **14**:1951.

Grosveld, F. G., and Spencer, J. H., 1977, The nucleotide sequence of two restriction fragments located in the gene *AB* region of bacteriophage S13, *Nucleic Acids Res.* **4**:2235.

Grosveld, F. G., Ojamaa, K. M., and Spencer, J. H., 1976, Fragmentation of bacteriophage S13 replicative form DNA by restriction endonucleases from *Hemophilus influenzae* and *Hemophilus aegyptius*, *Virology* 71:312.

Haegeman, G., and Fiers, W., 1978, Evidence for "splicing" of SV40 16 S mRNA, *Nature (London)* **273**:70.

Harbers, B., Delaney, A. D., Harbers, K., and Spencer, J. H., 1976, Nucleotide clusters in DNA. XI. Comparison of the sequences of the larger pyrimidine oligonucleotides of bacteriophage S13 and ϕX174 DNA, *Biochemistry* **15**:407.

Hayashi, M. N., and Hayashi, M., 1974, Fragment maps of ϕX174 RF DNA produced by restriction enzymes from *Haemophilus aphirophilus* and *Hemophilus influenzae* H-1, *J. Virol.* **14**:1142.

Hayashi, M., Fujimura, F. K., and Hayashi, M., 1976, Mapping of in vivo messenger RNAs for bacteriophage ϕX174, *Proc. Natl. Acad. Sci. USA* **73**:3519.

Hayes, S., and Szybalski, W., 1973, Control of short leftward transcripts from the immunity and *ori* regions in induced coliphage lambda, *Mol. Gen. Genet.* **126**:275.

Henry, T. J., and Pratt, D., 1969, The proteins of bacteriophage M13, *Proc. Natl. Acad. Sci. USA* **62**:800.

Hershey, A. D., 1971, *The Bacteriophage Lambda*, Cold Spring Harbor Laboratory, Cold Spring Harbor, N.Y.

Hershey, A. D., Burgi, E., and Ingraham, L., 1963, Cohesion of DNA molecules isolated from the phage lambda, *Proc. Natl. Acad. Sci. USA* **49**:748.

Horiuchi, K., and Zinder, N . D., 1976, Origin and direction of synthesis of bacteriophage f1 DNA, *Proc. Natl. Acad. Sci. USA* **73**:2341.

Horiuchi, K., Vovis, G. F., Enea, V., and Zinder, N. D., 1975, Cleavage map of bacteriophage f1: Location of the *Escherichia coli* B-specific modification sites, *J. Mol. Biol.* **95**:147.

Horwitz, M. S., 1976, Bidirectional replication of adenovirus type 2 DNA, *J. Virol.* **18**:307.

Howard, B. H., de Crombrugghe, B., and Rosenberg, M., 1977, Transcription in vitro of bacteriophage lambda 4 S RNA: Studies on termination and rho protein, *Nucleic Acids Res.* **4**:827.

Hsiang, M. W., Cole, R. D., Takeda, Y., and Echols, H., 1977, Amino acid sequence of cro regulatory protein of bacteriophage lambda, *Nature (London)* **270**:275.

Humayun, Z., 1977, DNA sequence of the end of the *CI* gene in bacteriophage λ, *Nucleic Acids Res.* **4**:2137.

Humayun, Z., Jeffrey, A., and Ptashne, M, 1977a, Completed DNA sequences and organization of repressor-binding sites in the operators of phage lambda, *J. Mol. Biol.* **112**:265.

Humayun, Z, Kleid, D., and Ptashne, M., 1977b, Sites of contact between λ operators and λ repressor, *Nucleic Acids Res.* **4**:1595.

Hutchison, C. A., III, and Edgell, M. H., 1971, Genetic assay for small fragments of bacteriophage ϕX174 DNA, *J. Virol.* **8**:181.

Jacob, E., and Hofschneider, P. H., 1969, Replication of the single-stranded DNA bacteriophage M13: Messenger RNA synthesis directed by M13 replicative form DNA, *J. Mol. Biol.* **46**:359.

Jacob, E., Jaenisch, R., and Hofschneider, P. H., 1973, Replication of the single-stranded DNA of bacteriophage M13; on the transcription in vivo of M13 RF, *Eur. J. Biochem.* **32**:432.

Jay, E., Bambara, R., Padmanabhan, R., and Wu, R., 1974, DNA sequencing large oligodeoxyribonucleotide fragments by mapping, *Nucleic Acids Res.* **1**:331.

Jazwinski, S. M., Lindeberg, A. A., and Kornberg, A., 1975a, The lipopolysaccharide receptor for bacteriophages φX174 and S13, *Virology* **66**:268.

Jazwinski, S. M., Lindeberg, A. A., and Kornberg, A., 1975b, The gene H spike protein of bacteriophages φX174 and S13. I. Functions in phage-receptor recognition and in transfection, *Virology* **66**:283.

Jazwinski, S. M., Marco, R., and Kornberg, A., 1975c, The gene H spike protein of bacteriophages φX174 and S13. II. Relation to synthesis of the parental replicative form, *Virology* **66**:294.

Jeng, Y., Gelfand, D., Hayashi, M., Shleser, R., and Tessman, E. S., 1970, The eight genes of bacteriophage φX174 and S13 and comparison of the phage specified proteins, *J. Mol. Biol.* **49**:521.

Jeppesen, P. G. N., Sanders, L., and Slocombe, P. M., 1976, A restriction cleavage map of φX174 DNA by pulse-chase labelling using *E. coli* DNA polymerase, *Nucleic Acids Res.* **3**:1323.

Kamen, R., Lindstrom, D. M., Shure, H., and Old, R. W., 1974, Virus specific RNA in cells productively infected or transformed by polyoma virus, *Cold Spring Harbor Symp. Quant. Biol.* **39**:187.

Kaptein, J. S., and Spencer, J. H., 1978, Nucleotide clusters in deoxyribonucleic acids: Sequence analysis of DNA using pyrimidine oligonucleotides as primers in the DNA polymerase I repair reaction, *Biochemistry* **17**:841.

Khoury, G., Howley, P., Brown, M., and Martin, M., 1974, The detection and quantitation of SV40 nucleic acid sequences using single-stranded SV40 DNA probes, *Cold Spring Harbor Symp. Quant. Biol.* **39**:147.

Khoury, G., Howley, P., Nathans, D., and Martin, M., 1975, Posttranscriptional selection of simian virus 40-specific RNA, *J. Virol.* **15**:433.

Kleid, D., Humayun, Z., Jeffrey, A., and Ptashne, M., 1976, Novel properties of a restriction endonuclease isolated from *Haemophilus parahaemolyticus*, *Proc. Natl. Acad. Sci. USA* **73**:293.

Klessig, D. F., 1977, Two adenovirus messenger RNAs have a common 5′ terminal leader sequence which is encoded at least 10 kilobases upstream from the main coding regions for these messengers, *Cell* **12**:9.

Konings, R. N. H., 1973, Synthesis of phage M13 specific proteins in a DNA-dependent cell-free system, *FEBS Lett.* **35**:155.

Konings, R. N. H., Hulsebos, T., and Van den Hondel, C. A., 1975, Identification and characterization of the in vitro synthesized gene products of bacteriophage M13, *J. Virol.* **15**:570.

Lai, C. J., and Nathans, D., 1974, Mapping temperature-sensitive mutants of simian virus 40: Rescue of mutants by fragments of viral DNA, *Virology* **60**:466.

Lai, C. J., and Nathans, D., 1975, A map of temperature-sensitive mutants of simian virus 40, *Virology* **66**:70.

Landy, A., and Ross, W., 1977, Viral integration and excision: Structure of the lambda *att* sites, *Science* **197**:1147.

Langeveld, S. A., van Mansfeld, A. D. M., Baas, P. D., Jansz, H. S., van Arkel, G. A., and Weisbeek, P. J., 1978, Nucleotide sequence of the origin of replication in bacteriophage φX174 RF DNA, *Nature (London)* **271**:417.

Lawley, P. D., and Brookes, P., 1963, Further studies on the alkylation of nucleic acids and their constituent nucleotides, *Biochem. J.* **89**:127.

Lazarides, E., Files, J. G., and Weber, K., 1974, Simian virus 40 structural proteins: Amino terminal sequence of the major capsid protein, *Virology* **60**:584.

Lebowitz, P., Kelly, T. J., Nathans, D., Lee, T. N., and Lewis, A. M., 1974, A colinear map relating the simian virus 40 (SV40) DNA segments of six adenovirus-SV40 hybrids to the DNA fragments produced by restriction endonuclease cleavage of SV40 DNA, *Proc. Natl. Acad. Sci. USA* **71**:441.

Lee, A. S., and Sinsheimer, R. L., 1974, A cleavage map of bacteriophage φX174 genome, *Proc. Natl. Acad. Sci. USA* **71**:2882.

Lee, F., Squires, C. L., Squires, C., and Yanofsky, C., 1976, Termination of transcription in vitro in the *Escherichia coli* tryptophan operon leader region, *J. Mol. Biol.* **103**:383.

Lehninger, A. L., 1970, *Biochemistry: The Molecular Basis of Cell Structure and Function*, 1st ed., Worth, New York.

Lewin, B., 1975, Units of transcription and translation: Sequence components of heterogeneous nuclear RNA and messenger RNA, *Cell* **4**:77.

Lewis, A. M., 1977, Defective and non-defective Ad2-SV40 hybrids, *Progr. Med. Virol.* **23**:96.

Lewis, J. B., Atkins, J. F., Anderson, C. W., Baum, P. R., and Gesteland, R. F., 1975, Mapping of late adenovirus genes by cell-free translation of RNA selected by hybridisation to specific DNA fragments, *Proc. Natl. Acad. Sci. USA* **72**:1344.

Lewis, J. B., Atkins, J. F., Baum, P. R., Solem, R., Gesteland, R. F., and Andersen, C. W., 1976, location and identification of the genes for adenovirus type 2 early polypeptides, *Cell* **7**:141.

Lillehaug, J. R., and Kleppe K., 1975, Effect of salts and polyamines on T4 polynucleotide kinase, *Biochemistry* **14**:1225.

Lin, N. S. C., and Pratt, D., 1974, Bacteriophage M13 gene 2 protein: Increasing its yield in infected cells, and identification and localization, *Virology* **61**:334.

Lindberg, V., and Sundquist, B., 1974, Isolation of messenger ribonucleoproteins from mammalian cells, *J. Mol. Biol.* **86**:451.

Ling, V., 1971, Partial digestion of ^{32}P-fd DNA with T4 endonuclease IV, *FEBS Lett.* **19**:50.

Ling, V., 1972a, Pyrimidine sequences from the DNA of bacteriophages fd, f1, and φX174, *Proc. Natl. Acad. Sci. USA* **69**:742.

Ling, V., 1972b, Fractionation and sequences of the large pyrimidine oligonucleotides from bacteriophage fd DNA, *J. Mol. Biol.* **64**:87.

Loewen, P. C., 1975, Determination of the sequences of 18 nucleotides from the 5′ end of the l-strand and 15 nucleotides from the 5′ end of the r-strand of T7 DNA, *Nucleic Acids Res.* **2**:839.

Loni, M. C., and Green, M., 1973, Detection of viral DNA sequences in adenovirus transformed cells by in situ hybridisation, *J. Virol.* **12**:1288.

Lyons, L. B., and Zinder, N. D., 1972, The genetic map of the filamentous bacteriophage f1, *Virology* **49**:45.

Maniatis, T., and Ptashne, M., 1973a Multiple repressor binding at the operators in bacteriphage λ, *Proc. Natl. Acad. Sci. USA* **70**:1531.

Maniatis, T., and Ptashne, M., 1973b, Structure of the λ operators, *Nature (London)* **246**:133.

Maniatis, T., Ptashne, M., and Maurer, R., 1973, Control elements in the DNA of bacteriophage λ, *Cold Spring Harbor Symp. Quant. Biol.* **38**:857.

Maniatis, T., Ptashne, M., Barrell, B. G., and Donelson, J., 1974, Sequence of a repressor-binding site in the DNA of bacteriophage λ, *Nature (London)* **250**:394.

Maniatis, T., Jeffrey, A., and Kleid, D., 1975, Nucleotide sequence of the rightward operator of phage λ, *Proc. Natl. Acad. Sci. USA* **72**:1184.

Marotta, C. A., Lebowitz, P., Dhar, R., Zain, B. S., and Weissman, S. M., 1974, Preparation of RNA transcripts of discrete segments of DNA, in: *Methods in Enzymology*, Vol. 29 (L. Grossman and K. Moldave, eds.), pp. 254–272, Academic Press, New York.

Mathews, M. B., 1975, Genes for VA-RNA in adenovirus 2, *Cell* **6**:223.

Maurer, R., Maniatis, T., and Ptashne, M., 1974, Promoters are in the operators in phage lambda, *Nature (London)* **249**:221.

Maxam, A., and Gilbert, W., 1977, A new method for sequencing DNA, *Proc. Natl. Acad. Sci. USA* **74**:560.

May, E., Maizel, J. G., and Salzman, N. P., 1977, Mapping of transcription sites of simian virus 40-specific late 16 S and 19 S mRNA by electron microscopy, *Proc. Natl. Acad. Sci. USA* **74**:496.

McDougall, J. K., Dunn, A. R., and Jones, K., 1972, In situ hybridisation of adenovirus RNA and DNA, *Nature (London)* **236**:346.

Meyer, B., Kleid, D., and Ptashne, M., 1975, λ repressor turns off transcription of its own gene, *Proc. Natl. Acad. Sci. USA* **72**:4785.

Middleton, J. H., Edgell, M. H., and Hutchison, C. A., III, 1972, Specific fragments of ϕX174 deoxyribonucleic acid produced by a restriction enzyme from *Haemophilus aegyptius*, endonuclease Z, *J. Virol.* **10**:42.

Miller, L. K., and Fried, M., 1976, Construction of the genetic map of the polyoma genome, *J. Virol.* **18**:824.

Model, P., and Zinder, N. D., 1974, In vitro synthesis of bacteriophage f1 proteins, *J. Mol. Biol.* **83**:231.

Mulder, C., Arrand, J. R., Delius, H., Keller, W., Petterson, U., Roberts, R. J., and Sharp, P. A., 1974, Cleavage maps from adenovirus types 2 and 5 by restriction endonuclease *Eco* RI and *Hpa*I, *Cold Spring Harb. Symp. Quant. Biol.* **39**:397.

Murray, K., and Murray, N. E., 1973, Terminal nucleotide sequences of DNA from temperate coliphages, *Nature New Biol. (London)* **243**:134.

Murray, K., and Old, R. W., 1974, The primary structure of DNA, *Progr. Nucleic Acid Res. Mol. Biol.* **14**:117.

Murray, K., Murray, N. E., and Bertani, G., 1975, Base changes in the recognition site for *ter* functions in lambdoid phage DNA, *Nature (London)* **254**:262.

Murray, K., Isaksson-Forsen, A. G., Challberg, M., and Englund, P., 1977, Symmetrical nucleotide sequences in the recognition sites for the *ter* function of bacteriophages P2, 299 and 186, *J. Mol. Biol.* **112**:471.

Nakashima, Y., and Konigsberg, W., 1974, Reinvestigation of a region of the fd bacteriophage coat protein sequence, *J. Mol. Biol.* **88**:598.

Nakashima, Y., Dunker, A. K., Marvin, D. A., and Konigsberg, W., 1974, The amino acid sequence of a DNA binding protein: The gene 5 product of fd filamentous bacteriophage, *FEBS Lett.* **40**:290.

Nathans, D., and Danna, K. J., 1972, Specific origin in SV40 DNA replication, *Nature (London) New Biol.* **236**:200.

Oakley, J. L., and Coleman, J. E., 1977, Structure of a promoter for T7 RNA polymerase, *Proc. Natl. Acad. Sci. USA* **74**:4266.

Oberg, B., Saborio, J., Persson, T., Everitt, E., and Philipson, L., 1975, Identification of the in vitro translation products of adenovirus mRNA by immunoprecipitation, *J. Virol.* **15**:199.

Ohe, K., and Weissman, S. M., 1970, Nucleotide sequence of an RNA from cells infected with adenovirus 2, *Science* **167**:879.

Okamoto, T., Sugimoto, K., Sugisaki, H., and Takanami, M., 1975, Studies of bacteriophage fd DNA. II. Localisation of RNA initiation sites on the cleavage map of the fd genome, *J. Mol. Biol.* **95**:33.

Okamoto, T., Sugimoto, K., Sugisaki, H., and Takanami, M., 1977, DNA regions essential for the function of a bacteriophage fd promoter, *Nucleic Acids Res.* **4**:2213.

Ortin, J., Scheidtmann, K.-H., Greenberg, R., Westphal, M., and Doerfler, W., 1977, Transcription of the genome of adenovirus type 12. III. Maps of transcription in productively infected human cells and in abortively infected and transformed hamster cells, *J. Virol.* **20**:355.

Padmanabhan, R., and Padmanabhan, R. V., 1977, Specific interaction of a protein(s) at or near the termini of adenovirus 2 DNA, *Biochem. Biophys. Res. Commun.* **75**:955.

Padmanabhan, R., Wu, R., and Calendar, R., 1974, Complete nucleotide sequence of the cohesive ends of bacteriophage P2 deoxyribonucleic acid, *J. Biol. Chem.* **249**:6197.

Pan, J., Reddy, V. B., Thimmappaya, B., and Weissman, S. M., 1977, Nucleotide sequence of the gene for the major structural protein of SV40 virus, *Nucleic Acids Res.* **4**:2539.

Paucha, E., Mellor, A., Harvey, R., Smith, A. E., Hewick, R. M., and Waterfield, M. D., 1978, Large and small tumor antigens from simian virus 40 have identical amino termini mapping at 0.65 map units, *Proc. Natl. Acad. Sci. USA* **75**:2165.

Philipson, L., 1977, Adenovirus gene expression—A model for mammalian cells, *FEBS Lett.* **74**:167.

Philipson, L., Pettersson, U., and Lindberg, U., 1975, *Molecular Biology of Adenoviruses*, Virology Monographs 14, Springer-Verlag, Vienna.

Pieczenik, G., Model, P., and Robertson, H. D., 1974, Sequence and symmetry in ribosome binding sites of bacteriophage f1 RNA, *J. Mol. Biol.* **90**:191.

Pirrotta, V., 1975, Sequence of the O_R operator of phage λ, *Nature (London)* **254**:114.

Pribnow, D., 1975a, Nucleotide sequence of an RNA polymerase binding site at an early T7 promoter, *Proc. Natl. Acad. Sci. USA* **72**:784.

Pribnow, D., 1975b, Bacteriophage T7 early promoters: Nucleotide sequences of two RNA polymerase binding sites, *J. Mol. Biol.* **99**:419.

Price, S. S., Schwing, J. M., and Englund, P. T., 1973, The 3′ terminal heptanucleotide sequence of the l strand of T7 deoxyribonucleic acid, *J. Biol. Chem.* **248**:7001.

Prives, C., Gilboa, E., Revel, M., and Winocour, E., 1977, Cell-free translation of simian virus 40 early messenger RNA coding for viral T antigen, *Proc. Natl. Acad. Sci. USA* **74**:457.

Proudfoot, N. J., 1977, Complete 3′ non-coding region sequences of rabbit and human β-globin messenger RNAs, *Cell* **10**:559.

Ptashne, M., Backman, K., Humayun, M. Z., Jeffrey, A., Maurer, R., Meyer, B., and Sauer, R. T., 1976, Autoregulation and function of a repressor in bacteriophage lambda, *Science* **194**:156.

Ravetch, J. V., Model, P., and Robertson, H. D., 1977a, Isolation and characterisation of the φX174 ribosome binding sites, *Nature (London)* **265**:698.

Ravetch, J. V., Horiuchi, K., and Zinder, N. D., 1977*b*, Nucleotide sequences near the origin of replication of bacteriophage f1, *Proc. Natl. Acad. Sci. USA* **74**:4219.

Ray, D. S., 1977, Replication of filamentous bacteriophages, in: *Comprehensive Virology*, Vol. 7 (H. Fraenkel-Conrat and R. R. Wagner, eds.), pp. 105–178, Plenum, New York.

Reddy, V. B., Dhar, R., and Weissman, S. M., 1978*a*, Nucleotide sequence of the genes for the SV40 proteins VP2 and VP3, *J. Biol. Chem.* **253**:621.

Reddy, V. B., Thimmappaya, B., Dhar, R., Subramanian, K. N., Zain, B. S., Pan, J., Ghosh, P. K., Celma, M. L., and Weissman, S. M., 1978*b*, The genome of simian virus 40, *Science* **200**:494.

Rekosh, D. M. K., Russell, W. C., Bellett, A. J. D., and Robinson, A. J., 1977, Identification of a protein linked to the ends of adenovirus DNA, *Cell* **11**:283.

Richardson, C. C., 1965, Phosphorylation of nucleic acid by an enzyme from T4 bacteriophage-infected *Escherichia coli*, *Proc. Natl. Acad. Sci. USA* **54**:158.

Richardson, C. C., 1971, Polynucleotide kinase from *Escherichia coli* infected with bacteriophage T4, in: *Procedures in Nucleic Acid Research 2* (G. L. Cantoni and D. R. Davies, eds.), pp. 815–828, Harper and Row, New York.

Ritchey, D. A., Thomas, C. A., Jr., MacHattie, L. A., and Wensink, P. C., 1967, Terminal repetition in non-permuted T3 and T7 bacteriophage DNA molecules, *J. Mol. Biol.* **23**:365.

Roberts, R. J., 1976, Restriction endonucleases, *CRC Crit. Rev. Biochem.* **4**:123.

Roberts, R., Arrand, J. R., and Keller, W., 1974, The length of the terminal repetition in adenovirus 2 DNA, *Proc. Natl. Acad. Sci. USA* **71**:3829.

Roberts, T. M., Shimatake, H., Brady, C. and Rosenberg, M., 1977, Sequence of *cro* gene of bacteriophage lambda, *Nature (London)* **270**:274.

Robertson, H. D., Barrell, B. G., Weith, H. L., and Donelson, J. E., 1973, Isolation and sequence analysis of a ribosome-protected fragment from bacteriophage φX174 DNA, *Nature (London) New Biol.* **241**:38.

Robertson, H. D., Dickson, E., and Dunn, J. J., 1977, A nucleotide sequence from a ribonuclease III processing site in bacteriophage T7 RNA, *Proc. Natl. Acad. Sci. USA* **74**:822.

Robinson, A. J., and Bellett, A. J. D., 1975, Complementary strands of CELO virus DNA, *J. Virol.* **15**:458.

Rosenberg, M., and Kramer, R. A., 1977, Nucleotide sequence surrounding a ribonuclease III processing site in bacteriophage T7 RNA, *Proc. Natl. Acad. Sci. USA* **74**:984.

Rosenberg, M., de Crombrugghe, B., and Musso, R., 1976, Determination of nucleotide sequences beyond the sites of transcriptional termination, *Proc. Natl. Acad. Sci. USA* **73**:717.

Roychoudhoury, R., Jay, E., and Wu, R., 1976, Terminal labeling and addition of homopolymer tracts to duplex DNA fragments by terminal deoxynucleotidyl transferase, *Nucleic Acids Res.* **3**:863.

Rozenblatt, S., Mulligan, R. C., Gorecki, M., Roberts, B. E., and Rich, A., 1976, Direct biochemical mapping of eukaryotic viral DNA by means of a linked transcription-translation cell-free system, *Proc. Natl. Acad. Sci. USA* **73**:2747.

Rundell, K., Collins, J. K., Tegtmeyer, P., Ozer, H. L., Lai, C. J., and Nathans, D., 1977, Identification of simian virus 40 protein A, *J. Virol.* **21**:636.

Russell, W. C., Skehel, J. J., and Williams, J. F., 1974, Characterisation of temperature-sensitive mutants of adenovirus type 5—Synthesis of polypeptides in infected cells, *J. Gen. Virol.* **24**:247.

Sadowski, P. D., and Bakyta, I., 1972, T4 endonuclease IV: Improved purification procedure and resolution from T4 endonuclease III, *J. Biol. Chem.* **247**:405.

Salser, W. A., 1974, DNA sequencing techniques, *Annu. Rev. Biochem.* **43**:923.

Salser, W., Fry, K., Brunk, C., and Poon, R., 1972, Nucleotide sequencing of DNA: Preliminary characterization of the products of specific cleavages at guanine, cytosine or adenine residues, *Proc. Natl. Acad. Sci. USA* **69**:238.

Salzman, N. P., and Khoury, G., 1974, Reproduction of papovaviruses, in: *Comprehensive Virology*, Vol. 3 (H. Fraenkel-Conrat and R. R. Wagner, eds.), pp. 63–141, Plenum, New York.

Sambrook, J., Sharp, P. A., and Keller, W., 1972, Transcription of SV40 DNA. I. Strand separation and hybridization of the separated strands to RNAs isolated from lytically infected and transformed cells. *J. Mol. Biol.* **70**:57.

Sambrook, J., Sugden, B., Keller, W., and Sharp, P. A., 1973, Transcription of SV40 DNA. III. Orientation of RNA synthesis and mapping of "early" and "late" species of viral RNA extracted from lytically infected cells, *Proc. Natl. Acad. Sci. USA* **70**:3711.

Sambrook, J., Williams, J., Sharp, P. A., and Grodzicker, T., 1975, Physical mapping of temperature-sensitive mutations of adenoviruses, *J. Mol. Biol.* **97**:369.

Sanger, F., and Couslon, A. R., 1975, A rapid method for determining sequences in DNA by primed synthesis with DNA polymerase, *J. Mol. Biol.* **94**:441.

Sanger, F., and Coulson, A. R., 1978, The use of thin acrylamide gel for DNA sequencing, *FEBS Lett.* **87**:107.

Sanger, F., Donelson, J. E., Coulson, A. R., Kössel, H., and Fischer, D., 1973, Use of DNA polymerase I primed by a synthetic oligonucleotide to determine a nucleotide sequence in bacteriophage f1 DNA, *Proc. Natl. Acad. Sci. USA* **70**:1209.

Sanger, F., Air, G. M., Barrell, B. G., Brown, N. L., Coulson, A. R., Fiddes, J. C., Hutchison, C. A., III, Slocombe, P. M., and Smith, M., 1977a, Nucleotide sequence of bacteriophage ϕX174 DNA, *Nature (London)* **265**:687.

Sanger, F., Nicklen, S., and Coulson, A. R., 1977b, DNA sequencing with chain-terminating inhibitors, *Proc. Natl. Acad. Sci. USA* **74**:5463.

Sanger, F., Coulson, A. R., Friedmann, T., Air, G. M., Barrell, B. G., Brown, N. L., Fiddes, J. C., Hutchison, C. A., III, Slocombe, P. M., and Smith, M., 1978, The nucleotide sequence of bacteriophage ϕX174, *J. Mol. Biol.* **125**:225.

Sato, S., Hutchison, C. A. III, and Harris, J. I., 1977, A thermostable sequence-specific endonuclease from *Thermus aquaticus*, *Proc. Natl. Acad. Sci. USA* **74**:542.

Schaller, H., Beck, E., and Takanami, M., 1978, Sequence and regulatory signals of the filamentous phage genome, in: *Single Stranded DNA Phage* (D. T. Denhardt, D. Dressler, and D. S. Ray, eds.), Cold Spring Harbor Laboratory, Cold Spring Harbor, N.Y.

Schaller, H., Gray, C., and Herrmann, K., 1975, Nucleotide sequence of an RNA polymerase binding site from the DNA of bacteriophage fd, *Proc. Natl. Acad. Sci. USA* **72**:737.

Schaller, H., Uhlmann, A., and Geider, K., 1976, A DNA fragment from the origin of single-strand to double-strand DNA replication of bacteriophage fd, *Proc. Natl. Acad. Sci. USA* **73**:49.

Scherer, G., Hobom, G., and Kössel, H., 1977, DNA base sequence of the Po promoter region of phage λ, *Nature (London)* **265**:117.

Schnös, M., and Inman, R. B., 1970, Position of branch points in replicating λ DNA, *J. Mol. Biol.* **51**:61.

Schwarz, E., Scherer, G., Hobom, G., and Kössel, H., 1978, Nucleotide sequence of *cro* cII and part of *O* gene in phage λ DNA, *Nature (London)* **272**:410.

Sedat, J. W., Ziff, E. B., and Galibert, F., 1976, Direct determination of DNA nucleotide sequences: Structures of large specific fragments of bacteriophage φX174 DNA, *J. Mol. Biol.* **107**:391.

Seeburg, P. H., and Schaller, H., 1975, Mapping and characterisation of promoters in bacteriophages fd, f1 and M13, *J. Mol. Biol.* **92**:261.

Seeburg, P. H., Nusslein, C., and Schaller, H., 1977, Interaction of RNA polymerase with promoters from bacteriophage fd, *Eur. J. Biochem.* **74**:107.

Shatkin, A. J., 1976, Capping of eukaryotic mRNAs, *Cell* **9**:645.

Shaw, D. C., Walker, J. E., Northrop, F. D., Barrell, B. G., Godson, G. N., and Fiddes, J. C., 1978, Gene K: a new overlapping gene in bacteriophage G4, *Nature (London)* **272**:510.

Shenk, T. E., Carbon, J., and Berg, P., 1976, Construction and analysis of viable deletion mutants of simian virus 40, *J. Virol.* **18**:664.

Shine, J., and Dalgarno, L., 1974, The 3′ terminal sequence of *Escherichia coli* 16 S ribosomal RNA: Complementarity to nonsense triplets and ribosome binding sites, *Proc. Natl. Acad. Sci. USA* **71**:1342.

Shulman, M. J., and Gottesman, M. E., 1973, Attachment site mutants of bacteriophage lambda, *J. Mol. Biol.* **81**:461.

Sigal, N., Delius, H., Kornberg, T., Gefter, M. L., and Alberts, B., 1972, A DNA-unwinding protein isolated from *E. coli:* Its interaction with DNA and with DNA polymerases, *Proc. Natl. Acad. Sci. USA* **69**:3537.

Sleigh, M. J., Topp, W. C., Hanich, R., and Sambrook, J. F., 1978, Mutants of SV40 with an altered small t protein are reduced in their ability to transform cells, *Cell* **14**:79.

Slocombe, P. M., 1977, Ph.D. Thesis, University of Cambridge.

Smith, A., Bayley, S., Wheeler, T., and Maizel, W., 1975, in: *In Vitro Transcription and Translation of Viral Genomes* (A. Haenni and G. Beard, eds.), pp. 331–338, Inserm, Paris.

Smith, L. H., and Sinsheimer, R. L., 1976, The in vitro transcription units of bacteriophage φX174. II. In vitro initiation sites of φX174 transcription, *J. Mol. Biol.* **103**:699.

Smith, M., Brown, N. L., Air, G. M., Barrell, B. G., Coulson, A. R., Hutchison, C. A., III, and Sanger, F., 1977, DNA sequence at the C-termini of the overlapping genes A and B in bacteriophage φX174, *Nature (London)* **265**:702.

Snell, D. T., and Offord, R. E., 1972, The amino acid sequence of the B protein of bacteriophage ZJ-2, *Biochem. J.* **127**:167.

Soeda, E., Miura, K., Nakaso, A., and Kimura, G., 1977, Nucleotide sequence around the replication origin of polyoma virus DNA, *FEBS Lett.* **79**:383.

Sogin, M. L., Pace, N. R., Rosenberg, M., and Weissman, S. M., 1976, Nucleotide sequence of a 5 S ribosomal RNA precursor from *Bacillus subtilis*, *J. Biol. Chem.* **251**:3480.

Steege, D., 1977, A ribosome binding site from the P_R RNA of bacteriophage lambda, *J. Mol. Biol.* **114**:559.

Steenbergh, P. H., Sussenbach, J. S., Roberts, R. J., and Jansz, H. S., 1975, The 3′terminal nucleotide sequences of adenovirus types 2 and 5 DNA, *J. Virol.* **15**:268.

Steitz, J. A., 1969, Polypeptide chain initiation: Nucleotide sequences of the three ribosomal binding sites in bacteriophage R17 RNA, *Nature (London)* **224**:957.

Steitz, J. A., and Jakes, K., 1975, How ribosomes select initiator regions in mRNA: Base pair formation between the 3' terminus of 16 S rRNA and the mRNA during initiation of protein synthesis in *Escherichia coli, Proc. Natl. Acad. Sci. USA* **72**:4734.

Stillman, B. W., Bellett, A. J. D., and Robinson, A. J., 1977, Replication of linear adenovirus DNA is not hairpin-primed, *Nature (London)* **269**:723.

Straus, S. E., Sebring, E. D., and Rose, J. A., 1976, Concatemers of alternating plus and minus strands are intermediates in adenovirus-associated virus DNA synthesis, *Proc. Natl. Acad. Sci. USA* **73**:742.

Subramanian, K. N., Dhar, R., and Weissman, S. M., 1977a, Nucleotide sequence of a fragment of SV40 DNA that contains the origin of DNA replication and specifies the 5' ends of "early" and "late" viral RNA. I. Mapping of the restriction endonuclease sites within the *Eco* RII-G fragment and strategy employed for its sequence analysis, *J. Biol. Chem.* **252**:333.

Subramanian, K. N., Dhar, R., and Weissman, S. M., 1977b, Nucleotide sequence of a fragment of SV40 DNA that contains the origin of DNA replication and specifies the 5' ends of "early" and "late" viral RNA. III. Construction of the total sequence of *Eco* RII-G fragment of SV40 DNA, *J. Biol. Chem.* **252**:355.

Subramanian, K. N., Dhar, R., Weissman, S. M., and Ghosh, P. K., 1977c, Nucleotide sequence of a fragment of SV40 DNA that contains the origin of DNA replication and specifies the 5' ends of "early" and "late" viral RNA. II. Sequences of T_1 and pancreatic ribonuclease digestion products of RNA transcripts prepared from subfragments of *Eco* RII-G, *J. Biol. Chem.* **252**:340.

Subramanian, K. N., Reddy, V. B., and Weissman, S. M., 1977d, Occurrence of reiterated sequences in an untranslated region of SV40 DNA determined by nucleotide sequence analysis, *Cell* **10**:497.

Suggs, S. V., and Ray, D. S., 1977, Replication of bacteriophage M13. XI. Localization of the origin for M13 single-strand synthesis, *J. Mol. Biol.* **110**:147.

Sugimoto, K., Okamoto, T., Sugisaki, H., and Takanami, M., 1975a, The nucleotide sequence of an RNA polymerase binding site on bacteriophage fd DNA, *Nature (London)* **253**:410.

Sugimoto, K., Sugisaki, H., Okamoto, T., and Takanami, M., 1975b, Studies on bacteriophage fd DNA. III. Nucleotide sequence preceding the RNA start-site on a promoter-containing fragment, *Nucleic Acids Res.* **2**:2091.

Sugimoto, K., Sugisaki, H., Okamoto, T., and Takanami, M., 1977, Studies on bacteriophage fd DNA. IV. The sequence of messenger RNA for the major coat protein gene, *J. Mol. Biol.* **111**:487.

Sugiura, M., Okamoto, T., and Takanami, M., 1969, Starting nucleotide sequences of RNA synthesised on the replicative form DNA of coliphage fd, *J. Mol. Biol.* **43**:299.

Sussenbach, J. S., and Kuijk, M. G., 1977, Studies on the mechanism of replication of adenovirus DNA. V. The location of termini of replication, *Virology* **77**:149.

Sussenbach, J. S., Tolun, A., and Pettersson, U., 1976, On the nature of the single-stranded DNA in replicating adenovirus type 5 DNA, *J. Virol.* **20**:532.

Szybalski, W., Bøvre, K., Fiandt, M., Guha, A., Hradecna, Z., Kumar, S., Lozeron, H. A., Maher, V. M., Nijkamp, H. J. J., Summers, W. C., and Taylor, K., 1969,

Transcriptional controls in developing bacteriophages, *J. Cell. Physiol.* **74**:33–70 (Suppl. 1).

Tabak, H., Griffith, J., Geider, K., Schaller, H., and Kornberg, A., 1974, Initiation of deoxyribonucleic acid synthesis. VII. A unique location of the gap in the M13 replicative duplex synthesised in vitro, *J. Biol. Chem.* **249**:3049.

Takanami, M., Okamoto, T., and Sugiura, M., 1970, The starting nucleotide sequences and size of RNA transcribed in vitro on phage DNA templates, *Cold Spring Harbor Symp. Quant. Biol.* **34**:179.

Takanami, M., Okamoto, T., and Sugiura, M., 1971, Termination of RNA transcription on the replicative form DNA of bacteriophage fd, *J. Mol. Biol.* **62**:81.

Takanami, M., Okamoto, T., Sugimoto, K., and Sugisaki, H., 1975, Studies on bacteriophage fd DNA. I. A cleavage map of the fd genome, *J. Mol. Biol.* **95**:21.

Takanami, M., Sugimoto, K., Sugisaki, H., and Okamoto, T., 1976, Sequence of promoter for coat protein gene of bacteriophage fd, *Nature* (*London*) **260**:297.

Tegtmeyer, P., Rundell, K., and Collins, J. K., 1977, Modification of simian virus 40 protein A, *J. Virol.* **21**:647.

Tessman, I., Tessman, E. S., Pollock, T. J., Borrás, M.-T., Puga, A., and Baker, R., 1976, Reinitiation mutants of gene B of bacteriophage S13 that mimic gene A mutants in blocking replicative form DNA synthesis, *J. Mol. Biol.* **103**:583.

Thimmappaya, B., and Weissman, S. M., 1977, The early region of SV40 DNA may have more than one gene, *Cell* **11**:837.

Tilghman, S. M., Tiemeier, D. C., Seidman, J. G., Peterlin, B. M., Sullivan, M., Maizel, J. V., and Leder, P., 1978, Intervening sequence of DNA identified in the structural portion of a mouse β-globin gene, *Proc. Natl. Acad. Sci. USA* **75**:725.

Tomizawa, J., Ohmori, H., and Bird, R. E., 1977, Origin of replication of colicin E1 plasmid DNA, *Proc. Natl. Acad. Sci. USA* **74**:1865.

Tooze, J. (ed.), 1973, *The Molecular Biology of Tumor Viruses*, Cold Spring Harbor Laboratory, Cold Spring Harbor, N.Y.

Tooze, J., and Sambrook, J. (eds.), 1974, *Selected Papers in Tumor Virology*, Cold Spring Harbor Laboratory, Cold Spring Harbor, N.Y.

Tu, C.-P. D., Roychoudhury, R., and Wu, R., 1976, Direct DNA sequence determination of a fragment of SV40 genome produced by restriction endonuclease *Hin*d (or *Hin*c II), *Fed. Proc.* **35**:1595.

Van den Hondel, C. A., and Schoenmakers, J. G. G., 1975, Studies on bacteriophage M13 DNA: Cleavage map of the M13 genome, *Eur. J. Biochem.* **53**:547.

Van den Hondel, C. A., and Schoenmakers, J. G. G., 1976, Cleavage maps of the filamentous bacteriophages M13, fd, f1 and ZJ-2, *J. Virol.* **18**:1024.

Van den Hondel, C. A., Weijers, A., Konings, R. N. H., and Schoenmakers, J. G. G., 1975, Studies on bacteriophage M13 DNA: Gene order of the M13 genome, *Eur. J. Biochem.* **53**:559.

Van den Hondel, C. A., Pennings, L., and Schoenmakers, J. G. G., 1976, Restriction-enzyme cleavage maps of bacteriophage M13: Existence of an intergenic region on the M13 genome, *Eur. J. Biochem.* **68**:55.

Van de Sande, J. H., Kleppe, K., and Khorana, H. G., 1973, Reversal of bacteriophage T4 induced polynucleotide kinase action, *Biochemistry* **12**:5050.

Van de Vliet, P. C., Zandberg, J., and Jansz, H. S., 1977, Evidence for a function of the adenovirus DNA-binding protein in initiation of DNA synthesis as in elongation of nascent DNA chains, *Virology* **80**:98.

Van de Voorde, A., Rogiers, R., Van Herreweghe, J., Van Heuverswyn, H., Volckaert, G., and Fiers, W., 1974, Deoxynucleotide substitution: A new technique for sequence analysis of RNA, *Nucleic Acids Res.* **1**:1059.

Van de Voorde, A., Contreras, R., Rogiers, R., and Fiers, W., 1976, The initiation region of the SV40 VP$_1$ gene, *Cell* **9**:117.

Van Heuverswyn, H., Van de Voorde, A., and Fiers, W., 1977, Nucleotide sequence of the SV40 DNA restriction fragment *Hin*d C–*Hap* 2, *Nucleic Acids Res.* **4**:1015.

Vereijken, J. M., Van Mansfeld, A. D. M., Baas, P. D., and Jansz, H. S., 1975, *Arthrobacter luteus* restriction endonuclease cleavage map of ϕX174 RF DNA, *Virology* **68**:221.

Volckaert, G., Min Jou, W., and Fiers, W., 1976, Analysis of ^{32}P-labeled bacteriophage MS2 RNA by a mini-fingerprinting procedure, *Anal. Biochem.* **72**:433.

Volckaert, G., Contreras, R., Soeda, E., Van de Voorde, A., and Fiers, W., 1977, Nucleotide sequence of simian virus 40 *Hin*d H restriction fragment, *J. Mol. Biol.* **110**:467.

Volckaert, G., van de Voorde, A., and Fiers, W., 1978, Nucleotide sequence of the simian virus 40 small-t gene, *Proc. Natl. Acad. Sci. USA* **75**:2160.

Vovis, G. F., Horiuchi, K., and Zinder, N. D., 1975, Endonuclease R Eco RII restriction of bacteriophage f1 DNA in vitro: Ordering of genes V and VII, location of an RNA promoter for gene VIII, *J. Virol.* **16**:674.

Walter, G., and Maizel, J. V., 1974, The polypeptides of adenovirus. IV. Detection of early and late virus-induced polypeptides and their distribution in subcellular fractions, *Virology* **57**:402.

Walz, A., and Pirrotta, V., 1975, Sequence of the P$_R$ promoter of phage λ, *Nature (London)* **254**:118.

Watson, J. D., 1972, Origin of concatameric T7 DNA, *Nature (London) New Biol.* **239**:197.

Weber, J., 1974, Absence of adenovirus specific repressor in adenovirus tumor cells, *J. Gen. Virol.* **22**:259.

Weber, J., Jelinek, W., and Darnell, J. E., Jr., 1977, The definition of a large viral transcription unit late in Ad 2 infection of HeLa cells: Mapping of nascent RNA molecules labelled in isolated nuclei, *Cell* **10**:611.

Webster, R. E., and Cashman, J. S., 1973, Abortive infection of *Escherichia coli* with the bacteriophage f1: Cytoplasmic membrane proteins and the f1 DNA-gene 5 protein complex, *Virology* **55**:20.

Weigel, P. H., Englund, P. T., Murray, K., and Old, R. W., 1973, The 3'terminal nucleotide sequences of bacteriophage λ DNA, *Proc. Natl. Acad. Sci. USA* **70**:1151.

Weingartner, B., Winnacker, E. L., Tolun, A., and Pettersson, U., 1976, Two complementary strand-specific termination sites for adenovirus DNA replication, *Cell* **9**:259.

Weinstock, R., Sweet, R., Weiss, M., Cedar, H., and Axel, R., 1978, Intragenic DNA spacers interrupt the ovalbumin gene, *Proc. Natl. Acad. Sci. USA* **75**:1299.

Weisbeek, P. J., Vereijken, J. M., Baas, P. D., Jansz, H. S., and Van Arkel, G. A., 1976, The genetic map of bacteriophage ϕX174 constructed with restriction enzyme fragments, *Virology* **72**:61.

Weisbeek, P. J., Borrias, W. E., Langeveld, S. A., Baas, P. D., and Van Arkel, G. A., 1977, Bacteriophage ϕX174: Gene A overlaps gene B, *Proc. Natl. Acad. Sci. USA* **74**:2504.

Weiss, B., and Richardson, C. C., 1967, The 5' terminal dinucleotides of the separated strands of T7 bacteriophage deoxyribonucleic acid, *J. Mol. Biol.* **23**:405.

Wickner, W., Brutlag, D., Schekman, R., and Kornberg, A., 1972, RNA synthesis initiates in vitro conversion of M13 DNA to its replicative form, *Proc. Natl. Acad. Sci. USA* **69**:965.

Williams, J. F., Gharpur, M., Ustacelebi, S., and McDonald, S., 1971, Isolation of temperature-sensitive mutants of adenovirus type 5, *J. Gen. Virol.* **11**:95.

Williams, J. F., Young, C. S., and Austin, P. E., 1974, Genetic analysis of human adenovirus type 5 in permissive and nonpermissive cells, *Cold Spring Harbor Symp. Quant. Biol.* **39**:427.

Wilner, B. I., 1969, *A Classification of the Major Groups of Human and Other Animal Viruses*, pp. 120–132, Burgess, Minneapolis.

Wolfson, J., and Dressler, D., 1972, Adenovirus-2 DNA contains an inverted terminal repetition, *Proc. Natl. Acad. Sci. USA* **69**:3054.

Wu, R., 1970, Nucleotide sequence analysis of DNA. I. Partial sequence of the cohesive ends of bacteriophage λ and 186 DNA, *J. Mol. Biol.* **51**:501.

Wu, R., and Kaiser, A. D., 1968, Structure and base sequence in the cohesive ends of bacteriophage lambda DNA, *J. Mol. Biol.* **35**:523.

Wu, R., and Taylor, E., 1971, Nucleotide sequence analysis of DNA. II. Complete nucleotide sequence of the cohesive ends of bacteriophage λ DNA, *J. Mol. Biol.* **57**:491.

Wu, R., Jay, E., and Roychoudhury, R., 1976, Nucleotide sequence analysis of DNA, *Methods Cancer Res.* **12**:87.

Wu, M., Roberts, R. J., and Davidson, N., 1977, Structure of the inverted terminal repetition of adenovirus type 2 DNA, *J. Virol.* **21**:766.

Yeng, Y., Gelfand, D., Hayashi, M., Shleser, R., and Tessman, E. S., 1970, The eight genes of bacteriophage ϕX174 and S13 and comparison of the phage-specified proteins, *J. Mol. Biol.* **49**:521.

Ysebaert, M., Thys, F., Van de Voorde, A., and Fiers, W., 1976, Nucleotide sequence of the restriction fragments *Hind* L and *Hind* M of SV40 DNA, *Nucleic Acids Res.* **3**:3409.

Zain, B. S., and Roberts, R. J., 1978, Characterization and sequence analysis of a recombination site in the hybrid virus Ad2$^+$ND$_1$, *J. Mol. Biol.* **120**:13.

Zain, B. S., Dhar, R., Weissman, S. M., Lebowitz, P., and Lewis, A. M., Jr., 1973, Preferred site for initiation of RNA transcription by *Escherichia coli* RNA polymerase within the simian virus 40 segment of the nondefective adenovirus–simian virus 40 hybrid viruses Ad2$^+$ND$_1$ and Ad2$^+$ND$_3$, *J. Virol.* **11**:682.

Zain, B. S., Thimmappaya, B., Dhar, R., and Weissman, S. M., 1978, Nucleotide sequences of DNA encoding the 3' ends of SV40 mRNA, *J. Biol. Chem.* **253**:1606.

Ziff, E. B., Sedat, J. W., and Galibert, F., 1973, Determination of the nucleotide sequence of a fragment of bacteriophage ϕX174 DNA, *Nature (London) New Biol.* **241**:34.

CHAPTER 5

Viral Membranes

Richard W. Compans

Department of Microbiology
University of Alabama Medical Center
Birmingham, Alabama 35294

and

Hans-Dieter Klenk

Institut für Virologie
Justus-Liebig-Universität Giessen
6300 Giessen, Germany

1. INTRODUCTION

Many animal viruses, as well as certain plant and bacterial viruses, possess a lipid-containing membrane termed the "viral envelope." For most of these viruses, the envelope is acquired by budding at a cellular membrane, and viral components become an integral part of this membrane during assembly. In this chapter, we review the extensive body of information that has been obtained recently on the fine structure, composition, and assembly processes of the enveloped animal viruses. The replication processes of these viruses have been reviewed in other volumes of this series (e.g., Volumes 3, 4, 10, and 11).

It has become increasingly apparent that viral membranes possess important advantages for studies of membrane structure and assembly; the simplicity of viral membranes in terms of protein composition is probably the most significant advantage for detailed studies of membrane structure. Many lipid-containing viruses are important human and animal pathogens, and their membrane proteins possess biologically important functions and immunological properties, which also provide much of the stimulus for research in this area of molecular virology.

Although significant differences in sizes and number of structural proteins occur among lipid-containing viruses, there are several features of membrane structure shared by all these viruses. These include the presence of a lipid bilayer, glycosylated proteins exposed on the external surface of the bilayer, and internal nonglycosylated proteins. The available evidence indicates that the viral genome codes for the protein components of viral membranes, whereas the lipids are derived from the host cell membrane. Carbohydrates, which are covalently linked to viral glycoproteins as well as glycolipids, are also probably specified by cellular enzymes, although some virus-specific modifications of carbohydrates have been identified.

2. METHODS FOR ANALYSIS OF VIRAL MEMBRANES

2.1. Proteins

Viral membrane proteins resemble proteins of other biological membranes in their solubility properties. While numerous methods have been employed for the study of viral proteins, some general experimental approaches which have been useful are those common to membrane proteins in general. Thus viral membrane proteins can be solubilized by detergents, and polyacrylamide gel electrophoresis in the presence of sodium dodecylsulfate (Summers et al., 1965) is the most widely used approach for analysis of the polypeptide constituents of enveloped viruses. Other useful general preparative procedures include gel filtration in the presence of guanidine hydrochloride (Lazarowitz et al., 1971; Fleissner, 1971) and isoelectric focussing in the presence of nonionic detergents (Hung et al., 1971). Standard procedures of protein chemistry, including compositional analysis, peptide mapping, and amino acid sequencing, have been applied to certain isolated viral membrane proteins, but much basic information remains to be obtained.

In addition to methods resulting in complete solubilization of virion components, other procedures for the analysis of viral structure rely on the isolation of substructures of the virion. Treatment of enveloped virions with nonionic detergents such as Triton X100 or Nonidet P40, or weak ionic detergents such as deoxycholate, results in solubilization of the viral envelope and release of the internal nucleoproteins. Separation of envelope and nucleocapsid proteins can usually then be achieved by centrifugation or phase separation procedures. Affinity chromatography on lectin columns (Hayman *et al.*, 1973) or ion exchange chromatography on phosphocellulose (Strand and August, 1973) has also been useful for isolation of viral glycoproteins.

A variety of approaches have been applied to determine the location of the structural proteins in enveloped viruses, as discussed in detail in sections on individual virus groups. Proteolytic digestion results in selective degradation of viral glycoproteins, which are located on the external surface of the lipid bilayer. The internal proteins remain intact after such treatment and can be isolated as components of glycoprotein-free particles surrounded by an intact lipid bilayer. The external proteins of the virion can also be selectively labeled by surface labeling procedures, including lactoperoxidase-catalyzed iodination, Schiff's base formation with pyridoxal phosphate followed by reduction with borotritide, or reaction with formylmethionylsulfone methylphosphate. Direct electron microscopic examination of subviral components has also frequently enabled their identification as specific structural components of the virion. Using these and other approaches, the location of the major structural polypeptides has been established for many different enveloped viruses. Further analysis of the structure of viral membranes will include identification of nearest-neighbor relationships among viral envelope proteins. Such studies have recently been undertaken using bifunctional cross-linking reagents (Garoff, 1974; Wiley *et al.*, 1977; Dubovi and Wagner, 1977).

2.2. Lipid Bilayer

Several biophysical methods have been employed to analyze the organization and physical properties of lipids in viral membranes. X-ray diffraction patterns of virus pellets or concentrated suspensions exhibit a series of concentric circular fringes; the separation and relative intensity of these fringes are related to the variation in electron density as a function of radius from the center of the particle. Fourier analysis of the diffraction data yields a profile of the radial electron density distribution, and the location of the lipid hydrocarbon phase is assumed to correspond to an observed deep minimum in electron density. It has been concluded that only a bilayer arrangement could account for the deep minimum in electron density distribution observed in viral envelopes (Harrison *et al.*, 1971). The proteins on the external surface of the bilayer are also represented in the electron density profiles.

Although it could be concluded that most of the region of the bilayer was occupied by lipid, the possibility of penetration of the bilayer by a small amount of protein probably cannot be excluded.

Electron spin resonance spectroscopy using spin label methods has also provided evidence for a bilayer structure in a variety of enveloped viruses (for review, see Landsberger *et al.*, 1978). This technique employs fatty acid or phospholipid derivatives containing a paramagnetic nitroxide ring, which are incorporated into the lipid bilayer. The resulting ESR spectra have provided evidence concerning the fluidity of lipid fatty acyl chains, as well as other properties of the environment and mobility of lipid molecules. Bilayer structures exhibit a characteristic flexibility gradient, in which the mobility of the fatty acyl chain progressively increases with distance from the polar head group (Hubbell and McConnell, 1971). Spin label ESR spectroscopy has also been used to determine the effects of changes in lipid and protein composition on lipid bilayer fluidity (Landsberger *et al.*, 1973; Landsberger and Compans, 1976) and to study aspects of virus–cell interaction (Maeda *et al.*, 1977).

Nuclear magnetic resonance studies of ^{13}C-labeled lipids incorporated into enveloped viruses have been employed to analyze the organization of the lipid phase (Stoffel and Bister, 1975). Measurements of spin lattice relaxation times have been carried out with whole virions labeled with ^{13}C incorporated into specific positions in lipids, and the results indicate a high degree of rigidity in the envelope structure.

Fluorescence depolarization measurements with probes incorporated into the lipid bilayer have been used to estimate the microviscosity of lipids in viral membranes (Moore *et al.*, 1976; Barenholz *et al.*, 1976). Fluorescent energy transfer from aromatic amino acid residues of viral proteins to a probe incorporated into the lipid bilayer has also been used to estimate the distance separating the donor and acceptor residues (Lenard *et al.*, 1974). Precise distances could not be calculated, however, since it is possible that more than one amino acid residue may be transfering energy to the probe. The precise location of fluorescent probes in viral membranes is not known either, although their solubility properties suggest that they are incorporated into the hydrocarbon phase of the bilayer.

The distribution of lipids between the internal and external monolayers of the lipid bilayer has been investigated by several approaches, including labeling of amino groups with [^{35}S]formylmethionylsulfone methyl phosphate (Gahmberg *et al.*, 1972*a*), treatment with phospholipases and phospholipid exchange proteins (Rothman *et al.*,

1976), and measurement of transfer of radioactive cholesterol from virions to lipid vesicles (Lenard and Rothman, 1976). The lipids of the outer monolayer are thought to be involved in these reactions and transfer processes; exchange of lipids between the inner and outer monolayers appears to be a very slow process. These approaches have indicated an asymmetrical distribution of lipids in viral membranes.

Several laboratories have investigated the origin of viral lipids by comparative compositional analyses of lipids of the viral envelope and those of the host cell and its plasma membrane. Either direct chemical determinations or radiolabeling with $^{32}PO_4$ has been employed to determine the distribution of phospholipids. The results of these studies, described in detail in the sections which follow, indicate that viral lipids are derived from the host cell membrane where virus assembly occurs.

2.3. Carbohydrates

Carbohydrates are covalently linked to viral glycoproteins as well as glycolipids. Identification of glycoproteins has generally been accomplished by specific labeling with sugar precursors; glucosamine and fucose have been employed most often because they are not converted extensively into other metabolites (Klenk et al., 1970a; Strauss et al., 1970). The carbohydrates of viral glycoproteins can also be labeled by exposure to galactose oxidase followed by reduction with tritiated sodium borohydride (Klenk et al., 1978). Further information about the size and structure of the oligosaccharides of viral glycoproteins has been obtained by digestion of the polypeptide backbone with pronase and analysis of the resulting glycopeptide components by gel filtration (Burge and Strauss, 1970). Digestion with specific glycosidases has provided some information of the sequence of sugars in viral oligosaccharides, as described in the sections which follow on rhabdoviruses and togaviruses. Other studies employed methylation of the constituent sugars followed by gas chromatographic analysis as described in the section on influenza virus. Valuable information on the carbohydrate moiety of the viral glycoproteins has been obtained from studies employing inhibitors of glycosylation, such as 2-deoxy-D-glucose, D-glucosamine (Klenk et al., 1972b), and tunicamycin (R. Schwarz et al., 1976; Leavitt et al., 1977; Nakamura and Compans, 1978a). Tunicamycin has been shown to inhibit the synthesis of lipid-bound precursors of the carbohydrate side chains (Takatsuki et al., 1975; Tkacz and Lampen, 1975), and evidence has been obtained that the other inhibitors act by a similar mechanism (R. Schwarz et al., 1977).

3. VIRAL MEMBRANE STRUCTURE AND ASSEMBLY

3.1. Arenaviruses

3.1.1. Classification, Morphology, Composition

The arenaviruses are a recently identified group of enveloped RNA-containing viruses (Pfau *et al.*, 1974). The members of the group include lymphocytic choriomeningitis virus (LCM), Lassa fever virus, and the Tacaribe complex of viruses (Amapari, Junin, Latino, Machupo, Parana, Pichinde, Tacaribe, and Tamiami viruses). Virions are essentially spherical particles which occur in sizes ranging from 50 to 300 nm in diameter. Distinct surface projections approximately 10 nm in length radiate from the viral envelope. A striking feature of arenavirus morphology is the presence of one or more distinct granules of approximately 20 nm diameter in the interior of virions as observed by thin-section electron microscopy (Dalton *et al.*, 1968; Murphy *et al.*, 1969, 1970). As described below, these granules have been identified biochemically as 80 S ribosomes incorporated into the virion during the assembly process. Although the presence of ribosomes is probably the most distinctive morphological characteristic of the virion, other aspects of virion morphology, including nucleocapsid structure and surface structure, are sufficient to distinguish arenaviruses from the other known groups of animal viruses. Further, ribosomes may not be present in all arenavirus particles (Vezza *et al.*, 1978).

It has been established that arenaviruses contain at least five RNA species, three of which are host cell derived 28 S, 18 S, and 4–6 S RNA species. Virus-specific RNAs of approximately 31 S and 22 S have been observed for several arenaviruses (Carter *et al.*, 1973; Pedersen, 1971, 1973; Anon *et al.*, 1976); in addition, a 15 S RNA species has also been reported for Pichinde (Farber and Rawls, 1975). Convincing evidence has been obtained that the 28 S and 18 S RNAs in arenavirus preparations originate from host cell derived ribosomes (Farber and Rawls, 1975). Whether the ribosomes are essential components of arenaviruses has not been established; however, recent results indicate that some arenaviruses lack significant amounts of the 18 S ribosomal RNA (Vezza *et al.*, 1977, 1978).

The virion proteins of Pichinde virus were the first to be characterized (Ramos *et al.*, 1972), and more recently structural proteins of several other arenaviruses have been identified including those of Junin virus (Martinez-Segovia and DeMitri, 1977), Tacaribe and Tamiami viruses (Gard *et al.*, 1977), and LCM virus (Buchmeier *et al.*, 1977). The available information indicates that all arenaviruses possess a major carbohydrate-free polypeptide of 66,000–72,000 daltons associated with the nucleocapsid, and one or more envelope glycoprotein species. Pichinde virions contain two glycoproteins with molecular weights of 38,000 and 64,000 (Ramos *et al.*, 1972; Vezza *et al.*, 1977). In contrast to earlier reports indicating that a glycoprotein of Pichinde virus was associated with the viral nucleocapsid (Ramos *et al.*, 1972), recent observations indicate that both glycoproteins of Pichinde virus are located on the surface of the virion, and neither is found as a component of the isolated nucleocapsid (Vezza *et al.*, 1977). In these studies it was observed that both glycoproteins of Pichinde virus are sensitive to digestion by pronase, which produces spikeless particles which contained the major nonglycosylated protein. Further, ribonucleoprotein complexes were isolated from detergent-disrupted virions; these contained the major nucleocapsid protein but were free of either glycoprotein. These results indicate that both glycoproteins of Pichinde virions are present as components of the surface spikes, as found with other enveloped viruses. The two Pichinde glycoproteins are present in approximately equimolar ratios (Vezza *et al.*, 1977). It remains to be determined whether they are present in the same or in different spike structures on the viral surface and whether they contain distinct amino acid sequences.

In contrast to the two glycoproteins of Pichinde virions, only a single glycoprotein size class was detected in Tacaribe or Tamiami virions; these had molecular weights of 44,000 and 42,000, respectively (Gard *et al.*, 1977). These glycoproteins were sensitive to proteolytic digestion with chymotrypsin, which produced spikeless particles containing the major nonglycosylated protein; thus the glycoproteins are located on the viral surface. Junin virions also contained a major glycoprotein of 38,000 daltons, but several additional minor glycoproteins were also reported (Martinez-Segovia and DeMitri, 1977).

Arenaviruses contain lipids as indicated by their inactivation by detergents or lipid solvents (Pfau *et al.*, 1974). Electron microscopic studies indicating the presence of a distinct unit membrane also strongly suggest that these are lipid-containing viruses (Dalton *et al.*, 1968; Murphy *et al.*, 1970). No data are available on viral lipid composition or on carbohydrate components present in arenavirus particles, other than the demonstration that glycosylated polypeptides can be selectively radiolabeled by sugar precursors such as glucosamine.

3.1.2. Biosynthesis and Assembly

Little information has been obtained on the biosynthesis of arenavirus proteins in infected cells. In BHK21 cells infected with

Tacaribe virus, synthesis of the major structural proteins could be detected above the background of host cell synthesis (Saleh and Compans, 1978). In addition to the major virion proteins, a virus-induced glycoprotein of ~70,000 daltons was synthesized in large amounts in infected cells; this glycoprotein was not detected in purified virions. It remains to be established whether it is a precursor of the 44,000-dalton virion glycoprotein, a distinct viral gene product, or a virus-induced host cell protein.

The process of morphogenesis of several arenaviruses in Vero cells was studied by Murphy *et al.* (1970). Virus particles form by budding at the plasma membrane in most instances, with occasional budding at intracytoplasmic membranes. Membrane changes characteristic of the viral envelope were observed in regions of the plasma membrane, and a distinct increase in density of the membrane was found in restricted areas large enough to form individual virions. Surface projections were present on the external surface of budding particles, and dense granules (ribosomes) were contained in the interior. In some cells a large proportion of the plasma membrane appears to be involved in the budding process.

No information is available on the molecular interactions involved in viral assembly. The internal nucleoproteins of arenavirions appear as convoluted strands when released from disrupted virions (Gard *et al.*, 1977; Vezza *et al.*, 1977). Most other enveloped viruses which contain strandlike or helical nucleoproteins also contain an internal membrane (M) protein which appears to be involved in assembly of the viral envelope. Since arenaviruses lack such a protein, the nucleoprotein and glycoproteins must determine the assembly process. Further information on the nature of the interactions between these components, as well as the arrangement of the nucleoprotein in the intact virion, is needed to provide insight into the process of virus assembly.

3.2. Bunyaviruses

The bunyaviridae include at least 150 distinguishable serological types, 87 of which were classified as the Bunyamwera supergroup of arboviruses (Murphy *et al.*, 1973, Porterfield *et al.*, 1976). They are clearly distinct from the togaviruses both in morphology and in molecular composition. The RNA genome of these viruses consists of three segments, which are contained within circular ribonucleoprotein complexes (Pettersson and von Bonsdorff, 1975; Bouloy *et al.*, 1974; Pettersson and Kääriäinen, 1973). In thin section, virus particles appear to be roughly spherical with a mean diameter of 100 nm, and a distinct unit membrane suggests a lipid bilayer structure in the envelope (von Bonsdorff and Pettersson, 1975).

Prominent large subunits have been seen by negative staining with uranyl acetate on the external surfaces of Uukuniemi virions (von Bonsdorff and Pettersson, 1975) but not of La Crosse virions (Obijeski *et al.*, 1976). The Uukuniemi morphological units resembled hollow cylinders 10–12 nm in diameter, with a central cavity of about 5 nm. The subunits were closely packed, and clustering as hexagonal arrays with frequent pentons (subunits surrounded by five neighboring units) was observed, suggesting icosahedral symmetry. A $T = 12$ surface lattice was observed in particles where vertex subunits were identified (von Bonsdorff and Pettersson, 1975).

Two glycoproteins with molecular weights of about 65,000 and 75,000 are present in Uukuniemi virions. Both glycoproteins are removed following protease treatment, which removes the surface subunits leaving pleiomorphic smooth surfaced particles (von Bonsdorff and Pettersson, 1975). Thus, like other enveloped viruses, both glycoproteins are located on the external surface of the virion. A small residual peptide was observed after proteolytic digestion, which may represent a protease-resistant segment of the glycoproteins. The virion nucleocapsid consists of RNA and a major nucleocapsid protein (N, 25,000 daltons). Like arenaviruses, the bunyaviruses possess neither an M protein nor an icosahedral nucleocapsid beneath the envelope, and it was therefore suggested (von Bonsdorff and Pettersson, 1975) that interactions between the surface glycoproteins may be important in viral assembly and maintenance of structural stability of the particles. The spikeless particles produced by protease treatment were markedly pleomorphic, which may reflect the role of the glycoproteins in determining the shape of the virion.

Although a similar number of polypeptide components are found in other bunyaviruses, the molecular weights of the components differ from those found for Uukuniemi virus. Three major and one minor protein have been found with four different members of the bunyavirus group (Obijeski *et al.*, 1976). In studies with La Crosse virus, two of the components, with estimated molecular weights of 120,000 and 34,000, were glycosylated, and the two glycoproteins were present in equimolar amounts. Nucleocapsids contained a major protein of 23,000 daltons, and a large protein (180,000 daltons) was present in small amounts in virions. Bromelain treatment removed both glycoproteins and yielded spikeless particles containing the two carbohydrate-free proteins. Lactoperoxidase-catalyzed iodination of intact virions also labeled the two glycoproteins and not the internal proteins, confirming that they are the only species on the external surface of the envelope. It is not known if the two glycoproteins are components of a single spike or form different spikes on the surface of the virion. Three or four polypeptides including two glycoproteins have also been detected for several other bunyaviruses (McLerran and Arlinghaus, 1973; Rosato *et al.*, 1974; White, 1975; Gentsch *et al.*, 1977).

Virtually nothing is known of the assembly process of bunyaviruses apart from the morphological demonstration of budding. Morphogenesis takes place at Golgi complex and endoplasmic reticulum membranes, within which virions accumulate (Murphy *et al.*, 1973). Precursor particles have not been detected in infected cells by electron microscopy, but the strandlike nucleoprotein structures are probably difficult to resolve in thin section. As discussed above, it has been suggested (von Bonsdorff and Pettersson, 1975) that lateral interactions between the glycoproteins of bunyaviruses may be important in the assembly process.

3.3. Coronaviruses

The coronavirus group of RNA viruses is defined by common morphological properties, the most distinctive being the presence of large club-shaped surface projections. The group includes viruses of diverse origins, and insufficient information is now available to determine whether these agents form a unified group in their chemical composition and replication processes. Some biochemical studies have been undertaken with several coronaviruses, including mouse hepatitis, avian infectious bronchitis, transmissible gastroenteritis virus of swine, and a human coronavirus OC43.

The structure of the murine coronavirus A59 has been studied in greatest detail (Sturman, 1977; Sturman and Holmes, 1977). A single nonglycosylated polypeptide of 50,000 daltons is located in the interior of the virion and is probably the structural subunit of the nucleocapsid. On the surface of the virion a number of glycoproteins are detected, but these do not all contain distinct amino acid sequences. A 23,000-dalton glycoprotein designated "E1" and a large glycoprotein designated "E2" appear to be two distinct envelope glycoproteins. E2 is observed in virions as a 180,000- or a 90,000-dalton glycoprotein; however, the two possess common tryptic peptides and the 180,000-dalton component is converted into a 90,000-dalton glycoprotein by trypsin treatment. Thus the 180,000-dalton component appears to be a precursor of the 90,000-

dalton component, or possibly of two cleavage products of similar elec-trophoretic mobility. Cleavage of the 180,000-dalton glycoprotein had little effect on viral infectivity (Sturman and Holmes, 1977).

The E2 glycoprotein appears to be degraded completely by the proteases bromelain or pronase, which produce particles lacking the sur-face spikes (Sturman, 1977). In contrast, only about 20% of E1 is removed by protease treatment, and a carbohydrate-free cleavage product of 18,000 daltons is produced (Sturman, 1977; Sturman and Holmes, 1977). It was suggested that the protease-resistant portion of E1 is buried within the lipid bilayer and that E2 forms the spike struc-ture projecting from the surface. This protease-resistant portion of E1 is significantly larger than protease-resistant glycoprotein fragments observed with other lipid-containing viruses. It is therefore conceivable that a large part of this molecule may extend through the bilayer, possibly forming a protein layer on the internal surface of the viral membrane, as suggested by Sturman (1977).

The E1 glycoprotein of murine coronavirus A59 displays unusual properties on SDS gel electrophoresis (Sturman, 1977). Heating to 100°C in the presence of SDS causes the formation of forms of E1 with lower electrophoretic mobility, and sulfhydryl-reducing agents enhance this aggregation.

Studies of polypeptides of other coronaviruses have revealed a larger number of components (Hierholzer et al., 1972; Garwes and Po-cock, 1975; Bingham, 1975), but it remains to be established how many of these are virus coded, and whether they contain distinct amino acid sequences. The proteins of the transmissible gastroenteritis virus of swine appear similar to those of murine A59 virions in several respects (Garwes and Pocock, 1975). The largest glycoprotein (200,000 daltons) was removed from virions by treatment with bromelain, and the surface projections were removed concomitantly, indicating that this glycoprotein forms the spike structure. Two low-molecular-weight glycoproteins (30,000 and 28,500) were resistant to protease treatment, as was a nonglycosylated polypeptide of molecular weight 50,000. Six or seven polypeptides including four glycoproteins were identified in preparations of the human coronavirus OC43 (Hierholzer et al., 1972). Two glycoproteins (molecular weights 104,000 and 15,000) were selec-tively removed by bromelain treatment and appeared to be components of the viral spikes, whereas other glycosylated and nonglycosylated pro-teins were resistant to protease.

These results indicate that the surface projections of three unre-lated coronaviruses apparently contain a high-molecular-weight glycoprotein. In both murine and porcine coronaviruses, one or two low-molecular-weight glycoproteins appear to be resistant to proteolytic digestion, in part or entirely, and probably penetrate extensively into the viral membrane. Further studies of the interactions between these glycoproteins, and between the envelope proteins and nucleocapsid, are needed to determine the arrangement of coronavirus proteins in the virion and the nature of their association with the viral membrane.

Electron microscopic studies of coronavirus-infected cells indicate that virus assembly occurs by budding at intracytoplasmic membranes, including endoplasmic reticulum and Golgi complex membranes (David-Ferreira and Manaker, 1965; Oshiro, 1973). Virions accumulate in large amount within such vacuoles and are thought to be released by fusion of the vacuolar membrane with the cell surface. At late stages, extensive regions of plasma membranes are observed with adherent virions, but budding at the plasma membrane is not generally observed (Oshiro, 1973).

3.4. Herpesviruses

3.4.1. Classification, Morphology, Composition

The herpesvirus group contains a large number of viruses, which have been isolated from a variety of animal hosts. Herpes simplex virus (HSV) has been the subject of intensive investigation, as have been certain herpesviruses of other species, notably pseudorabies, a porcine herpesvirus, and equine herpesvirus (EHV). The group is united by common morphological and biochemical properties, but little information is available concerning possible relationships between various herpesviruses. A similar number of structural polypeptides have been identified in HSV types 1 and 2, and EHV (Perdue *et al.*, 1974; Kemp *et al.*, 1974; Cassai *et al.*, 1975). Further, antigenic relationships between certain glycoproteins of HSV type 1 and type 2 have been shown by immune precipitation experiments (Spear, 1976). Detailed reviews of the structure and replication of herpesviruses include those of Roizman and Furlong (1974), O'Callaghan and Randall (1976), and Kaplan (1974).

Herpesviruses are large enveloped DNA-containing viruses with icosahedral nucleocapsids. Virions are usually 150–180 nm in diameter, with their icosahedral capsids measuring 100 nm in diameter. The capsid is a $T = 16$ structure with 162 capsomers. The envelope is a unit membrane structure when seen in thin sections, and spikelike surface projections about 8–10 nm in length can be resolved on the surface by negative staining (Wildy *et al.*, 1960; Epstein, 1962; O'Callaghan and Randall, 1976). Additional amorphous or fibrous material located between the capsid and envelope has been termed the "tegument" (Roizman and Furlong, 1974).

Herpesvirions are among the most complex of the enveloped viruses. Over 30 structural polypeptides ranging from 18,000 to 275,000 daltons have been identified in purified virions by SDS-polyacrylamide gel electrophoresis (Roizman and Furlong, 1974; O'Callaghan and Randall, 1976). Much information remains to be determined before the precise location of these proteins in the virion can be understood, but many have been localized as components of the capsid or envelope. Isolated nucleocapsids have been obtained by extraction from infected cells or detergent treatment of virions and their polypeptides compared with those of intact virions (Abodeely *et al.*, 1971; Robinson and Watson, 1971; Gibson and Roizman, 1974; Perdue *et al.*, 1974). At least six major proteins and several additional minor proteins are located in the capsid structure, all of which are nonglycosylated proteins.

Herpesvirions contain at least 13 glycoproteins, all of which appear to be components of the viral envelope (Roizman and Furlong, 1974; O'Callaghan and Randall, 1976). By analogy with other enveloped viruses, it is likely that all herpesvirus glycoproteins are exposed on the external surface of the virion, but this has not been definitively established. Some information on the location of virion glycoproteins was obtained by detergent solubilization and selective labeling by tritiated borohydride reduction of Schiff's bases formed between viral proteins and pyridoxal phosphate (Roizman and Furlong, 1974). Four major glycoproteins (VP7, 8, 17, and 18), ranging in size from approximately 60,000 to 130,000 daltons, appeared to be most readily labeled and most easily solubilized, suggesting that they are components present on the external surface of the virion. In addition, six major proteins and four minor proteins were detected as surface components of herpesvirions by lactoperoxidase-catalyzed iodination; most or all of these were glycosylated (Gupta and Rapp, 1977). Interestingly, several glycosylated as well as nonglycosylated envelope proteins of herpesvirions appear to be covalently linked to lipids, as shown by oil red O staining (Abodeely *et al.*, 1971) and specific incorporation of radioactive choline (Perdue *et al.*, 1974). The nature of the linkage of lipid to these proteins and its possible significance in terms of virus structure and assembly remain to be established. Sulfated structural glycoproteins are also present in herpesvirions (Kaplan and Ben Porat, 1976).

Limited information has been obtained about the lipids of herpesvirions. It is likely that the lipids are arranged in a bilayer corrresponding to the unit membrane in the viral envelope, although the arrangement of lipids has not been investigated. The lipid composition of herpesvirions was found to closely resemble that of the inner nuclear membrane, from which the virus buds, whereas it differed from that of the outer nuclear or cytoplasmic membranes (Ben Porat and Kaplan, 1971). Although most of the viral lipids appeared to be synthesized prior to infection, ^{32}P-labeled lipids synthesized after infection were preferentially incorporated from the inner nuclear membrane into virions (Ben Porat and Kaplan, 1971). Thus the incorporation of lipids into virions did not seem to occur solely by a random process. The essential role of the envelope lipids for infectivity was indicated by the inactivation of virions by phospholipase C (Spring and Roizman, 1968). Glycolipids of herpesvirions have been analyzed and found to be similar to those observed in infected cells (Brennan et al., 1976).

As described above, both glycoproteins and glycolipids are carbohydrate-containing components of herpesvirions. Glucosamine, galactosamine, galactose, mannose, fucose, and sialic acid have been identified as sugar constituents of the glycoproteins (Roizman and Furlong, 1974). The glycopeptides obtained by pronase digestion of virions or infected cell glycoproteins have been characterized by gel filtration, and up to five species with estimated molecular weights ranging from about 2000 to 10,000 were observed (Honess and Roizman, 1975). Two species with molecular weights of about 4300 and 6800 were the major glycopeptides obtained from glucosamine-labeled virions. The larger glycopeptides contained substantial amounts of sialic acid, which could be released by mild acid hydrolysis.

3.4.2. Synthesis and Assembly

Herpesvirus glycoproteins are synthesized with little or no involvement of proteolytic cleavage events (Honess and Roizman, 1973; Spear, 1976). Four immunologically distinct classes of major glycoproteins have been detected; three of these appear to be glycosylated in two discrete stages in infected cells, with partially and fully glycosylated forms that can be resolved by gel electrophoresis (Spear, 1976). Evidence for discrete stages of glycosylation was also obtained by analysis of oligosaccharide units of viral glycoproteins observed after pronase digestion (Honess and Roizman, 1975). In 15-min labeling periods viral glycoproteins contained small glucosamine-containing oligosaccharides of about 2000 daltons, which contained little or no fucose or sialic acid. The completed glycoproteins possess larger oligosaccharides containing fucose as well as sialic acid; only these glycoproteins are observed in virions.

The glycoproteins specified by herpesviruses are found in association with various cellular membranes, including smooth and rough endoplasmic reticulum and plasma membranes (Spear and Roizman, 1970; Spear et al., 1970; Heine et al., 1972). The role of those glycoproteins in virus replication is uncertain, although some may migrate to the inner nuclear membrane where envelopment occurs. In addition, they confer altered immunological properties on the plasma membrane, and may be responsible for herpesvirus-induced cell fusion (Roizman and Furlong, 1974; Ludwig et al., 1974). Virion glycoproteins differ from those present in the inner nuclear membrane of uninfected cells, indicating that host cell proteins are excluded from the envelope of budding virions, although they are not lost from the membrane after infection (Kaplan and Ben Porat, 1970).

As discussed above, the process of herpesvirus envelopment is usually observed at the inner nuclear membrane, particularly at early stages of infection (Darlington and Moss, 1969; Epstein, 1962; Fong et al., 1973; Schwartz and Roizman, 1969). Budding into nuclear or cytoplasmic vacuoles has also been observed. The inner nuclear membrane appears thickened in the region which becomes part of the envelope of the budding virion, presumably because of the presence of viral glycoproteins. By freeze-fracture electron microscopy, normal intramembranous particles were seen to be deleted from specific areas of the inner nuclear envelope in herpesvirus-infected cells, which may represent areas where cellular proteins are displaced by virus-specific proteins (Haines and Baerwald, 1976). Mature enveloped virus particles have been observed in cytoplasmic vacuoles or channels, which are thought to be involved in egress of virions from the nuclear envelope to the cell surface (Morgan et al., 1959; Darlington and Moss, 1969; Schwartz and Roizman, 1969).

Inhibition of glycosylation by 2-deoxyglucose or glucosamine inhibits production of infectious herpesvirus as well as the process of virus-induced cell fusion (Courtney et al., 1973; Gallaher et al., 1973; Ludwig et al., 1974; Knowles and Person, 1976). In the presence of these inhibitors, changes were observed in the electrophoretic mobility of viral glycoproteins, probably due to production of unglycosylated or partially glycosylated glycoproteins. Inhibition of herpesvirus replication by cytochalasin B may occur by a similar mechanism (Dix and Courtney, 1976). These inhibitors caused a greater inhibition of the production of infectious particles than of physical particles, and the virus particles produced contained aberrant glycoproteins (Courtney et al., 1973; Dix and Courtney, 1976). When radioactive 2-deoxyglucose was added to infected cells, it was found to be incorporated into herpesvirus-specific glycoproteins (Courtney et al., 1973).

3.5. Myxoviruses

3.5.1. Classification, Morphology, Composition

The orthomyxovirus group includes the influenza viruses of man and animals. Virions are roughly spherical particles ~100 nm in diameter, or filamentous forms of similar width but up to several micrometers in length. By negative staining, prominent surface spikes are seen, and a helical nucleocapsid is contained within the envelope (Horne et al., 1960; Hoyle et al., 1961; Waterson et al., 1961). Thin sections show a distinct unit membrane in the viral envelope, similar to the plasma membrane of the host cell. An additional electron-dense layer on the internal surface (Compans and Dimmock, 1969; Bächi et al., 1969) corresponds to the location of a nonglycosylated internal membrane protein, as described below. Several reviews are available concerning various aspects of influenza virus structure and replication (Schulze, 1973; Laver, 1973; White, 1974; Kilbourne, 1975; Palese, 1977), and a chapter on "Reproduction of Myxoviruses" is contained in Volume 4 of this series (Compans and Choppin, 1975).

The available information indicates that influenza virions consist of about 1–2% RNA, 70–75% protein, 20–24% lipid, and 5–8% carbohydrate (Ada and Perry, 1954; Frommhagen et al., 1959; Schäfer, 1959; Blough et al., 1967). The RNA genome consists of eight distinct single-stranded RNA species, each of which codes for one of the virus-specific polypeptides (Palese, 1977; Pons, 1976; Scholtissek et al., 1976; McGeoch et al., 1976). The virion polypeptides include two glycoproteins, the hemagglutinin and neuraminidase, which form distinct spikes on the external surface (Laver and Valentine, 1969; Webster and Darlington, 1969; Rott et al., 1970). A nucleocapsid subunit, a membrane-associated protein, and three minor high-molecular-weight proteins (P1,

P2, and P3) are internal components of the virion. In Table 1 a list of the envelope proteins of influenza virions along with their accepted designations, estimated molecular weights, and functions is presented.

Classification of influenza viruses is based on serological properties of the viral polypeptides. Three distinct serological types (A, B, and C) have been recognized, which show no immunological cross-reaction between any of their structural components. Both the hemagglutinin and neuraminidase antigens of type A viruses show extensive variation, and distinct serological subtypes have been identified which contain common internal antigens but have surface antigens which appear to be completely unrelated. The appearance of these new subtypes of type A viruses, with distinct surface antigens, is the cause of major pandemics of influenza. The antigenic subtypes of type A influenza viruses are designated according to the serological type of both their hemagglutinin (H) and neuraminidase (N). Four distinct subtypes, H_0N_1, H_1N_1, H_2N_2, and H_3N_2, have been identified among human influenza viruses between the first isolation in 1933 and the present time. Type A influenza viruses with hemagglutinin and neuraminidase antigens distinct from those of human influenza viruses have also been isolated from horses, swine, and birds. Only minor variation in immunological properties has been observed with influenza B viruses, and influenza C viruses have not been studied in detail.

3.5.2. Fine Structure and Arrangement of Envelope Components

The envelope of influenza virus has probably been studied in more detail than that of any other lipid-containing viruses. The recognized envelope components of influenza A and B viruses include a lipid

TABLE 1

Envelope Proteins of Influenza A Viruses

Protein	Designation	Molecular weight of polypeptide	Function
Hemagglutinin	HA	75,000–80,000	Binding to receptors
	HA1	50,000–55,000	
	HA2	25,000–30,000	
Neuraminidase	NA	55,000	Removal of neuraminic acid
Membrane Protein	M	26,000	Membrane structure and assembly

bilayer, external spikes consisting of the two glycoproteins hemagglutinin and neuraminidase, and an internal carbohydrate-free protein, the M protein. The hemagglutinin protein of influenza virus is probably the best-characterized viral envelope protein; there has been a longstanding interest in this protein because of its importance as the major antigen involved in immunity to influenza virus infection. A host-cell-derived carbohydrate antigen has also been detected in association with the viral envelope.

3.5.2a. The Hemagglutinin

Influenza virus was the first virus found to agglutinate erythrocytes (Hirst, 1941; McClelland and Hare, 1941); this has proved to be a convenient rapid assay for viruses of many different major groups. In the case of the influenza viruses, hemagglutination is caused by one of the envelope glycoproteins, termed the "hemagglutinin protein." When isolated from SDS-disrupted virus, the hemagglutinin protein was found to be a rodlike subunit ~14 nm in length and 4 nm in diameter (Laver and Valentine, 1969). In the absence of detergents, these glycoproteins were found in characteristic rosettelike aggregates, and it was suggested that one end of each spike may be hydrophobic and may be involved in binding to the viral envelope. End-on views of the hemagglutinin show a triangular shape (Laver, 1973; Griffith, 1975), and the size of the spike suggests that it may be composed of three identical polypeptide chains (see below).

The hemagglutinin spike may be composed of a 75,000-dalton glycoprotein species, designated "HA," or alternatively two cleavage products, designated "HA1" and "HA2" (~50,000 and ~25,000 daltons, respectively). The extent of cleavage of HA into HA1 and HA2 varies with the virus strain and cell type and the presence or absence of serum proteases (Lazarowitz et al., 1971, 1973a,b; Rifkin et al., 1972; Skehel, 1972; Stanley et al., 1973; Klenk et al., 1975). No cleavage of HA is necessary for virus assembly or receptor binding activity, and virions of some strains containing uncleaved HA are infectious (Lazarowitz et al., 1973a; Stanley et al., 1973), but subsequent studies have shown that the infectivity of virions is enhanced by proteolytic cleavage (Klenk et al., 1975; Lazarowitz and Choppin, 1975; Klenk et al., 1977b). It was observed that cleavage of HA into polypeptides of sizes similar to HA1 and HA2 could be accomplished by a variety of proteases; however, only cleavage by trypsinlike enzymes resulted in the formation of highly infectious virus (Lazarowitz and Choppin, 1975; Klenk *et al.*, 1977*b*). Activation of infectivity thus requires cleavage of a specific peptide bond with arginine or lysine in the carboxyl linkage. Dual infection experiments with different influenza virus strains demonstrated that the sensitivity or resistance of the hemagglutinin protein to cleavage is a structural property of each virus glycoprotein (Klenk *et al.*, 1977*b*).

The estimated molecular weight as well as the morphology of the intact hemagglutinin spike suggested that it was a trimer composed of three HA polypeptides, or three HA1-HA2 complexes (Laver, 1973; Griffith, 1975; Schulze, 1975*b*). Further evidence for a trimer structure was obtained by cross-linking experiments with dimethyl suberimidate (Wiley *et al.*, 1977), in which trimers of HA were demonstrated. The available estimates of the number of hemagglutinin polypeptides per virion (Compans *et al.*, 1970; White *et al.*, 1970; Skehel and Schild, 1971; Klenk *et al.*, 1972*a*; Schulze, 1972; Inglis *et al.*, 1976) indicate that 200–350 hemagglutinin spikes are present per particle. Tiffany and Blough (1970) calculated from electron microscopic measurements that a 100-nm-diameter particle possessed 550 spikes and an 80-nm-diameter particle 300 spikes, most of which are hemagglutinin proteins. Since virions occur in a range of sizes, no single value will apply to all virions in a population.

Treatment of influenza virus with the protease bromelain under certain conditions results in degradation of the HA1 polypeptide, producing smooth-surfaced spikeless particles which still contain HA2 (Compans *et al.*, 1970). Therefore, the HA2 segment of the hemagglutinin appears to interact closely with the lipid bilayer, whereas HA1 is located distally in the spike structure. On more extensive proteolytic digestion, HA2 is also cleaved (Schulze, 1970; Klenk *et al.*, 1972*a*) but a small peptide still remains associated with the envelope, which may represent a segment of the glycoprotein which penetrates into the lipid bilayer (Lenard *et al.*, 1976). Treatment of some influenza virus strains with bromelain results in solubilization of a segment of the spike consisting of HA1 as well as a cleavage product of HA2 that is about 5000 daltons smaller than the intact molecule (Skehel and Waterfield, 1975). These solubilized glycoproteins have been crystallized (Brand and Skehel, 1972), and the crystals were shown to exhibit erythrocyte-binding activity (Wiley, 1975). Comparison of the amino acid composition of the intact and bromelain-released glycoproteins indicated a preponderance of hydrophobic amino acids in the segment which is missing after bromelain cleavage (Skehel and Waterfield, 1975), suggesting that this may be a hydrophobic segment which may penetrate into the lipid bilayer. Since the N terminus of HA2 is unmodified by bromelain treatment, the hydrophobic segment must be located at the C-terminal end of the molecule. Comparison of the N-terminal amino acid sequences of HA1 and HA2 of various human subtypes of type A influenza viruses shows marked conservation of the sequence and a characteristic "palindrome sequence" of amino acids occurs at the N-terminal region of HA2 (Skehel and Waterfield, 1975). This sequence, which is located at the site of the HA polypeptide which is cleaved to form HA1 and HA2, is highly conserved among all influenza A viruses and may be important for recognition by the protease involved in cleavage. Alternatively, since virions with cleaved HA show enhanced infectivity, it is also possible that this region of the molecule undergoes a change in conformation and participates in some aspect of virus–cell interaction. The overall amino acid compositions of HA1 and HA2 subunits of the A_0/Bel strain of influenza virus were very similar, except that HA1 was higher in proline and lower in methionine than HA2 (Laver, 1971; Laver and Baker, 1972).

The hemagglutinin glycoprotein contains about 15–20% carbohydrate by weight (Laver, 1971; White, 1974; Schwarz and Klenk, 1974; Nakamura and Compans, 1978a). The carbohydrate composition is determined in large part by the host cell, and differences in electrophoretic mobilities are observed in glycoproteins from the same strain of virus grown in different host cells (Compans et al., 1970; Haslam et al., 1970; Schulze, 1970), which are due to differences in carbohydrate content of the glycoproteins (Schwarz et al., 1977; Nakamura and Compans, 1978b). An antigenic relationship has also been demonstrated between carbohydrate components obtained from chick allantoic cells and influenza virions grown in these cells (Laver and Webster, 1966).

Until recently, little information was available concerning the carbohydrate portion of the HA glycoprotein. About 80% of the carbohydrate attached to viral proteins was shown to be linked to HA; the glycosyl moieties were shown to be composed of glucosamine, mannose, galactose, and fucose at a molar ratio of 6:4:1:1, respectively, and the total carbohydrate of HA, determined by chemical means, was estimated to be approximately 12,000 daltons (Laver, 1971). Like all myxoviruses containing neuraminidase, influenza A and B viruses lack neuraminic acid. It was also found that HA2 of influenza A virions contains fucose, whereas HA2 of influenza B (GL1760) does not (Choppin et al., 1975). Recently the glycopeptides obtained by pronase digestion of influenza A viruses were characterized (Schwarz et al., 1977; Nakamura and Compans, 1978b). Both laboratories showed that HA possesses type I (oligosaccaride side-chain composed of glucosamine, mannose, galactose, and fucose) and type II (oligosaccharides composed of glucosamine and mannose) glycopeptides. Methylation studies indicated that fucose and galactose are exclusively present in terminal positions. Mannose and glucosamine are in part located in the periphery and in part in more central regions. The occurrence of 2,4-methyl mannose indicates that mannose may be involved in branch formation (Schwarz *et al.*, 1978*a*). Galactose is accessible to surface labeling reactions, such as the action of galactose oxidase followed by reduction with tritiated borohydride (Klenk *et al.*, 1978). The side chains are attached to the polypeptide by *N*-glycosidic linkages between *N*-acetylglucosamine and asparagine; *O*-glycosidic linkages do not exist (Keil *et al.*, 1978). The distribution of type I and type II oligosaccharides on HA1 and HA2 was shown to depend on the virus strain. Schwarz *et al.* (1977) showed that HA1 of an avian influenza virus possessed only type I glycopeptides, whereas both types I and II glycopeptides were shown to be present on HA2. However, Nakamura and Compans (1978*b*) using the WSN strain of influenza found that HA1 possessed both types I and II glycopeptides whereas HA2 contained only type I glycopeptides. Because of such strain differences, it has been suggested that specific amino acid sequences determine whether a type I or type II oligosaccharide is added at a particular site on the glycoprotein (Nakamura and Compans, 1978*b*).

The host cell type may also determine the type of oligosaccharide chains added to a given viral glycoprotein. Thus, although HA2 of WSN strain influenza virions grown in MDBK cells contained only type I glycopeptides, both types I and II glycopeptides were found in HA2 of WSN virions grown in CEF cells (Nakamura and Compans, in preparation).

Schwarz *et al.* (1977) showed that the type I HA glycopeptides of fowl plague and N influenza strains grown in chicken embryo fibroblasts (CEF) had a molecular weight of approximately 2600, whereas type II glycopeptides from the same source had a molecular weight of approximately 2000. The molecular weights of types I and II glycopeptides of the WSN strain of influenza virus grown in CEF cells were also found to be approximately this size (Nakamura and Compans, 1978*b*). HA glycopeptides of virus grown in MDBK cells were slightly larger in size than those of virus grown in CEF cells. Based on the estimated carbohydrate content (12,000 daltons) of the HA glycoprotein and the sizes of the types I and II glycopeptides of influenza virus grown in MDBK cells, it was estimated that HA2 contains a single type I glycopeptide whereas HA1 possesses two type I and one or two type II oligosaccharide side chains for the WSN strain (Nakamura and Compans, 1978*b*). However, out of five or six side chains present on the fowl plague virus hemagglutinin at least two (both types I and II) appear to be located on HA2 (Schwarz *et al.*, 1977).

Antigenic determinants which react with neutralizing antibody are present on the HA1 portion of the hemagglutinin glycoprotein (Eckert, 1973; Brand and Skehel, 1972; Laver *et al.*, 1974). Immunodiffusion tests with purified hemagglutinin subunits revealed two or three different antigenic determinants (Laver *et al.*, 1974) However, all of the antigenic determinants appeared to be on the same protein molecule, and only one species of hemagglutinin was observed in each virus type.

3.5.2b. The Neuraminidase

Enzymatic destruction of receptors on the surface of the erythrocyte by influenza virus provided the first evidence for a virus-associated enzyme (Hirst, 1942). The enzyme was subsequently identified as a neuraminidase (Klenk, 1955; Gottschalk, 1957). The fine structure and function of this enzyme have recently been reviewed (Bucher and Palese, 1975).

The morphology of purified neuraminidase subunits isolated from detergent-disrupted virions is quite distinct from that of the hemagglutinin spikes (Laver and Valentine, 1969; Webster and Darlington, 1969; Rott *et al.*, 1970). The neuraminidase has an oblong head measuring approximately 5 × 8.5 nm, from which a fiber ∼10 nm long extends. A small knob of ∼4 nm is present at the distal end. Like the hemagglutinin subunits, the neuraminidase proteins aggregate into characteristic rosettes in the absence of detergents, with the oblong heads located on the periphery of the rosettes. Therefore, the neuraminidase also appears to possess a hydrophobic end. Protease treatment removes the fiber and releases the oblong head which is still enzymatically active (Seto *et al.*, 1965; Drzeniek *et al.*, 1966*b*) and is seen as a square array of four 4-nm spherical subunits (Wrigley *et al.*, 1973). These observations suggest that the neuraminidase binds to the viral membrane by its hydrophobic end, with the fiber and oblong head projecting outward; however, it has not been possible to clearly resolve the arrangement of neuraminidase subunits on the envelopes of intact virions.

Biochemical evidence has also indicated a tetrameric structure for the intact spikes. The native structure appears to have a molecular weight of ∼200,000–250,000 (Drzeniek *et al.*, 1966*b*), and in the presence of SDS and reducing agents it is dissociated into four NA polypeptides of 55,000 daltons (Bucher and Kilbourne, 1972; Lazdins *et* *al.*, 1972; Kendal and Eckert, 1972). It has been suggested that two NA polypeptides are disulfide linked to form a dimer and that two dimers associate noncovalently to form a tetramer (Lazdins *et al.*, 1972). Several laboratories reported that two different neuraminidase polypeptides of similar molecular weights were present in the X7 recombinant of influenza virus (Webster, 1970; Bucher and Kilbourne, 1972; Lazdins *et al.*, 1972). However, most strains have been shown to possess a single NA polypeptide (Haslam *et al.*, 1970; Laver and Baker, 1972; Skehel and Schild, 1971; Gregoriades, 1972). The possibility that one of the two NA polypeptides in the X7 strain is a proteolytic cleavage product has therefore been considered (Lazdins *et al.*, 1972). Recently it has been shown by analysis of recombinant viruses that a single viral RNA segment codes for the neuraminidase polypeptide (Palese, 1977; Scholtissek *et al.*, 1976), further supporting the conclusion that a single polypeptide is present.

A high proportion of the carbohydrate of the neuraminidase is removed by trypsin treatment (Lazdins *et al.*, 1972; Allen *et al.*, 1977); this removes the fiber and leaves the terminal knob, which is still enzymatically active (Seto *et al.*, 1966).

The NA polypeptide possesses types I and II glycopeptides that appear to be similar to those of the HA polypeptide and both glycoproteins have a similar monosaccharide composition (Allen *et al.*, 1977; Schwarz *et al.*, 1977). Allen *et al.* (1977) and Keil *et al.* (1978) have obtained evidence that the glycopeptides of NA are linked to the polypeptide backbone through an *N*-acetylglucosamine–asparagine linkage.

Recently both the hemagglutinin and neuraminidase of influenza virions were shown to be sulfated glycoproteins (Compans and Pinter, 1975). The sulfate appears to be covalently linked to the oligosaccharide chains of viral glycoproteins (Nakamura and Compans, 1977, 1978*b*). Glycoproteins of enveloped viruses of all other major groups studied also are sulfated, whereas carbohydrate-free polypeptides are not (Pinter and Compans, 1975; Kaplan and Ben Porat, 1976).

The possible function of the neuraminidase in virus replication is discussed below.

3.5.2c. The Lipid Bilayer

The envelope of influenza virions is acquired by a process of budding at the plasma membrane (Murphy and Bang, 1952), and there is continuity between the unit membrane of the cell surface and that of the emerging virus particle (Bächi *et al.*, 1969; Compans and Dimmock, 1969). During this process of morphogenesis, the lipids of the viral envelope are acquired from those of the cellular plasma membrane. It is therefore likely that the arrangement of lipids in the viral envelope reflects that of the plasma membrane.

Evidence for a lipid bilayer structure in influenza virions has been obtained by electron spin resonance (ESR) spectroscopy using spin label methods (Landsberger *et al.*, 1971, 1973). Using stearic acid derivatives with nitroxide-containing functional groups located at different positions on the hydrocarbon chain, a flexibility gradient was observed in the viral envelope, which is characteristic of a lipid bilayer structure (McConnell and McFarland, 1972). When the functional group is located close to the polar head group, it is observed to be in a relatively rigid environment, and fluidity of the environment increases as the nitroxide group is located further down the hydrocarbon chain.

The composition of the virion includes 10–13% phospholipids, 6–8% cholesterol, and at least 1–2% glycolipids (Frommhagen *et al.*, 1959; Blough and Merlie, 1970; Klenk *et al.*, 1972a). In early studies it was demonstrated that prelabeled cellular lipids were incorporated into influenza virions and that the lipid composition resembled that of the host cell of origin (Wecker, 1957; Kates *et al.*, 1961). A part of the viral lipid may, however, also be newly synthesized after virus infection (Blough, 1974). Differences in fatty acid composition have been reported for various strains of influenza virus grown in ovo, primarily in the neutral lipid fraction (Tiffany and Blough, 1969a,b; Blough and Tiffany, 1973). Because of these differences, it has been proposed that viral envelope proteins determine the lipid composition by binding specific lipids; however, extensive and detailed analyses with other virus groups indicate that the viral lipid composition closely reflects that of the host cell plasma membrane and may be influenced by viral proteins only to a very limited extent (see sections on paramyxoviruses and togaviruses). Thus virions obtained from different host cell types contain the same protein components but may show marked differences in lipid composition, which parallel those of the host cell plasma membrane. These differences in lipid composition may result in viral membranes with differences in fluidity of the lipid bilayer as observed by ESR spectroscopy. Thus influenza virions grown in MDBK (bovine kidney) cells were observed to have a more rigid lipid bilayer than virions grown in BHK21 cells (Landsberger *et al.*, 1973). The higher cholesterol content in virions from MDBK cells was thought to be the major determinant of the increased lipid rigidity.

Recently the distribution of lipids between the inner and outer sides of the lipid bilayer of influenza virions has been investigated using phospholipases and phospholipid exchange proteins (Tsai and Lenard, 1975; Rothman *et al.*, 1976). Approximately 30% of the phospholipid was observed to be inaccessible to either phospholipase C digestion or the exchange protein. Nearly all of the phosphatidylinositol, about half of the phosphatidylcholine, 30% of the phosphatidylethanolamine, and 15–25% of sphingomyelin and phosphatidylserine were accessible to either treatment, and it was concluded that these lipids are exposed on the outer monolayer of the viral membrane. The population of lipid molecules which were exchanged in the reaction catalyzed by exchange protein was shown to be the same as that digested by phospholipase C (Rothman *et al.*, 1976). The phospholipid pools accessible to the exchange protein were stable, indicating that exchange between the inner and outer monolayer is extremely slow (a half-time in excess of 30 days for sphingomyelin and 10 days for phosphatidylcholine). The presence of amine-containing phospholipids on the external surface of influenza virions was suggested previously based on staining properties of the viral membrane (Choppin and Compans, 1975). The distribution of lipids in the viral membrane differs from that observed for human erythrocytes in this respect (Bretscher, 1972, 1973). Since less than half of the total phospholipid was observed to be present on the outer monolayer of influenza virions, it was suggested that there is a high glycolipid content on the external side of the bilayer (Rothman *et al.*, 1976). The presence of glycolipid carbohydrates on the external surface of the viral envelope has been demonstrated by binding of specific lectins to protease-treated particles devoid of glycoproteins (Klenk *et al.*, 1972*a*).

An exchange process between virions and lipid vesicles was used to investigate the distribution of cholesterol in the viral envelope (Lenard and Rothman, 1976). Exchange of labeled cholesterol occurred only after treatment with chymotrypsin, which degrades the viral glycoproteins. About half of the cholesterol was rapidly exchangeable, and appeared therefore to be present in the outer monolayer. The half-time for the equilibration of cholesterol between the inner and outer halves of the bilayer was estimated to be at least 13 days.

3.5.2d. The M Protein

The M protein was first identified as a distinct structural component by the use of proteolytic enzymes or detergents to selectively remove the surface glycoproteins of influenza virions (Compans *et al.*, 1970; Schulze, 1970; Skehel and Schild, 1971) which enabled the isolation of "spikeless" particles which lacked hemagglutinin and neuraminidase activities. Analysis of their polypeptide composition by SDS-polyacrylamide gel electrophoresis revealed that two major polypeptides were present. The larger of the major polypeptides had been previously identified as the nucleoprotein subunit, but the smaller (~26,000 daltons) was previously unrecognized as a viral structural component. It is now virtually certain that this major protein is associated with the inner surface of the viral envelope, and it has been designated as the M, or membrane, protein. The M protein is the smallest and most plentiful of the virion polypeptides, composing about 40% of the total virion protein by weight. Similar polypeptides have also been identified for other enveloped viruses (see sections on paramyxoviruses and rhabdoviruses).

Electron microscopic studies initially suggested the presence of a protein layer on the inner surface of the viral envelope. Thin sections of influenza virions showed an electron-dense layer on the internal surface of the unit membrane, which is not present on the normal cellular membrane (Apostolov and Flewett, 1969; Bächi *et al.*, 1969; Compans and Dimmock, 1969). It has been calculated that the M protein is present in sufficient quantity to form such a shell beneath the lipid bilayer (Compans *et al.*, 1972; Schulze, 1972). Further evidence for the location of the M protein was obtained by extraction of the lipids of glutaraldehyde or formaldehyde-fixed virions; the resulting particles exhibited a smooth-surfaced membrane surrounding the nucleocapsid, which corresponds to the M protein layer (Schulze, 1972; Reginster and Nermut, 1976). Iodination with chloramine T (Stanley and Haslam, 1971) and fluorescence transfer experiments (Lenard *et al.*, 1974) have also supported the conclusion that the M protein is located beneath the lipid bilayer and external to the viral ribonucleoprotein. The M protein is unaffected when intact virions are exposed to proteolytic enzymes (Compans *et al.*, 1970; Schulze, 1970; Klenk *et al.*, 1972a), and it is unreactive with labeling reagents specific for proteins on the external surface of the bilayer (Stanley and Haslam, 1971; Rifkin *et al.*, 1972), indicating that no part of the M protein penetrates through the lipid bilayer to the external surface of the envelope.

The M protein has been purified by gel filtration in the presence of guanidine hydrochloride (Lazarowitz *et al.*, 1971), acid chloroform–methanol extraction (Gregoriades, 1973), and precipitation after solubilization of virions with ammonium deoxycholate (Laver and Downie, 1976). The amino acid composition of the M protein of several strains of influenza virus has been determined (Laver and Baker, 1972; Gregoriades, 1973); M protein contained ~42% of polar amino acids, similar to the nucleoprotein subunit. Therefore, the overall composition of the M protein is not markedly hydrophobic, although the fact that it is selectively extracted in acid chloroform–methanol indicates hydrophobic properties. Isoelectric focusing of the influenza (A_0/WSN) M protein in the presence of NP40 or Triton X100 indicated an isoelectric point of pH 4.6 (Gregoriades, 1973).

The M proteins of various type A influenza viruses are closely related immunologically (Schild, 1972) as well as biochemically, as shown by peptide mapping procedures (Laver and Downie, 1976). A single tryptic peptide was observed to differ when the M proteins of Port Chalmers (H_3N_2) and BEL (H_0N_1) viruses were compared; all other tryptic peptides were indistinguishable. Influenza B viruses have M proteins which appear to be unrelated immunologically or biochemically to those of type A viruses (Schild, 1972; Laver and Downie, 1976). With type C influenza viruses, a major nonglycosylated polypeptide of 26,000–28,000 daltons is present (Kendal, 1975; Compans et al., 1977), which is thought to correspond to the M protein based on its resistance to protease and absence as a component of purified ribonucleoproteins.

Exposure of intact virions to [^{14}C]dansylchloride results in selective labeling of the M protein (Robertson et al., 1978). This observation suggested that the dansyl label became associated with the lipid bilayer, and labeled a portion of the protein which interacted with the bilayer. The dansyl label occurs exclusively on lysine residues; however, several cyanogen bromide peptides are labeled, and further understanding of the basis of the reaction will have to await a better understanding of the molecular structure of the protein.

Several laboratories have recently obtained evidence that the M protein is exposed on the surface of influenza virus infected cells, where it may act as a target for cytotoxic T lymphocytes (Braciale, 1977; Biddison et al., 1977; Ada and Yap, 1977). These observations will undoubtedly stimulate further investigation of the possible functional significance of this membrane association in virus replication and its importance in the immune response to influenza virus.

3.5.2e. Sulfated Glycosaminoglycans

The use of $^{35}SO_4$ as a label has revealed a sulfated component in virions migrating near the origin of SDS-polyacrylamide gels, which was previously unrecognized in studies using amino acid or sugar incorporation or procedures for staining of polypeptides (Compans and Pinter, 1975; Pinter and Compans, 1975). Prelabeling experiments indicate that this component is derived from the host cell (Compans and Pinter, 1975), and it appears likely to correspond to a host cell antigen originally described by Knight (1944, 1946) and subsequently found by others to be a sulfated glycosaminoglycan associated with influenza virions (Haukenes *et al.*, 1965; Howe *et al.*, 1967; Lee *et al.*, 1969). The host antigen has been purified from influenza virions grown in embryonated eggs and shown to be uronic and sialic acid-free sulfated glycosaminoglycan, similar in composition to the keratan sulfate group of acid glycosaminoglycans (Haukenes *et al.*, 1965; Lee *et al.*, 1969). The constituent sugars of this material differ from those of the viral glycoproteins by the presence of glucose and galactosamine and the absence of mannose (Schwarz *et al.*, 1978a).

The sulfated glycosaminoglycan is exposed on the surface of the virion, as it can be removed by treatment with proteolytic enzymes. However, it does not appear to be bound firmly to the virion glycoproteins, as a gentle extraction procedure using Triton X100 results in a quantitative separation of the glycoproteins and sulfated glycosaminoglycan (Compans and Pinter, 1975). Therefore, the glycosaminoglycan is either bound loosely to the glycoproteins or attached to the viral lipid directly. If the latter is the case, the binding appears to involve a peptide portion of the molecule, since trypsin treatment quantitatively removes these sulfated components from virions.

3.5.2f. Envelope Components of Influenza C Virus

There are marked similarities between the structural components of influenza A and B viruses; however, influenza C virions exhibit some distinct biochemical and morphological properties. These viruses are generally similar to other influenza viruses in particle size and shape, possession of a segmented genome, and morphology of the internal ribonucleoprotein (Ritchey *et al.*, 1976; Cox and Kendal, 1976; Compans *et al.*, 1977). The nucleoprotein subunit and M protein of influenza C virions also are similar to those of other influenza virions in size and relative amounts (Kendal, 1975; Compans *et al.*, 1977). The most distinctive feature of influenza C virions is their lack of detectable neuraminidase activity (Hirst, 1950; Kendal, 1975; Nerome *et al.*, 1976). A receptor-destroying enzyme is present in influenza C virions, but it does not cleave neuraminic acid from various substrates; the receptors for influenza A and C viruses on erythrocytes appear to be unrelated since both viruses possess receptor-destroying activity for their own receptor but lack activity against the receptor for the heterologous virus. In agreement with the lack of neuraminidase is the finding that influenza C virions contain neuraminic acid (Nerome *et al.*, 1976; Meier-Ewert *et al.*, 1978).

Three glycoprotein species have been detected in influenza C virions: a major glycoprotein of ~88,000 daltons and two minor glyco-proteins of ~66,000 and 26,000 daltons (Kendal, 1975; Compans *et al.*, 1977). The two smaller glycoproteins are linked by disulfide bonds (Meier-Ewert *et al.*, 1978), suggesting analogy to HA1 and HA2 of influenza A and B viruses; in the absence of reducing agents only a single glycoprotein peak of ~88,000 daltons is resolved. It is uncertain whether the larger virion glycoprotein seen in the presence of reducing agents is a result of incomplete conversion into the two smaller glyco-proteins by proteolytic cleavage or whether it is a distinct viral glyco-protein.

Glycoproteins of influenza C virions are frequently seen in a regular hexagonal arrangement on the surface of the virus (Apostolov *et al.*, 1970; Compans *et al.*, 1977). Such an arrangement is not a regular feature of influenza A viruses, although similar patterns have sometimes been reported.

3.5.3. Comparison of the Envelope Structure of Standard and Incomplete Influenza Virus

Noninfectious, hemagglutinating particles of influenza virus are produced upon serial undiluted passage [reviewed in Volume 4 of this series (Compans and Choppin, 1975)]. These particles are termed "incomplete virus" or "von Magnus" virus, since the phenomenon was first described by von Magnus (1954). Frequently incomplete virus is markedly pleomorphic (Rott and Schäfer, 1960; Lenard and Compans, 1975), and altered patterns of surface spikes have been reported (Moore *et al.*, 1962; Almeida and Waterson, 1970). A square array of spikes, observed on some large, pleomorphic particles (Almeida and Waterson, 1970), may represent areas enriched in neuraminidase subunits, which appear as square subunits when viewed end-on (Wrigley *et al.*, 1973).

The polypeptides of standard and incomplete virus of the A/WSN strain grown in MDBK cells were found to differ, in that incomplete virus possessed about twice the relative amount of glycoproteins, while the amount of NP protein was significantly decreased (Lenard and

Compans, 1975). The specific neuraminidase activity was also higher in incomplete virus. A subpopulation of incomplete virus with normal morphology showed the same alterations in protein composition as the large pleomorphic particles. These results indicate that the total amount of glycoproteins per unit area incorporated into the influenza viral membrane may vary with the growth conditions and does not play a primary role in determining viral size and shape. No differences were found in phospholipid content or composition between standard and incomplete virus, nor was any difference in membrane fluidity detected by ESR spectroscopy of spin-labeled virus (Lenard *et al.*, 1976), indicating that these properties of the viral membrane are not determined by the amount of viral glycoprotein present in the envelope. Since lipids of viral envelopes appear to be considerably more rigid than a lipid bilayer of the same composition that is devoid of viral protein (Landsberger and Compans, 1976), these results suggest that the M protein is the major determinant of membrane rigidity (Lenard *et al.*, 1976).

3.5.4. Functions of Influenza Virus Glycoproteins

3.5.4a. Adsorption to Receptors

In the case of enveloped viruses, glycoproteins located on the surface of the virion are the components involved in adsorption to cellular receptors, which may or may not be host cell glycoproteins. Hemagglutination by influenza virus has been studied as a model system for adsorption of a virus to receptors, and considerable information has been obtained. Adsorption to the erythrocyte occurs by the hemagglutinin spike binding to sialic acid-containing components on the cellular surface. The receptor molecule has been isolated from chick red blood cells, and it is a major glycoprotein which contains M and N blood group antigens. A detailed summary of the properties of this receptor is given by Schulze (1975*b*). Removal of sialic acid from the receptor molecule by neuraminidase prevents the agglutination of erythrocytes by influenza virus. Hemagglutination can also be inhibited by pretreating the virus with specific antibodies. As has been pointed out above, proteolytic cleavage of HA is not a precondition for hemagglutination, but it is necessary for complete infectivity. Thus it appears that, in addition to its role in adsorption, the hemagglutinin has another function in the infection process, and it has been suggested that it may be involved in penetration (Klenk *et al.*, 1975; Lazarowitz and Choppin,

1975). This notion is supported by the recent observation that the F protein of paramyxoviruses known to be responsible for penetration has a highly hydrophobic amino acid sequence at the N terminus of the F2 fragment (see section on paramyxoviruses) which exhibits almost complete homology with the N-terminal end of HA2 (Skehel and Waterfield, 1975). Thus both glycoproteins might have similar functions.

Antibody to the hemagglutinin protein of influenza virus will neutralize virus infectivity. The specific determinants of viral glycoproteins that are recognized by viral neutralizing antibodies have not been chemically characterized. It has been postulated that antibody molecules may recognize only determinants on the tip of the HA spike of the influenza virion (White, 1974). In reaching these conclusions, it has been assumed that the size of the antibody molecule precludes the possibility that it could make contact with any other part of the spike since the spaces between the spikes are too small for the immunoglobulin to interact with other regions. Electron mciroscopic observations (Lafferty and Oertilis, 1963) indicate that antibody molecules do interact with the tips of surface spikes, and analysis of the tryptic peptides of HA molecules isolated from closely related influenza strains has shown that they rarely differ by more than one or two peptides (Laver and Webster, 1973; Webster and Laver, 1972), suggesting that these strain differences are restricted to small regions or determinants of the HA spike.

The antigenic character exhibited by the glycoproteins of influenza virions is highly variable as evidenced by the many different strains of type A and B influenza. The HA and NA glycoproteins of influenza viruses are antigenically distinct, and they undergo antigenic changes independently of each other (Drzeniek et al., 1966b; Seto and Rott, 1966; Webster and Laver, 1967; Kilbourne et al., 1968). The antigenic changes that occur may be gradual, in which case the different virus strains are clearly related to each other with respect to both surface antigens. Antigenic changes of this nature are termed "antigenic drift," which is thought to result from the interplay of viral mutability and immunological selection (Webster and Laver, 1975). The presence of antibody of low avidity may select for single-step mutants, which have an altered amino acid in the key area of the antigenic determinant, giving rise to a new viral strain.

At intervals of 10–15 years sudden and complete changes in the determinants of type A influenza glycoproteins occur; the changes are such that the virus possess glycoproteins that appear completely distinct by peptide mapping and serological tests (Webster and Laver, 1975).

Dramatic changes in the antigenic determinants of the viral glycoproteins are termed "antigenic shifts," and it is these new viruses that cause worldwide influenza pandemics. It has been postulated that antigenic shift may occur because type A strains of human origin may undergo recombination with type A strains of avian or other animal origin. The antigenic determinants of the new HA or NA are sufficiently different that the human host does not possess immunity, and the virus gains a selective advantage. Interestingly, type B influenza viruses do not undergo antigenic shift. The reason for this may lie in the fact that type B influenza viruses have not been isolated from other animal species; thus it is probable that the type B viruses cannot undergo similar recombination events (for review, see Webster and Laver, 1975).

3.5.4b. Neuraminidase Activity

Several distinct functions have been proposed for this enzyme. It is postulated that neuraminidase-containing virus lodges in the upper respiratory tract and binds to mucin via the hemagglutinin. The glycosyl residues of mucin are terminated by sialic acid (N-acetylneuraminic acid) to which the hemagglutinin binds, and one role of neuraminidase may be to cleave the sialoglycoprotein bond, freeing the bound virion. It is presumed that in this way the virus is released and underlying cell receptors are exposed to which the hemagglutinin can attach (Davenport, 1976).

It is unlikely that neuraminidase is involved in an early event such as penetration because virions remain infectious after inhibition of the activity by specific antibody (Seto and Rott, 1966; Bucher and Palese, 1975). However, the possibility that neuraminidase participates in the release of the budding virion from the infected cell surface has gained support from several types of experiments. By using influenza strains that had different levels of enzyme activity, it was shown that virus strains having low activity were released from cells more slowly than strains with higher enzyme activity (Palese and Schulman, 1974). Further, in the presence of antibody to the viral neuraminidase, which inhibited enzyme activity, virions were formed, but release of virus into culture medium was inhibited (Seto and Rott, 1966; Compans *et al.*, 1969; Webster, 1970). When bacterial neuraminidase was added to the cultures, infectious virus was released from the cells. These studies, however, are complicated by the fact that bivalent antibody can cause cross-linking of virions to viral antigens on cell surfaces, and Becht *et*

al. (1971) reported that monovalent Fab fragments inhibited neuraminidase activity without affecting virus release.

More conclusive evidence for the function of the enzyme has been
obtained with temperature-sensitive mutants of influenza virus which
are defective in neuraminidase activity (Palese *et al.*, 1974). At nonpermissive temperature, no neuraminidase activity is detected; virus particles are produced by cells despite the fact that infectivity titers are
markedly reduced. However, the virus particles form large aggregates,
and in contrast to wild-type virions these particles contain sialic acid as
shown by colloidal iron hydroxide staining. Since influenza virions bind
to sialic acid residues, these results indicate that the mutant virus particles aggregate to each other because sialic acid is added to viral carbohydrates, and that the essential function of viral neuraminidase is to
remove or prevent the addition of such sialic acid. In support of this
conclusion, addition of bacterial neuraminidase to cells infected with
these mutants causes a marked enhancement of virus release.

Further evidence which supports this role for the neuraminidase
was obtained with a neuraminidase inhibitor, 2-deoxy-2,3-dehydro-*N*-
trifluoracetylneuraminic acid (FANA). Influenza virions grown in the
presence of FANA contain neuraminic acid on their envelopes and the
particles undergo extensive aggregation (Palese and Compans, 1976). A
marked reduction in virus yield is observed because of this aggregation,
and treatment with a purified neuraminidase results in enhancement of
progeny virus yields, apparently by disaggregation of virus. Thus viral
neuraminidase is not required for assembly of progeny virions but
appears to be essential for the removal of sialic acid from the surface of
the virion itself.

3.5.5. Biosynthesis of Envelope Components

3.5.5a. Proteins

The synthesis and assembly of influenza virus-specific polypeptides
can readily be analyzed in cell cultures because host cell polypeptide
synthesis is inhibited after infection. All of the virion polypeptides plus
a virus-specific nonstructural polypeptide (designated "NS") can be
identified by polyacrylamide gel electrophoresis. The time course of
synthesis varies with the specific virus strain and cell type (Lazarowitz
et al., 1971; Skehel, 1972; Klenk *et al.*, 1972*b*; Krug and Etkind, 1973;
Meier-Ewert and Compans, 1974; Inglis *et al.*, 1976; Lamb and
Choppin, 1976).

The intracellular location of viral polypeptide species has been determined using cell fractionation procedures. The HA polypeptide is always membrane associated, and the results of pulse-chase experiments suggest that it is synthesized on membrane-bound polyribosomes in the rough endoplasmic reticulum and that completed chains are transported to the smooth cytoplasmic membrane fraction and from there to the plasma membrane (Lazarowitz et al., 1971; Compans, 1973a; Klenk et al., 1974; Hay, 1974; Meier-Ewert and Compans, 1974). This scheme of intracellular migration is also supported by results indicating a progressive addition of sugars to the HA polypeptide (Compans, 1973b; Stanley et al., 1973; Klenk et al., 1978). Glucosamine is incorporated into HA polypeptides in the rough as well as the smooth membrane fraction, whereas fucose is present in smooth membranes but absent in the HA polypeptides in the rough membrane fraction (Compans, 1973b). Inhibition of protein synthesis by puromycin stops the incorporation of glucosamine almost immediately, whereas fucose is incorporated only after the completed HA polypeptide migrates to the smooth endoplasmic reticulum or Golgi complex membranes in the infected cell (Stanley et al., 1973). Incorporation of sulfate into HA polypeptides also occurs for up to 30 min after inhibition of protein synthesis (Nakamura and Compans, 1977). The initial glycosylation events involve en bloc transfer of the glucosamine–mannose cores of the side chains from a lipid precursor (Schwarz et al., 1977; Klenk et al., 1978). This transfer appears to be extremely rapid, possibly occurring on nascent chains (Klenk, 1974), since it is not possible to detect unglycosylated forms of the HA polypeptide by short pulse labeling (Compans, 1973a; Klenk et al., 1974). The site of cleavage of HA into HA1 and HA2 varies with the virus strain. With the WSN strain cleavage occurs at the plasma membrane (Lazarowitz et al., 1971), whereas the fowl plague virus cleavage occurs intracellularly in membranes of the endoplasmic reticulum (Klenk et al., 1974). Cleavage of HA is inhibited if the virus is grown in the presence of protease inhibitors or at reduced temperature (Klenk and Rott, 1973).

The NA polypeptide is present in small amounts in infected cells, and there is less information available on its intracellular location. The NA polypeptide is found along with HA in the smooth membrane fraction (Compans, 1973a; Klenk et al., 1974; Hay, 1974), and it appears to be one of the polypeptides to arrive rapidly at the plasma membrane (Lazarowitz et al., 1971; Hay, 1974). These data suggest that the steps in the synthesis and transport of HA and NA to the plasma membrane may be similar. Evidence has been obtained that the hemagglutinin is incorporated into discrete regions of the plasma membrane, whereas the neuraminidase is more dispersed (Hay, 1974).

The M protein, although the most abundant polypeptide in the virion, is synthesized in limited amounts in infected cells, and it has been suggested that the synthesis of M may be rate limiting for viral assembly (Lazarowitz *et al.*, 1971). In contrast to other viral polypeptides, the rate of synthesis of M increases late in the infectious cycle (Skehel, 1972; Meier-Ewert and Compans, 1974; Lamb and Choppin, 1976). The M protein is found associated with various cytoplasmic membrane fractions as well as the plasma membrane (Lazarowitz *et al.*, 1971; Compans, 1973a; Stanley *et al.*, 1973; Klenk *et al.*, 1974; Meier-Ewert and Compans, 1974; Hay, 1974). However, the behavior of M in pulse-chase experiments differs from the behavior of HA, in that no migration of M has been detected between various cellular compartments. M protein is inserted rapidly into the plasma membrane, and it has been suggested that this polypeptide may be synthesized on free polyribosomes and inserted into membranes after synthesis (Compans *et al.*, 1974; Hay, 1974). If this is the case, those molecules found in association with intracellular membranes may be by-products rather than intermediates in assembly. In cells infected at reduced temperature, synthesis of the M protein is selectively inhibited (Klenk and Rott, 1973), and this inhibition results in a block in virus maturation. Similarly, in abortive infection, as it occurs if fowl plague virus is grown in HeLa, L, or BHK cells, synthesis of M protein is suppressed, and virus particles are not formed. However, the lack of M protein has no effect on synthesis and processing of the hemagglutinin. Thus the envelope proteins are synthesized and processed by independent mechanisms (Lohmeyer *et al.*, 1977).

3.5.5b. Lipids

The available evidence suggests that the normal cellular processes of lipid biosynthesis are used to generate the lipids incorporated into the viral envelope. Prelabeling of cells with $^{32}PO_4$ before infection was used to demonstrate that preformed host cell lipids were utilized for virus assembly (Wecker, 1957). The lipids are acquired from the plasma membrane during budding and reflect closely the composition of the plasma membrane. The asymmetrical distribution of phospholipids and glycolipids also presumably reflects the distribution on the cell surface. The rate of synthesis of phospholipids was depressed late in the growth cycle in influenza virus infected cells (Blough and Weinstein, 1973), and it is likely that this may be a secondary effect of inhibition of cellular biosynthesis.

3.5.5c.   Carbohydrates

Because the genetic information in the viral RNA is accounted for by the known structural and nonstructural viral polypeptides, it is not possible for the virus to direct the synthesis of enzymes involved in carbohydrate biosynthesis. Host cell glycosyltransferases therefore appear to be utilized. Glycosylation of the viral glycoproteins can be detected by addition of radioactive sugars such as glucosamine and fucose to infected cells. It is not known whether carbohydrates present in viral glycolipids are preformed or newly synthesized after infection.

Inhibition of the glycosylation of viral glycoproteins has been reported using the sugars 2-deoxyglucose or glucosamine (Kilbourne, 1959; Gandhi *et al.*, 1972; Kaluza *et al.*, 1972; Klenk *et al.*, 1972*b*) or the antibiotic tunicamycin (R. Schwarz *et al.*, 1977; Nakamura and Compans, 1978*a*). Both the production of the normal HA polypeptide and that of neuraminidase activity are inhibited by these compounds, whereas there is little or no effect on synthesis of carbohydrate-free polypeptides. A new polypeptide designated "HA0" is detected in the presence of inhibitors (Klenk *et al.*, 1972*b*) which appears to be an unglycosylated or partially glycosylated form of the HA polypeptide. Glycosylation of the viral glycoproteins appears to influence their sensitivity to proteolytic cleavage. Thus the aberrant HA0 glycoproteins produced in the presence of glycosylation inhibitors are cleaved into more heterogeneous products resembling HA1 and HA2 (Klenk *et al.*, 1974; Nakamura and Compans, 1978*a*), and in fowl-plague-virus-infected cells treated with tunicamycin the unglycosylated hemagglutinin polypeptide is completely degraded (R. Schwarz *et al.*, 1976). HA0 appears to migrate from rough to smooth cytoplasmic membranes in the same manner as HA (Klenk *et al.*, 1974; Nakamura and Compans, 1978*a*) and in some virus–cell systems the maturation process occurs, although at a reduced level, in the presence of these inhibitors to yield virions containing aberrant glycoproteins (Compans *et al.*, 1974; Nakamura and Compans, 1978*a*). Therefore, full glycosylation is not a requirement for either intracellular migration or assembly of influenza viral glycoproteins into virions. The particles produced in the presence of inhibitors have low specific infectivity, however, indicating that glycosylation is probably essential for normal biological activity of the glycoproteins.

3.5.6. The Assembly Process

Influenza virus was the first virus to be shown to be released from infected cells by a process not involving lysis; virus particles emerged from the cell surface by budding into the extracellular space (Murphy and Bang, 1952). The emerging virions contain a unit membrane like that observed on the cellular plasma membrane, with modifications on the internal and external surfaces (Compans and Dimmock, 1969; Bächi et al., 1969). The external surface contains projections corresponding to the viral glycoproteins, whereas the internal surface shows an electron-dense layer which is thought to represent the internal membrane (M) protein. Viral envelope proteins appear to be incorporated into areas of membrane of normal morphology, which however exhibit specific adsorption of erythrocytes (Compans and Dimmock, 1969). After alignment of the internal viral components, budding occurs by an outfolding of the plasma membrane. Since virions contain little or no host cell proteins, these proteins must be excluded from regions of the cell surface where virus maturation occurs. There is little direct evidence for the nature of the macromolecular interactions involved in assembly that lead to domains on the cell surface from which host cell polypeptides are excluded. With influenza A viruses, there is little morphological evidence for direct interactions between glycoproteins, whereas the M protein appears to form a tightly packed shell with extensive protein–protein interactions. It therefore seems that lateral interactions between M protein molecules, together with transmembrane interactions between glycoproteins and M protein, are likely to be involved in assembly of the envelope.

Recent reports of the presence of actin in enveloped viruses have suggested the possibility that actin microfilaments may be involved in virus maturation (Wang et al., 1976). However, the assembly of influenza virions was not prevented by cytochalasin B (Griffin and Compans, 1978), despite the disruption of cellular microfilaments by the drug. Released virus yields were diminished in the presence of cytochalasin as a result of aggregation of virions at cell surfaces; it was found that this resulted from production of an inactive neuraminidase in the presence of the drug. When purified V. cholera neuraminidase was added to cytochalasin-treated cells, a marked enhancement of virus release was observed. Cytochalasin partially inhibits the glycosylation of influenza virus glycoproteins, which probably results in the formation of inactive neuraminidase.

3.6. Paramyxoviruses

3.6.1. Classification, Morphology, Composition

The paramyxoviridae family comprises three genera: paramyxovirus (paramyxovirus subgroup), morbillivirus (measles–distemper group), and pneumovirus (respiratory syncytial virus subgroup). Members of the paramyxovirus subgroup include a variety of human and animal viruses, such as Newcastle disease virus (NDV), mumps, and the parainfluenza viruses. The envelope of these viruses has hemagglutinating and neuraminidase activities. The measles–distemper group includes measles virus, canine distemper virus, and rinderpest virus. These viruses contain only hemagglutinin but no neuraminidase. The respiratory syncytial virus (RSV) subgroup includes RSV of man and cattle, and pneumonia virus of mice. These viruses have no neuraminidase activity and RSV has no hemagglutinating activity either. A common feature of almost all paramyxoviruses is their ability to induce cell fusion; RSV causes cell fusion whereas pneumonia virus of mice has not been reported to cause fusion.

Virions are usually spherical, 150 nm or more in diameter, but filamentous forms several micrometers long may be observed. Virions are composed of a helical nucleocapsid and an envelope with surface projections about 10 nm in length. The envelope of paramyxoviruses appears to be particularly flexible, and virus particles exhibit a high degree of pleomorphism.

Virus particles are composed of about 1% RNA, 70% protein, 20% lipid, and 6% carbohydrate (Klenk and Choppin, 1969a). The lipids, the carbohydrates, and about 70% of the total viral protein constitute the envelope (Compans and Choppin, 1967; Caliguiri et al., 1969). The carbohydrate is present in the form of glycoprotein (Klenk et al., 1970a), glycolipid (Klenk and Choppin, 1970b), and mucopolysaccharide (Pinter and Compans, 1975).

Detailed studies have been carried out on the envelopes of NDV and two parainfluenza viruses: Sendai virus and simian virus 5 (SV5). Less information is available on morbillivirus and pneumovirus envelopes, but there is increasing evidence that they follow the same general rules for structure, function, and biosynthesis. Reviews on paramyxovirus replication have been published in Volume 4 of this series (Choppin and Compans, 1975), and elsewhere (Kingsbury, 1973).

3.6.2. Fine Structure and Arrangement of Envelope Components

The paramyxovirus envelope is composed of a lipid bilayer, an inner carbohydrate-free protein (M protein), and external spikes consisting of glycoproteins. Table 2 presents a list of the envelope proteins, their estimated molecular weights, and functions.

The envelope can be disrupted and its components can be solubilized by detergents (Rott and Schäfer, 1960). The glycoprotein spikes and the M protein have different solubilities in detergent–salt solutions and can thus be separated from each other (Scheid et al., 1972). The spikes are removed from the virus particles by extensive protease treatment (Chen et al., 1971). It is not clear if the spikes completely penetrate the lipid layer and thus are able to directly interact with the M protein. Glucosamine, mannose, galactose, and fucose have been identified as carbohydrate constituents of the spike glycoproteins (Klenk et al., 1970a). By means of their carbohydrate complement the spikes are able to bind to phytoagglutinins (Becht et al., 1972).

Paramyxoviruses possess two different glycoprotein species, as was shown first with SV5 (Klenk et al., 1970a), Sendai virus (Content and Duesberg, 1970), and NDV (Mountcastle et al., 1971), and has been subsequently further substantiated with several other members of this group. The available evidence indicates that each glycoprotein species constitutes a distinct type of spike (Scheid et al., 1972; Seto et al., 1973; Shimizu et al., 1974). By means of gradient centrifugation (Scheid et al., 1972), affinity chromatography to agarose-bound fetuin (Scheid and Choppin, 1973), or isoelectric focussing (Shimizu et al., 1974), both types have been separated from each other and characterized in detail. From a comparison of the structural and functional data of all paramyxovirus glycoproteins analyzed to date (Table 2) the following picture emerges: One spike type consists of a glycoprotein which in the case of NDV, SV5, Sendai virus, and mumps virus has hemagglutinin and neuraminidase activities and has, therefore, been designated HN. With measles virus, this glycoprotein has only hemagglutinin activity, and with RSV it has none of these activities. The other type of spike is composed of glycoprotein F and with all viruses has cell-fusing and hemolytic activity. The data from which this general conclusion has been derived will now be discussed in more detail.

TABLE 2
Envelope Proteins of Paramyxoviruses[a]

Designation[b]	Paramyxovirus		Morbillivirus		Pneumovirus[c]	
	Molecular weight	Biological activity	Molecular weight	Biological activity	Molecular weight	Biological activity
HN	65,000–74,000	Hemagglutinin, neuraminidase	80,000	Hemagglutinin	48,000	Hemagglutinin[e]
F ⎰ F1,2	54,000–68,000 ⎱		62,000 ⎱		n.a.[g] ⎱	
⎨ F1	48,000–56,000 ⎬ Hemolysis and cell fusion		40,000[d] ⎬ Hemolysis and cell fusion		42,000 ⎬ Cell fusion[f]	
⎱ F2	10,000–16,000 ⎰		15,000 ⎰		n.a. ⎰	
M	40,000	—	37,000		27,000	—

[a] For references, see text.
[b] Nomenclature of Scheid and Choppin (1977).
[c] Localization and function of pneumovirus proteins have not been firmly established yet.
[d] This polypeptide is not glycosylated with measles virus.
[e] Hemagglutination is observed only with pneumonia virus of mice.
[f] Cell fusion is observed with pneumonia virus of mice.
[g] n.a., Not analyzed.

3.6.2a.   The Hemagglutinin–Neuraminidase Spike

In contrast to influenza virus which has hemagglutinin and neu-raminidase on distinct glycoprotein molecules, in paramyxoviruses both of these activities are associated with one glycoprotein species, the HN glycoprotein (Scheid *et al.*, 1972; Scheid and Choppin, 1973; Seto *et al.*, 1973; Tozawa *et al.*, 1973; Shimizu *et al.*, 1974). HN of Sendai virus, SV5, and NDV has a molecular weight in the range of 65,000–74,000 as determined by polyacrylamide gel electrophoresis in the presence of SDS and reducing agents. Under nonreducing condi-tions a dimer is observed, suggesting that the hemagglutinin–neuramini-dase spike is composed of two disulfide-linked HN glycopolypeptides (Scheid *et al.*, 1978). Chymotrypsin treatment of this spike yields a water-soluble protein with neuraminidase activity (Drzeniek and Rott, 1963) which contains the larger polypeptide fragment (HN-c1) as a disulfide-linked dimer (Scheid *et al.*, 1978). The other cleavage product(s) are lipophilic and contain that part of HN which anchors the spike in the virus membrane. Failure to detect an N-terminal amino acid on HN or HN-c1 suggests that the hydrophobic tail of HN contains the C terminus (Scheid *et al.*, 1978).

In some strains of NDV, an 82,000-dalton precursor to the HN glycoprotein designated "HNO" is incorporated into virions (Nagai *et al.*, 1976b; Nagai and Klenk, 1977). Such particles have reduced hemagglutinin and neuraminidase activities as will be described in detail below.

3.6.2b.   The Fusion Spike

The fusion spike is composed of glycoprotein F, which consists of two disulfide-linked fragments, F1 (MW 48,000–56,000) and F2 (MW 10,000–16,000). Under nonreducing conditions the two fragments are not separated from each other and migrate on polyacrylamide gels as a complex (MW 54,000–68,000) which has been designated "F1,2" (Table 2). The fragments are derived by proteolytic cleavage from a common precursor F0 (MW ~65,000) which under certain conditions is incorporated into NDV and Sendai virus particles (see below). Since only the cleavage product but not the uncleaved precursor is biologi-cally active, it could be clearly demonstrated that glycoprotein F is responsible for hemolysis and cell fusion (Homma and Ohuchi, 1973; Scheid and Choppin, 1974a; Shimizu *et al.*, 1974; Nagai *et al.*, 1976b). Similar conclusions have been drawn from a study using monospecific antibodies (Seto *et al.*, 1974). Of the two cleavage fragments only the larger one (F1) was first identified and was then designated "F" (Scheid and Choppin, 1974). Subsequently evidence has been obtained that a smaller cleavage fragment F2 is also present on the spike (Shimizu *et al.*, 1974; Homma *et al.*, 1975; Nagai *et al.*, 1976*a*), and recently this fragment has been isolated and characterized in some detail (Scheid and Choppin, 1977). With Sendai virus, SV5, and NDV, F1 as well as F2 is glycosylated, but F2 contains relatively more carbohydrates than F1. No free N terminus was detected on F0 or F2 of Sendai virus, whereas N-terminal phenylalanine was found on F1. This suggests that the order of the F0 polypeptide is X-NH-F2-Phe-F1-COOH. Analysis of the N-terminal sequence of the F1 polypeptide revealed a high degree of hydrophobicity and of homology among all three viruses (Scheid *et al.*, 1978; Gething *et al.*, 1978).

3.6.2c.   The Lipid Bilayer

Paramyxoviruses derive their lipids from the plasma membrane of the host, where maturation occurs. This concept is based to a large extent on a series of comparative lipid analysis of SV5 and isolated plasma membranes of different host cells (Klenk and Choppin, 1969*b*, 1970*a,b*). These studies demonstrated that all lipid species observed in the plasma membrane are also found in the viral envelope. The only exception are gangliosides, which because of the action of the viral neuraminidase are not incorporated into the virion. The envelope lipids are present in proportions typical for plasma membranes; i.e., there is a high cholesterol content with a molar ratio of cholesterol to phospholipid close to 1, and there are relatively high amounts of sphingomyelin and of glycolipids. The close similarity between the viral envelope and the plasma membrane is further emphasized when the patterns of the individual glycolipid species are analyzed which show distinct variations depending on the host cell. For instance, galactosyl-galactosyl-glucosyl-ceramide is found in rhesus monkey kidney cells and in virions grown in them, but not in bovine kidney (MDBK) cells or virus from MDBK cells (Klenk and Choppin, 1970*b*). Lipids of Sendai virus and of several strains of NDV grown *in ovo* have also been analyzed, and differences mainly in the fatty acid composition have been interpreted to demonstrate that the viral proteins have the ability to select preferentially certain lipid classes (Blough and Lawson, 1968; Tiffany and Blough, 1969*b*). However, the studies on SV5 described above clearly show that it is primarily the plasma membrane of the host cell that determines the lipid composition of the paramyxovirus envelope.

Electron spin resonance studies have provided evidence that the lipids of SV5 are found in bilayer structures with fluid lipid phases similar to those observed for other biological membranes (Landsberger *et al.*, 1973). All viral membranes were shown to be substantially more rigid than the corresponding host cell plasma membranes. Proteolytic removal of the glycoprotein spikes did not appreciably alter the fluidity of the lipid bilayer of the envelope. Thus it was concluded that the rigidity of viral membranes may be determined by the M protein and not by the viral glycoproteins. However, another factor in determining envelope rigidity was the lipid composition, since differences in the rigidity of different host cell membranes were reflected in the viral lipid bilayer.

3.6.2d. The M Protein

Like influenza and rhabdoviruses, paramyxoviruses possess two major nonglycosylated proteins. One of those is the nucleocapsid protein; the other one (MW ~40,000, Table 2) is associated with the viral membrane and has therefore been designated the M protein. The first evidence for a protein associated with the inner side of the lipid bilayer came from electron microscopic studies (see section on influenza viruses). This location was further substantiated by the observation that the M protein is resistant to protease treatment, which removes the spikes from the surface of intact virus particles (Chen *et al.*, 1971). The M protein is insoluble in water and nonionic detergents but can be solubilized by nonionic detergents in the presence of high salt. On the basis of these properties purification procedures have been developed, and chemical analysis revealed that the M protein of SV5 contains a high proportion of hydrophobic amino acids (Scheid *et al.*, 1972; McSharry *et al.*, 1975). The M protein has high affinity for membranes, as indicated by cell fractionation studies which revealed that it is present in infected cells only in membrane-containing fractions (Nagai *et al.*, 1976*a*; Lamb and Choppin, 1977).

3.6.2e. The Envelopes of Mumps, Measles, and Respiratory Syncytial Viruses

Mumps, measles, and respiratory syncytial viruses are by far not as well analyzed as Sendai virus, NDV, and SV5. The data on protein composition available to date (Table 2) suggest, however, that their envelopes are organized by the same general principles.

Mumps virus contains two glycoproteins. The larger one has been found to possess hemagglutinin and neuraminidase activities. Evidence has also been obtained for the presence of an M protein as judged by its solubility in Triton X100 and high-salt solution (Jensik and Silver, 1976).

The experimental evidence obtained in a series of studies on measles virus indicates that this virus also has two glycoproteins. One of these glycoproteins has a molecular weight of ~80,000 as indicated by polyacrylamide gel electrophoresis in the presence of mercapto-ethanol (Bussell *et al.*, 1974; Mountcastle and Choppin, 1977), whereas under nonreducing conditions it migrates as a dimer (Hardwick and Bussell, 1976). It resembles therefore the HN glycoprotein of Sendai virus in these properties. The other glycoprotein exhibits structural features typical for F. It is composed of two disulfide-linked fragments F1 and F2, and a precursor F0 has also been identified. In contrast to Sendai virus, SV5, and NDV, F1 appears to be unglycosylated with measles virus (Hardwick and Bussell, 1976; Mountcastle and Choppin, 1977; Scheid *et al.*, 1978). These data are compatible with immunological studies in which two distinct antigens have been identified, one with hemagglutinating and the other one with hemolytic activity (Norrby and Gollmar, 1975).

The polypeptides of RSV have also been analyzed by polyacryl-amide gel electrophoresis, but so far an association with biological activities has not been established. Two glycoproteins have been found, and there is suggestive evidence for an M protein (Wunner and Pringle, 1976).

3.6.3. Biogenesis and Assembly of the Envelope

The envelopes of paramyxoviruses are assembled on preformed cellular membranes, and the final step in assembly is a budding process at the plasma membrane. The available evidence, which is derived mainly from electron microscopic and cell fractionation studies and will be discussed in detail below, suggests that envelope maturation is a multistep process involving sequential incorporation of viral proteins into cellular membranes.

3.6.3a. Biosynthesis of Glycoproteins

Fractionation studies on cells infected with NDV (Nagai *et al.*, 1976*a*) and Sendai virus (Lamb and Choppin, 1977) have shown that the polypeptide chains of the glycoproteins are synthesized on the rough endoplasmic reticulum. The available evidence indicates that they migrate via the smooth endoplasmic reticulum and the Golgi apparatus to the plasma membrane.

In the course of migration, the polypeptides of the glycoproteins undergo posttranslational modifications. These involve, as can be assumed from analogy to influenza virus (see Section 3.5.5a), sequential glycosylation on the rough endoplasmic reticulum and on smooth membranes. Inhibitors of glycoprotein synthesis such as 2-deoxy-D-glucose (Scholtissek *et al.*, 1974; Hodes *et al.*, 1975) and tunicamycin (Takatsuki and Tamura, 1971) block paramyxovirus replication. There is evidence that the inhibitors interfere with glycosylation (H. D. Klenk, R. T. Schwarz, M. F. G. Schmidt, and K. Bortfeldt, manuscript in preparation) as has been demonstrated in the case of other enveloped viruses such as orthomyxoviruses or togaviruses (see Sections 3.5.5c and 3.10.3).

The other type of posttranslational modification which has been studied extensively with paramyxoviruses is proteolytic cleavage. Cleavage is involved in the biosynthesis of both envelope glycoproteins. As described above, the F1 and F2 subunits of glycoprotein F are derived from a common precursor F0. This precursor has been identified with Sendai virus (Homma and Ohuchi, 1973; Scheid and Choppin, 1974a), SV5 (Peluso *et al.*, 1977), measles virus (Scheid *et al.*, 1978), and a whole series of different strains of NDV (Samson and Fox, 1973; Hightower *et al.*, 1975; Nagai *et al.*, 1976a,b). Cleavage of F0 takes place on smooth internal membranes and on the plasma membrane (Nagai *et al.*, 1976b). With two strains of NDV, a precursor HNO has been observed which is converted, again by proteolytic cleavage, into glycoprotein HN (Nagai *et al.*, 1976a). It is not clear whether synthesis of HN0 is a general phenomenon occurring with all paramyxoviruses. However, suggestive evidence has been obtained by *in vitro* translation studies that HNO might be synthesized by another NDV strain in which the precursor cannot be detected if analyzed under *in vivo* conditions (Clinkscales *et al.*, 1977).

Cleavage is not required for virus assembly, but it is necessary for the expression of the biological activities of each glycoprotein, i.e., hemolysis and cell fusion in the case of F (Homma and Ohuchi, 1973; Scheid and Choppin, 1974a; Nagai *et al.*, 1976a) and hemagglutinating and neuraminidase activity in the case of HN (Nagai *et al.*, 1976a; Nagai and Klenk, 1977). As will be shown later, these activities reflect the role of the glycoproteins in the penetration process. It is therefore not surprising that virus particles with uncleaved precursors have reduced infectivity.

Whether cleavage occurs depends on the virus strain and on the host cell. Sendai virus (Homma and Ohuchi, 1973; Scheid and Choppin, 1974a) and certain strains of NDV (Nagai et al., 1976a) in appropriate host cells produce virus particles with one or both glycoproteins present in the inactive precursor form, whereas if grown in other host systems the virions are fully infectious and contain both glycoproteins in the cleaved form. This observation indicates that host enzymes, which are present in a given cell type and absent in another one, are responsible for cleavage. On the other hand, in a given host cell the glycoproteins of one NDV strain may be cleaved, whereas those of another one are not cleaved, and evidence has been presented that these variations in cleavage are based on structural differences of the glycoproteins (Nagai et al., 1976a).

Virus particles with uncleaved glycoproteins, which are obtained with Sendai virus and certain NDV strains, can be activated by in vitro treatment with proteases and provide suitable substrates to determine the specificity of these enzymes. It was found that the F glycoprotein of these viruses is cleaved and activated exclusively by trypsin (Scheid and Choppin, 1976; Nagai and Klenk, 1977). With Sendai virus, mutants with an altered protease sensitivity have been isolated that are not susceptible to trypsin but are activated by other enzymes such as chymotrypsin and elastase (Scheid and Choppin, 1976). In contrast to glycoprotein F0, which requires a specific protease, glycoprotein HNO was cleaved and activated by a series of enzymes of different specificities (Nagai and Klenk, 1977). Thus there is a striking difference in the susceptibility of the two glycoproteins to proteolytic enzymes, and it is reasonable to assume that HNO has a much higher chance to encounter an appropriate protease in a given host cell and that it is, therefore, more readily cleaved than F0. This might explain why, so far, HNO could be detected only with two NDV strains, whereas F0 has been observed with almost all paramyxoviruses analyzed.

3.6.3b.   Biosynthesis of the M Protein

The association of the M protein with membranes of infected cells and its incorporation into mature envelopes have been investigated in cell fractionation studies (Nagai et al., 1976b; Lamb and Choppin, 1977). The M protein was found to be incorporated into plasma membranes and into virions immediately after its synthesis. It appears that insertion of the M protein into the plasma membrane is one of the final steps in envelope assembly.

Evidence has been obtained with NDV that M is inserted into membrane regions which already contain glycoproteins (Nagai *et al.*, 1976*b*). The mechanism by which M recognizes such areas is not known. Direct interaction across the lipid bilayer between the envelope glycoproteins and the M protein has not been demonstrated with paramyxoviruses, but reconstitution studies with isolated components suggest that the M protein mediates the binding of the spikes to the nucleocapsid (Yoshida *et al.*, 1976).

The data described so far support the concept that incorporation of M into the envelope precursor results in the formation of mature envelope with morphologically distinct spikes appearing on the outer and nucleocapsid strands being attached to the inner side of the envelope. It is reasonable to assume that on its incorporation into the membrane the M protein serves as a binding site for the nucleocapsid (Shimizu and Ishida, 1975; McSharry *et al.*, 1971, 1975).

Little is known about the events that lead to the appearance of the spikes, but it has to be assumed that extensive rearrangement of the glycoproteins occurs. Recently evidence has been obtained that the rearrangement might involve patch formation. It has been found that the NDV glycoproteins that are incorporated into smooth membranes of infected cells have a high degree of mobility in the plane of the membrane and show random distribution, whereas in the mature envelope they have a low mobility and are aggregated in patches (Nagai *et al.*, 1975). Thus it appears that insertion of the M protein into the envelope and patch formation of the glycoproteins are closely linked events. However, it is not yet known whether patch formation is a precondition for attachment of M, or whether insertion of M promotes the aggregation of the glycoproteins.

3.6.3c. Budding

Our knowledge of the budding process is derived mainly from electron microscope and cell fractionation studies. As described in the preceding section, cell fractionation studies suggest that the immediate precursor to the viral envelope is a discrete patch of plasma membrane containing virus-specific proteins. The concept of patch formation is supported by electron microscopic studies which show that (1) a layer of surface projections covers the virus particle but is absent on the adjacent cell surface (Compans *et al.*, 1966), (2) ferritin-labeled antibody binds to the entire surface of the budding virions but not to adjacent cell membrane (Choppin *et al.*, 1971), and (3) neuraminic acid residues are present on the nonaltered cell surface but are absent on the budding virus particle (Klenk *et al.*, 1970*b*). Host cell polypeptides appear to be excluded from regions of membrane which give rise to virus particles as indicated by their absence in the mature virion.

An important feature of the assembly of the virus is that during the budding process the membrane of the viral envelope is continuous with and morphologically similar to the plasma membrane of the host cell. This suggests that the lipids in the unaltered plasma membrane are easily exchangeable by lateral diffusion with those in the budding virus particles. It is therefore not surprising that the lipids in the envelopes very closely resemble those of the host cell membrane.

There is thus good evidence that the viral envelope is derived from a patch of plasma membrane modified by the incorporation of virus-specific proteins. However, little is known about the mechanism which promotes protrusion of this patch to induce bud formation. Since the M protein and the nucleocapsid are the last virus-specific components to arrive in these patches, it is perhaps not unreasonable to assume that either one or both of these structures might be directly responsible for budding. In this respect, it is of interest to note that under certain conditions virus particles lacking nucleocapsid can be isolated (Rott *et al.*, 1963). This observation suggests that the M protein plays a more important role in the budding process than the nucleocapsid.

3.6.4. Biological Function of Envelope Glycoproteins

3.6.4a. Role in Initiation of Infection

The glycoproteins of paramyxoviruses play essential roles in the initiation of infection. HN appears to be responsible for adsorption and F is involved in penetration. This conclusion can be drawn from numerous studies on the function of these glycoproteins. Paramyxoviruses are particularly suitable for such studies for the following two reasons: (1) There are specific activities associated with each glycoprotein that can be easily measured and thus can serve as model reactions. (2) Virus particles with biologically inactive precursors are available that can be activated by *in vitro* treatment with specific proteases, e.g., strain Ulster of NDV HNO can be activated by chymotrypsin and F0 by trypsin. Thus the activity of each individual glycoprotein can be analyzed independently.

i. The HN Glycoprotein. The ability of paramyxoviruses to interact and agglutinate a wide spectrum of erythrocytes has been known for many years. That it is justified to use hemagglutination as a model reaction for adsorption is demonstrated by the observation described above that NDV particles with the biologically inactive precursor HN0 have a reduced infectivity (Nagai *et al.*, 1976*b*; Nagai and Klenk, 1977). This concept is also supported by the observation that a mutant of Sendai virus forms virions that lack the HN glycoprotein as well as infectivity (Portner *et al.*, 1975). Both of these findings demonstrate that HN is essential for infection.

The glycoprotein nature of the myxovirus receptor on erythrocytes and the essential role of neuraminic acid for its function have been known for many years (Klenk *et al.*, 1955). Since then much information has been accumulated on the receptor (for reviews, see Bächi *et al.*, 1977). There appears to be little specificity concerning the structure to which neuraminic acid is linked, because a whole series of different neuraminic acid containing glycoproteins have been shown to bind. Moreover, gangliosides are also active (Huang *et al.*, 1973; Haywood, 1975).

There is evidence that the same active center on the HN glycoprotein is responsible for hemagglutinating and neuraminidase activities. This is suggested by binding studies of a neuraminic acid analogue (Scheid and Choppin, 1974*b*) and by activation studies with proteases (Nagai and Klenk, 1977). The neuraminidase of paramyxoviruses has a broader substrate specificity than the enzyme of influenza viruses (Drzeniek, 1967; Huang and Orlich, 1972). As has been pointed out above, lipids and carbohydrates in the virus particle are determined largely by the host. The neuraminidase appears to be responsible for the only distinct virus-specific modification, i.e., the absence of neuraminic acid in glycoproteins and glycolipids (Klenk and Choppin, 1970*b*; Klenk *et al.*, 1970*a,b*). Whereas there is general agreement that hemagglutination reflects the role of the HN glycoprotein in adsorption, less is known about the biological significance of the enzymatic activity. It has been suggested that the neuraminidase may be important for virus release, but the evidence for this concept has been obtained mostly from studies with influenza virus (see Section 3.5.4b).

ii. The F glycoprotein. There is now wide agreement that the common principle underlying cell fusion and hemolysis is insertion of the viral envelope into the cell membrane by fusion. Experimental evidence for insertion and subsequent dispersion of envelope antigens in the plasma membrane has been obtained from electron microscopic studies (Hoyle, 1962; Howe and Morgan, 1969; Apostolov and Almeida, 1972; Bächi *et al.*, 1977). Hemolysis appears to require insertion of a highly permeable envelope in order to allow leakage of ions, swelling of the cells, and finally rupture and egress of hemoglobin (Shimizu *et al.*, 1976; Homma *et al.*, 1976). Cell fusion occurs if the envelope incorporated into the plasma membrane fuses with another cell. Hemolysis as well as cell fusion requires the presence of glycoprotein F in its cleaved form as outlined above. Since this glycoprotein is also necessary for infectivity, it is a fair assumption that envelope–membrane fusion is also the mechanism of paramyxovirus penetration.

Cell fusion and hemolysis have found wide application as model systems to study envelope–membrane fusion (for a review, see Hosaka and Shimizu, 1977), and recent studies suggest that the virus alters the structure of the lipid bilayer of the target cell membrane and that there is an exchange of lipid between the viral envelope and the cell membrane. Evidence for lipid exchange has been obtained by Hoyle (1962), who reported that radioactively labeled phospholipid was transferred from influenza virus to membrane vesicles prepared from virus-infected cells, and Drzeniek *et al.* (1966), who showed that lipid antigens were transferred from paramyxovirions into erythrocytes on exposure of cells to viruses. Recently lipid exchange mediated by NDV between cells in culture could be demonstrated by means of a fluorescent lipid probe (Huang, 1977).

Further insight into the molecular mechanism involved in the fusion process came from studies employing spin-labeled probes (Maeda *et al.*, 1975, 1977; Lyles and Landsberger, 1977). These studies suggest that first the envelope bilayer of the Sendai virion and the membrane of the erythrocyte are brought in close contact by the action of the HN glycoprotein. Subsequently the lipids of the cell membrane are destabilized and lipid intermixing between both bilayers occurs. For destabilization and lipid exchange glycoprotein F must be present in the cleaved form; virions devoid of F or virions containing the uncleaved form have very low activity. Similar results have been obtained by nuclear magnetic resonance studies of chick embryo cells exposed to NDV which also showed that the virus alters the bilayer structure of the target cell membrane and that this perturbation depends on cleavage of F (Klenk *et al.*, 1977a). The mechanism of the perturbation induced by glycoprotein F appears to be a biophysical rather than a biochemical event since the chemical composition of the membrane lipids is not changed in the fusion process (Elsbach *et al.*, 1969; Diringer and Rott, 1976). As has been pointed out above, the F protein has a highly hydrophobic region at the N terminus of the F1 segment, and it is tempting to speculate that this region might be responsible for the interaction with the target cell membrane.

3.6.4b.   Envelope Glycoproteins as Determinants of Host Range and Pathogenicity

It has been pointed out above that proteolytic cleavage of the viral glycoproteins is determined by the structure of these molecules as well as by the disposition of the appropriate enzymes by the host. Depending on the host cell and the virus strains, Sendai virus (Scheid and Choppin, 1976) and NDV (Nagai *et al.*, 1976*b*) form either infectious particles with cleaved glycoproteins or particles with reduced infectivity and uncleaved glycoproteins. Thus there are differences in host range, and these differences proved to be of high importance for the pathogenicity of NDV. Five virulent and five avirulent strains have been analyzed that were grown in five different host systems. For avirulent strains, only a few host systems were permissive, i.e., they produced infectious virus and allowed replication under multiple cycle conditions; most host cells were nonpermissive for these strains, i.e., they produced inactive virus and did not allow multiple cycle replication. In contrast, all host systems were permissive for virulent strains. It is a reasonable assumption that the wide host range of the virulent strains should facilitate spread of infection in the organism and thus promote outbreak of disease.

3.7.   Poxviruses

3.7.1.   Classification, Morphology, Composition

The poxviridae family comprises six different genera and several other members not yet allocated to a specific genus, such as molluscum contagiosum virus. Natural hosts are a wide range of vertebrates and invertebrates. Most of the information on structure and replication has been obtained from studies on vaccinia virus (genus orthopoxvirus). The replication of poxviruses has been reviewed in Volume 3 of this series (Moss, 1974).

Poxviruses are large, brick-shaped or ovoid particles 300–450 nm long and 170–260 nm wide. The chemical composition of vaccinia virus has been shown to be about 92% protein, 3% DNA, 5% lipid (1.2% cholesterol, 2.1% phospholipid, 1.7% neutral lipid), and 0.2.% non-DNA carbohydrates (Hoagland *et al.*, 1940; Smadel *et al.*, 1940; Zwartouw, 1964). Biochemical studies and electron microscopy have demonstrated that the external envelope of vaccinia virus meets all the criteria for biological membranes. Chemically it has been demonstrated to contain protein and lipid. Morphologically it possesses a trilaminar or unit membrane structure of the same width as that of cell membranes and exhibits tubular elements at the outer surface (Peters, 1956; Dales and Siminovitch, 1961; Nagington and Horne, 1962; Westwood *et al.*, 1964; Dales and Mosbach, 1968). A second membrane may be present in the core structure, but it has not been so well studied as the surface membrane (Morgan *et al.*, 1962; Easterbrook, 1966; Mitchiner, 1969).

3.7.2. Components of the Envelope

Because of the complexity of the virus structure, our knowledge on composition and architecture of the envelope is far from complete.

3.7.2a. Proteins

In vaccinia virions 20–30 polypeptides ranging in molecular weight between about 8000 and 200,000 have been identified by polyacrylamide gel electrophoresis (Holowczak and Joklik, 1967; Moss and Salzman, 1968; Katz and Moss, 1970; Moss and Rosenblum, 1972; Sarov and Joklik, 1972). Out of 28 carbohydrate-free polypeptides observed in whole virus in one of these studies, 17 have been found in cores that were prepared by treating virions with Nonidet P40 and 2-mercaptoethanol followed by iodoacetamide, sonication, and banding in sucrose density gradients. Five carbohydrate-free polypeptides appeared to be envelope proteins, since they were found to be located at or near the surface of the virus. This conclusion was based on their ability to react in situ with surface labeling agents and on the ability of chymotrypsin and Nonidet P40 to release them from virions (Sarov and Joklik, 1972). One of these five polypeptides (MW 58,000) appears to constitute the tubules at the surface of the virus (Stern and Dales, 1976).

In contrast to the apparently complex pattern of carbohydrate-free envelope proteins, the glycoprotein composition of vaccinia virus is relatively simple. Only one (Holowczak, 1970; Garon and Moss, 1971; Moss *et al.*, 1973) or perhaps two glycoproteins (Sarov and Joklik, 1972) could be identified in the virion. The vaccinia virus glycoprotein differs remarkably in its carbohydrate composition from the glycoproteins of other enveloped viruses, since glucosamine has been found to be

the only constituent sugar. Glycopeptides obtained after pronase digestion of virions grown in avian and mammalian cell lines were indistinguishable and a similar glycopeptide was not detected in uninfected
cells (Garon and Moss, 1971). The precise location of the glycoprotein
within the viral envelope or even within the virion is unknown.
Holowczak (1970) and Garon and Moss (1971) noted that a major portion of the glucosamine-labeled glycoprotein was removed from virions
by treatment with Nonidet P40 and a reducing agent. This procedure
was originally devised by Easterbrook (1966) to remove the viral
envelopes. The glycoprotein was also removed by tryptic digestion
under conditions in which the lipids were not removed, viral DNA was
not released, and no loss of plaque-forming units occurred (Moss *et al.*,
1973). These results, which would suggest that the glycoprotein is
located at the surface of the viral envelope, are difficult to reconcile
with the observations of Sarov and Joklik (1972), who reported that the
glycoproteins could not be removed by Nonidet P40 treatment in the
absence of reducing agents or by chymotrypsin and that the glycoproteins are not accessible to surface labeling agents.

3.7.2b. Lipids

The vaccinia virus envelope in its trilaminar structure resembles
cellular membranes and the envelopes of viruses that are assembled on
such membranes. Unlike the budding viruses, however, vaccinia does
not derive its lipid constituents by emerging from preexisting cellular
membranes but rather most probably by a process of autonomous self-
assembly within cytoplasmic "virus factories" (Dales and Mosbach,
1968). As a consequence of this mode of membrane biogenesis, the lipid
composition of vaccinia virus is distinct from that of the host cell
plasma membrane, notably with respect to a decreased amount of
phosphatidylethanolamine and the presence of much greater quantities
of an as yet unidentified phospholipid (Stern and Dales, 1974). Both
preformed and nascent phospholipids entered the virion during and
after particle maturation. *In vitro* transfer of phospholipids from
liposomes to virus was demonstrated in the presence of either beef heart
or HeLa cell phospholipid exchange protein, implying that such a protein may catalyze the *in vivo* transfer of phospholipid from endoplasmic
reticulum to assembling vaccinia envelopes (Stern and Dales, 1974).
Evidence has been obtained that virus infection affects the lipid
metabolism of the cell and that the resulting alterations in lipid composition are reflected in the host. Thus, after infection with vaccinia

virus, there is a shift in HeLa and L cells from complex to less complex glycolipids. Purified virus contains the same relative amounts of glycolipid as do the host cells whose composition has been altered by the infection. Evidence has been obtained that these changes may be the consequence of virus-mediated suppression of host protein synthesis, thereby affecting also the activity of enzymes involved in production of glycolipids (Anderson and Dales, 1978). Similarly, fowlpox virus has been found to contain significant amounts of squalene, which is a metabolic precursor of cholesterol and is not observed in the uninfected host cell (White *et al.*, 1968).

3.7.3. Biogenesis of the Envelope

The envelopes of vaccinia and other poxviruses are assembled *de novo* in cytoplasmic foci termed viroplasmic "matrices" or "factories." Such envelopes appear first within the factories and are not continuous with preexisting cellular membranes. The envelopes develop progressively from arc-shaped trilamellar structures, possessing an external coat of a closely packed layer of spicules. Ultimately they are formed into closed spheres enclosing immature forms of vaccinia. With time, progressive differentiation into a core and lateral bodies takes place inside the envelopes, while the external surface undergoes poorly understood morphological alterations, such as transformation in which spicules disappear and surface tubules appear (Dales and Mosbach, 1968). Rifampicin blocks the formation of virus particles at an early stage and membranes lacking the spicule layer accumulate within the cytoplasm. When rifampicin is removed, virtually all membranes become coated with spicules within 10 min (Moss *et al.*, 1969).

3.7.4. Virus-Induced Modifications of Cellular Membranes

Despite the apparent lack of involvement of the host plasma membrane in poxvirus assembly, there are indications that this structure is modified during virus replication. Alterations occurring early after infection are the appearance of virus-specific antigens at the cell surface (Miyamoto and Kato, 1968; Ueda *et al.*, 1969). Other modifications are hemagglutination and cell fusion. Interestingly, there is evidence that in some of these phenomena virus-specific proteins might be involved that are not structural components of the virions.

3.7.4a.   Hemagglutination

Vaccinia virus produces a hemagglutinin which is found only in infected cells, not in virions. It is a late antigen and is located at the cell surface (Ichihashi and Dales, 1971). The hemagglutinin might be identical with the major plasma membrane glycoprotein synthesized after infection, which is thought to be virus specific (Weintraub and Dales, 1974). Such nonstructural glycoproteins have been observed in relatively large amounts in membrane fractions of infected cells (Moss *et al.*, 1973) and have been found to differ from the glycoprotein present in the virus particle in electrophoretic mobility, size of the oligosaccharide, and carbohydrate composition (Garon and Moss, 1971).

3.7.4b.   Cell Fusion

Vaccinia virus induces cell fusion, which requires both DNA replication and protein synthesis, occurs only after mature particles have been assembled, and is not elicited from the outside by inoculum virus (Dales *et al.*, 1976). Cell fusion can be suppressed by antiserum prepared against isolated surface tubules of the virion. Such treatment also neutralizes virus infectivity (Stern and Dales, 1976). These observations support the concept derived from electron microscopic studies that the virus penetrates into the host cell by fusion of the envelope with the plasma membrane (Chang and Metz, 1976; Dales *et al.*, 1976). Moreover, these findings suggest that the fusing agent is located at the virus surface. It remains to be seen, however, whether this agent is the surface tubule itself or another component of the envelope.

3.8.   Rhabdoviruses

3.8.1.   Classification, Morphology, Composition

The rhabdoviridae family comprises the genus vesiculovirus, with the prototype vesicular stomatitis virus (VSV), and the genus lyssavirus, with the prototype rabies virus. Natural hosts of these viruses are vertebrates and arthropods. In addition, there are members of this family that multiply in plants.

Virions are usually bullet shaped, 130–300 nm long and 70 nm wide. They contain a long tubular nucleocapsid with helical symmetry that is surrounded by an envelope. They are composed of about 3–4% RNA, 65% protein, 20–25% lipid, and 3–13% carbohydrate (McSharry and Wagner, 1971a; Schneider and Diringer, 1976). The carbohydrate is present in the form of glycoprotein, glycolipid (Klenk and Choppin, 1971), and mucopolysaccharide (Pinter and Compans, 1975).

We will confine ourselves here to VSV, which is one of the best-studied enveloped viruses, and to rabies virus. Various aspects of rhabdovirus structure and replication have been reviewed previously in Volume 4 of this series (Wagner, 1975) and elsewhere (Emerson, 1976; Schneider and Diringer, 1976).

3.8.2. Fine Structure and Arrangement of Envelope Components

The rhabdovirus envelope is composed of a lipid bilayer, one or two inner carbohydrate-free M proteins, and external spikes consisting of a single glycoprotein designated G. Table 3 presents a list of the envelope proteins of VSV and rabies virus.

The envelope proteins of VSV have been separated from the nucleocapsid by treatment with deoxycholate (Kang and Prevec, 1969; Cartwright et al., 1970), digitonin (Wagner et al., 1969), hydrochloric acid at pH 1.5 (Mudd, 1973), or Triton X100 in the presence of 0.3 M NaCl (Emerson and Wagner, 1972). In low-ionic-strength solution, Triton X100 (Kelley et al., 1972) and other nonionic detergents, such as Nonidet P40 (Arstila, 1973; Cartwright et al., 1970) and Triton N101 (Dietzschold et al., 1974), solubilize selectively the G protein of VSV. Similarly, the glycoproteins of rabies virus have been solubilized by the

TABLE 3
Envelope Proteins of Rhabdoviruses

Vesicular stomatitis virus Indiana serotype		Rabies virus			
		HEP flury strain		PM strain	
Designation[a]	Molecular weight[a]	Designation[a]	Molecular weight[b]	Designation[a]	Molecular weight[c]
G	69,000	G	80,000	G1	78,000
				G2	65,000
M	29,000	M2	25,000	M2	22,000

[a] Wagner et al. (1972b).
[b] Sokol et al. (1971).
[c] Neurath et al. (1972).

action of Triton X100 and purified from contaminating proteins by isoelectric focusing (Schneider and Diringer, 1976).

Although the rhabdovirus envelope is composed predominantly of virus-specific proteins, there is evidence that host cell proteins are incorporated at levels too low to be detected by biochemical means. Thus the L-cell histocompatibility antigen has been found in VSV purified from these cells (Hecht and Summers, 1972).

3.8.2a. The Spikes

Rhabdoviruses are covered with closely spaced glycoprotein spikes that are approximately 10 nm in length as shown by electron microscopic studies. The spikes can be removed by proteases, such as trypsin (Cartwright *et al.*, 1970; Schloemer and Wagner, 1974), and in intact virions only the spike glycoprotein can be labeled by surface labeling agents (Eger *et al.*, 1975). The available evidence indicates that the spikes are composed of a single glycoprotein species termed the "G protein." With VSV it has a molecular weight of approximately 69,000 (Table 3). With rabies virus, occasionally two glycoprotein peaks, G1 and G2 (Table 3), can be observed on polyacrylamide gels, which, however, appear to be modifications of the same species. The proportions of G1 and G2 varied depending on the virus strain, the virus preparation, and storage (Sokol *et al.*, 1971; Neurath *et al.*, 1972). This suggests that the lower-molecular-weight component G2 is a degradation product of the high-molecular-weight component G1.

The glycoproteins of rhabdoviruses are amphipathic like those of other enveloped viruses. After protease treatment of VSV a fragment of the G protein was demonstrated to be associated with the intact virion (Mudd, 1974). More recently Schloemer and Wagner (1975*b*) have isolated a small nonglycosylated portion of the protein from the envelope of protease-treated VSV virions. The fragment was found to have a molecular weight of 5200, approximately equivalent to 50 amino acids. Amino acid analysis showed that there was a preponderence of hydrophobic amino acids. The hydrophobic fragment of the G protein is long enough to penetrate the lipid bilayer. Conclusive evidence for such penetration has not been obtained, but cross-linking experiments with glutaraldehyde suggest that interactions may occur between G proteins and the internal M proteins (Brown *et al.*, 1974).

The carbohydrates linked to the G protein of VSV have been studied in detail. The glycoprotein is 9–10% carbohydrate by weight and has been found to contain mannose, galactose, *N*-acetylglucosamine, and neuraminic acid as the major sugar components with lesser amounts of N-acetylgalactosamine and fucose (McSharry and Wagner, 1971b). The presence of N-acetylgalactosamine would imply O-glyco-sidic linkages of carbohydrate chains to the polypeptide. However, such linkages have not been observed in the G protein, and in recent analyses N-acetylgalactosamine could indeed not be detected (Hunt and Sum-mers, 1976b).

The attachment of the oligosaccharide to the polypeptide is most probably via a β-N-glycosidic linkage between asparagine and N-acetylglucosamine. This conclusion is based on the susceptibility of the oligosaccharide to endo-β-N-acetylglucosaminidase and to strong alkali and its resistance to mild alkaline hydrolysis, which would cleave O-gly-cosidic bonds involving serine and threonine (Moyer et al., 1976).

The carbohydrate side chains of the VSV glycoprotein have been characterized in quite some detail. Analysis of the glycopeptides obtained by pronase digestion followed by gel chromatography revealed that there is only one type of side chain (Moyer et al., 1976). From the size of the pronase glycopeptides (MW 3000–3400), the molecular weight of the glycoprotein, and the amount of carbohydrate present in the glycoprotein, it has been calculated that the G protein contains only two carbohydrate side chains (Etchison and Holland, 1974a,b; McSharry and Wagner, 1971b).

Analysis of the tryptic glycopeptides of the G protein of VSV showed that the oligosaccharides are attached at two specific sites (Robertson et al., 1976). These sites are apparently strongly conserved, since tryptic glycopeptides were indistinguishable in wild-type VSV and in a mutant which had been chosen by repeated selection for ther-molability and resistance to neutralizing (anti-G) antibody, and therefore presumably possessed multiple alterations in its G protein (Robertson and Summers, 1977).

The structure of the oligosaccharide side chain resembles the struc-tures of influenza virus and togavirus glycoproteins in possessing a core structure of mannose and N-acetylglucosamine followed by branches containing additional residues of N-acetylglucosamine, galactose, and terminal fucose and neuraminic acid (Etchison et al., 1977). The oli-gosaccharide is sulfated, but the attachment site of the sulfate is not clear (Pinter and Compans, 1975). The presence of neuraminic acid on the envelope of VSV has been demonstrated by treating the virus with colloidal iron hydroxide, which stains neuraminic acid residues (Klenk et al., 1970b). The oligosaccharide side chains lack neuraminic acid when VSV is grown in mosquito cells, because these cells lack neuraminosyl-transferase (Schloemer and Wagner, 1975b). Previous studies had also shown that the size and composition of the carbohydrate moieties are variable, depending on the cell type in which the virions were grown (Burge and Huang, 1970; Etchison and Holland, 1974a). Likewise, the sequence of the carbohydrate within the glycosyl side chains may exhibit cell dependence (Moyer and Summers, 1974).

3.8.2b. The Lipid Bilayer

The lipids of VSV are composed of phospholipids and neutral lipids with high ratios of cholesterol to phospholipid and of sphingolipids to glycerophospholipids. The lipid composition of the virions reflects, but does not exactly mimic, the lipid composition of the host cell plasma membrane (McSharry and Wagner, 1971a). In virions grown in BHK 21-F cells, relatively large amounts of hematoside are observed, which is also the predominant glycolipid of the host cell (Klenk and Choppin, 1971). A similar lipid pattern has been found in rabies virus (Diringer et al., 1973).

The lipids are present in the envelope as a bilayer. This has been demonstrated with VSV by electron spin resonance studies using spin labels (Landsberger and Compans, 1976) and by ^{13}C nuclear magnetic resonance (Stoffel and Bister, 1975; Stoffel et al., 1976). Neuraminidase treatment of intact and spikeless particles of VSV grown in BHK cells converted gangliosides into neuraminic acid-free glycolipids, demonstrating that these were present exclusively on the outer surface of the viral bilayer (Stoffel et al., 1975). Treatment of VSV grown in BHK cells with a nonpenetrating reagent showed that only 36% of the phosphatidylethanolamine was available for reaction and was therefore present on the outer surface (Fong et al., 1976).

The envelope lipids of VSV are derived from the host and reflect compositional differences of the host. Such differences are paralleled by physical changes of the envelope (Landsberger and Compans, 1976). Envelope rigidity, however, is also dependent on the envelope proteins. Landsberger and Compans (1976) have observed that when the glycoproteins of VSV are removed by proteases the envelope becomes more fluid, indicating that the viral glycoproteins may contribute to the rigidity of the envelope. However, Landsberger and Compans postulated also that the major effect on bilayer fluidity is exerted by the M protein, since the fluidity of the lipid bilayer is altered only slightly when the G protein is removed by proteases, whereas vesicles prepared from extracted viral lipids were much more fluid than lipids in virions. Moore et al. (1976) and Barenholz et al. (1976) have shown that the envelope of VSV has a higher microviscosity than the plasma membranes from which the virus budded. The increased viscosity was attributed in part to the insertion of the hydrophobic regions of the glycoproteins into the envelope bilayer. Stoffel and Bister (1975) using NMR spectra of ^{13}C-labeled lipids also demonstrated that the envelope lipids of VSV are highly rigid, due either to lipid–lipid or to lipid–protein interactions. In general, it may be concluded therefore that the glycoprotein does interact with the lipid bilayer and may affect the rigidity of the membrane to some extent, but that the M protein may be of equal or greater importance in determining membrane rigidity.

3.8.2c. The M Protein

Only one type of M protein is found in VSV. Rabies virus has been reported to possess two different types of this protein (M1 and M2), but there is no evidence that M1 is really an envelope protein. The M protein is located on the inner side of the lipid bilayer as indicated by its resistance to protease treatment of the intact virus particle (Cartwright *et al.*, 1970; McSharry *et al.*, 1971; Schloemer and Wagner, 1974) and its inaccessibility to surface labeling agents (Eger *et al.*, 1975). The amino acid composition of the M protein of VSV has been analyzed, and no unusual distributions have been found (Moore *et al.*, 1974).

The M protein of VSV is antigenic (Cartwright *et al.*, 1970*b*) and monospecific antibodies against purified M protein clearly demonstrated that it is an antigen distinct from the G protein and the nucleocapsid protein (Dietzschold *et al.*, 1974). The anti-M serum does not neutralize the infectivity of virions but reacts specifically with the M protein in either Ouchterlony or complement fixation assays.

3.8.3. Biogenesis and Assembly of the Envelope

Maturation of the rhabdovirus envelope is a multistep process involving sequential incorporation of viral proteins into preformed cellular membranes. In general, the envelope appears to be assembled by mechanisms similar to those that have been observed with ortho- and paramyxoviruses (see Sections 3.5.6 and 3.6.3).

3.8.3a. Biosynthesis of the Glycoprotein

The G protein of VSV is synthesized on membrane-bound ribosomes (Grubman *et al.*, 1974; Morrison and Lodish, 1975; Wirth *et al.*, 1977), and glycoproteins are always found associated with intracellular or plasma membranes but are never free in the cytoplasm (Wagner *et al.*, 1972*a*; Hunt and Summers, 1976). Pulse-chase experiments have shown that during and shortly after biosynthesis the glycoprotein is associated with the rough endoplasmic reticulum. At later times it is associated with a smooth cytoplasmic membrane fraction and finally, after about 20 min, it appears at the plasma membrane (David, 1973; Lafay, 1974; Hunt and Summers, 1976*a*; Knipe *et al.*, 1977*a*). With *ts* mutants of complementation group V of VSV the G protein is arrested at the nonpermissive temperature at the rough endoplasmic reticulum. Budding of virions occurs only when the block in migration to smooth membranes is released by a shift to the permissive temperature. Thus there is a correlation between the migration of the G protein and virus assembly (Lafay, 1974; Knipe *et al.*, 1977*b*).

Further insight into the relationship between polypeptide synthesis, insertion into membranes, and glycosylation of the G protein is obtained from studies analyzing the translation of this protein in a cell-free system. The protein which is synthesized in the presence of endoplasmic reticulum membranes appears to be about 2000 daltons larger than that prepared in the absence of membranes. This extra material probably represents carbohydrate as shown by its susceptibility to digestion by endoglycosidases, and by the fact that protein synthesized in the presence of membranes binds concanavalin A, while that prepared in the absence of membranes does not (Katz *et al.*, 1977; Toneguzzo and Ghosh, 1977, 1978). Further, the glycoprotein produced in the presence of membranes is inaccessible to proteolytic digestion, except for about 5% of the total protein, which has been found by peptide analysis to comprise the C terminus of the polypeptide chain (Katz *et al.*, 1977; Toneguzzo and Ghosh, 1978). Membranes must be added before peptide chain synthesis is about 15% complete in order for glycosylation and proper insertion to occur (Rothman and Lodish, 1977; Toneguzzo and Ghosh, 1978). This shows that initiation of polypeptide synthesis can precede membrane binding. These observations are in agreement with the "signal hypothesis" according to which polypeptide synthesis is initiated by the synthesis of a short amino acid sequence at the N terminus that is responsible for attachment of the protein to and transport through the membrane (Blobel and Dobberstein, 1975).

The available evidence suggests that in the *in vitro* system the carbohydrates are attached to the polypeptide as two distinct entities which correspond to the cores of the two oligosaccharide side chains of the molecule (see above) (Rothman and Lodish, 1977). The inability to detect intermediates containing a smaller number of sugar residues suggests that each core is added in a single step presumably by transfer from lipid intermediates. Pulse-chase experiments in infected cells cannot distinguish between the time course of incorporation of amino acids and core sugars to the completed glycoprotein, indicating that the cores are added in the course of, or promptly on completion of, the polypeptide chain. Fucose, galactose, and neuraminic acid are added later during processing. The oligosaccharide is completed before the protein arrives at the cell surface (Knipe *et al.*, 1977*c*). Similar conclusions on the mechanisms involved in glycosylation have been drawn previously from studies with influenza virus (Compans, 1973*b*; Klenk *et al.*, 1974, 1978).

Glycosylation of the G protein of VSV can be inhibited by tunicamycin, also supporting the concept that lipid intermediates are involved in this reaction. Virus particles are not produced under these conditions, but the unglycosylated G protein is synthesized and appears to be stable in the cell (Leavitt *et al.*, 1977).

3.8.3b. Biosynthesis of the M Protein

The M protein is synthesized independently from the G protein and by different mechanisms. It is synthesized on soluble ribosomes, and is found largely in the cytoplasm without being strictly bound to cellular membranes. The M protein is rapidly incorporated into the plasma membrane, where it appears in pulse chase experiments already after 2 min (Knipe *et al.*, 1977*a*). The M protein is also more rapidly and efficiently incorporated into virions than the G protein (Lafay, 1974).

3.8.3c. Envelope Assembly

The available evidence presented above suggests that, on arrival of the G protein at the site of assembly, the M protein and subsequently the nucleocapsid associate with this area. Assembly occurs usually by budding from cellular membranes. The budding site of VSV is in most instances the plasma membrane, but occasionally maturation at intracellular membranes has been observed. The New Jersey strain of this virus was observed to bud primarily from plasma membranes of L or Vero cells, and almost entirely at intracytoplasmic membranes of pig kidney cells (Zee *et al.*, 1970). This report indicated that the site of maturation of a specific virus type may vary depending on the host cell.

Several sites of virus assembly have also been observed with rabies virus. In cell cultures, virus budding regularly occurs at the plasma membrane and within the cytoplasm from preexisting membranes of the endoplasmic reticulum (Hummeler et al., 1967; Matsumoto and Kawai, 1969). Virus assembly at de novo-synthesized membranes in or near the matrix as described by Hummeler et al. (1967) seems to be a rarer event which possibly is virus strain dependent (Schneider and Diringer, 1976). Budding from the Golgi complex has been observed in cultivated mammalian neurons (Matsumoto et al., 1974).

3.8.4. Biological Function of the Envelope Glycoprotein

It is reasonable to assume that rhabdovirus glycoproteins are involved in the initiation of infection, like the glycoproteins of other enveloped viruses such as myxoviruses. Thus spikeless VSV particles which have been produced by treatment with proteolytic enzymes were shown to be non infectious. Infectivity was restored, however, when these particles were reconstituted with purified G protein isolated from the same virus strain or from a different serotype. Antibody directed against the homologous G protein used for reconstitution effectively neutralized the virus, but antibody directed against the serotype of the spikeless particle was ineffective in neutralization if glycoproteins from a different serotype were used for reconstitution (Bishop et al., 1975).

The G protein may be involved in the adsorption process. This is suggested by the observation that VSV (Arstila et al., 1969; Arstila, 1972) as well as rabies virus (Halonen et al., 1968) are able to agglutinate goose erythrocytes and that, at least in the case of VSV, the G protein has been identified as the hemagglutinin (Arstila, 1973).

Little is known about how rhabdoviruses penetrate the plasma membrane. Evidence has been presented that VSV may penetrate by a fusion process (Heine and Schneitman, 1971), and, in appropriate cells, this virus may induce cell fusion (Takehara, 1975). However, it is not clear whether the G protein plays a direct role in this process.

Antibody against the G protein will neutralize the infectivity of VSV, and vaccination of mice with purified G protein effectively protects them against challenge with infective virions (Dietzschold et al., 1974). The antibody to G protein of VSV is type specific and forms the basis for division of this virus into serotypes (Kang and Prevec, 1969). The G protein of rabies virus is also responsible for induction of virus neutralizing antibodies (Schneider et al., 1973; Wiktor et al., 1973) and for conferring immunity to animals against a lethal challenge infection (Atanasiu et al., 1974).

3.9. Retroviruses: C-Type Particles

The retrovirus group includes viruses found in various avian and mammalian species, with the murine and avian C-type viruses being the best-studied members. The viruses have a distinctive appearance and are unique among RNA viruses in replicating through a DNA intermediate. Although most of the viruses are oncogenic, certain nononcogenic viruses such as visna and progressive pneumonia viruses of sheep also possess the morphological and biochemical characteristics of the group. A number of reviews are available which provide more details of the structure and replication process of these viruses (Bolognesi, 1974; Bauer, 1974; Bader, 1974; Shapiro and August, 1976; Vogt, 1977; Eisenman and Vogt, 1978).

3.9.1. Envelope Components

3.9.1a. Surface Proteins and Glycoproteins

One or two glycoproteins have been recognized as virus-specific components on the external surface of the viral envelope. Avian RNA tumor viruses, including Rous sarcoma virus (RSV) and avian myeloblastosis virus (AMV), possess two glycoproteins with apparent molecular weights of 85,000 and 37,000, designated "gp85" and "gp37," respectively (Hung et al., 1971; Rifkin and Compans, 1971; Bolognesi et al., 1972). Murine leukemia viruses (MuLVs), including Rauscher, Moloney, and Friend leukemia viruses, possess a single major glycoprotein of molecular weight ~70,000, designated "gp70" (Moroni, 1972; August et al., 1974). In many preparations, two closely adjacent bands designated "gp69" and "gp71" have been observed (Strand and August, 1973), whereas in other systems only a single component has been identified. However, the two MuLV glycoprotein bands cannot be distinguished by peptide mapping (Elder et al., 1977), and it is therefore likely that a single functional type of glycoprotein is present, with possible minor differences in size or charge due to heterogeneity upon secondary modifications. Minor glycoproteins of molecular weight 45,000–52,000 have also been identified in murine leukemia virus preparations (Moroni, 1972; Moenning et al., 1974; Pinter and Compans, 1975; Marquardt et al., 1977), and their possible origin is discussed below.

Both glycoproteins of avian RNA tumor viruses, as well as gp70 of murine leukemia viruses, are located on the external surface of the viral envelope. This has been demonstrated by proteolytic digestion experiments, in which the glycoproteins were selectively removed, leaving smooth-surfaced particles which still contained the internal carbohydrate-free viral proteins (Rifkin and Compans, 1971; Witter et al., 1973). In addition, surface labeling procedures resulted in selective labeling of the glycoproteins (Robinson et al., 1971; Witte et al., 1973; McLellan and August, 1976). The glycoproteins can be isolated in the form of rosettelike aggregates after detergent treatment, which morphologically resemble aggregates of the projections on the viral envelope (Bolognesi et al., 1972). Further, the fact that these isolated glycoproteins possess the type-specific antigens of the virus which react with neutralizing antibody (Duesberg et al., 1970; Tozawa et al., 1970; Bolognesi et al., 1972) indicates their location on the surface of the virion.

Evidence has been obtained that the two glycoproteins of avian RNA tumor viruses, gp85 and gp37, are distinct gene products (Mosser et al., 1977) linked by disulfide bonds (Leamnson and Halpern, 1976). The resulting complex has an electrophoretic mobility slightly less than that of gp85, and it appears to consist of one molecule each of gp85 and gp37. As discussed below, these two glycoproteins also appear to be synthesized as a single large precursor molecule (England et al., 1977). Recently, an additional carbohydrate-free polypeptide has been resolved in murine leukemia virus preparations, which also appears to be located on the external surface of the viral envelope and is designated p15(E) (Ikeda et al., 1975; Ihle et al., 1976; Famulari et al., 1976; Van Zaane et al., 1976). This protein tends to aggregate in the absence of detergents and is found in the void volume using gel filtration in guanidine hydrochloride. It can be resolved from an internal virion polypeptide of similar electrophoretic mobility by high pH discontinuous SDS gel electrophoresis (Famulari et al., 1976). Recent studies with Moloney murine leukemia virus (Leamnson et al., 1977) indicate that gp70 and p15(E) are also linked by disulfide bonds. While it is uncertain whether this is the case in all murine leukemia viruses, it is likely that p15(E) is associated with gp70, and it may play a role in binding of the spike structure to the viral envelope. The association of gp70 and p15(E) is also suggested by recent observations that they are synthesized in the form of a common precursor polypeptide (Famulari et al., 1976; Witte and Weismann, 1976; Van Zaane et al., 1976).

The exact size of the spike structure of RNA tumor viruses and the number of polypeptide chains which compose the spikes have not been determined. Bolognesi et al. (1972) have suggested that gp37 of AMV forms the spike and gp85 is located as peripheral knob in the spike structure. Sedimentation of RSV glycoproteins in sucrose gradients in the presence of Tween 20 resolved peaks at 9 S and 12 S, and it was suggested that these consisted of two or three disulfide-linked complexes of gp85 plus gp37 (Leamnson and Halpern, 1976). However, it is uncertain whether either of these corresponds to the native spike structure. The major glycoproteins of Friend leukemia virus, after release from virions by osmotic shock, sedimented as a single peak at 4.05 S, corresponding to a molecular weight of 58,000 (Moennig et al., 1974). Thus, under these conditions, MuLV glycoproteins appear to be released from virions as individual glycoprotein molecules.

It is apparent that the glycoproteins of RNA tumor viruses can be dissociated easily from the viral envelope by a variety of conditions, which are not generally feasible for isolation of glycoproteins of other virus groups. This is particularly true for murine leukemia viruses, in which release of glycoproteins has been demonstrated using osmotic shock, freeze-thawing, ultrasonication, and the use of chaotropic agents (Moenning et al., 1974; Strand and August, 1976; Marquardt et al., 1977). The glycoprotein (gp70) preparations obtained appeared free of detectable levels of p15(E), suggesting that no covalent linkage existed between these envelope proteins. These observations indicate that the nature of the interactions which bind RNA tumor virus glycoproteins to the viral membrane may differ from those observed with other enveloped viruses. There may be a weak interaction between gp70 and p15(E), so that gp70 is readily dissociated from the envelope whereas the interaction of p15(E) with the bilayer may resemble that observed with hydrophobic segments of other viral glycoproteins.

As discussed above, a minor glycoprotein of 45,000–52,000 daltons has been observed in many murine leukemia virus preparations. Several possibilities have been suggested for the origin of this component. Marquardt et al. (1977) have isolated both gp70 and gp45 from Rauscher leukemia virus and compared their carbohydrate content. Their data suggest that gp70 contains about 32% of carbohydrate by weight and that gp45 contains 6–7%; both glycoproteins appeared to have polypeptide chains of about 45,000 daltons. On the other hand, it has recently been observed that brief trypsin treatment results in conversion of gp70 to a glycoprotein of 45,000–52,000 daltons (Krantz et al., 1977; Kemp et al., 1978), suggesting that the minor glycoprotein is a proteolytic cleavage product of gp70. It has also been suggested that the minor glycoprotein may represent host-cell-coded H-2 antigen (Bubbers and Lilly, 1977). Whether a single mechanism will account for the results obtained in various virus–cell systems remains to be established. In the case of avian C-type viruses, tryptic peptide analysis has demonstrated that gp37 is not a cleavage product of gp85 (Mosser *et al.*, 1977), whereas similar experiments with murine viruses show that gp45 and gp70 have common peptide species (Elder *et al.*, 1977). Thus it appears that there is no analogy between the minor glycoproteins of murine and avian viruses.

The glycoproteins of avian C-type viruses define the viral host range as well as the classification into subgroups based on interference and neutralization properties (Vogt and Ishizaki, 1966; Ishizaki and Vogt, 1966; Tozawa *et al.*, 1970). The major glycoprotein of murine C-type viruses also is essential for binding to cellular receptors (DeLarco and Todaro, 1976). Proteolytic digestion of the surface glycoproteins inactivates the infectivity of both avian and murine C-type viruses (Rifkin and Compans, 1971; Witter *et al.*, 1973). A hemagglutination assay for mouse leukemia viruses requires the presence of intact glycoproteins on the viral surface (Witter *et al.*, 1973).

Comparisons of tryptic peptides of gp70 molecules isolated from a large number of murine C-type viruses reveal extensive strain differences (Kennel, 1976; Elder *et al.*, 1977). Further, gp70 molecules isolated from different tissues of the same mouse strains also showed differences, suggesting that modifications of a prototype gene may occur during differentiation. On the other hand, murine C-type viruses with similar host range also showed similarities in gp70 primary structure.

3.9.1b. Lipid Bilayer

The lipids of RNA tumor viruses are arranged in a bilayer structure, as shown by electron spin resonance spectra of spin-labeled fatty acid derivatives incorporated into Rauscher leukemia virus (Landsberger *et al.*, 1972). Lipids were shown to compose about 20% of the mass of Rous sarcoma virions (Quigley *et al.*, 1971). The lipid composition of the virus was shown to be similar to that of the cellular plasma membrane, and enveloped viruses of several major groups were all found to have very similar lipids when grown in the same host cell (Rao *et al.*, 1966; Quigley *et al.*, 1971). However, the content of phosphatidylcholine in the virion was lower, and that of sphingomyelin and phosphatidylethanolamine was higher, than in the plasma membrane, and the ratio of cholesterol to phospholipid was also significantly higher in the virion than in the plasma membrane (Quigley *et al.*, 1972). It was suggested that these compositional differences might result from preferential budding of virus particles at sites which differ in composition from the average composition of the overall isolated membrane.

3.9.1c. Internal Membrane Proteins

At least four or five carbohydrate-free polypeptides are present as internal components of C-type viruses, and it is uncertain whether one or more of these is closely associated with the viral envelope. The core structure appears to be an icosahedral capsid (Nermut *et al.*, 1972) which contains the viral RNA as well as two major proteins (Bolognesi *et al.*, 1973). One or more additional internal proteins (10,000 and 19,000 daltons in the case of avian and 12,000 daltons in murine viruses) are not found in isolated core structures, and it has been suggested that these polypeptides are associated with the envelope or located between the core and the viral membrane (Bolognesi *et al.*, 1973; Stromberg *et al.*, 1974). Both the p10 polypeptide of AMV and p12 of MuLV are selectively labeled with dansyl chloride, which suggests that they are exposed on or near the surface of the virion (Bolognesi *et al.*, 1973). Further information is needed to determine the exact location of the various internal polypeptide components of C-type viruses.

3.9.1d. Carbohydrate Components

The oligosaccharides of glycoproteins of various RSV strains have been characterized by gel filtration after extensive pronase digestion (Lai and Duesberg, 1972). A single broad peak, with an estimated molecular weight of 3900–5100, was observed. The glycopeptides in viruses obtained from transformed cells were consistently larger than those obtained from nontransformed cells; such differences were observed in viruses of various RSV subgroups. The structure of the oligosaccharide groups has been partially characterized, and they have been shown to contain glucosamine, mannose, galactose, and sialic acid (Krantz *et al.*, 1976).

Host cell derived mucopolysaccharide components also appear to be present in avian and murine RNA tumor viruses (Lai and Duesberg, 1972; Pinter and Compans, 1975). The polysaccharide components as well as the major and minor glycoproteins of murine C-type viruses are sulfated; the ratio of sulfate to glucosamine appears to be 3 times higher in the minor glycoprotein (gp52) than in gp70 (Pinter and Compans, 1975). The possible significance of this glycoprotein sulfation, as well as the presence of host-cell-derived mucopolysaccharides in virions, remains to be investigated.

Evidence has been presented which indicates that the carbohydrate components are not required for several biological activities of RNA tumor virus glycoproteins, including their antigenic determinants, interference properties, or ability to adsorb neutralizing antibodies, as shown by retention of these properties after removal of about 70% of the carbohydrate with a mixture of glycosidases (Bolognesi *et al.*, 1975; Schäfer *et al.*, 1977). However, indirect hemagglutination activity by the glycoprotein was inactivated by the glycosidase treatment.

3.9.2. Synthesis and Assembly of Envelope Components

3.9.2a. Identification of Viral Proteins in Infected Cells

Unlike many cytocidal viruses, productive infection by RNA tumor viruses occurs without marked effects on cellular biosynthesis, and virus-specific proteins compose a minor fraction of the proteins being synthesized in infected cells. Immunoprecipitation and gel electrophoresis have therefore been employed to detect newly synthesized radiolabeled viral proteins. In initial studies, it was demonstrated that the internal virion proteins are synthesized as a single precursor molecule which is subsequently cleaved to yield the virion structural proteins (Vogt and Eisenmann, 1973; Vogt *et al.*, 1975; Naso *et al.*, 1975; Van Zaane *et al.*, 1975). More recently, it has been demonstrated that the envelope proteins are also synthesized in the form of a precursor molecule. In the murine leukemia viruses, the major external proteins gp70 and p15(E) are found as a precursor of about 85,000 daltons (Famulari *et al.*, 1976; Naso *et al.*, 1976; Witte *et al.*, 1977). Antiserum to either gp70 or p15(E) could precipitate the precursor protein, and it was converted to the two virion proteins in pulse chase experiments. In cells infected with avian C-type particles, a 90,000-dalton precursor has been identified using antiserum to the virion glycoprotein gp85 (England *et al.*, 1977). In pulse-chase experiments, this precursor appears to be cleaved to yield both gp85 and gp37. It has also been reported that a 70,000-dalton precursor, thought to represent incompletely glycosylated gp85, could be identified in infected cells (Halpern *et al.*, 1974; Moelling and Hayami, 1977) but this species was not observed in other studies (England *et al.*, 1977).

Some information on the intracellular location of MuLV glycoproteins and their precursors has been obtained by Witte *et al.* (1977). The precursor glycoprotein was predominant in a high-density cytoplasmic membrane fraction, whereas fractions of lower density contained increasing amounts of gp70 and a component believed to be p15(E).

None of the precursor molecules appeared accessible to reagents which label the external surface of the cell, indicating that cleavage to yield gp70 occurred prior to or simultaneously with the appearance of the glycoproteins on the cell surface. The precursor glycoproteins also appear to lack an appreciable amount of sialic acid, which is added prior to arrival of glycoprotein on the cell surface. Studies of the kinetics of appearance of newly synthesized viral proteins into mature virions (Fleissner *et al.*, 1975; Witte and Weissman, 1976) have indicated that core proteins are incorporated rapidly into virions, whereas there is a significant delay before envelope glycoproteins are incorporated. This may reflect intracellular events involved in secondary modification and transport of the glycoproteins to the cell surface. Further, the results indicate that a large intracellular pool of glycoproteins is available for continued incorporation into virions over a long time period.

3.9.2b. Assembly and Maturation of Virions

Formation of progeny virions occurs by budding at the cell membrane. In contrast to most other virus groups, preformed nucleocapsid or core structures are not generally observed in the cytoplasm; rather, formation of the nucleocapsid occurs by a process of progressive enlargement as the budding particle emerges. Crescent-shaped core structures are observed during the process of budding. No information is available on the precise molecular interactions which occur during budding. A structural alteration in C-type viruses also occurs after their release from the infected cell, which involves condensation of the core structure and has been termed the "maturation process." Comparison of the RNA and polypeptide profiles of rapidly harvested virions with those obtained after longer intervals indicates differences in both the RNA and proteins (Canaani *et al.*, 1973; Cheung *et al.*, 1972). The mechanism and significance of this phenomenon is not understood; however, newly formed virions possess higher infectivity (Smith, 1974), indicating that the "maturation" process may not be beneficial for the virions.

3.9.2c. Assembly of Spikeless Particles

Both morphological and biochemical evidence has been obtained which demonstrates that spikeless particles lacking viral glycoproteins can be produced by cells infected with avian C-type virus mutants deficient in the gene coding for envelope protein (Scheele and Hanafusa, 1971; DeGiuli *et al.*, 1975; Halpern *et al.*, 1976). These observations indicate that glycoproteins are not required for assembly and release of progeny virus particles. It is, however, uncertain whether some portion of the spike is present in these particles. The particles thus obtained are noninfectious (Weiss, 1969; Hanafusa *et al.*, 1976) and appear similar to particles from which glycoproteins have been removed by proteolytic digestion. Formation of particles lacking glycoproteins has not been generally observed with other groups of enveloped viruses.

3.9.2d.   Effects of Inhibitors

The effects of several inhibitors of glycosylation on assembly and release of RNA tumor viruses have been described. Three inhibitors, glucosamine, 2-deoxy-D-glucose, and tunicamycin, have been employed; based on results with other viruses it is likely that only the last is completely effective in preventing glycosylation of virion glycoproteins. Glucosamine was observed to inhibit the release of infectious Rous sarcoma virus as well as physical particles as measured by [^{3}H]uridine incorporation (Hunter *et al.*, 1974). The effects of 2-deoxyglucose on Kirsten murine leukemia sarcoma virus also included inhibition of the formation of infectious progeny virions; however, release of physical particles did not appear to be impaired (Prochownik *et al.*, 1975). The protein components of such particles appeared to be markedly different from those of normal virions. Tunicamycin did not prevent the release of physical particles of Rous sarcoma virus and the resulting particles appeared to completely lack glycoproteins (Schwarz *et al.*, 1976), thus resembling the noninfectious spikeless particles produced by defective deletion mutants of RSV. These results support earlier observations indicating that glycoproteins are not required for the assembly process of C-type virus particles.

3.9.2e.   Aberrant Particles Produced by Virus Mutants

A temperature-sensitive mutant of RSV designated LA334 possesses a defect in replication which leads to the production of aberrant virus particles (Hunter and Vogt, 1976; Hunter *et al.*, 1976; Friis *et al.*, 1976; Rohrschneider *et al.*, 1976). The particles bud atypically and are more heterogeneous in size and density than wild-type virions. Evidence has been obtained that the defect in this mutant leads to aberrant cleavage of the precursor to the internal proteins of the virion (Hunter *et al.*, 1976; Rohrschneider *et al.*, 1976). However, immunoferritin staining of viral glycoproteins was also markedly reduced on the external surface of budding particles, suggesting that the alteration in internal proteins may affect the incorporation of glycoproteins into the viral membrane.

A number of physiologically distinct temperature-sensitive mutants of MuLV have been examined by electron microscopy (Yeger *et al.*, 1976), and the results indicate that the maturation process can be blocked at several discrete stages. These include mutants blocked at the stage of formation of a slight outfolding of the plasma membrane, with an underlying crescent of core material, and other mutants blocked at a point near the termination of the budding process in which an almost completely formed core can be seen. Other mutants produce complete virus particles of aberrant morphology. The precise definition of the biochemical lesions in these mutants should provide new insight into the events in C-type virus assembly.

3.10.   Togaviruses

3.10.1.   Classification, Morphology, Composition

The togaviridae family comprises four genera: alphavirus (previously known as arboviruses of group A), flavivirus (previously known as arboviruses of group B), rubivirus, and pestivirus. All alphaviruses and probably all flaviviruses multiply in arthropods as well as vertebrates.

Virions are spherical, with a diameter of 40–70 nm. They contain an icosahedral nucleocapsid that is surrounded by an envelope with spikes about 7 nm in length. Alphaviruses are composed of about 6% RNA, 60% protein, 6% carbohydrate, and 30% lipid (Pfefferkorn and Hunter, 1963a; Strauss *et al.*, 1970; Laine *et al.*, 1973).

Of the many members of the togavirus family, Semliki forest virus (SFV) and Sindbis virus have been studied in most detail as far as structure and replication are concerned. We will therefore concentrate here on these two viruses which are both alphaviruses. In addition, some data will be reported on flaviviruses.

3.10.2. Fine Structure and Arrangement of Envelope Components

The envelope of alphaviruses consists of a lipid layer studded with spikes that are composed of glycoproteins. There is a high degree of organization as shown by surface analysis of negatively stained Sindbis virus. Evidence has been obtained that the glycoproteins are organized as 240 trimers clustering in a $T = 4$ icosahedral surface lattice (von Bonsdorff and Harrison, 1975). Alphaviruses do not possess a carbohydrate-free membrane (M) protein at the inner side of the lipid bilayer as do other enveloped viruses, such as rhabdoviruses and myxoviruses. It is reasonable to assume that, with the alphaviruses, the function of the M protein is exerted by the core protein. Flavivirus, however, appears to contain a nonglycosylated envelope protein (MW $\sim$7000–9000) that might be comparable to the M protein (Table 4).

The togavirus envelope can be disintegrated by detergents, and the action of Triton X100, sodium dodecylsulfate, and sodium deoxycholate on SFV has been studied extensively. The solubilization process begins with binding of detergents to the virus, then it proceeds with increasing detergent concentration to lysis of the membrane, solubilization into lipid–protein–detergent complexes, and finally complete delipidization of the proteins (Helenius and Söderlund, 1973; Becker et al., 1975; Helenius et al., 1976). Thus the envelope proteins of SFV and Sindbis virus have been purified by chromatography on hydroxylapatite in the presence of SDS (Garoff et al., 1974) or on

TABLE 4

Envelope Proteins of Togaviruses

Alphaviruses		Flaviviruses	
Designation[a]	Molecular weight[b]	Designation[c]	Molecular weight[d]
E1	$\sim$50,000		
E2	$\sim$50,000	E	53,000–58,000
E3[e]	10,000		
——		M	7000

[a] Baltimore et al. (1976).
[b] Schlesinger et al. (1972), Garoff et al. (1974), Ivanic (1974), Pedersen et al. (1974).
[c] Trent (1977).
[d] Shapiro et al. (1971), Stollar (1969), Trent and Qureshi (1971), Westaway (1975), Westaway and Reedman (1969).
[e] Occurs only in SFV.

DEAE-cellulose in the presence of Triton X100 (Burke and Keegstra, 1976). Other isolation procedures employed preparative isoelectric focusing in the presence of Triton X100 (Dalrymple *et al.*, 1976) and sucrose gradient centrifugation in the presence of sodium deoxycholate (Helenius *et al.*, 1976).

3.10.2a. The Spikes

The spikes of togaviruses are composed of glycoproteins. Whereas flaviviruses contain only one glycoprotein, three species (E1, E2, E3) have been observed in alphaviruses (Table 4). E1 and E2, which both have molecular weights around 50,000, appear to be regularly present in the virion and have been observed with Eastern equine encephalitis, Semliki forest, Sindbis, Venezuelan equine encephalitis, and Western equine encephalitis viruses (Schlesinger *et al.*, 1972; Garoff *et al.*, 1974; Ivanic, 1974; Pedersen *et al.*, 1974). The smallest glycoprotein, E3 (MW ~10,000), which is highly glycosylated, has been observed only in SFV, not in other alphaviruses. Using cross-linking agents and immunoprecipitation with specific antisera, evidence has been obtained that the spike structure of SFV is a trimer containing one each of E1, E2, and E3 (Garoff, 1974).

That the glycoproteins form the spikes at the virus surface can be demonstrated by surface labeling techniques (Gahmberg *et al.*, 1972*a*; Sefton *et al.*, 1973), by treatment with proteolytic enzymes, which results in the formation of spikeless particles from which the glycoproteins have been removed (Calberg-Bacq and Osterrieth, 1966; Compans, 1971), and by the agglutinability of the virus with concanavalin A (Oram *et al.*, 1971; Birdwell and Strauss, 1973).

The envelope glycoproteins are amphipathic molecules. Whereas amino acid analysis of the whole glycoprotein does not show a significantly higher proportion of hydrophobic amino acids (Garoff *et al.*, 1974; Burke and Keegstra, 1976), evidence has been obtained for small hydrophobic regions. After proteolytic treatment of virions, these regions remain as fragments of the glycoproteins in the bilayer (Gahmberg *et al.*, 1972*b*). Both E1 and E2 contain such peptides, which are rich in hydrophobic amino acids (Utermann and Simons, 1974). Through these hydrophobic segments the isolated membrane glycoproteins are able to aggregate into star-shaped oligomers or rosettes (Mussgay and Rott, 1964; Simons *et al.*, 1973; Helenius and von Bonsdorff, 1976) and to bind detergents such as Triton X100 and deoxycholate (Helenius and Simons, 1972, 1975; Utermann and Simons, 1974; Becker *et al.*, 1975).

Through the hydrophobic segments, the spikes are anchored in the lipid bilayer. The fact that the SFV glycoproteins can be cross-linked to the nucleocapsid by dimethyl suberimidate suggests that at least one of the glycoproteins spans the bilayer (Garoff and Simons, 1974). Treatment of Sindbis virus with formaldehyde results in cross-linking of envelope proteins to the nucleocapsid, suggesting that with this virus the glycoproteins span the lipid layer, too (Brown *et al.*, 1974).

The carbohydrate moieties of the SFV and Sindbis virus glycoproteins have been isolated after pronase digestion and their sugar composition has been determined (Burge and Huang, 1970; Burge and Strauss, 1970; Strauss *et al.*, 1970; Sefton and Keegstra, 1974; Keegstra *et al.*, 1975; Burke and Keegstra, 1976; Mattila *et al.*, 1976). Side chains of type A (nomenclature of Johnson and Clamp, 1971), containing glucosamine, mannose, galactose, fucose and neuraminic acid, and side chains of type B, containing only glucosamine and mannose, have been found. E1 and E2 of Sindbis virus contain one A-type and one B-type side chain while SFV contains one or two A-type side chains in E1 and E3, and one A- and two or three B-type chains in E2.

Sequential degradation of the oligosaccharide side chains with exo- and endoglycosidases has been carried out, and the structures for the A chains of SFV which appear to be heterogenous have been deduced (Pesonen and Renkonen, 1976; Renkonen *et al.*, 1976). The largest A chains are present on E3 and appear to be to be the most exposed ones on the intact virus, because they react most readily with neuraminidase and galactose oxidase (Luukkonen *et al.*, 1977a). With Sindbis virus, the A-type oligosaccharide of E2 appears to be the most exposed one, because it is the only side chain which can be removed by glycosidase treatment of intact virions (McCarthy and Harrison, 1977).

Virions which lack neuraminic acid in their envelope proteins, either after enzymatic removal or when grown in mosquito cells, retain their infectivity and hemagglutinating activity (Kennedy, 1974; Stollar *et al.*, 1976). Even the subterminal glucosamine and galactose residues may be lacking without decreased biological activity, suggesting that the glucosamine–mannose core of the A-type oligosaccharide is sufficient for these activities (Schlesinger *et al.*, 1976).

The available evidence indicates that the primary polypeptide structure of the envelope proteins determines the number and type of the oligosaccharide chains, which are added, however, by cellular enzymes (Burge and Huang, 1970; Grimes and Bruge, 1971; Sefton,

1976). Thus there are host-dependent variations in the oligosaccharides (Keegstra *et al.*, 1975; Schlesinger *et al.*, 1976; Stollar *et al.*, 1976).

3.10.2b. The Lipid Bilayer

Thirty-seven percent of the alphavirus envelope consists of lipids (Laine *et al.*, 1973). The main components are phospholipid and cholesterol. The lipids are derived from the host cell (Pfefferkorn and Hunter, 1963*b*), and the composition resembles that of the plasma membrane of the host (Renkonen *et al.*, 1971, 1972*a,b*). This is true also for the fatty acid composition within the different phospholipid classes (Laine *et al.*, 1972) and for the glycolipids (Renkonen *et al.*, 1971; Hirshberg and Robbins, 1974). The host-dependent lipid variation is particularly striking when virions grown in mammalian and mosquito cells are compared. There was nearly 50% change in phospholipid head group composition, and an even larger overall change if the nature of the linkage between the hydrocarbon chain and the glycerol moieties was also taken into account (Luukkonen *et al.*, 1976). Further, cholesterol is present in 5–6 times higher amounts in SFV from BHK than from mosquito cells, although the ratio of phospholipid to protein is similar in particles from both sources (Luukkonen *et al.*, 1977*b*). The stability of the virion may depend to some extent on the lipid composition (Sly *et al.*, 1976).

The lipids in the alphavirus envelope form a bilayer as demonstrated by X-ray diffraction studies on Sindbis virus (Harrison *et al.*, 1971). Electron spin resonance studies also indicated a bilayer structure (Sefton and Gaffney, 1974). The bilayer appears to be asymmetrical. Treatment of SFV from mosquito cells with a nonpenetrating reagent suggested that the outer layer possessed relatively more ceramide phosphoethanolamine and less phosphatidylethanolamine than the inner layer (Luukkonen *et al.*, 1976). Furthermore, neuraminidase treatment of intact and spikeless particles of Sindbis virus completely removed neuraminic acid from gangliosides, demonstrating that these were present exclusively on the outer surface of the viral bilayer (Stoffel and Sorgo, 1976).

Less than 10% of the bilayer is occupied by the penetrating segment of the envelope glycoproteins (Harrison *et al.*, 1971). Nevertheless, the envelope proteins appear to stabilize the organization of the lipids in the bilayer, since the microviscosity is higher in the presence of the envelope proteins or hydrophobic fragments than in liposomes made of viral lipids or in cell membranes (Sefton and Gaffney, 1974; Hughes and Pedersen, 1975; Moore *et al.*, 1976).

3.10.3. Biogenesis and Assembly of the Envelope

The structural proteins of alphavirus are translated from 26 S mRNA (Cancedda *et al.*, 1974*b*; Clegg and Kennedy, 1974*b*, 1975*a,b,c*; Simmons and Strauss, 1974*b*; Wengler *et al.*, 1974; Glanville *et al.*, 1976*a*). The 26 S RNA polysomes are membrane bound (Kennedy, 1972; Wirth *et al.*, 1977), as is the synthesis of structural proteins (Friedman, 1968*a*). The structural proteins appear to be translated as a polyprotein with a molecular weight of 130,000–140,000 (Schlesinger and Schlesinger, 1973; Keränen and Kääriäinen, 1975; Lachmi *et al.*, 1975; Kaluza, 1976; Kaluza *et al.*, 1976). Evidence has been obtained with SFV by sequential labeling that the core protein is translated first followed by the envelope proteins in the order E3, E2, and E1 (Clegg, 1975; Clegg and Kennedy, 1975*b,c*; Lachmi and Kääriäinen, 1976).

The capsid protein is cleaved from the nascent polyprotein *in vivo* (Burke, 1975; Strauss and Strauss, 1976) and *in vitro* (Cancedda *et al.*, 1974*a,b*; Clegg and Kennedy, 1974*b*; Wengler *et al.*, 1974; Glanville and Ulmanen, 1976), probably immediately after the ribosome has finished the translation of the sequences coding for capsid protein (Clegg, 1975; Söderlund, 1976). The cleavage enzyme might be virus specific, as suggested by mixed infection experiments with Sindbis *ts* mutants (Scupman *et al.*, 1977). The cleavage between the envelope proteins takes place at a time when most of the polyprotein has been translated (Söderlund, 1976). The products of this cleavage are the envelope protein E1 and a common precursor to E2 and E3 (MW 62,000–68,000) designated "p62," "NSP68," "NVP68," or "PE2" (Schlesinger and Schlesinger, 1973; Simons *et al.*, 1973*b*; Garoff *et al.*, 1974; Lachmi *et al.*, 1975).

The envelope proteins are transferred from the endoplasmic reticulum to the plasma membrane and finally into released virus (Richardson and Vance, 1976). In the plasma membrane the envelope proteins of Sindbis virus can be demonstrated as early as 2 hr after infection (Birdwell and Strauss, 1974). Studies with *ts* mutants of Sindbis virus suggest that both E1 and PE2 are incorporated into the plasma membrane, where subsequently cleavage of PE2 takes place. In wild-type virus, cleavage of PE2 can be prevented by antiserum against E1, suggesting that both glycoproteins are closely associated with each other at the outside of the plasma membrane (Bracha and Schlesinger, 1976b; Smith and Brown, 1977).

Valuable information on glycosylation mechanisms has been obtained from studies in which this reaction has been blocked. In the presence of specific inhibitors such as 2-deoxy-D-glucose (Kaluza et al., 1973; Scholtissek et al., 1975; Schmidt et al., 1976), D-glucosamine (Duda and Schlesinger, 1975), 2-fluorohexoses (Schmidt et al., 1976), and tunicamycin (Schwarz et al., 1976; Leavitt et al., 1977; Ogura et al., 1977) and in glucose-free medium (Kaluza, 1975), the envelope glycoproteins and their immediate precursors are synthesized in an unglycosylated form. Studies on Sindbis virus have shown that, after release of the block, carbohydrate is not attached to these unglycosylated polypeptides. Furthermore, under normal conditions unglycosylated Sindbis virus glycoproteins are not found in the infected cell. From these and other observations it has been concluded that glycosylation is initiated on the nascent polypeptide chain before release from the polysomes (Sefton, 1977). However, glycosylation appears to take place after cleavage of E1 and PE2, since the common precursor of both proteins (MW ~100,000) (Strauss et al., 1969; Schlesinger and Schlesinger, 1973) has been reported to be carbohydrate free (Sefton and Burge, 1973). This first step of glycosylation probably involves the transfer of the cores of the oligosaccharides consisting of glucosamine and mannose (MW ~1800) (Sefton, 1977) from a lipid intermediate to the polypeptide as suggested by glycosylation studies in a cell-free system (Krag and Robbins, 1977). Similar results have also been obtained by in vitro glycosylation of SFV proteins (Schwarz et al., 1978b).

The addition of the distal sugars such as glucosamine, galactose, and neuraminic acid takes place later after about 20 min (Sefton, 1977). At this stage part of the the mannose residues are probably removed from the "core" before addition of the distal sugars (Sefton and Burge, 1973).

The unglycosylated form of the precursor p62 is metabolically stable. A possible explanation for this observation is that cleavage requires proper glycosylation (Kaluza, 1975, 1976). Antibodies specified against the envelope glycoproteins react readily with the glycosylated precursor p62, but only poorly with its unglycosylated form. Thus glycosylation appears to be necessary for the proper antigenic configuration of the glycoprotein (Kaluza, 1976).

Little is known about the biosynthesis of the envelope proteins of flaviviruses. Tentative evidence for posttranslational processing has been presented in the case of the glycoprotein of Kunjin virus, but the nature of this processing is unclear (Westaway and Shaw, 1977).

3.10.4. Morphogenesis of the Envelope

In mammalian cells alphaviruses mature usually by budding from the plasma membrane (Acheson and Tamm, 1967; Erlandson *et al.*, 1967; Bykovsky *et al.*, 1969; Waite *et al.*, 1972). Prior to budding the nucleocapsid aligns under the plasma membrane. It has been proposed that because of transmembrane interaction between the glycoproteins and the core protein the spikes are arrested in patches, whereas host proteins are excluded from these areas by lateral movement, and that this mechanism initiates budding (Garoff and Simons, 1974). The interaction between spikes and nucleocapsid cannot be highly specific, since phenotypic mixing occurs with alphaviruses (Burge and Pfefferkorn, 1966; Lagwinska *et al.*, 1975).

In mosquito cells alphaviruses mature at intracellular membranes by budding into vacuoles, which release the virus particles into the medium by fusing with the cell membrane (Whitfield *et al.*, 1971; Gliedman *et al.*, 1975).

Flavivirus are usually found in association with internal membranes of the infected cells. However, there is conclusive evidence neither that this is the site of assembly nor that assembly takes place by budding (for references, see Schlesinger, 1977).

3.10.5. Biological Activities of the Envelope

Alphaviruses and flaviviruses have hemagglutinating capacity (Clarke and Casals, 1958). Titrations are usually carried out on goose erythrocytes. It is reasonable to assume that the spikes are responsible for this activity. This has been demonstrated with Sindbis virus and SFV, where hemagglutinating activity was found to be associated specifically with glycoprotein E1 (Dalrymple *et al.*, 1976; Helenius *et al.*, 1976). Also in Venezuelan equine encephalitis virus the hemagglutinin seems to be only one of the envelope proteins (Pederson and Eddy, 1974).

Flaviviruses, particularly primary isolates of dengue virus, induce significant fusion and syncytium formation in cultures of *Aedes albopictus* cells (Paul *et al.*, 1969). This effect occurs several days after infection and therefore represents fusion from within. Thus fusion appears to depend on membrane alterations occurring late in infection and might be associated with incorporation of viral glycoproteins into the cell membrane. Similar observations have been made in another togavirus which appears to be neither an alpha- nor a flavivirus (Igarashi *et al.*, 1976).

4. CONCLUSIONS

4.1. Viral Membrane Structure

Recent models of membrane structure include the fluid lipid bilayer–globular protein mosaic in which membrane proteins are free to migrate in the plane of the membrane, as well as models in which extensive lateral interaction between protein subunits fixes the location of these proteins in the membrane. The general features of the fluid mosaic model have been supported by morphological, biochemical, and biophysical observations on various membrane systems. Knowledge concerning the composition and arrangement of membrane components of lipid-containing viruses has emerged in parallel with similar studies on cellular membranes. Aspects of both a fluid mosaic model and protein subunit model apply to some features of viral envelope structures. Viral envelopes possess a lipid membrane with glycoproteins and glycolipids exposed on the external surface and carbohydrate-free proteins in the interior. Cell surface membranes are similar in asymmetry with respect to localization of all carbohydrate constituents on the external surfaces. Viral glycoproteins appear to be amphipathic globular proteins, as have been proposed in the fluid mosaic model for cellular membrane glycoproteins. Recently evidence has been obtained for asymmetrical distribution of various phospholipid classes between the internal and external sides of the bilayer in both cellular and viral membranes. Amine-containing phospholipids are preferentially located on the internal surface and phosphatidylcholine and sphingomyelin on the external surface. The origin of this asymmetry is an interesting problem for future investigation.

A variety of biophysical methods, including X-ray diffraction, electron spin resonance, nuclear magnetic resonance, differential calorimetry, and fluorescence polarization spectroscopy have been applied to analyze the structure of the lipid phase of viral and cellular membranes. The results have indicated that a lipid bilayer structure is universally present as the fundamental matrix of all biological membranes. The fluidity of viral lipids, as indicated by spin label probes, appears to be significantly less than that of corresponding host cell membranes or vesicles prepared from extracted viral lipids. These observations, along with data indicating that viral membrane fluidity is affected only slightly by variation in glycoprotein content or by proteolytic digestion of the surface glycoproteins, have suggested that internal membrane proteins (M proteins) are primary determinants of viral membrane rigidity in myxoviruses, paramyxoviruses, and rhabdoviruses. The M proteins of these viruses are major proteins that appear to form a continuous layer of protein subunits on the internal surface of the lipid bilayer. Interactions between M proteins and viral nucleocapsids (and probably viral glycoproteins as well) are undoubtedly important features in the specificity of viral membrane assembly.

An important distinction is made in the fluid mosaic model between "peripheral" and "integral" membrane proteins, which differ with respect to their modes of interaction with the lipid bilayer. Integral proteins are those considered to be at least partially embedded in the lipid phase and to be associated with membranes by strong hydrophobic interactions. Generally they are not dissociated from membranes unless drastic conditions such as detergent treatment are used. Peripheral proteins appear to be associated with the surface of the membrane, possibly by electrostatic interactions, and are dissociated by conditions such as changes in ionic strength or use of chelating agents. Viral glycoproteins generally appear to be integral membrane proteins with a strong hydrophobic association with the bilayer. Evidence for partial penetration of the bilayer by a hydrophobic segment of the glycoprotein has been obtained for certain viruses, in which residual hydrophobic peptides remain associated with the lipid phase after extensive proteolytic digestion. Individual virus groups may differ in this respect, however. The major glycoprotein of C-type retroviruses appears more loosely associated with the bilayer, being released by procedures such as osmotic shock or freezing and thawing. The precise nature of the interaction of internal viral membrane (M) proteins with the bilayer has not been investigated. These proteins may resemble cellular proteins which associate with the cytoplasmic surfaces of the membranes, such as the protein termed "spectrin" on the inner surface of the erythrocyte which has properties of a peripheral membrane protein. Spectrin forms fibrous aggregates, and similar structures are seen with isolated viral M proteins. Such proteins may be involved in transmembrane interactions with surface glycoproteins, and phenomena such as antibody- or lectin-mediated patching or capping of surface glycoproteins are therefore influenced by such internal membrane proteins.

It is evident from the above comments that viral envelopes and cellular membranes are similar with respect to important features of the arrangement and properties of molecular components. Certain aspects of viral membrane structure may differ from the fluid mosaic model of cellular plasma membrane organization, however. The ability of certain cell surface proteins to undergo lateral diffusion in the plane of the membrane is a well-established and important finding in support of the fluid mosaic model. Whether viral membrane proteins are able to

undergo such lateral diffusion is uncertain in the case of surface glycoproteins, and unlikely in the case of M proteins because of their location in a tightly packed layer, probably with extensive lateral interaction. Whether virion glycoproteins may be restricted in lateral mobility
because of transmembrane interactions with internal proteins has not
been firmly established for most virus groups.

It is likely that extensive lateral protein–protein interactions may
also occur in specialized regions of cellular membranes, such as junc-
tional complexes. Such interactions could occur at three levels:
extracellularly, on the internal side of the bilayer, or in the hydrocarbon
phase. No evidence has been obtained for the latter type of interaction
between viral membrane proteins, and the available data from
proteolytic digestion of glycoproteins and freeze fracture electron
microscopy suggest that it is unlikely that enough protein is present in
the hydrocarbon phase for such interaction. Lateral interactions
between envelope proteins may occur predominantly on the external
surface of the virion for viruses in which glycoproteins comprise a
large percentage of the total structural protein (e.g., togaviruses,
bunyaviruses), whereas with other groups such as the myxo- and
paramyxoviruses such interactions may occur at the level of the M protein on the internal surface of the bilayer.

4.2. Biogenesis and Assembly of the Envelope

The envelopes of many viruses are assembled on preformed
cellular membranes. In most instances assembly takes place by budding
from the plasma membrane, although occasionally other cellular
membranes serve as budding sites. Envelope maturation is a multistep
process involving sequential incorporation of viral proteins into cellular
membranes.

Viral glycoproteins are always bound to cellular membranes; they
do not appear free in the cytoplasm. Translation takes place on the
rough endoplasmic reticulum, and there is some evidence suggesting
that a "signal sequence" at the N terminus of the nascent polypeptide
chain directs attachment of the polyribosome to specific structures in
the endoplasmic reticulum, which in turn facilitate transmembrane
passage of the polypeptide into the lumen of the canaliculi. Subsequently the glycoproteins migrate via smooth endoplasmic reticulum
and Golgi complex to the plasma membrane, where budding takes
place. In the course of migration the polypeptides undergo posttranslational modifications, such as glycosylation and proteolytic cleavage.

The biosynthesis of the carbohydrate side chains of the glycoproteins occurs in a stepwise manner, with different saccharide residues added in distinct cellular compartments. Glycosylation is initiated at the rough endoplasmic reticulum on the nascent polypeptide chain as has been observed first with influenza virus and subsequently with toga and rhabdoviruses. The available evidence indicates that, at this stage, oligosaccharides containing glucosamine and mannose are transferred *en bloc* from a polyisoprenol derivative to the polypeptide. Fucose, galactose, and neuraminic acid appear to be attached later after migration of the glycoprotein to the smooth endoplasmic reticulum and the Golgi apparatus. The process of glycosylation does not appear to play an important role in determining the intracellular migration of viral glycoproteins. Although this has been suggested as a possible function for carbohydrate components of glycoproteins, the available data using inhibitors of glycosylation suggest that, at least with myxo- and oncornaviruses, it is possible to inhibit the glycosylation process without preventing the migration of the glycoproteins to the cell surface. The glycosylation site and the type of the carbohydrate side chains appear to be determined by the primary structure of the polypeptide. On the other hand, the side chain may exhibit host-dependent variations. Host-specific carbohydrate sequences may in turn be modified by virus-specific enzymes, such as the myxovirus neuraminidase. Thus the carbohydrate moiety of viral glycoproteins is the result of a complex interaction of virus- and host-specific factors.

Formation of precursors that are subsequently cleaved by proteolysis appears to be a fairly common event in the biogenesis of the envelope glycoproteins. Cleavage is involved in the processing of the influenza hemagglutinin, of both paramyxovirus glycoproteins, of the envelope glycoproteins of togaviruses, and of the envelope proteins of oncornaviruses. It is particularly interesting that cleavage was always found to be paralleled by induction of biological activity, if it was possible to obtain the precursor relatively free of its cleavage products. This has been observed with both glycoproteins of paramyxoviruses and with the hemagglutinin of influenza virus. With myxoviruses it could be demonstrated that strain-specific differences exist in the susceptibility of the glycoproteins to proteolytic enzymes. Furthermore, circumstantial evidence has been obtained that these enzymes are host-specific proteases and that a given protease may be present in some host cells but not in others. Thus proteolytic cleavage depends on the structure of the viral glycoprotein as determined by the viral genome as well as on the disposition of the appropriate enzyme by the host. It has also been shown that activation by proteolytic cleavage may be an important factor in determining host range and pathogenicity of a virus.

One of the final steps in envelope assembly appears to be the insertion of a carbohydrate-free protein such as the M protein of myxo- and rhabdoviruses or the core protein of alphaviruses. The M protein was found to be incorporated immediately after its synthesis into regions of the plasma membrane which already contain viral glycoproteins. The mechanism by which M recognizes such areas might be interaction with the glycoproteins that penetrate the membrane. However, so far only with some viruses reasonable evidence has been obtained that the glycoproteins span the membrane. Also, the interaction between the proteins cannot be very specific, since phenotypic mixing occurs between the envelope proteins of viruses belonging to a large variety of groups. An important feature of the assembly of the virus is that during the budding process the membrane of the viral envelope is continuous with and morphologically similar to the plasma membrane of the host cell. This suggests that the lipids in the unaltered plasma membrane area easily exchangeable by lateral diffusion with those in the budding virus particle. It is therefore not surprising that the lipids in the envelopes closely resemble those of the host cell membrane. There is thus good evidence that the viral envelope is derived from a patch of plasma membrane modified by the incorporation of virus-specific proteins. Little is known about the mechanism by which host proteins are excluded from this area. The budding process itself is not fully understood, either. However, the observation that budding does not occur under conditions where all envelope components are synthesized except the M protein suggests that this protein plays an important role.

ACKNOWLEDGMENTS

Research by R. W. C. was supported by Grants No. AI12680 and CA18611 from the USPHS, PCM78-09207 from the National Science Foundation, and VC149C from the American Cancer Society. Research by H.-D. K. was supported by the Deutsche Forschungsgemeinschaft (Sonderforschungsbereich 47, Virologie).

We are grateful to Janet K. Shafiey for invaluable assistance in preparing the manuscript.

We thank Dr. R. Rott for a critical reading of the manuscript, and Drs. M. Kemp and R. Friis for helpful comments. We also thank Drs. J. T. August, D. P. Bolognesi, E. Fleissner, J. Lenard, R. W. Schlesinger, and P. Spear for reprints and preprints of their publications.

5. REFERENCES

Abodeely, R. A., Palmer, E., Lawson, L. A., and Randall, C. C., 1971, The proteins of enveloped and de-enveloped equine abortion (herpes) virus and the separated envelope, *Virology* **44**:146.

Acheson, N. H., and Tamm, I., 1976, Replication of Semliki Forest virus: An electron microscopic study, *Virology* **32**:123.

Ada, G. L., and Perry, B. T., 1954, The nucleic acid content of influenza virus, *Aust. J. Exp. Biol. Med. Sci.* **32**:453.

Ada, G. L., and Yap, K. L., 1977, Matrix protein expressed at the surface of cells infected with influenza viruses, *Immunochemistry* **14**:643.

Allen, A. K., Skehel, J. J., and Yuferov, V., 1977, The amino acid and carbohydrate composition of the neuraminidase of B/Lee/40 influenza virus, *J. Gen. Virol.* **37**:625.

Almeida, J. D., and Waterson, A. P., 1970, Two morphological aspects of influenza virus, in: *The Biology of Large RNA Viruses* (R. D. Barry and B. W. J. Mahy, eds.), pp. 27–51, Academic Press, New York.

Anderson, R., and Dales, S., 1978, Biogenesis of poxviruses: Glycolipid metabolism in vaccinia-infected cells. *Virology* **84**:108.

Anon, M. C., Grau, O., Martinez Segovia, Z. M., and Franze-Ferandez, M. T., 1976, RNA composition of Junin virus, *J. Virol.* **18**:833.

Apostolov, K., and Almeida, J. D., 1972, Interaction of Sendai (HVJ) virus with human erythrocytes: A morphological study of haemolysis and cell fusion, *J. Gen. Virol.* **15**:227.

Apostolov, K., and Flewett, T. H., 1969, Further observations on the structure of influenza viruses A and C, *J. Gen. Virol.* **4**:365.

Apostolov, K., Flewett, T. H., and Kendall, A. P., 1970, Morphology of influenza A, B, C, and infectious bronchitis virus (IBV) virions and their replication, in: *The Biology of Large RNA Viruses* (R. D. Barry and B. W. J. Mahy, eds.), pp. 3–26, Academic Press, New York.

Arstila, P., 1972, Two hemagglutinating components of vesicular stomatitis virus, *Acta Pathol. Microbiol. Scand.* **80**:33.

Arstila, P., 1973, Small-sized hemagglutinin of vesicular stomatitis virus released spontaneously with Nonidet P40, *Acta Pathol. Microbiol. Scand.* **81**:27.

Arstila, P., Halonen, P. E., and Salmi, G., 1969, Hemagglutinin of vesicular stomatitis virus, *Arch. Ges. Virusforsch.* **27**:198.

Atanasiu, P., Tsiang, H., Perrin, P., Favre, S., and Sisman, J., 1974, Extraction d'un antigène soluble (glycoprotéine) par le Triton X100, *Ann. Microbiol.* **125B**:539.

August, J. T., Bolognesi, D. T., Fleissner, E., Gilden, R. V., and Nowinski, R., 1974, A proposed nomenclature for the virion proteins of oncogenic RNA viruses, *Virology* **60**:595.

Bächi, T., Gerhard, W., Lindenmann, J., and Mühlethaler, K., 1969, Morphogenesis of influenza A virus in Ehrlich ascites tumor cells as revealed by thin-sectioning and freeze-etching, *J. Virol.* **4**:769.

Bächi, T., Deas, J. E., and Howe, C., 1977, Virus–erythrocyte interactions, in: *Virus Infection and the Cell Surface*, Vol. 2 of *Cell Surface Reviews* (G. Poste and G. L. Nicolson, eds.), pp. 83–128, North-Holland, Amsterdam.

Bader, J. P., 1974, Reproduction of RNA tumor viruses, *Comp. Virol.* **4**:253.

Baltimore, D., Burke, D. C., Horzinek, M. C., Huang, A. S., Kääriäinen, L., Pfefferkorn, E. R., Schlesinger, M. J., Schlesinger, S., Schlesinger, R. W., and Scholtissek, C., 1976, Proposed nomenclature for alphavirus polypeptides, *J. Gen. Virol.* **30**:273.

Barenholz, Y., Moore, N. F., and Wagner, R. R., 1976, Enveloped viruses as model membrane systems: Microviscosity of vesicular stomatitis virus and host cell membranes, *Biochemistry* **15**:3563.

Bauer, H., 1974, Virion and tumor cell antigens of C-type RNA tumor viruses, *Adv. Cancer Res.* **20**:273.

Becht, H., Hämmerling, U., and Rott, R., 1977, Undisturbed release of influenza virus in the presence of univalent antineuraminidase antibodies, *Virology* **46**:337.

Becht, H., Rott, R., and Klenk, H.-D., 1972, Effect of concanavalin A on cells infected with enveloped viruses, *J. Gen. Virol.* **14**:1.

Becker, R., Helenius, A., and Simons, K., 1975, Solubilization of the Semliki Forest virus membrane with sodium dodecyl sulfate, *Biochemistry* **14**:1835.

Ben Porat, T., and Kaplan, A. S., 1971, Phospholipid metabolism of herpesvirus-infected and uninfected rabbit kidney cells, *Virology* **45**:252.

Ben Porat, T., and Kaplan, A. S., 1972, Studies on the biogenesis of herpesvirus envelope, *Nature (London)* **235**:165.

Biddison, W. E., Doherty, P. C., and Webster, R. G., 1977, *J. Exp. Med.* **146**:690.

Bingham, R. W., 1975, The polypeptide composition of avian infectious bronchitis virus, *Arch. Virol.* **49**:207.

Birdwell, C. R., and Strauss, J. H., 1973, Agglutination of Sindbis virus and of cells infected with Sindbis virus by plant lectins, *J. Virol.* **11**:502.

Birdwell, C. R., and Strauss, J. H., 1974, Replication of Sindbis virus. IV. Electron microscope study of the insertion of viral glycoproteins into the surface of infected chick cells, *J. Virol.* **14**:366.

Bishop, D. H. L., Repik, P., Obijeski, J. F., Moore, N. F., and Wagner, R. R., 1975, Restitution of infectivity to spikeless vesicular stomatitis virus by solubilized viral components, *J. Virol.* **16**:75.

Bittman, R., Majuk, Z., Honig, D. S., Compans, R. W., and Lenard, J., 1976, Permeability properties of the membrane of vesicular stomatitis virions, *Biochim. Biophys. Acta.* **433**:63.

Blobel, G., and Dobberstein, B., 1975, Transfer of proteins across membranes. I. Presence of proteolytically processed and unprocessed nascent immunoglobulin light chains on membrane-bound ribosomes of murine myeloma, *J. Cell Biol.* **67**:835.

Blough, H. A., 1974, Newly synthesized lipids incorporated into influenza virus membranes, *Nature (London)* **251**:333.

Blough, H. A., and Lawson, D. E. M., 1968, The lipids of paramyxoviruses: A comparative study of Sendai and Newcastle disease virus, *Virology* **36**:286.

Blough, H. A., and Merlie, J., 1970, The lipids of incomplete influenza virus, *Virology* **40**:685.

Blough, H. A., and Tiffany, J. M., 1973, Lipids in viruses, *Adv. Lipid Res.* **11**:267.

Blough, H. A., and Weinstein, D. B., 1973, Effect of influenza virus infection on lipid metabolism and chick embryo fibroblasts, in: *Biology of the Fibroblast* (E. Kulonen and J. Pikkarainen, eds.), pp. 303–308, Academic Press, London.

Blough, H. A., Weinstein, D. B., Lawson, D. E. M., and Kodicek, E., 1967, *Virology* **33**:459.

Bolognesi, D. P., 1974, Structural components of RNA tumor viruses, *Adv. Virus Res.* **19**:315.

Bolognesi, D. P., Bauer, H., Gelderblom, H., and Huper, G., 1972, Polypeptides of avian RNA tumor viruses. IV. Components of the viral envelope, *Virology* **47**:551.

Bolognesi, D. P., Luftig, R., and Shapper, J. H., 1973, Localization of RNA tumor virus polypeptides. I. Isolation of further virus substructures, *Virology* **56**:549.

Bolognesi, D. P., Collins, J. J., Leis, J. P., Moennig, V., Schäfer, W., and Atkinson, P. H., 1975, Role of carbohydrate in determining the immunochemical properties of the major glycoproteins (gp71) of Friend murine leukemia viruses, *J. Virol.* **16**:1453.

Bouloy, M., Krams-Czden, S., Horodmiceanu, F., and Hannoun, C., 1974, Three-segment RNA genome of Lumbo virus (bunyavirus), *Intervirology* **2**:173.

Bracha, M., and Schlesinger, M. J., 1976, Defects in RNA$^+$ temperature-sensitive mutants of Sindbis virus and evidence for a complex of PE2-E1 viral glycoproteins, *Virology* **74**:441.

Braciale, T. J., 1977, Immunologic recognition of influenza virus-infected cells. II. Expression of influenza A matrix protein on the infected cell surface and its role in recognition by cross-reactive cytotoxic T cells, *J. Exp. Med.* **146**:673.

Brand, C. M., and Skehel, J. J., 1972, Crystalline antigen from the influenza virus envelope, *Nature (London) New Biol.* **238**:145.

Brennen, J. P., Steiner, S. M., Courtney, P. J., and Skelly, J., 1976, Metabolism of galactose in herpes simplex virus-infected cells, *Virology* **69**:216.

Bretscher, M., 1972, Asymmetrical lipid bilayer structure for biological membranes, *Nature (London) New Biol.* **236**:11.

Bretscher, M., 1973, Membrane structure: Some general principles, *Science* **181**:622.

Brown, F., Smale, C. J., and Horzinek, M. C., 1974, Lipid protein organization in vesicular stomatitis and Sindbis viruses, *J. Gen. Virol.* **22**:455.

Bubbers, J. E., and Lilly, F., 1977, Selective incorporation of H-2 antigenic determinants into Friend virus particles, *Nature (London)* **266**:459.

Bucher, D. J., and Kilbourne, E. D., 1972, A$_2$(N$_2$) neuraminidase of the X-7 influenza virus recombinant: Determination of molecular size and subunit composition of the active unit, *J. Virol.* **10**:60.

Bucher, D., and Palese, P., 1975, The biologically active proteins of influenza virus: Neuraminidase, in: *The Influenza Virus and Influenza* (E. D. Kilbourne, ed.), p. 83, Academic Press, New York.

Buchmeier, M. J., Gee, S. R., and Rawls, W. E., 1977, Antigens of Pichinde virus. I. Relationship of soluble antigens derived from infected BHK-21 cells to the structural components of the virion, *J. Virol.* **22**:175.

Burge, B. W., and Huang, A. S., 1970, Comparison of membrane protein glycopeptides of Sindbis virus and vesicular stomatitis virus, *J. Virol.* **6**:176.

Burge, B. W., and Pfefferkorn, E. R., 1966, Phenotypic mixing between group A arboviruses, *Nature (London)* **210**:1397.

Burge, B. W., and Strauss, J. H., 1970, Glycopeptides of the membrane glycoprotein of Sindbis virus, *J. Mol. Biol.* **47**:449.

Burke, D. C., 1975, Processing of alphavirus proteins in infected cells, *Med. Biol.* **53**:352.

Burke, D. J., and Keegstra, K., 1976, Purification and composition of the proteins from Sindbis virus grown in chick and BHK cells, *J. Virol.* **20**:676.

Bussell, R. H., Waters, D. J., Seals, M. K., and Robinson, W. S., 1974, Measles, canine distemper and respiratory syncytial virions and nucleocapsids: A comparative study of their structure polypeptide and nucleic acid composition, *Med. Microbiol. Immunol.* **160**:105.

Bykovsky, A. F., Yershov, F. I., and Zhdanov, V. M., 1969, Morphogenesis of Venezuelan equine encephalomyelitis virus, *J. Virol.* **4**:496.

Calberg-Bacq, C. M., and Osterrieth, P. M., 1966, Morphological modifications of Semliki Forest virus after treatment with pronase, *Acta Virol. Prague* **10**:266.

Caliguiri, L. A., Klenk, H.-D., and Choppin, P. W., 1969, The proteins of the parainfluenza virus SV5. I. Separation of virion polypeptides by polyacrylamide gel electrophoresis, *Virology* **39**:460.

Canaani, E., Helm, K. V. D., and Duesberg, P., 1973, Evidence for 30–40 S RNA as precursor of the 60–70 S RNA of Rous sarcoma virus, *Proc. Natl. Acad. Sci. USA* **70**:401.

Cancedda, R., Swanson, R., and Schlesinger, M. J., 1974a, Effects of different RNAs and components of the cell-free system on in vitro synthesis of Sindbis viral proteins, *J. Virol.* **14**:652.

Cancedda, R., Swanson, R., and Schlesinger, M. J., 1974b, Viral proteins formed in a cell-free rabbit reticulocyte system programmed with RNA from a temperature-sensitive mutant of Sindbis virus, *J. Virol.* **14**:664.

Carter, M. F., Biswal, N., and Rawls, W. E., 1973, Characterization of the nucleic acid of Pichinde virus, *J. Virol.* **11**:61.

Cartwright, B., Talbot, P., and Brown, F., 1970, The proteins of biologically active subunits of vesicular stomatitis virus, *J. Gen. Virol.* **7**:267.

Cassai, E. N., Sarmiento, M., and Spear, P. G., 1975, Comparison of the virion proteins specified by herpes simplex virus types 1 and 2, *J. Virol.* **16**:1327.

Chang, A., and Metz, D. H., 1976, Further investigations on the mode of entry of vaccinia virus into cells, *J. Gen. Virol.* **32**:275.

Chen, C., Compans, R. W., and Choppin, P. W., 1971, Parainfluenza virus surface projections: Glycoproteins with hemagglutinin and neuraminidase activities, *J. Gen. Virol.* **11**:53.

Cheung, K. S., Smith, R. E., Stone, M. P., and Joklik, W. K., 1972, Comparison of immature (rapid harvest) and mature Rous sarcoma virus particles, *Virology* **50**:851.

Choppin, P. W., and Compans, R. W., 1975, Reproduction of paramyxoviruses, in: *Comprehensive Virology*, Vol. 4 (H. Fraenkel-Conrat and R. R. Wagner, eds.), pp. 95–178, Plenum Press, New York.

Choppin, P. W., Klenk, H.-D., Compans, R. W., and Caliguiri, L. A., 1971, The parainfluenza virus SV5 and its relationship to the cell membrane, in: *Perspectives in Virology*, Vol. VII (M. Pollard, ed.), pp. 127–156, Academic Press, New York.

Choppin, P. W., Lazarowitz, S. G., and Goldberg, A. R., 1975, Studies on proteolytic cleavage and glycosylation of the hemagglutinin of influenza A and B viruses, in: *Negative Strand Viruses* (R. D. Barry and B. W. J. Mahy, eds.), pp. 105–119, Academic Press, New York.

Clarke, D.-H., and Casals, J., 1958, Techniques for hemagglutination and hemagglutination-inhibition with arthropod-borne viruses, *Am. J. Trop. Med. Hyg.* **7**:561.

Clegg, J. C. S., 1975, Sequential translation of capsid and membrane protein genes in arbovirus-infected cells, *Nature (London)* **254**:454.

Clegg, J. C. S., and Kennedy, S. I. T., 1974, In vitro synthesis of structural proteins of Semliki Forest virus directed by isolated 26 S RNA from infected cells, *FEBS Lett.* **42**:327.

Clegg, J. C. S., and Kennedy, S. I. T., 1975a, Translation of Semliki Forest virus intracellular 26 S RNA: Characterization of the products synthesized in vitro, *Eur. Mol. Biol.* **53**:175.

Clegg, J. C. S., and Kennedy, S. I. T., 1975b, Initiation of synthesis of the structural proteins of Semliki Forest virus, *J. Mol. Biol.* **97**:401.

Clegg, J. C. S., and Kennedy, S. I. T., 1975c, Translation of the genes for the structural proteins of alphaviruses, *Med. Biol.* **53**:383.

Clinkscales, C. W., Bratt, M. A., and Morrison, T. G., 1977, Synthesis of Newcastle disease virus polypeptides in a wheat germ cell-free system, *J. Virol.* **22**:97.

Compans, R. W., 1971, Location of the glycoprotein in the membrane of Sindbis virus, *Nature (London) New Biol.* **229**:114.

Compans, R. W., 1973a, Influenza virus proteins. II. Association with components of the cytoplasm, *Virology* **51**:56.

Compans, R. W., 1973b, Distinct carbohydrate components of influenza virus glycoproteins in smooth and rough cytoplasmic membranes, *Virology* **55**:541.

Compans, R. W., and Choppin, P. W., 1967, Isolation and properties of the helical nucleocapsid of the parainfluenza virus SV5, *Proc. Natl. Acad. Sci. USA* **57**:541.

Compans, R. W., and Choppin, P. W., 1975, Reproduction of myxoviruses, in: *Comprehensive Virology*, Vol. 4 (H. Fraenkel-Conrat and R. R. Wagner, eds.), pp. 179–252, Plenum Press, New York.

Compans, R. W., and Dimmock, N. J., 1969, An electron microscopic study of single-cycle infection of chick embryo fibroblasts by influenza virus, *Virology* **39**:499.

Compans, R. W., and Pinter, A., 1975, Incorporation of sulfate into influenza virus glycoproteins, *Virology* **66**:151.

Compans, R. W., Holmes, K. V., Dales, S., and Choppin, P. W., 1966, An electron microscopic study of moderate and virulent virus–cell interactions of the parainfluenza virus SV5, *Virology* **30**:411.

Compans, R. W., Dimmock, N. J., and Meier-Ewert, H., 1969, Effect of antibody to neuraminidase on the maturation and hemagglutinating activity of an influenza virus A$_2$, *J. Virol.* **4**:528.

Compans, R. W., Klenk, H.-D., Caliguiri, L. A., and Choppin, P. W., 1970, Influenza virus proteins. I. Analysis of polypeptides of the virion and identification of spike glycoproteins, *Virology* **42**:880.

Compans, R. W., Landsberger, F. R., Lenard, J., and Choppin, P. W., 1972, Structure of the membrane of influenza virus, in: *International Virology 2* (J. L. Melnick, ed.), pp. 130–132, S. Karger, Basel.

Compans, R. W., Meier-Ewert, H., and Palese, P., 1974, Assembly of lipid-containing viruses, *J. Supramol. Struct.* **2**:496.

Compans, R. W., Bishop, D. H. L., and Meier-Ewert, H., 1977, Structural components of influenza C virions, *J. Virol.* **21**:658.

Content, J., and Duesberg, P., 1970, Electrophoretic distribution of the proteins and glycoproteins of influenza virus and Sendai virus, *J. Virol.* **6**:707.

Courtney, R. J., Steiner, S. M., and Benyesh-Melnick, M., 1973, Effects of 2-deoxy-D-glucose on herpes simplex virus replication, *Virology* **52**:447.

Cox, N. J., and Kendal, A. P., 1976, Presence of a segmented single-stranded RNA genome in influenza C virus, *Virology* **74**:239.

Dales, S., and Mosbach, E. H., 1968, Vaccinia as a model for membrane biogenesis, *Virology* **35**:564.

Dales, S., and Siminovitch, I., 1961, The development of vaccinia virus in strain L cells as examined by electron microscopy, *J. Biophys. Biochem. Cytol.* **10**:475.

Dales, S., Stern, W., Weintraub, S. B., and Huima, T., 1976, Genetically controlled surface modifications by poxvirus influencing cell–cell and cell–virus interactions, in: *Cell Membrane Receptors for Viruses, Antigens and Antibodies, Polypeptide Hormones, and Small Molecules* (R. F. Beers, Jr., and E. G. Bassett, eds.), pp. 253–270, Raven Press, New York.

Dalrymple, J. M., Schlesinger, S., and Russell, P. K., 1976, Antigenic characterization of two Sindbis envelope glycoproteins separated by isoelectric focusing, *Virology* **69**:93.

Dalton, A. J., Rowe, W. P., Smith, G. H., Wilsnack, R. W., and Pugh, W. E., 1968, Morphological and cytochemical studies on lymphocytic choriomeningitis virus, *J. Virol.* **2**:1465.

Darlington, R. W., and Moss, L. H., 1969, The envelope of herpes virus, *Progr. Med. Virol.* **11**:16.

Davenport, F. M., 1976, Influenza virus, in: *Viral Infections of Humans* (A. S. Evans, ed.), pp. 273–296, Plenum Press, New York.

David, A. E., 1973, Assembly of the vesicular stomatitis virus envelope: Incorporation of viral polypeptides into the host cell plasma membrane, *J. Mol. Biol.* **76**:135.

David-Ferreira, J. F., and Manaker, R. A., 1965, An electron microscope study of the development of a mouse hepatitis virus in tissue culture cells, *J. Cell Biol.* **24**:57.

DeGiuli, C., Kawai, S., Dales, S., and Hanafusa, H., 1975, Absence of surface projections on some noninfectious forms of RSV, *Virology* **66**:253.

DeLarco, J., and Todaro, G. J., 1976, Membrane receptors for murine leukemia viruses: Characterization using the purified viral envelope glycoprotein, gp71, *Cell* **8**:365.

Dietzschold, B., Schneider, L. G., and Cox, J. H., 1974, Serological characterization of the three major proteins of vesicular stomatitis virus, *J. Virol.* **19**:1.

Diringer, H., and Rott, R., 1976, Metabolism of preexisting lipids in baby hamster kidney cells during fusion from within, induced by Newcastle disease virus, *Eur. J. Biochem.* **65**:155.

Diringer, H., Kulas, H.-P., Schneider, L. G., and Schlumberger, H. D. 1973, The lipid composition of rabies virus, *Z. Naturforsch.* **28c**:90.

Dix, R. D., and Courtney, R. J., 1976, Effects of cytochalasin B on herpes simplex virus type 1 replication, *Virology* **70**:127.

Drzeniek, R., 1973, Viral and bacterial neuraminidase, *Curr. Top. Microbiol. Immunol.* **59**:35.

Drzeniek, R., and Rott, R., 1963, Abspaltung einer neuraminidase-haltigen Komponente aus Newcastle disease virus (NDV), *Z. Naturforsch.* **18b**:1127.

Drzeniek, R., Saber, M. S., and Rott, R., 1966a, Veränderung der Erythrozytenoberfläche durch Newcastle disease virus. II. Auftreten eines Forssman und eines Mononucleose"-Antigens an Newcastle disease virus-behändelten Erythrozyten, *Z. Naturforsch.* **21b**:254.

Drzeniek, R., Seto, J. T., and Rott, R., 1966b, Characterization of neuraminidase from myxoviruses, *Biochim. Biophys. Acta* **128**:547.

Dubovi, J. E., and Wagner, R. R., 1977, Spatial relationships of the proteins of vesicular stomatitis virus: Induction of reversible oligomers by cleavable protein cross-linkers and oxidation, *J. Virol.* **22**:900.

Duda, E., and Schlesinger, M. J., 1975, Alterations in Sindbis viral envelope proteins by treating BHK cells with glucosamine, *J. Virol.* **15**:416.

Duesberg, P. H., Martin, G. S., and Vogt, P. K., 1970, Glycoprotein components of avian and murine RNA tumor viruses, *Virology* **41**:631.

Easterbrook, K. B., 1966, Controlled degradation of vaccinia virus in vitro: An electron microscopic study, *J. Ultrastruct. Res.* **14**:484.

Eckert, E. A., 1973, Properties of an antigenic glycoprotein isolated from influenza virus hemagglutinin, *J. Virol.* **11**:183.

Eger, R., Compans, R. W., and Rifkin, D. B., 1975, The organization of the proteins of vesicular stomatitis virions: Labeling with pyridoxal phosphate, *Virology* **66**:610.

Eisenman, R. M., and Vogt, V. M., 1978, The biosynthesis of oncovirus proteins, *Biochim. Biophys. Acta* **473**:187.

Elder, J. H., Jensen, F. C., Bryant, M. L., and Lerner, R. A., 1977, Polymorphism of the major envelope glycoprotein (gp70) of murine C-type viruses: Virion associated and differentiation antigens encoded by a multi-gene family, *Nature* (*London*) **267**:23.

Elsbach, P., Holmes, K. V., and Choppin, P. W., 1969, Metabolism of lecithin and virus-induced cell fusion, *Proc. Soc. Exp. Biol. Med.* **130**:903.

Emerson, S. U., 1976, Vesicular stomatitis virus: Structure and function of virion components, *Curr. Top. Microbiol. Immunol.* **73**:1.

Emerson, S. U., and Wagner, R. R. 1972, Dissociation and reconstitution of the transcriptase and template activities of vesicular stomatitis B and T virions, *J. Virol.* **10**:297.

England, J. M., Bolognesi, D. P., Dietzschold, B., and Halpern, M. S., 1977, Evidence that a precursor glycoprotein is cleaved to yield the major glycoprotein of avian tumor virus, *J. Virol.* **21**:810.

Epstein, M. A., 1962, Observations on the fine structure of mature herpes simplex virus and on the composition of its nucleoid, *J. Exp. Med.* **115**:1.

Erlandson, R. A., Babcock, V. I., Southam, C. M., Bailey, R. B., and Shipkey, F. H., 1976, Semliki Forest virus in HEp2 cell cultures, *J. Virol.* **1**:996.

Etchison, J. R., and Holland, J. J., 1974a, Carbohydrate composition of the membrane glycoprotein of vesicular stomatitis virus, *Virology* **60**:217.

Etchison, J. R., and Holland, J. J., 1974b, Carbohydrate composition of the membrane glycoprotein of vesicular stomatitis virus grown in four mammalian cell lines, *Proc. Natl. Acad. Sci. USA* **71**:4011.

Etchison, J. R., Robertson, J. S., and Summers, D. F., 1977, Partial structural analysis of the oligosaccharide moieties of the vesicular stomatitis virus glycoprotein by sequential chemical and enzymatic degradation, *Virology* **78**:375.

Famulari, N. G., Buchhagen, D. L., Klenk, H.-D., and Fleissner, E., 1976, Presence of murine leukemia virus envelope proteins gp70 and p15 (E) in a common polyprotein of infected cells, *J. Virol.* **20**:501.

Farber, F. E., and Rawls, W. E., 1975, Isolation of ribosome-like structures from Pichinde virus, *J. Gen. Virol.* **26**:21.

Fleissner, E., 1971, Chromatographic separation and antigenic analysis of proteins of the oncornaviruses, *J. Virol.* **8**:778.

Fleissner, E., Ikeda, H., Tund, J.-S., Vitetta, E. S., Tress, E., Hardy, W., Jr., Stockert, E., Boyse, E. A., Pincus, T., and O'Donnell, P., 1975, Characterization of murine leukemia virus-specific proteins, *Cold Spring Harbor Symp. Quant. Biol.* **34**:1057.

Fong, B. S., Hunt, R. C., and Brown, J. C., 1976, Asymmetric distribution of phosphatidylethanolamine in the membrane of vesicular stomatitis virus, *J. Virol.* **20**:658.

Fong, C. K. Y., Tenser, R. B., Hsiung, G. D., and Gross, P. A., 1973. Ultrastructural studies of the envelopment and release of guinea pig herpes-like virus in cultured cells, *Virology* **52**:468.

Friedman, R. M., 1968, Protein synthesis directed by an arbovirus, *J. Virol.* **2**:26.

Friis, R. R., Ogura, H., Gelderblom, H., and Halpern, M. S., 1976, The defective maturation of viral progeny with a temperature sensitive mutant of avian sarcoma virus, *Virology* **73**:259.

Frommhagen, L. H., Knight, C. A., and Freeman, N. K., 1959, The ribonucleic acid, lipid and polysaccharide constituents of influenza virus preparations, *Virology* **8**:176.

Gahmberg, C. G., Simons, K., Renkonen, O., and Kääriäinen, L., 1972*a*, Exposure of proteins and lipids in the Semliki Forest virus membrane, *Virology* **50**:259.

Gahmberg, C. G., Uterman, G., and Simons, K., 1972*b*, The membrane proteins of Semliki Forest virus have a hydrophobic part attached to the viral membrane, *FEBS Lett.* **28**:179.

Gallaher, W. R., Levitan, D. B., and Blough, H. A., 1973, Effect of 2-deoxy-D-glucose on cell fusion induced by Newcastle disease and herpes simplex viruses, *Virology* **55**:193.

Gandhi, S. S., Stanley, P., Taylor, J. M., and White, D. O., 1972, Inhibition of influenza viral glycoprotein synthesis by sugars, *Microbios* **5**:41.

Gard, G. P., Vezza, A. C., Bishop, D. H. L., and Compans, R. W., 1977, Structural proteins of Tacaribe and Tamiami virions, *Virology* **83**:84.

Garoff, H., 1974, Cross-linking of the spike glycoproteins in Semliki Forest virus with dimethylsuberimidate, *Virology* **62**:385.

Garoff, H., and Simons, K., 1974, Location of the spike glycoproteins in the Semliki Forest virus membrane, *Proc. Natl. Acad. Sci. USA* **71**:3988.

Garoff, H., Simons, K., and Renkonen, O., 1974, Isolation and characterization of the membrane proteins of Semliki Forest virus, *Virology* **61**:493.

Garon, C. F., and Moss, B., 1971, Glycoprotein synthesis in cells infected with vaccinia virus. II. A glycoprotein component of the virion, *Virology* **46**:233.

Garwes, D. J., and Pocock, D. H., 1975, The polypeptide structure of transmissible gastroenteritis virus, *J. Gen. Virol.* **29**:25.

Gentsch, J., Bishop, D. H. L., and Obijeski, J. F., 1977, The virus particle nucleic acids and proteins of four bunyaviruses, *J. Gen. Virol.* **34**:257.

Gething, M. J., White, J. M., and Waterfield, M. D., 1978, The purification and structural characterization of the fusion factor of Sendai virus, *Top. Infect. Dis.* **3**:213.

Gibson, B., and Roizman, B., 1974, Proteins specified by herpes simplex virus. X. Staining and radiolabeling properties of B-capsid and virion proteins in polyacrylamide gels, *J. Virol.* **13**:155.

Glanville, N., and Ulmanen, I., 1976, Biological activity of in vitro synthesized protein: Binding of Semliki Forest virus capsid protein to the large ribosomal subunit, *Biochem. Biophys. Res. Commun.* **71**:393.

Glanville, N., Morser, J., Uomala, P., and Kääriäinen, L., 1976, Simultaneous translation of structural and nonstructural proteins from Semliki Forest virus RNA in
two eukaryotic systems in vitro, *Eur. J. Biochem.* **64**:167.

Gliedman, J. B., Smith, J. F., and Brown, D. T., 1975, Morphogenesis of Sindbis virus
in cultured *Aedes albopictus* cells, *J. Virol.* **16**:913.

Gottschalk, A., 1957, Neuraminidase: The specific enzyme of influenza virus and
Vibrio cholerae, Biochim. Biophys. Acta **23**:645.

Gregoriades, A., 1972, Isolation of neuraminidase from the WSN strain of influenza
virus, *Virology* **49**:333.

Gregoriades, A., 1973, The membrane protein of influenza virus: Extraction from virus
and infected cell with acidic chloroform–methanol, *Virology* **54**:369.

Griffin, J., and Compans, R., 1978, Effects of cytochalasin B on the maturation of
enveloped viruses, Abst. ASM Meet., p. 257.

Griffith, I. P., 1975, The fine structure of influenza virus, in: *Negative Strand Viruses*
(R. D. Barry and B. W. J. Mahy, eds.), p. 121, Academic Press, New York.

Grimes, W. J., and Burge, B. W., 1971, Modification of Sindbis virus glycoprotein by
host-specified glycosyl transferase, *J. Virol.* **7**:309.

Grubman, M. J., Ehrenfeld, E., and Summers, D. F., 1974, In vitro synthesis of proteins by membrane-bound polyribosomes from vesicular stomatitis virus-infected
HeLa cells, *J. Virol.* **19**:560.

Gupta, P., and Rapp, F., 1977, Identification of virion polypeptides in hamster cells
transformed by herpes simplex virus type 1, *Proc. Natl. Acad. Sci. USA* **74**:372.

Haines, H., and Baerwald, R. J., 1976, Nuclear membrane changes in herpes simplex
virus-infected BHK-21 cells as seen by freeze-fracture, *J. Virol.* **17**:1038.

Halonen, P. E., Murphy, F. A., Fields, B. N., and Reese, D. R., 1968, Hemagglutination of rabies and some other bullet-shaped viruses, *Proc. Soc. Exp. Biol.*
127:1037.

Halpern, M. S., Bolognesi, D. P., and Friis, R. R., 1976, Viral glycoprotein synthesis
studied in an established line of Japanese quail embryo cells infected with Bryan
high titer strain of Rous sarcoma virus, *J. Virol.* **18**:504.

Hanafusa, T., Hanafusa, H., Metroka, C. E., Haguard, W. S., Rettenmier, C. W.,
Sawyer, R. C., Dougherty, R. M., and DiStefano, H. S., 1976, Pheasantvirus: A
new class of ribodeoxy virus, *Proc. Natl. Acad. Sci. USA* **73**:1333.

Hardwick, J. M., and Bussell, R. H., 1976, Glycoproteins of measles virus under
reduced and nonreduced conditions, *Abstr. Am. Soc. Microbiol.*, p. 232.

Harrison, S. C., David, A., Jumblatt, J., and Darnell, J. E., 1971, Lipid and protein
organization in Sindbis virus, *J. Mol. Biol.* **60**:523.

Haslam, E. A., Hampson, A. W., Radiskevics, I., and White, D. O., 1970, The
polypeptides of influenza virus. III. Identification of the hemagglutinin, neuraminidase, and nucleocapsid proteins, *Virology* **42**:566;

Haukenes, G., Harboe, A., and Mortensson-Egnund, K., 1965, A uronic and sialic acid
free chick allantoic mucopolysaccharide sulphate which combines with influenza
virus HI-antibody to host material, *Acta Pathol. Microbiol. Scand.***64**:534.

Hay, A. J., 1974, Studies on the formation of the influenza virus envelope, *Virology*
60:398.

Hayman, M. J., Skehel, J. J., and Crumpton, M. J., 1973, Purification of virus glycoproteins by affinity chromatography using *Lens culinaris* phytohemagglutinin,
FEBS Lett. **29**:185.

Haywood, A., 1975, Model membranes and Sendai virus: Surface–surface interaction, in: *Negative Strand Viruses* (B. W. J. Mahy and R. D. Barry, eds.), pp. 923–928, Academic Press, London.

Hecht, T. T., and Summers, D. F., 1972, Effect of vesicular stomatitis virus infection on the histocompatibility antigen of L cells, *J. Virol.* **10**:578.

Heine, J. W., and Schnaitman, C. A., 1971, Entry of vesicular stomatitis virus into L cells, *J. Virol.* **8**:786.

Heine, J. W., Spear, P. G., and Roizman, B., 1972, The proteins specified by herpes simplex virus. VI. Viral proteins in the plasma membrane, *J. Virol.* **9**:431.

Helenius, A., and Simons, K., 1972, The binding of detergents to lipophilic and hydrophilic proteins, *J. Biol. Chem.* **247**:3656.

Helenius, A., and Simons, K., 1975, Solubilization of membranes by detergents, *Biochim. Biophys. Acta* **415**:29.

Helenius, A., and Soderlund, H., 1973, Stepwise dissociation of the Semliki Forest virus membrane with Triton X-100, *Biochim. Biophys. Acta* **307**:287.

Helenius, A., and von Bonsdorff, C.-H., 1976, Semliki Forest virus membrane proteins: Preparation and characterization of spike complexes soluble in detergent-free medium, *Biochim. Biophys. Acta* **436**:895.

Helenius, A., Fries, E., Garoff, H., and Simons, K., 1976, Solubilization of the Semliki Forest virus membrane with sodium deoxycholate, *Biochim. Biophys. Acta* **436**:319.

Hierholzer, J. C., Palmer, E. L., Whitfield, S. G., Kaye, H. S., and Dowdle, W. R., 1972, Protein composition of coronavirus OC 43, *Virology* **48**:516.

Hightower, L. E., Morrison, T. G., and Bratt, M. A., 1975, Relationships among the polypeptides of Newcastle disease virus, *J. Virol.* **16**:1599.

Hirschberg, C. G., and Robbins, P. W., 1974, The glycolipids and phospholipids of Sindbis virus and their relation to the lipids of the host cell plasma membrane, *Virology* **61**:602.

Hirst, G. K., 1941, The agglutination of red cells by allantoic fluid of chick embryos infected with influenza virus, *Science* **94**:22.

Hirst, G. K., 1942, Adsorption of influenza hemagglutinins and virus by red blood cells, *J. Exp. Med.* **76**:195.

Hirst, G. K., 1950, The relationship of the receptors of a new strain of virus to those of the mumps-NDV-influenza group, *J. Exp. Med.* **91**:177.

Hirst, G. K., and Pons, M. W., 1973, Mechanism of influenza virus recombination. II. Virus aggregation and its effect on plaque formation by so-called noninfectious virus, *Virology* **56**:620.

Hoagland, C. L., Smadel, J. E., and Rivers, T. M., 1940, Constituents of elementary bodies of vaccinia. I. Certain basic analysis and observations on lipid components of the virus, *J. Exp. Med.* **71**:737.

Hodes, D. S., Schnitzer, T. J., Kalica, A. R., Camargo, E., and Chanock, R. M., 1975, Inhibition of respiratory syncytial, parainfluenza 3, and measles viruses by 2-deoxy-D-glucose, *Virology* **63**:201.

Holowczak, J. A., 1970, Glycopeptides of vaccinia virus. I. Preliminary characterization and hexosamine content, *Virology* **42**:87.

Holowczak, J. A., and Joklik, W. K., 1967, Studies on the proteins of vaccinia virus. I. Structural proteins of virions and cores, *Virology* **33**:726.

Homma, M., and Ohuchi, M., 1973, Trypsin action on the growth of Sendai virus in tissue culture cells. III. Structural difference of Sendai virus grown in eggs and tissue culture cells, *J. Virol.* **12**:1457.

Homma, M., Tozawa, H., Shimizu, K., and Ishida, N., 1975, A proposal for designation of Sendai virus proteins, *Jpn. J. Microbiol.* **19**:467.

Homma, M., Shimizu, K., Shimizu, Y. K., and Ishida, N., 1976, On the study of Sendai virus hemolysis. I. Complete Sendai virus lacking in hemolytic activity, *Virology* **71**:41.

Honess, R. W., and Roizman, B., 1973, Proteins specified by herpes simplex virus. XI. Identification and relative molar rates of synthesis of structural and nonstructural herpesvirus polypeptides in the infected cell, *J. Virol.* **12**:1347.

Honess, R. W., and Roizman, B., 1975, Proteins specified by herpes simplex virus, *J. Virol.* **16**:1308.

Horne, R. W., Waterson, A. P., Wildy, P., and Farnham, A. E., 1960, The structure and composition of the myxoviruses. I. Electron microscope studies of the structure of the myxovirus particles by negative staining techniques, *Virology* **11**:79.

Hosaka, Y., and Shimizu, K., 1977, Cell fusion by Sendai virus, in: *Virus Infection and the Cell Surface*, Vol. 2 of *Cell Surface Reviews* (G. Poste and G. L. Nicolson, eds.), pp. 129–156, North-Holland, Amsterdam.

Howe, C., and Morgan, C., 1969, Interactions between Sendai virus and human erythrocytes, *J. Virol.* **3**:70.

Howe, C., Lee, L. T., Harboe, A., and Haukenes, G., 1967, Immunochemical study of influenza virus and associated host tissue components, *J. Immunol.* **98**:543.

Hoyle, L., 1962, The entry of myxoviruses into the cell, *Cold Spring Harbor Symp. Quant. Biol.* **27**:113.

Hoyle, L., Horne, R. W., and Waterson, A. P., 1961, The structure and composition of the myxoviruses. II. Components released from the influenza virus particle by ether, *Virology* **13**:448.

Huang, R. T. C., 1977, Transfer of glycolipid between membranes of tissue culture cells, using dansylcerebroside as a model, *Z. Naturforsch.* **32c**:379.

Huang, R. T. C., and Orlich, M., 1972, Substrate specificities of the neuraminidase of Newcastle disease virus and fowl plague virus, *Z. Physiol. Chem.* **353**:318.

Huang, R. T. C., Rott, R., and Klenk, H.-D., 1973, On the receptor for influenza viruses. I. Artificial receptor for influenza virus, *Z. Naturforsch.* **28c**:342.

Hubbell, W. L., and McConnell, H. M., 1971, Molecular motion in spin-labeled phospholipids and membranes, *J. Am. Chem. Soc.* **93**:314.

Hughes, F., and Pedersen, C. E., 1975, Paramagnetic spin label interactions with the envelope of a group A arbovirus: Lipid organization, *Biochim. Biophys. Acta* **394**:102.

Hummeler, K., Koprowski, H., and Wiktor, T. J., 1967, Structure and development of rabies virus in tissue culture, *J. Virol.* **1**:152.

Hung, P. P., Robinson, H. L., and Robinson, W. S., 1971, Isolation and characterization of proteins from Rous sarcoma virus, *Virology* **43**:251.

Hunt, L. A., and Summers, D. F., 1976a, Association of vesicular stomatitis virus proteins with HeLa cell membranes and released virus, *J. Virol.* **20**:637.

Hunt, L. A., and Summers, D. F., 1976b, Glycosylation of vesicular stomatitis virus glycoprotein in virus-infected HeLa cells, *J. Virol.* **20**:646.

Hunter, E., Friis, R. R., and Vogt, P. K., 1974, Inhibition of avian sarcoma virus replication by glucosamine, *Virology* **58**:449.

Hunter, E., Hayman, M. J., Rongey, R. W., and Vogt, P. K., 1976, An avian sarcoma virus mutant which is temperature-sensitive for virion assembly, *Virology* **69**:35.

Ichihashi, Y., and Dales, Y., 1971, Biogenesis of poxviruses: Interrelationship between hemagglutinin production and polykaryocytosis, *Virology* **46**:533.

Igarashi, A., Harrap, A. A., Casals, J., and Stollar, V., 1976, Morphological, biochemical and serological studies on a viral agent (CFA) which replicates and causes fusion of Aedes albopictus (Singh) cells, *Virology* **74**:174.

Ihle, J. M., Hanna, M. G., Jr., Schäfer, W., Hunsmann, G., Bolognesi, D. P., and Huper, G., 1975, Polypeptides of mammalian oncornaviruses. III. Localization of p15 and reactivity with natural antibody, *Virology* **63**:60.

Ihle, J. N., Lee, J. C., Collins, J. J., Fischinger, P. J., Pazmino, N. H., Moenning, V., Schäfer, W., Hanna, M. G., and Bolognesi, D. P., 1976, Characterization of the immune response to the major glycoprotein (gp71) Friend leukemia virus. II. Response in C57BL/6 mice, *Virology* **75**:88.

Ikeda, H., Hardy, W. J., Tress, E., and Fleissner, E., 1975, Chromatographic separation and antigenic analysis of proteins of the oncornaviruses V. Identification of a new murine viral protein, *J. Virol.* **16**:53.

Inglis, S. C., Carroll, A. R., Lamb, R. A., and Mahy, B. W. J., 1976, Polypeptides specified by the influenza virus genome, *Virology* **74**:489.

Ishizaki, R., and Vogt, P. K., 1966, Immunological relationships among envelope antigens of avian tumor viruses, *Virology* **30**:375.

Ivanic, S., 1974, Identification of two envelope proteins of Semliki Forest virus before and after treatment with Triton X-100, *Arch. Ges. Virusforsch.* **44**:164.

Jensik, S. C., and Silver, S., 1976, Polypeptides of mumps virus, *J. Virol.* **17**:363

Johnson, I., and Clamp, J. R., 1971, The oligosaccharides of human type L immunoglobulin M (macroglobulin), *Biochem. J.* **123**:739.

Joseph, B. S., and Oldstone, M. B. A., 1974, Antibody-induced redistribution of measles virus antigens on the cell surface, *J. Immunol.* **113**:1205.

Kaluza, G., 1975, Effect of impaired glycosylation on the biosynthesis of Semliki Forest virus glycoproteins, *J. Virol.* **16**:602.

Kaluza, G., 1976, Early synthesis of Semliki Forest virus-specific proteins in infected chicken cells, *J. Virol.* **19**:1.

Kaluza, G., Scholtissek, G., and Rott, R., 1972, Inhibition of the multiplication of enveloped RNA viruses by glucosamine and 2-deoxy-D-glucose, *J. Gen. Virol.* **14**:251.

Kaluza, G., Schmidt, M. F. G., and Scholtissek, C., 1973, Effect of 2-deoxy-D-glucose on the multiplication of Semliki Forest virus and the reversal of the block by mannose, *Virology* **54**:179.

Kaluza, G., Kraus, A. A., and Rott, R., 1976, Inhibition of cellular protein synthesis by simultaneous pretreatment of host cells with fowl plague virus and actinomycin D: A method for studying early protein synthesis of several RNA viruses, *J. Virol.* **17**:1.

Kang, C. Y., and Prevec, L., 1969, Proteins of vesicular stomatitis virus. I. Polyacrylamide gel analysis of viral antigens, *J. Virol.* **3**:404.

Kaplan, A. S., 1974, *The Herpes Viruses*, Academic Press, New York.

Kaplan, A. S., and Ben-Porat, T., 1970, Synthesis of proteins in cells infected with herpesvirus. VI. Characterization of proteins of the viral membrane, *Proc. Natl. Acad. Sci. USA* **66**:799.

Kaplan, A. S., and Ben-Porat, T., 1976, Synthesis of proteins in cells infected with herpes virus. XI. Sulfated, structural glycoproteins, *Virology* **70**:561.

Kates, M., Allison, A. C., Tyrrell, D. A., and James, A. T., 1961, Lipids of influenza virus and their relation to those of the host cell, *Biochim. Biophys. Acta* **52**:455.

Katz, E., and Moss, B., 1970, Formation of a vaccinia virus structural polypeptide from a higher molecular weight precursor: Inhibition by rifampicin, *Proc. Natl. Acad. Sci. USA* **66**:677.

Katz, F. V., Rothman, J. E., Leingappa, V. R., Blobel, G., and Lodish, H. R., 1977, Membrane assembly in vitro: Synthesis, glycosylation, and asymmetric insertion of a transmembrane protein, *Proc. Natl. Acad. Sci. USA* **74**:3278.

Keegstra, K., Sefton, B., and Burke, D., 1975, Sindbis virus glycoproteins: Effect of the host cell on the oligosaccharide, *J. Virol.* **16**:613.

Keil, W., Klenk, H.-D., and Schwarz, R. T., 1978, Charakterisierung des Bindungstyps zwischen dem Kohlenhydrat-und Proteinanteil von Influenzavirus-glykoproteinen, *Z. Physiol. Chem.* **359**:283.

Kelley, J. M., Wagner, R. R., and Emerson, S. U., 1972, The glycoprotein of vesicular stomatitis virus is the antigen that gives rise to and reacts with neutralizing antibody, *J. Virol.* **10**:1231.

Kemp, M. C., Perdue, M. L., Rogers, H. W., O'Callaghan, D. J., and Randall, C. C. 1974, Structural polypeptides of the hamster strain of equine herpes virus type 1: Products associated with purification, *Virology* **61**:361.

Kemp, M. C., Wise, K. S., Edlund, L. E., Acton, R. T., and Compans, R. W., 1978, Origin of minor glycoproteins of murine leukemia viruses. *J. Virol.* **28**:84.

Kendal, A. P., 1975, A comparison of "influenza C" with prototype myxoviruses: Receptor-destroying activity, neuraminidase and structural polypeptides, *Virology* **65**:87.

Kendal, A. P., and Eckert, E. A., 1972, The preparation and properties of ^{14}C-carboxyamidomethylated subunits from A₂/1957 influenza neuraminidase, *Biochim. Biophys. Acta* **258**:484.

Kennedy, S. I. T., 1972, Isolation and identification of the virus-specified RNA species found on membrane-bound polyribosomes of chick embryo cells infected with Semliki Forest virus, *Biochem. Biophys. Res. Commun.* **38**:1254.

Kennedy, S. I. T., 1974, The effect of enzymes on structural and biological properties of Semliki Forest virus, *J. Gen. Virol.* **23**:129.

Kennel, S. J., 1976, Purification of a glycoprotein from mouse ascites fluid by immunoaffinity chromatography which is related to the major glycoprotein of murine leukemia viruses, *J. Biol. Chem.* **251**:6197.

Keranen, S., and Kääriäinen, L., 1975, Proteins synthesized by Semliki Forest virus and its 16 temperature-sensitive mutants, *J. Virol.* **16**:388.

Kilbourne, E. D., 1959, Inhibition of influenza virus multiplication with a glucose antimetabolite (2-deoxy-D-glucose), *Nature (London)* **183**:271.

Kilbourne, E. D., 1975, *The Influenza Viruses and Influenza*, Academic Press, New York.

Kilbourne, E. D., Laver, W. G., Shulmann, J. L., and Webster, R. G., 1968, Antiviral activity of antiserum specific for an influenza virus neuraminidase, *J. Virol.* **2**:28.

Kingsbury, D. W., 1973, Paramyxovirus replication, *Curr. Top. Microbiol. Immunol.* **59**:1.

Klenk, E., Faillard, H., and Lempfried, H., 1955, Über die enzymatische Wirkung von Influenzavirus, *Z. Physiol. Chem.* **301**:235.

Klenk, H.-D., 1974, Viral envelopes and their relationship to cellular membranes, *Curr. Top. Microbiol. Immunol.* **68**:29.

Klenk, H.-D., and Choppin, P. W., 1969a, Chemical composition of the parainfluenza virus SV5, *Virology* **37**:155.

Klenk, H.-D., and Choppin, P. W., 1969b, Lipids of plasma membranes of monkey and hamster kidney cells and of parainfluenza virions grown in these cells, *Virology* **38**:255.

Klenk, H.-D., and Choppin, P. W., 1970a, Plasma membrane lipids and parainfluenza virus assembly, *Virology* **40**:939.

Klenk, H.-D., and Choppin, P. W., 1970b, Glycosphingolipids of plasma membranes of cultured cells and an enveloped virus (SV5) grown in these cells, *Proc. Natl. Acad. Sci. USA* **66**:57.

Klenk, H.-D., and Choppin, P. W., 1971, Glycolipid content of vesicular stomatitis virus grown in baby hamster kidney cells, *J. Virol.* **7**:416.

Klenk, H.-D., and Rott, R., 1973, Formation of influenza virus proteins, *J. Virol.* **11**:823.

Klenk, H.-D., Caliguiri, L. A., and Choppin, P. W., 1970a, The proteins of the parainfluenza virus SV5. II. The carbohydrate content and glycoproteins of the virion, *Virology* **42**:473.

Klenk, H.-D., Compans, R. W., and Choppin, P. W., 1970b, An electron microscopic study of the presence or absence of neuraminic acid in enveloped viruses, *Virology* **42**:1158.

Klenk, H.-D., Rott, R., and Becht, H., 1972a, On the structure of the influenza virus envelope, *Virology* **47**:579.

Klenk, H.-D., Scholtissek, C., and Rott, R., 1972b, Inhibition of glycoprotein biosynthesis of influenza virus by D-glucosamine and 2-deoxy-D-glucose, *Virology* **49**:723.

Klenk, H.-D., Wöllert, W., Rott, R., and Scholtissek, C., 1974, Association of influenza virus proteins with cytoplasmic fractions, *Virology* **57**:28.

Klenk, H.-D., Rott, R., Orlich, M., and Blödorn, J., 1975, Activation of influenza A viruses by trypsin treatment, *Virology* **68**:426.

Klenk, H.-D., Nagai, Y., Rott, R., and Nicolau, C., 1977a, The structure and function of paramyxovirus glycoproteins, *Med. Microbiol. Immunol.* **164**:35.

Klenk, H., Rott, R., and Orlich, M. 1977b, Further studies on the activation of influenza virus by proteolytic cleavage of the hemagglutinin, *J. Gen. Virol.* **36**:151.

Klenk, H.-D., Schwarz, R. T., Schmidt, M. F. G., and Wollert, W., 1978, The structure and biosynthesis of the carbohydrate moiety of the influenza virus hemagglutinin, *Top. Infect. Dis.* **3**:83.

Knight, C. A., 1944, A sedimentable component of allantoic fluid and its relationship to influenza viruses, *J. Expl. Med.* **30**:83.

Knight, C. A., 1946, Precipitin reactions of highly purified influenza viruses and related materials, *J. Expl. Med.* **83**:281.

Knipe, D. M., Baltimore, D., and Lodish, H. F., 1977a, Separate pathways of maturation of the major structural proteins of vesicular stomatitis virus, *J. Virol.* **21**:1128.

Knipe, D. M., Baltimore, D., and Lodish, H. F., 1977b, Maturation of viral proteins in cells infected with temperature-sensitive mutants of vesicular stomatitis virus, *J. Virol.* **21**:1149.

Knipe, D. M., Lodish, H. F., and Baltimore, D., 1977c, Localization of two cellular forms of the vesicular stomatitis viral glycoprotein, *J. Virol.* **21**:1121.

Knowles, R. W., and Person, S., 1976, Effects of 2-deoxyglucose, glucosamine, and mannose on cell fusion and the glycoproteins of herpes simplex virus, *J. Virol.* **18**:644.

Krag, S. S., and Robbins, P. W., 1977, Sindbis envelope proteins as endogenous acceptors in reactions of guanosine diphosphate-(^{14}C)mannose with preparations of infected chicken embryo fibroblasts, *J. Biol. Chem.* **252**:2621.

Krantz, M. J., Lee, Y. C., and Hung, P. P., 1976, Characterization and comparison of the major glycoprotein from three strains of Rous sarcoma virus, *Arch. Bioch. Biophys.* **174**:66.

Krantz, M. J., Strand, M., and August, J. T., 1977, Biochemical and immunological characterization of the major envelope glycoprotein gp69/71 and degradation fragments from Rauscher leukemia virus, *J. Virol.* **22**:804.

Krug, R. M., and Etkind, P. R., 1973, Cytoplasmic and nuclear virus-specific proteins in influenza virus-infected MDCK cells, *Virology* **56**:334.

Lachmi, B., and Kääriäinen, L., 1976, Sequential translation of nonstructural proteins in cells infected with a Semliki Forest virus mutant, *Proc. Natl. Acad. Sci. USA* **73**:1936.

Lachmi, B., Glanville, N., Keranen, S., and Kääriäinen, L., 1975, Tryptic peptide analysis of nonstructural and structural precursor proteins from Semliki Forest virus mutant-infected cells, *J. Virol.* **16**:1615.

Lafay, F., 1974, Envelope proteins of vesicular stomatitis virus: Effect of temperature-sensitive mutations in complementation groups III and IV, *J. Virol.* **14**:1120.

Lafferty, K. J., and Oertilis, S., 1963, The interaction between virus and antibody III. Examination of virus–antibody complexes with the electron microscope, *Virology* **21**:91.

Lagwinska, E., Stewart, C. C., Adless, C., and Schlesinger, S., 1975, Replication of lactic dehydrogenase virus and Sindbis virus in mouse peritoneal macrophages: Induction of interferon and phenotypic mixing, *Virology* **65**:204.

Lai, M. M., and Duesberg, P. H., 1972, Differences between the envelope glycoproteins and glycopeptides of avian tumor viruses released from transformed and from nontransformed cells, *Virology* **50**:359.

Laine, R., Kettunen, M.-L., Gahmberg, C. G., Kääriäinen, L., and Renkonen, O., 1972, Fatty chains of different lipid classes of Semliki Forest virus and host cell membranes, *J. Virol.* **10**:433.

Laine, R., Soderlund, H., and Renkonen, O., 1973, Chemical composition of Semliki Forest virus, *Intervirology* **1**:110.

Lamb, R. A., and Choppin, P. W., 1976, Synthesis of influenza virus proteins in infected cells: Translation of viral polypeptides, including three P polypeptides, from RNA produced by primary transcription, *Virology* **74**:504.

Lamb, R. A., and Choppin, P. W., 1977, The synthesis of Sendai virus polypeptides in infected cells. II. Intracellular distribution of polypeptides, *Virology* **81**:371.

Landsberger, F. R., and Compans, R. W., 1976, Effect of membrane proteins on the lipid bilayer structure: A spin label ESR study of vesicular stomatitis virus, *Biochemistry* **15**:2356.

Landsberger, F. R., Lenard, J., Paxton, J., and Compans, R. W., 1971, Spin label ESR study of the lipid-containing membrane of influenza virus, *Proc. Natl. Acad. Sci. USA* **68**:2579.

Landsberger, F. R., Compans, R. W., Choppin, P. W., and Lenard, J., 1973, Organization of the lipid phase in viral membranes: Effects of independent variation of the lipid and the protein composition, *Biochemistry* **12**:4498.

Landsberger, F. R., Lyles, D. S., and Choppin, P. W., 1978, Enveloped viruses: Their structure and interaction with cells, in: *Negative Strand Viruses and the Host Cell* (R. D. Barry and B. W. J. Mahy, eds.), Academic Press, New York.

Laver, W. G., 1971, Separation of two polypeptide chains from the hemagglutinin subunit of influenza virus, *Virology* **45**:275.

Laver, W. G., 1973, The polypeptides of influenza virus, *Adv. Virus Res.* **18**:57.

Laver, W. G., and Baker, N., 1972, Amino acid composition of polypeptides from influenza virus particles, *J. Gen. Virol.* **17**:61.

Laver, W. G., and Downie, J. C., 1976, Influenza virus recombination. 1. Matrix protein markers and segregation during mixed infection, *Virology* **70**:105.

Laver, W. G., and Valentine, R. C., 1969, Morphology of the isolated hemagglutinin and neuraminidase subunits of influenza virus, *Virology* **38**:105.

Laver, W. G., and Webster, R. G., 1966, The structure of influenza viruses. IV. Chemical studies of the host antigen, *Virology* **30**:104.

Laver, W. G., and Webster, R. G., 1972, Studies on the origin of pandemic influenza. II. Peptide maps of the light and heavy polypeptide chains from the hemagglutinin subunits of A_2 influenza viruses isolated before and after the appearance of Hong Kong influenza, *Virology* **48**:445.

Laver, W. G., Downie, J. C., and Webster, R. G., 1974, Studies on antigenic variation of influenza virus: Evidence for multiple antigenic determinants on the hemagglutinin subunits of A/Hong Kong/68 (H_3N_2) virus and the A/England/72 strains, *Virology* **59**:230.

Lazarowitz, S. G., and Choppin, P. W., 1975, Enhancement of the infectivity of influenza A and B viruses by proteolytic cleavage of the hemagglutinin polypeptide, *Virology* **68**:440.

Lazarowitz, S. G., Compans, R. W., and Choppin, P. W., 1971, Influenza virus structural and nonstructural proteins in infected cells and their plasma membranes, *Virology* **46**:830.

Lazarowitz, S. G., Compans, R. W., and Choppin, P. W., 1973*a*, Proteolytic cleavage of the hemagglutinin polypeptide of influenza virus: Function of the uncleaved polypeptide HA, *Virology* **52**:199.

Lazarowitz, S. G., Goldberg, A. R., and Choppin, P. W., 1973*b*, Proteolytic cleavage by plasmin of the HA polypeptide of influenza virus: Host cell activation of serum plasminogen, *Virology* **56**:172.

Lazdins, I., Haslam, E. A., and White, D. O., 1972, The polypeptides of influenza virus. VI. Composition of the neuraminidase, *Virology* **49**:758.

Leamnson, R. N., and Halpern, M. S., 1976, Subunit structure of the glycoprotein complex of avian tumor virus, *J. Virol.* **18**:956.

Leamnson, R. N., Shander, M. H. M., and Halpern, M. S., 1977, A structural protein complex in Moloney leukemia virus, *Virology* **76**:437.

Leavitt, R., Schlesinger, R., and Kornfeld, S., 1977, Tunicamycin inhibits glycosylation and multiplication of Sindbis and vesicular stomatitis viruses, *J. Virol.* **21**:375.

Lee, L. T., Howe, C., Meyer, K., and Choi, H. U., 1969, Quantitative precipitin analysis of influenza virus host antigen and of sulfated polysaccharides of chicken embryonic allantoic fluid, *J. Immunol.* **102**:1144.

Lenard, J., and Compans, R. W., 1974, The membrane structure of lipid-containing viruses, *Biochim. Biophys. Acta* **344**:51.

Lenard, J., and Compans, R. W., 1975, Polypeptide composition of incomplete influenza virus, *Virology* **65**:418.

Lenard, J., and Rothman, J. E. 1976, Transbilayer distribution and movement of cholesterol and phospholipid in the membrane of influenza virus, *Biochemistry* **73**:391.

Lenard, J., Landsberger, F. R., Wong, C. Y., Choppin, P. W., and Compans, R. W., 1974, Organization of lipid and protein in viral membranes: Spin label and fluorescent probe studies, in: *Negative Strand Viruses* (R. D. Barry and B. W. J. Mahy, eds.), pp. 823–833, Academic Press, New York.

Lenard, J., Tsai, D. K., Compans, R. W., and Landsberger, F. R., 1976, Observations on the membrane organization of standard and incomplete influenza grown in MDBK cells, *Virology* **71**:389.

Lohmeyer, J., Talens, L. T., and Klenk, H.-D., 1977, Biosynthese der Membrankomponenten des Influenzavirus im abortiven Zyklus, *Z. Physiol. Chem.* **358**:271.

Ludwig, H., Becht, H., and Rott, R., 1974, Inhibition of herpes virus-induced cell fusion by concanavalin A, antisera, and 2-deoxy-D-glucose, *J. Virol.* **14**:307.

Luukkonen, A., Kääriäinen, L., and Renkonen, O., 1976, Phospholipids of Semliki Forest virus grown in cultured mosquito cells, *Biochim. Biophys. Acta* **450**:109.

Luukkonen, A., Gahmberg, C. G., and Renkonen, O., 1977a, Surface labeling of Semliki Forest virus glycoproteins using galactose-oxidase, *Virology* **76**:55.

Luukkonen, A., von Bonsdorff, C.-H., and Renkonen, O., 1977b, Characterization of Semliki Forest virus grown in mosquito cells: Comparison with the virus from hamster cells, *Virology* **78**:331.

Lyles, D. S., and Landsberger, F. R., 1977, Sendai virus-induced hemolysis: Reduction in heterogeneity of erythrocyte lipid bilayer fluidity, *Proc. Natl. Acad. Sci USA* **74**:1918.

Maeda, T., Asano, A., Ohki, K., Okada, Y., and Ohnishi, S.-I., 1975, A spin-label study on fusion of red blood cells induced by hemagglutinating virus of Japan, *Biochemistry* **14**:3736.

Maeda, T., Asano, A., Okada, Y., and Ohnishi, S.-I., 1977, Transmembrane phospholipid motions induced by F glycoprotein in hemagglutinating virus of Japan, *J. Virol.* **21**:232.

Majuk, Z., Bittman, R., Landsberger, F. R., and Compans, R. W., 1977, Effects of filipin on the structure and biological activities of enveloped viruses, *J. Virol.* **24**:883.

Marquardt, H., Gilden, R. V., and Oroszlan, S., 1977, Envelope glycoproteins of Rauscher murine leukemia virus: Isolation and chemical characterization, *Biochemistry* **16**:710.

Martinez-Segovia, Z. M., and DeMitri, M. I., 1977, Junin virus structural proteins, *J. Virol.* **21**:579.

Matsumoto, S., and Kawai, A., 1969, Comparative studies on development of rabies virus in different host cells, *Virology* **39**:449.

Matsumoto, S., Schneider, L. G., Kawai, A., and Yonezawa, T., 1974, Further studies on the replication of rabies and rabies-like viruses in organized cultures of mammalian neural tissues, *J. Virol.* **19**:981.

Mattila, K., Luukkonen, A., and Renkonen, O., 1976, Protein-bound oligosaccharides of Semliki Forest virus, *Biochim. Biophys. Acta* **419**:435.

McCarthy, M., and Harrison, S. C., 1977, Glycosidase susceptibility: A probe for the distribution of glycoprotein oligosaccharides in Sindbis virus, *J. Virol.* **23**:61.

McClelland, L., and Hare, R., 1941, The adsorption of influenza virus by red cells and a new in vitro method of measuring antibodies for influenza virus, *Can. Pub. Health J.* **32**:530.

McConnell, H. M., and McFarland, B. G., 1972, The flexibility gradient in biological membranes, *Ann. N.Y. Acad. Sci.* **195**:207.

McGeoch, D., Fellner, P., and Newton, C., 1976, Influenza virus genome consists of eight distinct RNA species, *Proc. Natl. Acad. Sci. USA* **73**:3045.

McLellan, W. L., and August, J. T., 1976, Analysis of the envelope of Rauscher murine oncornavirus: In vitro labeling of glycopeptides, *J. Virol.* **20**:627.

McLerran, C. J., and Arlinghaus, R. B., 1973, Structural components of a virus of the California encephalitis complex: La Crosse virus, *Virology* **53**:247.

McSharry, J. J., and Wagner, R. R., 1971*a*, Lipid composition of purified vesicular stomatitis viruses, *J. Virol.* **7**:59.

McSharry, J. J., and Wagner, R. R., 1971*b*, Carbohydrate composition of vesicular stomatitis virus, *J. Virol.* **7**:412.

McSharry, J. J., Compans, R. W., and Choppin, P. W., 1971, Proteins of vesicular stomatitis virus and phenotypically mixed vesicular stomatitis–simian virus 5 virions, *J. Virol.* **8**:722.

McSharry, J. J., Compans, R. W., Lackland, H., and Choppin, P. W., 1975, Isolation and characterization of the non-glycosylated membrane protein and a nucleocapsid complex from the paramyxovirus SV5, *Virology* **67**:365.

Meier-Ewert, H., and Compans, R. W., 1974, Time course of synthesis and assembly of influenza virus proteins, *J. Virol.* **14**:1083.

Meier-Ewert, H., Compans, R. W., Bishop, D. H. L., and Herrler, G., 1978, in: *Negative Strand Viruses and the Host Cell* (R. D. Barry and B. W. J. Mahy, eds.), pp. 127–133, Academic Press, New York.

Miller, G. L., Lauffer, M. A., and Stanley, W. M., 1944, Electrophoretic studies on PR8 influenza virus, *J. Exp. Med.* **80**:549.

Mitchiner, M. B., 1969, The envelope of vaccinia and of viruses: An electron-cytochemical investigation, *J. Gen. Virol.* **5**:211.

Miyamoto, H., and Kato, S., 1968, Immune hemadsorption by cells infected with poxvirus, *Biken J.* **11**:343.

Moelling, K., and Hayami, M., 1977, Analysis of precursors to the envelope glycoproteins of avian RNA tumor viruses in chicken and quail cells, *J. Virol.* **22**:598.

Moennig, V., Frank, H., Hunsmann, G., Schneider, Il, and Schäfer, W., 1974, Properties of mouse leukemia viruses. VII. The major viral glycoprotein of Friend leukemia virus. Isolation and physicochemical properties, *Virology* **61**:100.

Moore, D. H., Davies, M. C., Levine, S., and Englert, M. E., 1962, Correlation of structure with infectivity of influenza virus, *Virology* **17**:470.

Moore, N. F., Kelley, J. M., and Wagner, R. R., 1974, Envelope proteins of vesicular stomatitis virions: Accessibility to iodination, *Virology* **61**:292.

Moore, N. F., Barenholz, Y., and Wagner, R. R., 1976, Microviscosity of togavirus membranes studied by fluorescence depolarization: Influence of envelope proteins and the host cell, *J. Virol.* **19**:126.

Morgan, C., Rose, H. M., Holden, M., and James, E. P., 1959, Electron microscopic observations on the development of herpes simplex virus, *J. Exp. Med.* **110**:643.

Morgan, C., Rifkin, R. A., and Rose, H. M., 1962, The use of ferritin-conjugated antibodies in electron microscopic studies of influenza and vaccinia viruses, *Cold Spring Harbor Symp. Quant. Biol.* **27**:57.

Moroni, C., 1972, Structural proteins of Rauscher leukemia virus and Harvey sarcoma virus, *Virology* **47**:1.

Morrison, T. G., and Lodish, H. F., 1975, Site of synthesis of membrane and non-membrane proteins of vesicular stomatitis virus, *J. Biol. Chem.* **250**:6955.

Moss, B., 1974, Reproduction of poxviruses, in: *Comprehensive Virology*, Vol. 3 (H. Fraenkel-Conrat and R. R. Wagner, eds.), pp. 405–474, Plenum Press, New York.

Moss, B., and Rosenblum, E. N., 1972, Hydroxylapatite chromatography of protein–sodium dodecyl sulfate complexes: A new method for the separation of polypeptide subunits, *J. Biol. Chem.* **247**:5194.

Moss, B., and Salzman, N. P., 1968, Sequential protein synthesis following vaccinia virus infection, *J. Virol.* **2**:1016.

Moss, B., Rosenblum, E. N., Katz, E., and Grimley, P. M., 1969, Rifampicin: A specific inhibitor of vaccinia virus assembly, *Nature (London)* **224**:1280.

Moss, B., Rosenblum, E. N., and Garon, C. F., 1973, Glycoprotein synthesis in cells infected with vaccinia virus. III. Purification and biosynthesis of the virion glycoprotein, *Virology* **55**:143.

Mosser, A. C., Montelaro, R. C., Rueckert, R. R., 1977, Proteins of Rous-associated virus type 61: Polypeptide stoichiometry and evidence that glycoprotein gp37 is not a cleavage product of gp85, *J. Virol.* **23**:1079.

Mountcastle, W. E., and Choppin, P. W., 1977, A comparison of the polypeptides of four measles virus strains, *Virology* **78**:463.

Mountcastle, W. E., Compans, R. W., and Choppin, P. W., 1971, Proteins and glycoproteins of paramyxoviruses: A comparison of Simian virus 5, Newcastle disease virus and Sendai virus, *J. Virol.* **7**:47.

Moyer, S. A., and Summers, D. F., 1974, Vesicular stomatitis virus envelope glycoprotein alterations induced by host cell transformation, *Cell* **2**:63.

Moyer, S. A., Tsang, J. M., Atkinson, P. H., and Summers, D. F., 1976, Oligosaccharide moieties of the glycoprotein of vesicular stomatitis virus, *J. Virol.* **18**:167.

Mudd, J. A., 1973, Effects of pH on the structure of vesicular stomatitis virus, *Virology* **55**:546.

Mudd, J. A., 1974, Glycoprotein fragment associated with vesicular stomatitis virus after proteolytic digestion, *Virology* **62**:573.

Murphy, F. A., Webb, P. A., Johnson, K. M., and Whitfield, S. G., 1969, Morphological comparison of Machupo with lymphocytic choriomeningitis virus: Basis for a new taxonomic group, *J. Virol.* **4**:535.

Murphy, F. A., Webb, P. A., Johnson, K. M., Whitfield, S. G., and Chappell, W. A., 1970, Arenoviruses in vero cells: Ultrastructural studies, *J. Virol.* **6**:507.

Murphy, F. A., Whitfield, S. G., Webb, P. A., and Johnson, K. M., 1973, Ultrastructural studies of arenaviruses, in: *Lymphocytic Choriomeningitis Virus and Other Arenaviruses* (F. Lehmann-Grube, ed.), pp. 273–285, Springer, Berlin.

Murphy, J. S., and Bang, F. B., 1952, Observations with the electron microscope on cells of the chick chorio-allantoic membrane infected with influenza virus, *J. Exp. Med.* **95**:259.

Mussgay, M., and Rott, R., 1964, Studies on the structure of a hemagglutinin component of a group A arbovirus (Sindbis), *Virology* **23**:573.

Nagai, Y., and Klenk, H.-D., 1977, Activation of precursors to both glycoproteins of NDV by proteolytic cleavage, *Virology* **77**:125.

Nagai, Y., Yoshida, T., Yoshii, S., Maeno, K., and Matsumoto, T., 1975, Modification of normal cell surface by smooth membrane preparations from BHK-21 cells infected with Newcastle disease virus, *Med. Microbiol. Immunol.* **161**:175.

Nagai, Y., Klenk, H.-D., and Rott, R., 1976*a*, Proteolytic cleavage of the viral glycoproteins and its significance for the virulence of Newcastle disease virus, *Virology* **72**:494.

Nagai, Y., Ogura, H., and Klenk, H.-D., 1976*b*, Studies on the assembly of the envelope of Newcastle disease virus, *Virology* **69**:523.

Nagington, J., and Horne, R. W., 1962, Morphological studies of orf and vaccinia viruses, *Virology* **16**:248.

Nakamura, K., and Compans, R. W., 1977, The cellular site of sulfation of influenza virus glycoproteins, *Virology* **79**:381.

Nakamura, K., and Compans, R. W., 1978*a*, Effects of glucosamine, 2-deoxy-D-glucose and tunicamycin on glycosylation, sulfation and assembly of influenza virus glycoproteins, *Virology* **84**:303.

Nakamura, K., and Compans, R. W., 1978*b*, Glycopeptide components of influenza viral glycoproteins, *Virology* **86**:432.

Naso, R. B., Arcement, L. J., and Arlinghaus, R. B., 1975, Biosynthesis of Rauscher leukemia viral proteins, *Cell* **4**:31.

Naso, R. B., Arcement, L. J., Karshin, W. L., Jamjoom, G. A., and Arlinghaus, R. B., 1976, A fucose-deficient glycoprotein precursor to Rauscher leukemia virus gp69, 71, *Proc. Natl. Acad. Sci. USA* **73**:2326.

Nermut, M. V., Frank, H., and Schäfer, W., 1972, Properties of mouse leukemia virus. III. Electron microscopic appearance as revealed after conventional preparation techniques as well as freeze-drying and freeze-etching, *Virology* **49**:345.

Nerome, K., Ishida, M., and Nakayama, M., 1976, Absence of neuraminidase from influenza C virus, *Arch. Virol.* **50**:241.

Neurath, A. R., Vernon, S. K., Dobkin, M. B., and Rubin, B. A., 1972, Characterization of subviral components resulting from treatment of rabies virus with tri-(*n*-butyl) phosphate, *J. Gen. Virol.* **14**:33.

Norrby, E., and Gollmar, Y., 1975, Identification of measles virus-specific hemolysis-inhibiting antibodies separate from hemagglutination-inhibiting antibodies, *Infect. Immun.* **11**:231.

Obijeski, J. F., Bishop, D. H. L., Murphy, F. A., and Palmer, E. L., 1976, The structural proteins of La Crosse virus, *J. Virol.* **19**:985.

O'Callaghan, D. J., and Randall, C. C., 1976, Molecular anatomy of herpesviruses: Recent studies, *Progr. Med. Viol.* **22**:152.

Ogura, H., Schmidt, M. F. G., and Schwarz, R. T., 1977, Effect of tunicamycin on the morphogenesis of Semliki Forest virus and Rous sarcoma virus, *Arch. Virol.* **55**:155.

Oram, J. D., Ellwood, D. C., Appleyard, G., and Stanley, J. C., 1971, Agglutination of an arbovirus by concanavalin A, *Nature (London) New Biol.* **233**:50.

Oshiro, L. S., 1973, Coronaviruses, in: *Ultrastructure of Animal Viruses and Bacteriophages* (A. J. Dalton and F. Haguenau, eds.), pp. 331–335, Academic Press, New York.

Palese, P., 1977, The genes of influenza virus, *Cell* **10**:1.

Palese, P., and Compans, R. W., 1976, Inhibition of influenza virus replication in tissue culture by 2-deoxy-2,3-dehydro-*N*-trifluoroacetylneuraminic acid (FANA): Mechanism of action, *J. Gen. Virol.* **33**:159.

Palese, P., and Schulman, J. L., 1974, Isolation and characterization of influenza virus recombinants with high and low neuraminidase activity: Use of 2-(3'-methoxyphenyl) N-acetylneuraminic acid to identify clone populations, *Virology* **57**:227.

Palese, P., Tobita, K., Ueda, M., and Compans, R. W., 1974, Characterization of temperature sensitive influenza virus mutants defective in neuraminidase, *Virology* **61**:397.

Paul, S. D., Singh, K. R. P., and Bhat, U. K. M., 1969, A study of the cytopathic effect of arboviruses on cultures from *Aedes albopictus* cell line, *Indian J. Med. Res.* **57**:339.

Pedersen, I. R., 1971, Lymphocytic choriomeningitis virus RNAs, *Nature (London) New Biol.* **234**:112.

Pedersen, I. R., 1973, Different classes of ribonucleic acid isolated from lymphocytic choriomeningitis virus, *J. Virol.* **11**:416.

Pedersen, C. E., and Eddy, G. A., 1974, Separation, isolation, and immunological studies of the structural proteins of Venezuelan equine encephalomyelitis virus, *J. Virol.* **14**:740.

Pedersen, C. E., Marker, S. C., and Eddy, G. A. 1974, Comparative electrophoretic studies on the structural proteins of selected group A arboviruses, *Virology* **60**:312.

Peluso, R. W., Lamb, R. A., and Choppin, P. W., 1977, Polypeptide synthesis in SV5-infected cells, *J. Virol.* **23**:177.

Perdue, M. L., Kemp, M. C., Randall, C. C., and O'Callaghan, D. J., 1974, Studies of the molecular anatomy of the L-M cell strain of equine herpes virus type 1: Proteins of the nucleocapsid and intact virion, *Virology* **59**:201.

Pesonen, M., and Renkonen, O., 1976, Serum glycoprotein-type sequence of monosaccharides in membrane glycoproteins of Semliki Forest virus, *Biochim. Biophys. Acta* **455**:510.

Peters, D., 1956, Morphology of resting vaccinia virus, *Nature (London)* **178**:1453.

Pettersson, R., and Kääriäinen, L., 1973, The ribonucleic acids of Uukuniemi virus, a non-cubical tick-borne arbovirus, *Virology* **56**:608.

Pettersson, R., and von Bonsdorff, C.-H., 1975, Ribonucleoproteins of Uukuniemi virus are circular, *J. Virol.* **15**:386.

Pfau, C. J., Bergold, G. H., Casals, J., Johnson, K. M., Murphy, F. A., Pedersen, I. R., Rawls, W. P., Webb, P. A., and Weissenbacher, M. C., 1974, Arenaviruses, *Intervirology* **4**:207.

Pfefferkorn, E. R., and Hunter, H. S., 1963a, Purification and partial chemical analysis of Sindbis virus, *Virology* **20**:443.

Pfefferkorn, E. R., and Hunter, H. S., 1963b, The source of the ribonucleic acid and phospholipid of Sindbis virus, *Virology* **20**:446.

Pinter, A., and Compans, R. W., 1975, Sulfated components of enveloped viruses, *J. Virol.* **16**:859.

Pons, M. W., 1976, A re-examination of influenza single- and double-stranded RNAs by gel electrophoresis, *Virology* **69**:789.

Porterfield, J. S., Casals, J., Shumakov, M. P., Gaidamovich, S. Y., Hannoun, C., Holmes, I. H., Horzinek, M. C., Mussgay, M., Oker-Blom, N, and Russell, P. K., 1976, Bunyaviruses and bunyaviridae, *Intervirol* **6**:13.

Portner, A., Scroggs, R. A., Marx, P. A., and Kingsbury, D. W., 1975, A temperature-sensitive mutant of Sendai virus with an altered hemagglutinin–neuraminidase polypeptide: Consequence for virus assembly and cytopathology, *Virology* **67**:179.

Prochownik, E. V., Panem, S., and Kirsten, W. H., 1975, Biological and physical modifications of a murine oncornavirus by 2-deoxy-glucose, *J. Virol.* **15**:1323.

Quigley, J. P., Rifkin, D. B., and Reich, E., 1971, Phospholipid composition of Rous sarcoma virus, host cell membranes and other enveloped RNA viruses, *Virology* **46**:106.

Quigley, J. P., Rifkin, D. B., and Compans, R. W., 1972, Isolation and characterization of ribonucleoprotein substructures from Rous sarcoma virus, *Virology* **50**:65.

Ramos, B. A., Courtney, R. J., and Rawls, W. E., 1972, Structural proteins of Pichinde virus, *J. Virol.* **10**:661.

Rao, P. R., Bonar, R. A., and Beard, J. W., 1966, Lipids of the BAI strain A avian tumor virus and of the myeloblast host cell, *Exp. Mol. Pathol.* **5**:374.

Reginster, M., and Nermut, M. V., 1976, Preparation and characterization of influenza virus cores, *J. Gen. Virol.* **31**:211.

Renkonen, O., Kääriäinen, L., Simons, K., and Gahmberg, C. G., 1971, The lipid class composition of Semliki Forest virus and of plasma membranes of the host cells, *Virology* **36**:318.

Renkonen, O., Gahmberg, C. G., Simons, K., and Kääriäinen, L., 1972a, The lipids of the plasma membrane and endoplasmic reticulum from cultured baby hamster kidney cells (BHK-21), *Biochim. Biophys. Acta* **255**:66.

Renkonen, O., Kääriäinen, L., Gahmberg, C. G., and Simons, K., 1972b, Lipids of Semliki Forest virus and host cell membranes, in: *Current Trends in the Biochemistry of Lipids* (J. Ganguly and R. M. S. Smellie, eds.), pp. 407–422, Academic Press, New York.

Renkonen, O., Pesonen, M., and Mattila, K., 1976, Oligosaccharides of the membrane glycoproteins of Semliki Forest virus, in: *Structure of Biological Membranes* (L. Abrahamson and I. Pascher, eds.), pp. 409–423, Plenum Press, New York.

Richardson, C. D., and Vance, D. E., 1976, Biochemical evidence that Semliki Forest virus obtains its envelope from the plasma membrane of the host cell, *J. Biol. Chem.* **251**:5544.

Rifkin, D. B., and Compans, R. W., 1971, Identification of the spike proteins of Rous sarcoma virus, *Virology* **46**:485.

Rifkin, D. B., Compans, R. W., and Reich, E., 1972, A specific labeling procedure for proteins on the outer surface of membranes, *J. Biol. Chem.* **247**:6432.

Ritchey, M. B., Palese, P., and Kilbourne, E. D., 1976, RNAs of influenza A, B, and C viruses, *J. Virol.* **18**:738.

Robertson, B. H., Bhown, A. S., Compans, R. W., and Bennett, J. C., 1978, in: *Negative Strand Viruses and the Host Cell* (R. D. Barry and B. W. J. Mahy, eds.), pp. 213–219, Academic Press, New York.

Robertson, J. S., and Summers, D. F., 1977, Glycosylation of the glycoprotein of a thermolabile mutant of vesicular stomatitis virus, *J. Supramol. Struct. Suppl.* **1**:5.

Robertson, J. S., Etchison, J. R., and Summers, D. F., 1976, Glycosylation sites of vesicular stomatitis virus glycoprotein, *J. Virol.* **19**:871.

Robinson, D. J., and Watson, D. H., 1971, Structural proteins of herpes simplex virus, *J. Gen. Virol.* **10**:163.

Robinson, W. S., and Robinson, H. L., 1971, Envelope proteins of the avian tumor viruses, in: *Membrane Research* (C. Fred Fox, ed.), pp. 187–203, Academic Press, New York.

Rohrschneider, J. M., Diggelmann, H., Ogura, H., Friis, R. R., and Bauer, H., 1976, Defective cleavage of a precursor polypeptide in a temperature sensitive mutant of avian sarcoma virus, *Virology* **75**:177.

Roizman, B., and Furlong, D., 1974, The replication of herpesviruses, in: *Comprehensive Virology*, Vol. 3 (H. Fraenkel-Conrat and R. R. Wagner, eds.), pp. 229–403, Plenum Press, New York.

Roizman, B., and Spear, P. G., 1971, The role of herpesvirus glycoproteins in the modification of membranes of infected cells, in: *Nucleic Acid–Protein Interactions: Nucleic Acid Synthesis in Viral Infection* (D. W. Ribbons, J. F. Woessner, and J. Schultz, eds.), pp. 435–455, North-Holland, New York.

Rosato, R. R., Dalrymple, J. M., Brandt, W. E., Cardiff, R. D., and Russell, P. K., 1974, Biophysical separation of major arbovirus serogroups, *Acta Virol.* **18**:25.

Rothman, J. E., and Lodish, H. F., 1977, Synchronised transmembrane insertion and glycosylation of a nascent membrane protein, *Nature (London)* **269**:775.

Rothman, J. E., Tsai, D. K., Dawidowicz, E. A., and Lenard, J., 1976, Transbilayer phospholipid asymmetry and its maintenance in the membrane of influenza virus, *Biochemistry* **15**:2361.

Rott, R., and Schäfer, W., 1960, Research on the hemagglutinizing non-infectious particles of influenza virus. 1. The production of "incomplete forms" of the virus of the classical fowl plague (Von Magnus phenomenon), *Z. Naturforsch.* **15b**:691.

Rott, R., Frank, H., and Schäfer, W., 1961, Isolierung und Eigenschaften der hemagglutinierenden Komponente des Virus der Newcastle disease, *Z. Naturforsch.* **16b**:625.

Rott, R., Reda, I. M., and Schäfer, W., 1963, Charakterisierung der verschiedenen, nach Infekten mit Newcastle disease Virus auftretenden, nichtinfektiosen, hemagglutinierenden Teilchen, *Z. Naturforsch.* **18b**:188.

Rott, R., Drzeniek, R., Saber, S., and Reichert, E., 1966, Blood group substances, Forssman and mononucleosis antigen in lipid-containing RNA viruses, *Arch. Ges. Virusforsch.* **19**:273.

Rott, R., Drzeniek, R., and Frank, H., 1970, On the structure of influenza viruses, in: *The Biology of Large RNA Viruses* (R. D. Barry and B. W. J. Mahy, eds.), pp. 74–85, Academic Press, London.

Rutter, G., and Mannweiler, K., 1976, Antibody-induced redistribution of virus antigens on the surface of influenza virus-infected cells, *J. Gen. Virol.* **33**:321.

Saleh, F., and Compans, R. W., 1978, Polypeptide synthesis in Tacaribe virus-infected cells, *Abstr. Annu. Meet. Am. Soc. Microbiol.*, p. 249.

Samson, A. C. R., and Fox, C. F., 1973, Precursor protein for Newcastle disease virus, *J. Virol.* **12**:579.

Sarov, I., and Joklik, W. K., 1972, Studies on the nature and location of the capsid polypeptide of vaccinia virions, *Virology* **50**:579.

Schäfer, W., 1959, The comparative chemistry of infective virus particles and of other virus-specific products: Animal viruses, in: *The Viruses*, Vol. 1 (F. M. Burnet and W. M. Stanley, eds.), pp. 475–504, Academic Press, New York.

Schäfer, W., Fischinger, P. J., Collins, J. J., and Bolognesi, D. P., 1977, Role of carbohydrate in biological functions of Friend murine leukemia virus gp71, *J. Virol.* **21**:35.

Scheele, C. M., and Hanafusa, H., 1971, Proteins of helper-dependent RSV, *Virology* **45**:401.

Scheid, A., and Choppin, P. W., 1973, Isolation and purification of the envelope proteins of Newcastle disease virus, *J. Virol.* **11**:263.

Scheid, A., and Choppin, P. W., 1974*a*, Identification and biological activities of paramyxovirus glycoproteins: Activation of cell fusion, hemolysis and infectivity by proteolytic cleavage of an inactive precursor of Sendai virus, *Virology* **57**:475.

Scheid, A., and Choppin, P. W., 1974b, The hemagglutinating and neuraminidase (HN) protein of a paramyxovirus: Interaction with neuraminic acid in affinity chromatography, *Virology* **62**:125.

Scheid, A., and Choppin, P. W., 1976, Protease activation mutants of Sendai virus: Activation of biological properties by specific proteases, *Virology* **69**:277.

Scheid, A., and Choppin, P. W., 1977, Two disulfide-linked polypeptide chains constitute the active F protein of paramyxoviruses, *Virology* **80**:54.

Scheid, A., Caliguiri, L. A., Compans, R. W., and Choppin, P. W., 1972, Isolation of paramyxovirus glycoproteins: Association of both hemagglutinating and neuraminidase activities with the larger SV5 glycoproteins, *Virology* **50**:640.

Scheid, A., Graves, M. C., Silver, S. M., and Choppin, P. W., 1978, Studies on the structure and function of paramyxovirus proteins, in: *Negative Strand Viruses and the Host Cell* (B. W. J. Mahy and R. D. Barry, eds.), pp. 181–193, Academic Press, New York.

Schlesinger, M. J., and Schlesinger, S., 1973, Large-molecular-weight precursors of Sindbis virus proteins, *J. Virol.* **11**:1013.

Schlesinger, M. J., Schlesinger, S., and Burge, B. W., 1972, Identification of a second glycoprotein in Sindbis virus, *Virology* **47**:539.

Schlesinger, R. W., 1977, Dengue virus, in: *Virology Monographs* (S. Gard and C. Hallauer, eds.), Springer-Verlag, New York.

Schlesinger, S., Schlesinger, M. J., and Burge, B. W., 1972, Defective virus particles from Sindbis virus, *Virology* **48**:615.

Schlesinger, S., Gottlieb, C., Feil, P., Gelb, N., and Kornfeld, S., 1976, Growth of enveloped RNA viruses in a line of chinese hamster ovary cells with deficient *N*-acetyl-glucosaminyltransferase activity, *J. Virol.* **17**:239.

Schloemer, R. H., and Wagner, R. R., 1974, Sialoglycoprotein of vesicular stomatitis virus: Role of the neuraminic acid in infection, *J. Virol.* **14**:270.

Schloemer, R. H., and Wagner, R. R., 1975a, Mosquito cells infected with vesicular stomatitis virus yield unsialylated virions of low infectivity, *J. Virol.* **15**:1029.

Schloemer, R. H., and Wagner, R. R., 1975b, Association of vesicular stomatitis virus glycoprotein with membranes: Isolation and characterization of a lipophilic fragment of the glycoprotein, *J. Virol.* **16**:237.

Schmidt, M. F. G., Schwarz, R. T., and Scholtissek, C., 1976a, Interference of nucleoside diphosphate derivatives of 2-deoxy-D-glucose with the glycosylation of virus-specific glycoproteins in vivo, *Eur. J. Biochem.* **70**:55.

Schmidt, M. F. G., Schwarz, R. T., and Ludwig, H., 1976b, Fluorosugars inhibit biological properties of different enveloped viruses, *J. Virol.* **18**:819.

Schneider, L. G., and Diringer, H., 1976, Structure and molecular biology of rabies virus, *Curr. Top. Microbiol. Immunol.* **75**:153.

Schneider, L. G., Dietzschold, B., Dierks, R. E., Matthaeus, W., Enzmann, P.-H., and Strohmaier, K., 1973, The rabies group-specific ribonucleoprotein (RNP) antigen and a test system for grouping and typing of rhabdoviruses, *J. Virol.* **11**:748.

Scholtissek, C., Rott, R., Hau, G., and Kaluza, G., 1974, Inhibition of the multiplication of vesicular stomatitis and Newcastle disease virus by 2-deoxy-D-glucose, *J. Virol.* **13**:1186.

Scholtissek, C., Kaluza, G., Schmidt, M. F. G., and Rott, R., 1975, Influence of sugar derivatives on glycoprotein synthesis of enveloped viruses, in: *Negative Strand Viruses*, Vol. 2 (B. W. J. Mahy and R. D. Barry, eds.), pp. 669–683, Academic Press, New York.

Scholtissek, C., Harms, E., Rohde, W., Orlich, M., and Rott, R., 1976, Correlation between RNA fragments of fowl plague virus and their corresponding gene functions, *Virology* **74**:332.

Schulze, I. T., 1970, The structure of influenza virus. I. The polypeptides of the virion, *Virology* **42**:890.

Schulze, I. T., 1972, The structure of influenza virus. II. A model based on the morphology and composition of subviral particles, *Virology* **47**:181.

Schulze, I. T., 1973, Structure of the influenza virion, *Adv. Virus Res.* **18**:1.

Schulze, I. T., 1975a, Effects of sialylation on the biological activities of the influenza virion, in: *Negative Strand Viruses* (R. D. Barry and B. W. J. Mahy, eds.), pp. 161–175, Academic Press, New York.

Schulze, I. T., 1975b, The biologically active proteins of influenza virus: The hemagglutinin, in: *The Influenza Viruses and Influenza* (E. D. Kilbourne, ed.), pp. 53–82, Academic Press, New York.

Schwartz, J., and Roizman, B., 1969, Concerning the egress of herpes simplex virus from infected cells: Electron microscopic observations, *Virology* **38**:42.

Schwarz, H., Hunsmann, G., Moenning, V., and Schäfer, W., 1976, Properties of mouse leukemia virus. VI. Immunoelectron microscopic studies on viral antigens on the cell surface, *Virology* **69**:169.

Schwarz, R. T., and Klenk, H.-D., 1974, Inhibition of glycosylation of influenza virus hemagglutinin, *J. Virol.* **14**:1023.

Schwarz, R. T., Rohrschneider, J. M., and Schmidt, M. F. G., 1976, Suppression of glycoprotein formation of Semliki Forest, influenza, and avian sarcoma virus by tunicamycin, *J. Virol.* **19**:782.

Schwarz, R. T., Schmidt, M. F. G., Anwer, U., and Klenk, H. D., 1977, Carbohydrates of influenza virus. I. Glycopeptides derived from viral glycoproteins after labeling with radioactive sugars, *J. Virol.* **23**:217.

Schwarz, R. T., Fournet, B., Montreuil, J., Rott, R., and Klenk, H.-D., 1978a, The carbohydrates of influenza virus. II. Gas chromatographic analysis of glycopeptides derived from viral glycoproteins and mucopolysaccharides, *Arch. Virol.* **56**:251.

Schwarz, R. T., Schmidt, M. F. G., and Lehle, L., 1978b, In vitro glycosylation of Semliki Forest- and influenza virus glycoproteins and its suppression by nucleotide 2-deoxy-sugar, *Eur. J. Biochem.* **85**:163.

Scupman, R. K., Jones, K. J., Sagik, B. P., and Bose, H. R., 1977, Virus-directed post-translational cleavage in Sindbis virus-infected cells, *J. Virol.* **22**:568.

Sefton, B. M., 1976, Virus-dependent glycosylation, *J. Virol.* **17**:85.

Sefton, B. M., 1977, Immediate glycosylation of Sindbis virus membrane proteins, *Cell* **10**:659.

Sefton, B. M., and Burge, B. W., 1973, Biosynthesis of the Sindbis virus carbohydrates, *J. Virol.* **12**:1366.

Sefton, B. M., and Gaffney, B. J., 1974, Effect of the viral proteins on the fluidity of the membrane lipids in Sindbis virus, *J. Mol. Biol.* **90**:343.

Sefton, B. M., and Keegstra, K., 1974, Glycoproteins of Sindbis virus: Preliminary characterization of the oligosaccharides, *J. Virol.* **14**:522.

Sefton, B. M., Wickus, G. G., and Burge, B. W., 1973, Enzymatic iodination of Sindbis virus proteins, *J. Virol.* **11**:730.

Seto, J. T., and Rott, R., 1966, Functional significance of sialidase during influenza virus multiplication, *Virology* **30**:731.

Seto, J. T., Drzeniek, R., and Rott, R., 1966, Isolation of low molecular weight sialidase (neuraminidase) from influenza virus, *Biochim. Biophys. Acta* **123**:402.
Seto, J. T., Becht, H., and Rott, R., 1973, Isolation and purification of surface antigens
from disrupted paramyxoviruses, *Med. Microbiol. Immunol.* **159**:1.
Seto, J. T., Becht, H., and Rott, R., 1974, Effect of specific antibodies on biological
function of the envelope components of Newcastle disease virus, *Virology* **61**:354.
Shapiro, S. Z., and August, J. T., 1976, Proteolytic cleavage events in oncornavirus
protein synthesis, *Biochim. Biophys. Acta Cancer Rev.*
Shapiro, D., Brandt, W. E., Cardiff, R. D., and Russell, P. K., 1971, The proteins of
Japanese encephalitis virus, *Virology* **44**:108.
Shimizu, K., and Ishida, N., 1975, The smallest protein of Sendai virus: Its candidate
function of binding nucleocapsid to envelope, *Virology* **67**:427.
Shimizu, K., Shimizu, Y. K., Kohama, T., and Ishida, N., 1974, Isolation and
characterization of two distinct types of HVJ (Sendai virus) spikes, *Virology* **62**:90.
Simmons, D. T., and Strauss, J. H., 1974, Translation of Sindbis virus 26 S RNA and
49 S RNA in lysates of rabbit reticulocytes, *J. Mol. Biol.* **86**:397.
Simons, K., Keranen, S., and Kääriäinen, L., 1973, Identification of a precursor of one
of the Semliki Forest virus membrane proteins, *FEBS Lett.* **29**:87.
Skehel, J. J., 1972, Polypeptide synthesis in influenza virus-infected cells, *Virology*
49:23.
Skehel, J. J., and Schild, G. C., 1971, The polypeptide composition of influenza A
viruses, *Virology* **44**:396.
Skehel, J. J., and Waterfield, M. D., 1975, Studies on the primary structure of the
influenza virus hemagglutinin, *Proc. Natl. Acad. Sci. USA* **72**:93.
Sly, W. S., Lagwinska, E., and Schlesinger, S., 1976, Enveloped virus acquires
membrane defect when passaged in fibroblasts from I-cell disease patients, *Proc.
Natl. Acad. Sci. USA* **73**:2443.
Smadel, J. E., Lavin, G. I., and Dubos, R. J., 1940, Some constituents of elementary
bodies of vaccinia virus, *J. Exp. Med.* **71**:373.
Smith, J. F., and Brown, D. T., 1977, Envelopment of Sindbis virus: Synthesis and
organization of protein in cells infected with wild type and maturation defective
mutants, *J. Virol.* **22**:662.
Smith, R. E., 1974, High specific infectivity avian RNA tumor viruses, *Virology* **60**:543.
Soderlund, H., 1976, The post-translational processing of Semliki Forest virus
structural polypeptide in puromycin treated cells, *FEBS Lett.* **63**:56.
Sokol, F., Stancek, D., and Koprowski, H., 1971, Structural proteins of rabies virus, *J.
Virol.* **7**:241.
Spear, P. G., 1976, Membrane proteins specified by herpes simplex viruses. I. Identifi-
cation of four glycoprotein precursors and their products in type 1-infected cells, *J.
Virol.* **17**:991.
Spear, P. G., and Roizman, B., 1970, Protein specified by herpes simplex virus. IV. Site
of glycosylation and accumulation of viral membrane proteins, *Proc. Natl. Acad.
Sci. USA* **66**:730.
Spear, P. G., Keller, J. M., and Roizman, B., 1970, Proteins specified by herpes sim-
plex virus, *J. Virol.* **5**:123.
Spring, S. B., and Roizman, B., 1968, Herpes simplex virus products in productive and
abortive infection. III. Differentiation of infectious virus derived from nucleus and
cytoplasm with respect to stability and size, *J. Virol.* **2**:979.

Stanley, P., and Haslam, E. A., 1971, The polypeptides of influenza virus. V. Localization of polypeptides in the virion by iodination techniques, *Virology* **46**:764.

Stanley, P., Gandhi, S. S., and White, D. O., 1973, The polypeptides of influenza virus. VII. Synthesis of the hemagglutinin, *Virology* **53**:92.

Stern, W., and Dales, S., 1974, Biogenesis of vaccinia: Concerning the origin of the envelope phospholipids, *Virology* **62**:293.

Stern, W., and Dales, S., 1976, Biogenesis of vaccinia: Isolation and characterization of a surface component that elicits antibody suppressing infectivity and cell–cell fusion, *Virology* **75**:232.

Stoffel, W., and Bister, K., 1975, ^{13}C Nuclear magnetic resonance studies on the lipid organization of enveloped virions (vesicular stomatitis virus), *Biochemistry* **14**:2841.

Stoffel, W., and Sorgo, W., 1976, Asymmetry of the lipid-bilayer of Sindbis virus, *Chem. Phys. Lipids* **17**:324.

Stoffel, W., Anderson, R., and Stahl, J., 1975, Studies on the asymmetric arrangement of membrane-lipid-enveloped virions as a model system, *Z. Physiol. Chem.* **356**:1123.

Stoffel, W., Bister, K., Schneider, C., and Tunggal, B., 1976, ^{13}C NMR studies of the membrane structure of enveloped virions (vesicular stomatitis virus), *Z. Physiol. Chem.* **357**:905.

Stollar, V., 1969, Studies on the nature of dengue viruses. IV. The structural proteins of type 2 dengue virus, *Virology* **39**:426.

Stollar, V., Stollar, B. D., Koo, R., Harrap, K. A., and Schlesinger, R. W., 1976, Sialic acid contents of Sindbis virus from vertebrate and mosquito cells: Equivalence of biological and immunological viral properties, *Virology* **69**:104.

Strand, M., and August, J. T., 1973, Structural proteins of oncogenic ribonucleic acid viruses: Interspec II, A new interspecies antigen, *J. Biol. Chem.* **248**:5627.

Strand, M., and August, J. T., 1976, Structural proteins of ribonucleic acid tumor viruses, *J. Biol. Chem.* **251**:559.

Strauss, J. H., and Strauss, E. G., 1976, Togaviruses, in: *The Molecular Biology of Animal Viruses* (D. P. Nayak, ed.), pp. 111–166, Marcel Dekker, New York.

Strauss, J. H., Burge, B. W., and Darnell, J. E., 1969, Sindbis virus infection of chick and hamster cells: Synthesis of virus-specific proteins, *Virology* **37**:367.

Strauss, J. H., Jr., Burge, B. W., and Darnell, J. E., Jr., 1970, Carbohydrate content of the membrane protein of Sindbis virus, *J. Mol. Biol.* **47**:437.

Stromberg, K., Hurley, N. E., Davis, N. L., Rueckert, R. R., and Fleissner, E., 1974, Structural studies of avian myeloblastosis virus: Comparison of polypeptides in virion and core components by dodecyl sulfate polyacrylamide gel electrophoresis, *J. Virol.* **13**:513.

Sturman, L. S., 1977, Characterization of a coronavirus. I. Structural proteins: Effects of preparative conditions on the migration of proteins in polyacrylamide gels, *Virology* **77**:637.

Sturman, L. S., and Holmes, K. V., 1977, Characterization of a coronavirus. II. Glycoproteins of the viral envelope: Tryptic peptide analysis, *Virology* **77**:650.

Summers, D. F., Maizel, J. V., Jr., and Darnell, J. E., 1965, Evidence for virus-specific noncapsid proteins in poliovirus-infected HeLa cells, *Proc. Natl. Acad. Sci. USA* **54**:509.

Takatsuki, A., and Tamura, G., 1971, Tunicamycin, a new antibiotic. III. Reversal of antiviral activity of tunicamycin by aminosugars and their derivatives, *J. Antibiot.* **24**:224.

Takatsuki, A., Khono, K., and Tamura, G., 1975, Inhibition of biosynthesis of polyisoprenol sugars in chick embryo microsomes by tunicamycin, *Agr. Biol. Chem.* **39**:2089.

Takehara, M., 1975, Polykaryocytosis induced by vesicular stomatitis virus infection in BHK-21 cells, *Arch. Virol.* **49**:297.

Tiffany, J. M., and Blough, H. A., 1969a, Myxovirus envelope proteins: A directing influence on the fatty acids of membrane lipids, *Science* **163**:573.

Tiffany, J. M., and Blough, H. A., 1969b, Fatty acid composition of three strains of Newcastle disease virus, *Virology* **37**:492.

Tiffany, J., and Blough, H., 1970, Models of structure of the envelope of influenza virus, *Proc. Natl. Acad. Sci. USA* **65**:1105.

Tkacz, D. S., and Lampen, J. O., 1975, Tunicamycin inhibition of biosynthesis of polyisoprenol sugars in chick embryo microsomes by tunicamycin, *Biochem. Biophys. Res. Commun.* **65**:248.

Toneguzzo, F., and Ghosh, H. P., 1977, Synthesis and glycosylation in vitro of glycoprotein of vesicular stomatitis virus, *Proc. Natl. Acad. Sci. USA* **74**:1516.

Toneguzzo, F., and Ghosh, H. P., 1978, In vitro synthesis and insertion into membranes of vesicular stomatitis virus membrane glycoprotein, *Proc. Natl. Acad. Sci. USA* **75**:715.

Tozawa, H., Bauer, H., Graf, T., and Gelderblom, H., 1970, Strain specific antigen of the avian leukosis sarcoma virus group, *Virology* **40**:530.

Tozawa, W., Watanabe, M., and Ishida, N., 1973, Structural components of Sendai virus: Serological and physico-chemical characterization of hemagglutinin subunit associated with neuraminidase activity, *Virology* **55**:242.

Trent, D. W., 1977, Antigenic characterization of flavivirus structural proteins separated by isoelectric focusing, *J. Virol.* **22**:608.

Trent, D. W., and Qureshi, A. A., 1971, Structural and nonstructural proteins of Saint Louis encephalitis virus, *J. Virol.* **7**:379.

Tsai, K. H., and Lenard, J., 1975, Asymmetry of influenza virus membrane bilayer demonstrated with phospholipase C, *Nature (London)* **225**:554.

Ueda, V., Ito, M., and Tagaya, I., 1969, A specific surface antigen induced by poxvirus, *Virology* **38**:180.

Uterman, G., and Simons, K., 1974, Studies on the amphipathic nature of the membrane proteins in Semliki Forest virus, *J. Mol. Biol.* **85**:569.

Van Zaane, D., Gielkens, A. L. J., Dekker-Michielsen, M. J. A., and Bloemers, H. P. J., 1975, Virus-specific precursor polypeptides in cells infected with Rauscher leukemia virus, *Virology* **67**:544.

Van Zaane, D., Dekker-Michielsen, M. J. A., and Bloemers, H. P. J., 1976, Virus-specific precursor polypeptides in cells infected with Rauscher leukemia virus: Synthesis, identification, and processing, *Virology* **75**:113.

Vezza, A. C., Gard, G. P., Compans, R. W., and Bishop, D. H. L., 1977, Structural components of the arenavirus Pichinde, *J. Virol.* **23**:776.

Vezza, A. C., Clewley, J. P., Gard, G. P., Abraham, N. Z., Compans, R. W., and Bishop, D. H. L., 1978, The virion RNA species of the arenaviruses Pichinde, Tacaribe and Tamiami, *J. Virol.* **26**:485.

Vogt, P. K., 1977, Genetics of RNA tumor viruses. in: *Comprehensive Virology*, Vol. 9 (H. Fraenkel-Conrat and R. R. Wagner, eds.), pp. 341–455, Plenum Press, New York.

Vogt, P. K., and Ishizaki, R., 1966, Patterns of viral interference in the avian leukosis and sarcoma complex, *Virology* **30**:368.

Vogt, V. M., and Eisenman, R., 1973, Identification of a large polypeptide precursor of avian oncornavirus proteins, *Proc. Natl. Acad. Sci. USA* **70**:1734.

Vogt, V. M., Eisenman, R., and Diggelman, H., 1975, Generation of avian myeloblastosis virus structural proteins by proteolytic cleavage of a precursor polypeptide, *J. Mol. Biol.* **96**:471.

von Bonsdorff, C. H., and Harrison, S. C., 1975, Sindbis virus glycoproteins form a regular icosahedral surface lattice, *J. Virol.* **16**:141.

von Bonsdorff, C. H., and Pettersson, R., 1975, Surface structure of Uukuniemi virus, *J. Virol.* **16**:1296.

von Magnus, P., 1954, Incomplete forms of influenza virus, *Adv. Virus Res.* **2**:59.

Wagner, R. R., 1975, Reproduction of rhabdoviruses, in: *Comprehensive Virology*, Vol. 4 (H. Fraenkel-Conrat and R. R. Wagner, eds.), Plenum, New York.

Wagner, R. R., Schnaitman, T. C., Snyder, R. M., and Schnaitman, C. A., 1969, Protein composition of the structural components of vesicular stomatitis virus, *J. Virol.* **3**:611.

Wagner, R. R., Kiley, M. P., Snyder, R. M., and Schnaitman, C. A., 1972a, Cytoplasmic compartmentalization of the protein and ribonucleic acid species of vesicular stomatitis virus, *J. Virol.* **9**:672.

Wagner, R. R., Prevec, L., Brown, F., Summers, D. F., Sokol, F., and McLead, R., 1972b, Classification of rhabdovirus proteins: A proposal, *J. Virol.* **10**:1228.

Waite, M. R. F., Brown, D. T., and Pfefferkorn, E. R., 1972, Inhibition of Sindbis virus release by media of low ionic strength: An electron microscope study, *J. Virol.* **10**:537.

Wang, E., Wolf, B. A., Lamb, R. A., Choppin, P. W. and Goldberg, A. R., 1976, The presence of actin in enveloped viruses, in: *Cell Motility* (R. Goldman, T. Pollard, and J. Rosenbaum, eds.), p. 589, Cold Spring Harbor Press, New York.

Waterson, A. P., Rott, R., and Schäfer, W., 1961, The structure of fowl plague virus and virus N, *Z. Naturforsch.* **16b**:154.

Webster, R. G., 1970, Estimation of the molecular weights of the polypeptide chains from the isolated hemagglutinin and neuraminidase subunits of influenza viruses, *Virology* **40**:643.

Webster, R. G., and Darlington, R. W., 1969, Disruption of myxoviruses with Tween 20 and isolation of biologically active hemagglutinin and neuraminidase subunits, *J. Virol.* **4**:182.

Webster, R. G., and Laver, W. G., 1967, Preparation and properties of antibody directed specifically against the neuraminidase of infleunza virus, *J. Immunol.* **99**:49.

Webster, R. G., and Laver, W. G., 1972, Studies on the origin of pandemic influenza I. Antigenic analysis of A_2 influenza viruses isolated before and after the appearance of Hong Kong influenza using antisera to the isolated hemagglutinin subunits, *Virology* **48**:433.

Webster, R. G., and Laver, W. G., 1975, Antigenic variation of influenza viruses, in: *The Infleunza Viruses and Influenza* (E. D. Kilbourne, ed.), pp. 270–314, Academic Press, New York.

Wecker, E., 1957, Die Verteilung von ^{32}P in Virus der klassischen Geflügelpest bei verschiedenen Markierungsverfahren, *Z. Naturforsch.* **12b**:208.

Wengler, G., Beato, M., and Hackemack, B.-A., 1974, Translation of 26 S virus-specific RNA from Semliki Forest virus-infected cells in vitro, *Virology* **61**:120.

Weintraub, S., and Dales, S., 1974, Biogenesis of poxviruses: Genetically controlled modifications of structural and functional components of the plasma membrane, *Virology* **60**:96.

Weiss, R. A., 1969, The host range of Bryan strain RSV synthesized in the absence of helper virus, *J. Gen. Virol.* **5**:511.

Westaway, E. G., 1975, The proteins of Murray Valley encephalitis virus, *J. Gen. Virol.* **27**:283.

Westaway, E. G., and Reedman, B. M., 1969, Proteins of group B arbovirus Kunjin, *J. Virol.* **4**:688.

Westaway, E. G., and Shaw, M., 1977, Proteins and glycoproteins specified by the flavivirus Kunjin, *Virology* **80**:309.

Westwood, J. C. N., Harris, W. J., Zwartouw, H. T., Titmuss, D. H. J., and Appleyard, G., 1964, Studies on the structure of vaccinia virus, *J. Gen. Microbiol.* **34**:67.

White, A. B., 1975, Structural polypeptides of California encephalitis virus, BFS-283, *Arch. Virol.* **49**:281.

White, D. O., 1974. Influenza viral proteins: Identification and synthesis, *Curr. Top. Microbiol. Immunol.* **63**:1.

White, D. O., Taylor, J. M., Haslam, E. A., and Hampson, A. W., 1970, The polypeptides of influenza virus and their biosynthesis, in: *The Biology of Large RNA Viruses* (R. D. Barry and B. W. J. Mahy, eds.), pp. 602–618, Academic Press, London.

White, H. B., Powell, S. S., Gafford, L. G., and Randall, C. C., 1968, The occurrence of squalene in lipid of fowlpox virus, *J. Virol. Chem.* **243**:4517.

Whitfield, S. G., Murphy, F. A., and Sudia, W. D., 1971, Eastern equine encephalomyelitis virus: An electron microscopic study of *Aedes triseriatus* (Say) salivary gland infection, *Virology* **43**:110.

Wiktor, T. J., Gyorgy, E., Schlumberger, H. D., Sokol. F., and Koprowski, H., 1973, Antigenic properties of rabies virus components, *J. Immunol.* **110**:269.

Wildy, P., Russell, W. C., and Horne, R. W., 1960, The morphology of herpes virus, *Virology* **12**:204.

Wiley, D. C., 1975, Crystalline hemagglutinin from influenza virus, *International Virology 3* (abstr.), p. 265.

Wiley, D. C., Skehel, J. J., and Waterfield, M., 1977, Evidence from studies with cross-linking reagent that the haemagglutinin of influenza virus is a trimer, *Virology* **79**:446.

Wirth, D. F., Katz, F., Small, B., and Lodish, H., 1977, How a single-stranded Sindbis virus mRNA directs the synthesis of one soluble protein and two integral membrane glycoproteins, *Cell* **10**:253.

Witte, O. N., and Weissman, I. L., 1976. Oncornavirus budding: Kinetics of formation and utilization of viral membrane glycoprotein, *Virology* **69**:464.

Witte, O. N., Weissman, I. L., and Kaplan, H. S., 1973, Structural characteristics of some murine RNA tumor viruses studied by lactoperoxidase iodination, *Proc. Natl. Acad. Sci. USA* **70**:36.

Witte, O. N., Tsukamoto-Adey, A., and Weissman, I. L., 1977, Cellular maturation of oncornavirus glycoproteins: Topological arrangement of precursor and product forms in cellular membranes, *Virology* **76**:539.

Witter, R., Frank, H., Moennig, V., Hunsmann, G., Lange, J., and Schäfer, W., 1973, Properties of mouse leukemia viruses. IV. Hemagglutination assay and characterization of hemagglutinating surface components, *Virology* **54**:330.

Wrigley, N. G., Skehel, J. J., Charlwood, P. A., and Brand, C. M., 1973, The size and shape of influenza virus neuraminidase, *Virology* **51**:525.

Wunner, W. H., and Pringle, C. R., 1976, Respiratory syncytial virus proteins, *Virology* **73**:228.

Yagi, M. J., and Compans, R. W., 1977, Structural components of mouse mammary tumor virus. I. Polypeptides of the virion, *Virology* **76**:751.

Yeger, H., and Kalnins, 1976, Electron microscopy of mammalian type-C RNA viruses: Use of conditional lethal mutants in studies of virion maturation and assembly, *Virology* **74**:459.

Yoshida, T., Nagai, Y., Yoshii, S., Maeno, K., and Matsumoto, T., 1976, Membrane (M) protein of HVJ (Sendai virus): Its role in virus assembly, *Virology* **71**:143.

Zee, Y. C., Hackett, A. J., and Talens, L., 1970, Vesicular stomatitis virus maturation sites in six different host cells, *J. Gen. Virol.* **7**:95.

Zwartouw, H. T., 1964, The chemical composition of vaccinia virus, *J. Gen. Microbiol.* **34**:115.

Adenovirus Structural Proteins

Harold S. Ginsberg

Columbia University College of Physicians and Surgeons
New York, New York 10032

1. INTRODUCTION

Eons ago a wise man might have asked: Can there evolve for study a poisonous, infectious particle, to be termed a "virus," having the following characteristics: (1) it should be architecturally developed to provide a stable structure; (2) it should be easily propagated and obtainable in large quantities; and (3) its subunits should be readily isolated in native form? Adenoviruses appear to provide one example of an evolutionary triumph that yields a solution to the problem posed. Adenovirus icosahedral structure furnishes nature's representation of the architects' presentation of the most stable geometric sphere; adenoviruses are easily propagated and many species can be readily isolated and purified in their native state.

It is the objective of this chapter to summarize the essential data* that permit a generalized consideration of the viral structural proteins in terms of their chemical, physical, and immunological characteristics; their role in the formation of the virion; and their biological functions.

---

* This chapter does not pretend to be an exhaustive review of the literature. The papers quoted have been selected on the basis of priority, most direct applicability to a point being developed, clarity of data, prejudice, or any combination of these factors. The author apologizes for his prejudices, which he hopes will not be found unbridled, and for any omissions owing to oversight.

Analyses of the reproduction of adenoviruses (Philipson and Lindberg, 1974) and their genetic properties (Ginsberg and Young, 1977) are set forth in other volumes in this series.

Viral capsomers are composed of several protomers joined through noncovalent bonds which are generally stronger than those bonds that assemble capsomers into capsids. Nevertheless, in most viruses the intracapsomeric bonds are too weak to permit intact, native capsomers to be soluble in aqueous fluids. In sharp contrast, the major adenovirus capsid proteins (i.e., hexons and pentons, as well as dissociated fibers) are formed from several protomers through such noncovalent bonds that the native multimeric proteins can be isolated from either purified virions (Wilcox and Ginsberg, 1963a) or the large pool of excess proteins (Klemperer and Pereira, 1959; Philipson, 1960; Wilcox and Ginsberg, 1961). These capsomers isolated from cellular pools are morphologically (Wilcox et al., 1963; Valentine and Pereira, 1965; Norrby, 1966a) and immunologically (Wilcox and Ginsberg, 1963a; Valentine and Pereira, 1965) indistinguishable from their virion counterparts. This unique property of the adenovirus capsid structural proteins has stimulated extensive studies of their chemical and physical structures, their immunological properties, and their biological functions.

2. CLASSIFICATION

The family of adenoviruses has been formed to group together those viruses with closely similar physical and chemical characteristics (Enders et al., 1956; Pereira et al., 1963). Many species of warm-blooded animals serve as hosts for adenoviruses, so that to date 31 human, 27 simian, ten bovine, eight avian, four porcine, two canine, two murine, one ovine, and one opposum immunological types have been described. In addition to their common physical and chemical properties, adenoviruses, except for the avian species, show a close immunological relationship, which is mediated primarily through the hexon capsid protein (Klemperer and Pereira, 1959; Wilcox and Ginsberg, 1961). The penton base also shows considerable cross-reactivity (Wilcox and Ginsberg, 1961; Waddell and Norrby, 1969; Pettersson and Höglund, 1969), although its extent has not been broadly tested.

Human adenoviruses have also been placed into subgroups according to their agglutination of monkey or rat erythrocytes (Rosen, 1969) and their oncogenic potential in newborn hamsters (Huebner et al., 1965). Based on these criteria, adenoviruses of humans are divided into four subgroups, and, although the nomenclature differs, each group has the same viral constituents. The validity of this subgroup classification is strengthened by the findings that viruses of the same subgroup have similar DNA base compositions (Piña and Green, 1965) and a high degree of homology between the nucleic acids of two related viruses (Lacy and Green, 1964, 1965, 1967; Piña and Green, 1968; Garon et al., 1973). It is noteworthy that viruses belonging to the same subgroups also show other similarities, which, however, have not yet been completely explored. For example, viruses of subgroups I (types 3, 7, 11, 14, 16, and 21) and II (types 8, 10, 13, 15, 19, etc.) have fibers only 9–13 nm in length (Norrby, 1968a, 1969a) whereas members of subgroup III (types 1, 2, 5, and 6) have rather long fibers of 23–31 nm. Viruses of subgroup III, which has been termed "subgroup C" (Huebner et al., 1965), replicate to yields as high as 10^4 pfu per cell whereas viruses of subgroup IV (types 12, 18, and 31), which have also been termed "subgroup A" according to their oncogenic potential (Huebner et al., 1965), present a yield of only $10^{2.5}$–$10^{3.0}$ pfu per cell. Viruses of subgroup I (Huebner's subgroup B) most commonly produce epidemics in man (Ginsberg, 1957) whereas viruses of subgroup III (types 1, 2, 5, and 6) are most frequently associated with latent infections of tonsils and adenoids (Ginsberg, 1957; Schlesinger and Strohl, 1962).

3. THE VIRION

3.1. Chemical Composition

These viruses, which initially seemed simple, consist of 11.6–13.5% DNA (Green, 1962; Piña and Green, 1965), depending on the viral type, the rest being protein, of which less than 1% is glycosylated (Ishibasi and Maizel, 1974b).

3.1.1. DNA

Each virion contains one linear, double-stranded DNA molecule of 20–25 × 10^6 daltons (Green et al., 1967; van der Eb et al., 1969). Just as the molecular weight of the DNA varies, the guanine plus cytosine content also varies from 47% to 61%, depending on viral type. Each strand of the molecule contains terminal nucleotide sequences that are inverted repetitions, like the adeno-associated virus DNA (Koczot et al., 1973), so that when the viral DNA is denatured both strands form single-stranded circles through hydrogen bonds between the complementary ends (Garon *et al.*, 1973; Wolfson and Dressler, 1972). The function of this unique DNA structure is unclear, however, since circular forms of replicating DNA have not been detected (Sussenbach *et al.*, 1972; Pettersson, 1973; Ellens *et al.*, 1974). Within the virion, however, the viral DNA may exist in a circular form mediated via one of the internal virion core proteins, since when the virion is artificially disrupted with sodium dodecylsulfate (SDS) a circular nucleoprotein structure is released (Robinson *et al.*, 1973). But it is also possible that the DNA is a linear structure coiled within the virion and that the circular form is an artifact of extraction: with virion disruptions, each "sticky" terminal protein, which is covalently linked to the 5' end of each viral DNA strand (Rekosh, 1977), associates with the other.

The fine structure of the viral DNA has been described in other volumes of this series (Philipson and Lindberg, 1974; Ginsberg and Young, 1977), as well as in Chapters 4 and 7 of this volume.

3.1.2.   Viral Proteins

The virion proteins (Fig. 1), which make up 87–89% of the particles' mass, consist of 10–14 unique species (Maizel *et al.*, 1968a; Anderson *et al.*, 1973; Everitt *et al.*, 1973; Ishibashi and Maizel, 1974a): five proteins (hexon, penton base, fiber, and two internal proteins, V and VII) comprise more than 90% of the total protein. Extracts of infected cells also contain at least eight to ten additional virus-induced, probably virus-coded, proteins (Fig. 1), which are not structural components of the virion; at least three of these proteins (pVI, pVII, and pVIII), however, are precursors of virion subunits (Anderson *et al.*, 1973; Ishibashi and Maizel, 1974a). Of the nonstructural proteins, only the 72K protein, a single-strand-specific DNA binding protein (van der Vliet and Levine, 1973), has been identified with a biological function, i.e., initiation of viral DNA replication (Ginsberg *et al.*, 1974; van der Vliet *et al.*, 1975). The so-called 100K protein, which is also a nonstructural protein, appears to be associated with hexon morphogenesis (Dragon and Ginsberg, in preparation).

Only the fiber protein is glycosylated (Ishibashi and Maizel, 1974a), but several of the proteins, including the structural protein IIIa, the 72K protein, and the 100K protein, are phosphorylated (Russell *et al.*, 1972). The fiber (protein IV) was also reported to be phosphorylated (Russell *et al.*, 1972), but this finding appears to be an error caused by the difficulty of separating fiber from protein IIIa (Russell, personal communication).

3.2. Architecture

X-ray crystallographic studies and electron microscopic observations with negative staining techniques suggested that the capsids of naked spherical viruses were composed of identical repeating subunits to form an isometric solid with rotational symmetry (Crick and Watson, 1956; Caspar and Klug, 1962). Such symmetry is present in three classes of polyhedral solids: tetrahedrons, octahedrons, and icosahedrons. These forms place specific restrictions on the structural characteristics of the subunits from which the solid can be assembled, but all must be composed of different capsomers at the corners and in the triangular faces of the polyhedrons. All of the face capsomers can be hexons, i.e., surrounded by six neighbors, although it is not essential that they be hexomers (see Sections 6.3 and 6.4); but the corner capsomers have different symmetry requirements, and it has been considered that they must be composed of three protomers for tetrahedrons, four for octahedrons, and five for icosahedrons (Caspar and Klug, 1962). In view of the fact that adenovirus hexons are formed from only three polypeptide chains (see Section 6.4) it seems unnecessary that the pentons, for example, consist of five protomers. Since electron microscopic examination revealed the structure and symmetry of the adenovirus capsid so clearly (Horne *et al.*, 1959), it was readily recognized to be an icosahedron with 5:3:2 rotational symmetry (Horne *et al.*, 1959; Smith *et al.*, 1965a). Indeed, all spherical polyhedral viruses are believed to be icosahedrons (Caspar and Klug, 1962). Morphologically, the adenovirus viron is more complex than predicted for naked isometric viruses (Crick and Watson, 1956). The capsid (Fig. 2) consists of 252 capsomers. The faces and edges of the 20 triangular facets are formed from 240 hexons, which compose the major structural viral protein (about 60% of the virion's mass). Each hexon is surrounded by six neighbors, hence its name (Ginsberg *et al.*, 1966), and therefore exhibits local 6-fold symmetry. All hexons, however, do not have identical intercapsomeric relationships: at each vertex, five hexons, the so-called peripentonal hexons (Prage *et al.*, 1970), surround a penton (Ginsberg *et al.*, 1966) so that each peripentonal hexon establishes one set of noncovalent bonds with a penton and another set with the six neighboring face hexons. The 180 face hexons

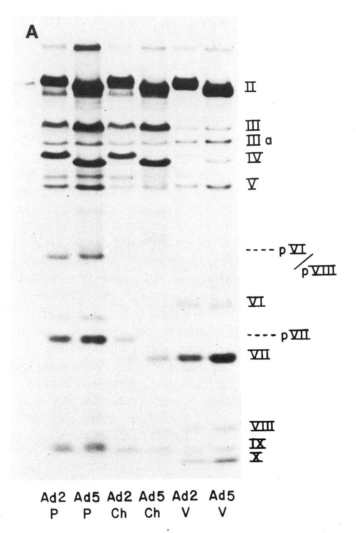

Fig. 1.   Comparison of the polypetides of type 2 and type 5 adenoviruses following separation by electrophoresis in SDS-polyacrylamide gel (PAGE). A: Comparison of types 2 and 5 proteins after a 30-min label with [35S]methionine, after a 60-min chase in unlabeled medium following a 30-min pulse, and in purified virions. The 35S label was added 20 hr after infection. B: Diagrammatic presentation of the virus-specific proteins observed in extract of cells 20 hr after infection and in purified virions.

appear to establish groups of nine in which each hexon has identical bonding forces, and the group has local 3-fold symmetry. Accordingly, when virions are gently disrupted by SDS, heat, or pyridine (Smith *et al.*, 1965*a*; Russell *et al.*, 1971; Prage *et al.*, 1970) in a hydrophobic environment, the "groups of nine" hexons (nonomers) are readily

B

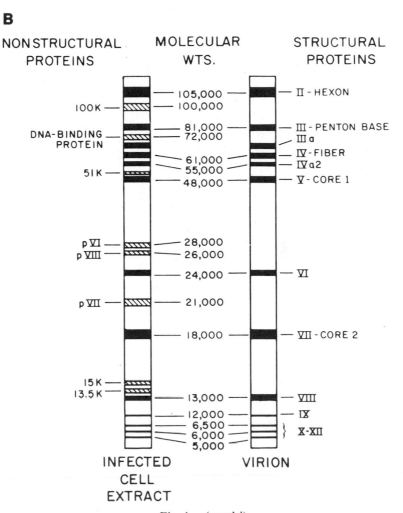

NONSTRUCTURAL   MOLECULAR   STRUCTURAL
     PROTEINS   WTS.   PROTEINS

—— 105,000 ——   II - HEXON
100K ——   —— 100,000 ——

—— 81,000 ——   III - PENTON BASE
DNA-BINDING ——   —— 72,000 ——   IIIa
     PROTEIN
—— 61,000 ——   IV - FIBER
51K ——   —— 55,000 ——   IVa2
—— 48,000 ——   V - CORE 1

pVI ——   —— 28,000 ——
pVIII ——   —— 26,000 ——

—— 24,000 ——   VI

pVII ——   —— 21,000 ——

—— 18,000 ——   VII - CORE 2

15K ——
13.5K ——   —— 13,000 ——   VIII
—— 12,000 ——   IX
—— 6,500 ——   } X-XII
—— 6,000 ——
—— 5,000 ——

INFECTED   VIRION
CELL
EXTRACT

Fig. 1.   (cont'd)

released. The pentons which are at each axis of 5-fold symmetry are unique structures consisting of a base capsomer and a protruding fiber (Valentine and Pereira, 1965). The fiber length is variable depending on the viral type (Norrby, 1969a).

Beneath the capsid is a core which consists of two "internal" proteins and a 55,000-dalton protein covalently linked to the 5' terminus of each DNA strand (Rekosh et al., 1977). Since the DNA consists of 64–67 kilobases, it can potentially code for 20–40 average proteins (14% of its nucleotide sequences is not encoded for translation). Fifteen to 20 virus-specific proteins, virion and nonvirion, have thus far been

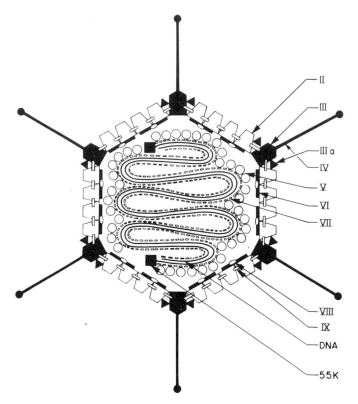

Fig. 2.   Model of an adenovirus particle showing the presumptive architectural relationships of the structural proteins and the nucleoprotein core in the virion.

identified, although it is still uncertain whether all the proteins detected
are primary gene products.

Morphologically, the viral capsid appears to contain three distinct
multimeric proteins. Using a more discriminating biophysical technique, SDS-polyacrylamide gel electrophoresis (Davis, 1964; Maizel,
1966; Loening, 1967), from ten to 14 protein bands (Fig. 1) may be
detected (Maizel *et al.*, 1968*a*; Everitt *et al.*, 1973; Anderson *et al.*, 1973;
Ishibashi and Maizel, 1974*a*). Those corresponding to the major capsid
and core proteins have been identified, but in addition several other
proteins are constituents of the viral capsid (Maizel *et al.*, 1968*b*; Prage
et al., 1970; Everitt *et al.*, 1973). Three of these peptides (VI, VIII, and
IX) have been consistently isolated in association with hexons (Everitt
et al., 1973, 1975); peptide IX is always found in association with the
groups of nine hexons (Everitt *et al.*, 1973). Several minor proteins (X,
XI, and XII) are frequently noted, but their location is unknown, their
quantity is inconsistent, and it is possible that they are degradation

products of identical virion structures. Where known, the chemical and physical structures, the function, and the immunological characteristics of all the viral structural proteins will be discussed in detail.

4. SYNTHESIS OF VIRAL PROTEINS

A brief discussion of the synthesis of the viral proteins is essential for an analysis of viral protein structure and assembly, although a detailed consideration of the biosynthesis of adenovirus-specific macromolecules is the subject of a chapter in another volume of this series (Philipson and Lindberg, 1974).

Synthesis of early virus-specific proteins, translated from transcripts of the infecting viral DNA, is essential for replication of viral DNA (Wilcox and Ginsberg, 1963b). And production of the progeny DNA (Fig. 3) is mandatory to make late transcripts and late viral proteins (Flanagan and Ginsberg, 1962; Thomas and Green, 1969; Lucas and Ginsberg, 1971; Carter and Ginsberg, 1976). Although viral DNA is replicated and transcribed in the nucleus, viral proteins, like host nuclear proteins, are made on cytoplasmic polyribosomes (Velicer and Ginsberg, 1968). The late viral proteins, which are primarily virion structural proteins, are synthesized on polyribosomes of 180–200 S (Thomas and Green, 1966; Velicer and Ginsberg, 1968) and require 1–2 min for production and release of a polypeptide (Horwitz et al., 1969;

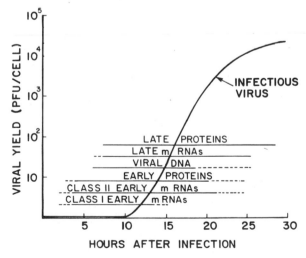

Fig. 3.   Schematic representation of the sequential biosynthetic events during replication of type 5 adenovirus.

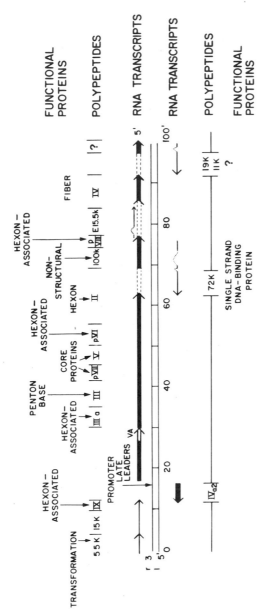

Fig. 4. Map of the type 2 adenovirus genome indicating the origins of transcripts that are processed into mRNAs. The viral proteins produced and their functions where known are also given. It should be noted that four widely separated regions on both strands of the genome give rise to early transcripts (——→). All but one of the late mRNAs arise from a primary transcript (——➤) which is initiated 16 map units from the left end of the rightward-reading strand (r) and terminates close to the 3′ end of the DNA; each of the processed mRNAs has three leaders derived from the primary transcript between positions 16.8 and 27, and therefore only one mRNA is produced from each primary transcript.

Velicer and Ginsberg, 1970). Kinetic data suggest that, after completion, the polypeptide chains are rapidly transported into the nuclei for assembly into multimeric structures and immunological maturation (Velicer and Ginsberg, 1970). Under unusual circumstances, however, when transport is hindered, hexons at least can undergo morphogenesis and assembly in the cytoplasm (Kauffman and Ginsberg, 1976). Indeed, polypeptide chains can assemble *in vitro* when synthesized in a cell-free extract of infected cells (Wilhelm and Ginsberg, 1972).

Viral proteins can also be faithfully translated *in vitro* from selected mRNAs (Eron *et al.*, 1974; Anderson *et al.*, 1974; Öberg *et al.*, 1975). Using specific segments of the type 2 adenovirus genome, prepared with bacterial restriction endonucleases, it has been possible to select late mRNAs transcribed from each identified portion of the genome and to translate the mRNAs *in vitro* (Lewis *et al.*, 1975). This novel approach has permitted identification of characteristic proteins as being primary gene products as well as the formulation of a biophysical map of the viral genome (Fig. 4). According to these considerations, all except the minor structural proteins X–XII noted in Fig. 1 have been identified as viral gene products (Lewis *et al.*, 1975, 1976; see also Chapter 7 of this volume).

The viral structural proteins, which are all translated from late mRNAs except for protein IX (Persson *et al.*, 1978), can first be detected 4–5 hr after initiation of DNA replication (Fig. 3), 10–11 hr after infection (Wilcox and Ginsberg, 1963*b*; Russell *et al.*, 1967*a*). When measured by immunological techniques, the major capsid proteins are sequentially detected: hexon, fiber, and penton base (Russell *et al.*, 1967*a*). However, the more sensitive techniques of SDS-polyacrylamide gel electrophoresis and autoradiography of labeled peptide chains reveal that all of the late proteins are synthesized at approximately the same time but that the hexon protein is produced in the greatest quantity and therefore is the most easily detected (Anderson *et al.*, 1973; Russell and Skehel, 1972).

5. PURIFICATION OF ADENOVIRUS STRUCTURAL PROTEINS: A CRITIQUE

Accurate characterization of a protein requires that it be rigorously purified. Therefore, to obtain reliable physical and chemical properties of a protein, the protein to be examined must be freed of contaminating materials and purified to homogeneity. This elementary but overriding principle is followed closely by enzymologists but often not properly attended to by virologists. A review of the literature describing the properties of adenovirus structural proteins reveals how loosely the basic dicta of purification have been followed. The procedures devised for rigorous purification of adenovirus proteins had to consider separation both from host and from other viral components. Cellular membranes, nuclear and cytoplasmic, were a recognized problem, which was generally solved by extracting the infected cell homogenate with the fluorocarbon Freon 112 (FCl_2C-CCl_2F) or Genetron ($F_2ClC-CCl_2F$). This procedure primarily precipitates cellular lipoproteins and lipopolysaccharides, constituents of membranes. When a viral protein is synthesized in association with membranes, and firmly bound to them, such as the nonstructural T antigen in type 12 adenovirus-infected cells (Gilead and Ginsberg, 1965), more vigorous procedures (e.g., organic solvents) must be used to obtain purified protein, or it will be lost in the fluorocarbon interface. Ion exchange chromatography, usually with DEAE-cellulose (Klemperer and Pereira, 1959; Philipson, 1960; Wilcox and Ginsberg, 1961; Horuna et al., 1961), has been a potent procedure for separating viral proteins from each other as well as from host macromolecules. Some investigators have depended on repeated cycles of chromatography on the same ion exchange material (e.g., DEAE-cellulose) for purification, which offers some increased purification, but is of limited value in comparison to utilizing a chromatographic material with different characteristics [e.g., hydroxylapatite (Levine and Ginsberg, 1967)]. Even more effective purification is attained if the investigator employs one or more additional procedures based on different physical principles than chromatography. Preparative polyacrylamide gel electrophoresis (Pettersson et al., 1967; Winters et al., 1970; Stinski and Ginsberg, 1975), liquid film electrophoresis (Boulanger et al., 1969), isoelectric focusing (Pettersson et al., 1967; Wadell, 1970; Dorsett and Ginsberg, 1975), and crystallization (Pereira et al., 1968; Mautner and Pereira, 1971; Franklin et al., 1971; Cornick et al., 1971) have been successfully employed for the appropriate proteins. These procedures must also be used with caution; for example, hexons are insoluble at their isoelectric point (Pettersson et al., 1967; Ginsberg, unpublished), so that purification by isoelectric focusing in an ampholyte gradient presents the hazard of precipitation with impurities and difficulties in collecting.

A number of simple ancillary procedures have been useful adjuncts in separation of viral proteins from host and viral macromolecules: (1) methanol precipitation at pH 4.0 in the cold (Wilcox and Ginsberg, 1963a; Köhler, 1965), (2) differential protein precipitation with ammonium sulfate (Levine and Ginsberg, 1967), (3) separation of viral proteins from nucleic acid by nuclease hydrolysis (Lawrence and Ginsberg, 1967) and streptomycin precipitation (Levine and Ginsberg, 1967), and (4) separation of the soluble viral proteins from virions and cellular aggregates by rate zonal centrifugation (Lawrence and Ginsberg, 1967) or exclusion chromatography on 4% agarose (Pettersson *et al.*, 1967).

Regardless of the purification method employed, however, reliable characterization of the product requires that the degree of purity be established. Not even crystallization of a protein is a guarantee of purity. Purity can be determined by the following critical procedures: (1) analytical ultracentrifugation, (2) analytical polyacrylamide gel electrophoresis, preferably at two widely separated pHs, (3) SDS-polyacrylamide gel electrophoresis, (4) isotope dilution in which a uniformly labeled uninfected cell homogenate is added to the infected cell sap prior to purification, and (5) immunological procedures. No single procedure listed is an absolute criterion of purity, and a combination of these techniques is recommended.

6. THE HEXON

The hexon is the major structural protein of the virion and makes up about 53% of the virion's mass. Since the native hexon protein can be readily obtained in large quantities, its structure, as a model viral protein, has been more thoroughly studied than that from any other animal virus. The hexon is made in considerable excess, and only about 10% of that synthesized is assembled into virions (Ginsberg and Dixon, 1961; Green, 1962; Wilcox and Ginsberg, 1963*b*). However, the nonassembled hexons, which are present in the pool of "soluble antigens," appear to be immunologically and structurally the same as those in virions (Wilcox and Ginsberg, 1963*a*; Wilcox *et al.*, 1963). The majority of physical and chemical studies therefore have been pursued with the nonassembled viral subunits.

6.1. Morphology

When electron microscopic examinations of negatively stained adenovirus particles were initially made, the capsomers were described as spheres (Horne *et al.*, 1959; Valentine and Pereira, 1965). Study of purified hexons and hexons from disrupted type 5 virions, however, revealed capsomers with polygonal rodlike structures of about 8.0 nm in the largest dimension and with a central hole of about 2.5 nm (Wilcox *et al.*, 1963). Elegant high-resolution electron microscopy associated with negative staining, as well as advanced techniques of shadowing (after freeze-drying) and freeze etching, has permitted fine structure analysis of the hexons' morphology (Nermut, 1975). According to Nermut's observations (1975), as well as those of others (Horne and Wildy, 1963; Horne, 1962; Wilcox *et al.*, 1963), the hexon is clearly not a sphere; its shape is closest to a truncated, triangular prism (Fig. 5) with a base of 8.5 × 9.9 nm and a narrower top of about 7.5 nm in diameter (Nermut, 1975). The central hole is 2.5–3.5 nm at the top and 1.0–1.5 nm at the base; frequently the channel does not appear to traverse the hexon completely. Occasionally, in negatively stained

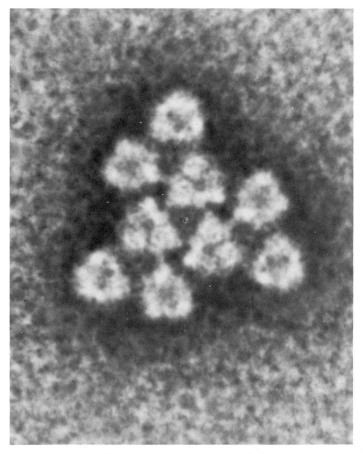

Fig. 5.   Electron micrograph of a group of nine purified type 5 hexons seen in the right-handed configuration (a 3-fold rotation). The three subunits and the small central hole are clearly seen (~2,000,000×). Kindly supplied by M. V. Nermut.

preparations, the hexons can be seen to be composed of three subunits which seem to be arranged more compactly at the base than at the top (Nermut, 1975). The complex subunit structure may confer the local symmetry on the hexon trimers which appear to aggregate via corner-to-edge into groups of nine hexons (Smith *et al.*, 1965a; Laver *et al.*, 1968; Prage *et al.*, 1970; Pereira and Wrigley, 1974; Nermut, 1975). In rotationally filtered electron micrographs, hexons display 3-fold symmetry (Crowther and Franklin, 1972). Moreover, hexons can form planar crystals in which they show 3-fold symmetry (Pereira and Wrigley, 1974). Despite their apparent triangular shape, the hexons assembled into the faces of capsids have local 6-fold symmetry relative to neighboring hexons (Ginsberg *et al.*, 1966).

6.2. Immunological Characteristics

As the predominant viral protein, both in the virion and in the infected cell sap, the hexon protein serves as a major antigenic reactant, inducing a complex immunological response. Following infection or immunization of animals, antibodies appear that detect antigenic determinants unique for each adenovirus type, i.e., type-specific, and determinants that cross-react with hexons of all mammalian adenoviruses, i.e., family cross-reactive (Wilcox and Ginsberg, 1961, 1963c; Köhler, 1965; Norrby and Wadell, 1969; Norrby *et al.*, 1969a,b). The responsible type-specific and cross-reacting antigenic determinants have been termed "ϵ" and "α," respectively (Köhler, 1965). As a reflection of the greater chemical similarities between hexons of viruses belonging to the same subgroup (Stinski and Ginsberg, 1975), the immunological cross-reactivity is comparably greater between closely related adenovirus than between viruses from different subgroups. For example, antibody to purified type 5 (subgroup III) hexon immuno-precipitated 70–75% of type 2 (subgroup III) hexon protein but only about 30–35% of the type 3 (subgroup I) hexon protein (Stinski and Ginsberg, 1975). The differences in degree of reactivity between hexon types within the same subgroup and between hexons of types belonging to different subgroups have been referred to as "intra- and intersubgroup specificities" (Philipson and Pettersson, 1973), but actual distinctions in antibody populations have not been demonstrated by cross-adsorption or other methods.

Immunological reactions may also serve as topological probes of the viral protein structures. Thus it is striking that the family cross-reactive hexon antibodies do not react with hexons assembled into virions (Wilcox and Ginsberg, 1963a; Smith et al., 1965b; Norrby et al., 1969a) but combine with the soluble hexons, whereas type-specific antibodies react with both the virion-assembled hexons and the soluble oligomeric proteins (Wilcox and Ginsberg, 1963c; Pereira and Laver, 1970). As a consequence of its reaction with virion hexons, type-specific antibodies neutralize viral infectivity (Wilcox and Ginsberg, 1963c; Kjellen and Pereira, 1968; Pereira and Laver, 1970), whereas cross-reacting hexon antibodies do not reduce infectivity except for some very closely related virus such as types 15 and 29 (Norrby, 1969c). These findings indicate that specified but different regions of the hexon protein contain the ϵ and α antigenic determinants, that only the type-specific (ϵ) determinant is exposed when the hexon is situated in the virion capsid, that the ϵ determinant is also available in soluble hexons, and that the cross-reacting α determinant can only react with antibodies when in the nonvirion form. Chemical data (discussed in Section 6.3) support these conclusions. Further evidence that the type-specific and cross-reactive antibodies are distinct was gained from the demonstration that the cross-reactive antibodies can be adsorbed from sera without disturbing the type-specific antibody titer (Wilcox and Ginsberg, 1963c; Köhler, 1965).

Further evidence of the hexon immunological structure was obtained using proteolytic enzymes to note their effect on the type-specific and family cross-reactive antigenic determinants (Pettersson, 1971). Chymotrypsin, subtilisin, or papain digests 20–50% of the type 2, 3, or 5 hexon protein and removes family antigenic determinants, but these enzymatic digestions do not detectably reduce the type specificity (Pettersson, 1971). These data imply that either the type-specific determinants reside in a portion of the hexon protein that is resistant to proteolysis by the enzymes used or they are not available to the enzymes when hexons are free in solution. Furthermore, trypsin does not affect either the immunological reactivity or physical structure of the hexon, although the assembled polypeptide chains are cleaved in several places (Pettersson, 1971; Pereira and Skehel, 1971).

The usual array of immunological reactions can be employed to assay the type-specific and cross-reactive antibodies. Neutralization of viral infectivity, however, is the most direct and discriminating method to titrate type-specific antibodies. Although there has been some conflicting evidence (Wilcox and Ginsberg, 1963a; Pettersson et al., 1967; Pettersson, 1971), the data are clear that purified hexon protein serves as the major antigen, but not the only antigen, for production of adenovirus type-specific neutralizing antibodies. The hexon proteins of all adenovirus types, however, may not be equally capable of inducing neutralizing antibodies since reports indicate that hexons from types 3, 4, 5, and 9 (Wilcox and Ginsberg, 1963a; Wadell, 1970) are excellent antigens for neutralizing antibodies whereas type 2 hexons are much less effective (Pettersson *et al.*, 1967; Wadell, 1970). The evidence available suggests that at least two populations of hexons distinguishable by charge differences may be found in type 2- and 5-infected cells and that only one of these forms may effectively induce type-specific antibodies (Pettersson, 1971; H. S. Ginsberg, P. Dorsett, and K. Coll, unpublished data). Evidence to be discussed below (Section 6.3) suggests that the two forms of excess pool hexons may be artifacts created by either intracellular proteolytic enzyme activity or enzymes inadvertently added during purification [e.g., chymotrypsin activity in most DNase preparations (Pereira and Skehel, 1971; H. S. Ginsberg, P. Dorsett, and K. Coll, unpublished data)].

6.3.   Chemical Characteristics

Amino acid analyses of types 2, 3, and 5 hexons, which have been carried out in several laboratories with similar results (Biserte *et al.*, 1966, Pettersson *et al.*, 1967; Boulanger *et al.*, 1969; Laver, 1970; Pettersson, 1971; Ginsberg, 1971), do not reveal any unusual features (Table 1). It is striking, however, that the hexons tested have relatively large numbers of amino acid residues capable of generating hydrophobic bonds which probably confer the marked stability to its multimeric structure. Initially, it was reported that hexons do not possess half-cystines (Pettersson *et al.*, 1967; Boulanger *et al.*, 1969; Laver, 1970), but free sulfhydryl groups were shown to be present when sulfhydryl interchange was noted on denaturation of the hexons (Ginsberg, 1971) and when appropriately denatured hexons were examined with more sensitive analytical methods [i.e., incorporation of [^{14}C]cysteine into type 7 hexons (Neurath *et al.*, 1970), analysis of performic acid oxidized type 2 hexons (Pettersson, 1971), and carboxymethylation with ^{14}C-labeled iodoacetate upon 6.0 M guanidine-HCl disruption of type 2 and 5 hexons (Jörnvall *et al.*, 1975; Dorsett and Ginsberg, unpublished data)]. The type 2, 3, and 5 hexons contain 0.5–0.8 mole % half-cystine, or about five to seven cysteines per polypeptide chain which has a total of approximately 749–850 amino acid residues (Ginsberg, 1971; Petterson, 1971; Jörnvall *et al.*, 1975).

The N-terminal amino acid of type 2 hexon appears to be blocked (Laver, 1970; Pettersson, 1971; Jörnvall *et al.*, 1974), although earlier

TABLE 1
Amino Acid Analyses of Type 2, 3, and 5
Adenovirus Hexons

Amino acid	Moles per 100 moles amino acid		
	Type 2[a]	Type 3[a]	Type 5[b]
Lysine	4.16	4.02	4.8
Histidine	1.40	1.65	1.7
Arginine	4.61	4.92	4.8
Aspartic acid	14.41	14.58	14.0
Threonine	7.03	8.25	7.0
Serine	6.84	6.80	6.5
Glutamic acid	9.49	8.31	9.5
Proline	6.08	6.14	6.3
Glycine	6.76	6.43	6.9
Alanine	7.10	6.82	6.8
Valine	5.69	6.02	4.9
Methionine	2.72	2.95	2.7
Isoleucine	3.55	3.85	4.0
Leucine	7.70	7.29	8.0
Tyrosine	5.61	5.46	5.4
Phenylalanine	4.44	5.01	5.0
Tryptophan	1.65	ND[c]	1.3
Half-cystine	0.76	0.48	0.55

[a] Pettersson (1971).
[b] Ginsberg (1971) (analysis by Dr. Preston H. Dorsett).
[c] Not detected.

reports suggested that arginine (Biserte *et al.*, 1968) or lysine (Boulanger *et al.*, 1969) was the N-terminal amino acid. (It is likely that minor contaminants of the hexon led to these conflicting data.) Jörnvall *et al.* (1974) showed that the N-terminal amino acid is acetylated and that the terminal peptide, obtained after chymotryptic and thermolytic cleavage, has the sequence acetyl-alanine-threonine-proline-serine. Similar analyses of hexons from other adenovirus types have not yet been made.

The overall amino acid compositions of the type 2, 3, and 5 hexons do not significantly differ (Table 1), although it is clear by their unique chromatographic characteristics on DEAE-cellulose and on hydroxylapatite columns that they have significant charge differences (Wilcox and Ginsberg, 1961; Norrby, 1968*b*; Pettersson, 1971; Stinski and Ginsberg, 1975). Moreover, their differing immunological reactivities (discussed above, Section 6.2) sharply point out their variations in chemical structure. These differences in physical and immunological properties must reflect differences in amino acid sequences. The complete amino acid sequence has not been identified for any hexon protein as yet, although sequencing of about 25% of the type 2 hexon protein has been accomplished (Jörnvall *et al.*, 1974). Peptide maps, however, have detected the expected significant differences between the type 2 and 5 hexons (Pereira and Laver, 1970) and among the hexons of types 2, 3, and 5 (Stinski and Ginsberg, 1975). A comparison of tryptic peptide maps of type 2 and 5 hexons revealed clear-cut differences, although it was not possible to make quantitative estimates of the differences since the methods employed detected only 50–60% of the theoretical number of peptides present in the hexon protein (Pereira and Laver, 1970). Comparison of the peptides generated by cyanogen bromide cleavage of hexon proteins at the methionine residues ("CNBr peptides") permitted a crude quantitative comparison of the protein structures (Stinski and Ginsberg, 1975). Twenty-six to 30 CNBr peptides were displayed on coelectrophoresis of ^{3}H- and ^{14}C-labeled hexon peptides from two types (Fig. 6), using a polyacrylamide gel isoelectric focusing technique. Approximately two-thirds of the CNBr peptides coelectrophoresed when the more closely related type 2 and 5 hexons (both are members of subgroup III) were examined, whereas when type 2 or 5 hexons were compared with the CNBr peptides of type 3 (subgroup I) only about one-third of the peptides had identical isoelectric points. Since the peptides were of small size and were maintained in 8 M urea during isoelectric focusing, the peptides should not have had any secondary structure. Thus coelectrophoresis of two peptides suggests identical amino acid content and possibly identical amino acid sequence. These data further imply that about one-third of the protein structure of each of the three hexon types is constant in its amino acid content, that even between closely related types (e.g., type 2 and 5 hexons) about one-third of the amino acid sequences differ, and that members of the same subgroup have extensive regions that are similar. Tryptic peptide maps of type 2 and 5 hexons show about the same amount of similarity (Pereira and Laver, 1970).

Radioautographic analyses of tryptic and cyanogen bromide peptide profiles permitted an estimation of the molecular weight of the polypeptide chains as well as an evaluation whether the monomers are identical. According to this sensitive technique, the type 5 hexon protein, which generates 26–30 CNBr peptides (Stinski and Ginsberg, 1975) and 80–85 tryptic peptides (Ginsberg, Dorsett, and Coll, unpublished data), is composed of three identical polypeptide chains of approximately 100,000–110,000 daltons each. This estimated size, which is significantly smaller than that for the type 2 hexon (Maizel *et al.*, 1968*b*), is consistent with the values obtained by SDS-polyacrylamide gel electrophoresis

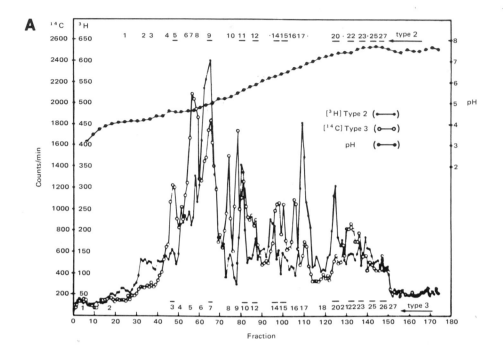

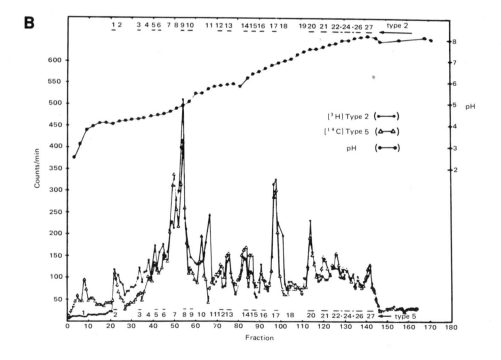

(Fig. 1) (Kauffman, 1976; Kauffman and Ginsberg, 1976) and exclusion chromatography in 5–6 M guanidine hydrochloride (Jörnvall *et al.*, 1975; Ginsberg, Dorsett, and Coll, unpublished data), both of which are physical methods (see Section 6.5).

Conflicting data have been reported on the molecular weights of the hexon polypeptide chains of type 2 and 5 hexons measured with SDS-polyacrylamide gel electrophoresis (Maizel *et al.*, 1968a; Pettersson, 1970) and exclusion chromatography using Sepharose columns equilibrated with guanidine hydrochloride (Pettersson, 1970; Ginsberg, 1971). These conflicts may now be largely resolved by the findings that (1) hexons of types 2 and 5 have significantly different-sized polypeptide chains (Kauffman, 1976); (2) the infected cells contain hexons that have different electrophoretic charges as noted by polyacrylamide gel electrophoresis under nondenaturing conditions (Pettersson, 1971); (3) the so-called "slow"- and "fast"-migrating soluble hexons (Pettersson, 1971) differ electrophoretically from hexons isolated from purified virions (Ginsberg, Dorsett, and Coll, unpublished data); (4) all three classes of hexons are indistinguishable by immunological reactions or size determinations (Ginsberg, Dorsett, and Coll, unpublished data); (5) tryptic peptide maps do not distinguish between "fast"- and "slow"-migrating hexons but show the virion hexon to have three to five more peptides (Ginsberg, Dorsett, and Coll, unpublished data); (6) exclusion chromatography indicates that the type 5 virion hexons consist of polypeptide chains of about 95,000 daltons, whereas "fast" hexons yield a polypeptide chain of about 70,000 daltons, and the "slow" hexons present polypeptide chains of approximately 70,000 and 23,000 daltons (Ginsberg and Coll, unpublished data). These data suggest that, in addition to the natural differences between type 2 and 5 hexons, the reported differences in sizes of polypeptide chains result from the varying degrees of artifactual proteolytic cleavages of soluble hexons (Pereira and Skehel, 1971) after their assembly and that the strength of bonds holding the folded monomers in the capsomers is sufficiently great to prevent disruption or even detectable distortion of the hexons.

Accordingly, there is now general agreement that the hexon

Fig. 6.   Patterns of oligopeptides obtained by cleavage of type 2, 3, and 5 adenovirus hexons with cyanogen bromide (CNBr) and separated by isoelectrophoresis in polyacrylamide gels. A: Coisoelectrophoresis of ^{3}H-labeled type 2 and ^{14}C-labeled type 5 hexon CNBr peptides. B: Coisoelectrophoresis of ^{3}H-labeled type 2 and ^{14}C-labeled type 3 hexon CNBr peptides. Peptide numbering is based on bands in parallel gels detected by Coomasie brilliant blue staining; numbered bands marked with bar indicate peptides with identical pI values. From Stinski and Ginsberg (1975).

polypeptide chains have an average molecular mass of approximately 120,000 daltons for type 2 adenovirus (Maizel *et al.*, 1968*a*; Horowitz *et al.*, 1970; Franklin *et al.*, 1971; Grütter and Franklin, 1974) and 105,000 daltons for type 5 adenovirus (Cornick *et al.*, 1971; Kauffman, 1976; Stinski and Ginsberg, 1975).

6.4. Physical Characteristics

The large yields and high degree of purity obtained with native hexons from type 2 and 5 adenoviruses have made possible detailed physical characterization of this major viral protein. The hexon of type 2 adenovirus has been most extensively studied, and therefore the most precise measurements are available with this protein. From the physical characteristics obtained by analytical untracentrifugation, the molecular weight of the type 2 hexon was calculated to be 355,000–363,000 (Pettersson *et al.*, 1967). The molecular weight according to crystal density measurement was calculated as 362,000–413,000 (Franklin *et al.*, 1971). Just as the molecular weight of the type 5 hexon's polypeptide chains is lower than that of polypeptide chains from type 2 when measured by SDS-polyacrylamide gel analysis (Kauffman, 1976) or gel exclusion chromatography (Pettersson, 1971; Ginsberg, Dorsett, and Coll, unpublished data), Cornick *et al.* (1973) showed that the molecular weight of native type 5 hexons is less than that of type 2 when calculated from measurement of crystal density. According to these measurements the molecular weight of the type 5 hexon is 282,000–315,000 (Cornick *et al.*, 1973). The sedimentation coefficients ($s_{20,w}$) of the type 2 and 5 hexons are 13 S (Grütter and Franklin, 1974) and 12.15 S (Levine and Ginsberg, 1967), respectively, which also demonstrates the differences in their sizes.

Hexons of type 2 and 5 adenoviruses have been crystallized (Pereira *et al.*, 1968; Franklin *et al.*, 1971; Cornick *et al.*, 1971) and were found to be isomorphous even though different methods of crystallization were used. The type 5 crystals examined were described as tetrahedral (Pereira *et al.*, 1968; Cornick *et al.*, 1971) whereas the type 2 crystals were shown as rhombic dodecahedral crystals (Franklin *et al.*, 1971). These differences in crystal morphology appear to reflect differences in methods of crystallization (Cornick *et al.*, 1971; Franklin *et al.*, 1971) rather than basic differences in the hexon proteins. The crystals of both types belong to the cubic space group P2,3 with $a =$ 15 nm (Cornick *et al.*, 1971; Franklin *et al.*, 1971). These studies indicate that the hexon is composed of three asymmetrical units: the molecular weight of the type 2 asymmetrical unit is 120,000 (Franklin *et al.*, 1971; Grütter and Franklin 1974); and the molecular weight of the type 5 asymmetrical unit is 96,000–105,000 (Cornick *et al.*, 1971; 1973). Thus the asymmetrical unit is equivalent to the hexon protomer, and the molecular weights for the type 2 and 5 hexons according to X-ray diffraction studies are 360,000–402,000 (Franklin *et al.*, 1971; Grütter and Franklin, 1974) and 288,000–315,000 (Cornick *et al.*, 1973), respectively.

Using small-angle X-ray scattering analysis, Tejg-Jensen *et al.* (1972) found that the type 2 hexon in solution has a length of 12.5 nm and a radius of gyration of 4.7 nm; this cross-section has a radius of gyration of 3 nm. These results imply that the hexon molecule in solution is cylindrical or prismatic, as described from electron microscopic examination (Wilcox *et al.*, 1963; Nermut, 1975).

6.5.　Genes Affecting Hexon Structure and Function

Genetic and physical mapping studies using conditionally lethal, temperature-sensitive (*ts*) mutants revealed that at least two genes control hexon structure and development and that precise folding is required for functional utilization of the hexon trimers. Thus mutations in the hexon gene result in at least three disparate phenotypes (Luciw and Ginsberg, 1979): (1) One set of mutants at the nonpermissive temperature produces hexon polypeptides but these cannot effectively fold into mature hexons [e.g., H5*ts10* (Russell, *et al.*, 1974)]. (2) A second set of *ts* mutants (e.g., H5*ts147*) folds the polypeptide into 12 S hexons which react with antibodies directed against either native hexons or denatured polypeptide chains (Luciw and Ginsberg, 1979). The affected hexons, however, cannot be transported into the nucleus (Kauffman and Ginsberg, 1976). (3) A third set of mutants (H5*ts135*) is exemplified by assembly of hexons that are physically and immunologically indistinguishable from wild-type hexons; they are transported into the nucleus but they cannot be assembled into capsids (Ensinger and Ginsberg, 1972; Luciw and Ginsberg, 1979).

A group of independent mutations in the gene for the late, nonstructural "100K" protein also phenotypically affects hexon expression (Lewis *et al.*, 1975; Mautner *et al.*, 1975). These mutants, exemplified by H5*ts116* (Ensinger and Ginsberg, 1972) and H5*ts1* (Williams *et al.*, 1974), cannot form hexon trimers at the nonpermissive temperature, although presumably only the 100K protein is directly affected. These data suggest that the 100K protein is required for assembly of the polypeptide chains into hexons, perhaps as a "scaffold-ing" protein for hexon, or that the nonstructural 100K protein modifies the hexon polypeptide chains to permit appropriate hexon development.

6.6.   Model of Hexon Structure

The variety of immunological, biochemical, and physical tech-niques employed in studying the hexon have yielded extensive data from which to suggest a model of the hexon's structure. The restraints imposed by the known properties of the hexon demand that the three polypeptide chains fold so that regions generating strong hydrophobic bonds interact to form a stable structure; that the unique regions of the polypeptide chains which confer type specifity be exposed on the hexon's outer surface when assembled in virions; that the constant regions of the polypeptide chains, which confer family antigenic cross-reactivity, be covered when hexons are assembled in a capsid but be exposed when hexons are freed from the capsid's constraints; and that the hexon have a trimeric form which is adequately flexible to permit stable interaction with six surrounding capsomers and smaller capsid

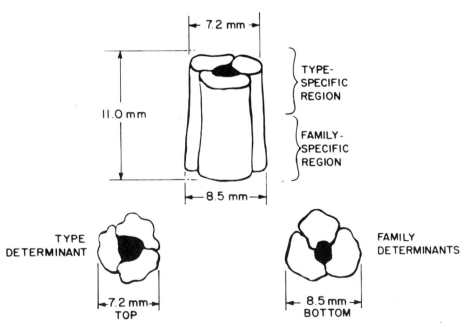

Fig. 7.   Proposed model of structure of adenovirus hexon. The model was formulated to take into account characteristics determined by electron microscopic, chemical, physical, and immunological measurements.

proteins (see below). Figure 7 presents a schematic model, modified from that suggested by Nermut (1975), which fits the above known characteristics.

7. THE PENTON

At each of the 12 vertices of the adenovirus icosahedral virion is a complex structure, the penton, which consists of a base capsomer and a projecting fiber. Pentons, as well as free fibers, are found in abundance in cell extracts, but the penton base is relatively unstable and therefore not detected, or found in small amounts in a free, soluble form.

7.1. General Description

For characterization, pentons have been purified from infected cell extracts by procedures similar to those used to separate hexons and free fibers (Levine and Ginsberg, 1967; Norrby, 1968b; Pettersson and Höglund, 1969). Pentons have also been obtained by disruption of purified virions (Wilcox and Ginsberg, 1963a; Prage et al., 1970), or by their release from purified virions, without disruption of the viral capsid, with 8% pyridine (Pettersson and Höglund, 1969), or by dialysis against distilled water (Laver et al., 1969). The recovery of pentons is low compared to that of hexons or fibers, however, regardless of the purification procedure employed.

The type 2 and 5 pentons have sedimentation coefficients of about 10.5–10.9 (Pettersson and Höglund, 1969; Wadell et al., 1969; Velicer and Ginsberg, 1970). Pettersson and Höglund (1969) calculated the molecular weight of the type 2 penton to be 370,000–400,000, depending on the analytical ultracentrifugation technique employed, and Wadell (1970) estimated the molecular weight of the type 5 penton to be 485,000–505,000, based on gel filtration and ultracentrifugation methods. As will be seen below (Section 7.2), this latter figure seems more appropriate when the sum of the molecular weights of the fiber and base subunits is considered.

Noncovalent bonds must join the penton's base and fiber since they can be dissociated by 2.5 M guanidine-HCl (Norrby and Skaaret, 1967), 33% formamide (Neurath et al., 1968), or 8% pyridine (Pettersson and Höglund, 1969). Physical methods can then be used to separate the penton bases (also called "vertex capsomers") from fibers so that the proteins can be characterized.

7.2. Penton Base

7.2.1. Morphology

The vertex capsomers of all adenoviruses examined appear to have the same general morphology and size. Penton bases have been described as spherical or globular (Valentine and Pereira, 1965; Pettersson and Höglund, 1969) or even pentagonal in outline (Pettersson and Höglund, 1969). However, they are best described as a cone or a truncated pyramid which is tapered proximally (Wadell et al., 1969; Laver et al., 1969a). The outer diameter of the base is 6–9 nm, and the length is 5.5–8 nm (Pettersson and Höglund, 1969). Occasionally the penton bases are seen to have a central cavity about 2.5 nm in diameter.

7.2.2. Physicochemical Characteristics

The penton base has a sedimentation coefficient of approximately 9 S (Velicer and Ginsberg, 1970) and is composed of polypeptide chains of 70,000–85,000 daltons (types 2 and 5 have been examined) (Maizel et al., 1968b; Pettersson and Höglund, 1969; Anderson et al., 1973; Ishibashi and Maizel, 1974a; Kauffman, 1976). No precise data are yet available to permit a determination of the number of polypeptide chains per penton base and of whether their primary structures are identical. Indeed, although amino acid analyses have been made on intact pentons (fibers and bases) (Pettersson and Höglund, 1969), none has yet been reported for purified vertex capsomers.

7.3. Fiber

Fibers may be found in three configurations: at vertices of virions, as the projections of free pentons (i.e., the vertex capsomers), and as free fibers in the viral excess antigen pool of infected cells. In any one of these forms, their morphology appears identical (Wilcox et al., 1963; Valentine and Pereira, 1965; Pettersson et al., 1968). Purified fibers have also been crystallized into needle-shaped crystals up to 50 μm long, which are seen in a highly ordered helical form when examined by electron microscopy (Mautner and Pereira, 1971).

7.3.1. Morphology

The fiber consists of a shaft which terminates in a knob 4–6 nm in diameter (Wilcox *et al.*, 1963; Valentine and Pereira, 1965). The shaft appears as a threadlike structure about 2 nm in diameter (Wilcox *et al.*, 1963; Valentine and Pereira, 1965; Pettersson *et al.*, 1968) and varies in length depending on the viral type. But viruses within a single subgroup have fibers of comparable length: subgroup I, 9–11 nm; subgroup II, 12–13 nm; subgroup III, 23–31 nm; subgroup IV, 28–31 nm (Norrby, 1969*a*; Norrby *et al.*, 1969*b*). The somewhat unique type 4 adenovirus, a member of subgroup III according to hemagglutination reactions (Rosen, 1960), has fibers of intermediate length, 17–18 nm (Norrby *et al.*, 1969*b*).

7.3.2. Physicochemical Characteristics

Unfortunately, the fibers of few types have been studied by physical methods. The fibers of types 2 and 5, examined by analytic ultracentrifugation determinations, were shown to have sedimentation coefficients ($s_{20,w}$) of 5.8–6.2 (Levine and Ginsberg, 1967; Pettersson *et al.*, 1968; Wadell *et al.*, 1969). The molecular weight of purified fibers, determined by the sedimentation equilibrium method of Yphantis (1964), indicated that the type 2 and 5 adenovirus fibers have average molecular weights of 207,000 (Sundquist *et al.*, 1973*b*) and 178,000 (Dorsett and Ginsberg, 1975), respectively. The differences in molecular weight of the two types reflect the smaller size of the type 5 fiber polypeptide chains; these differences in polypeptide chains are seen to be most striking when the denatured fiber proteins are electrophoresed in parallel on slab SDS-polyacrylamide gels (Fig. 1). According to the SDS-polyacrylamide gel method for measuring the molecular weight of adenovirus polypeptides (Shapiro *et al.*, 1967), the type 2 fiber polypeptide has been reported as 70,000 (Anderson *et al.*, 1973) or 60,000–65,000 (Ishibashi and Maizel, 1974*b*) and the type 5 fiber polypeptide has been estimated to be 61,000 (Dorsett and Ginsberg, 1975). According to molecular weights calculated from amino acid analyses (Table 2), the fiber polypeptide of type 2 virus is 64,000 (Sundquist *et al.*, 1973*b*) and the type 5 fiber is 61,000 (Dorsett and Ginsberg, 1975). These data in aggregate imply that the fiber is composed of three polypeptide chains of similar or identical molecular weights and that the molecular weight of the type 2 fiber is

TABLE 2

Amino Acid Analyses of Fiber Proteins from Type 2 and 5 Adenoviruses

Amino acid	Moles per 100 moles amino acid	
	Type 2[a]	Type 5[b]
Lysine	6.0	6.1
Histidine	0.8	1.2
Arginine	1.6	1.4
Aspartic acid	12.8	12.2
Threonine	11.0	11.4
Serine	12.1	8.1
Glutamic acid	7.2	6.3
Proline	5.2	4.4
Glycine	9.5	8.9
Alanine	7.1	8.1
Valine	5.4	5.9
Methionine	1.2	1.3
Isoleucine	5.2	4.5
Leucine	9.6	13.3
Tyrosine	2.1	2.3
Phenylalanine	2.2	3.8
Tryptophan	1.2	1.1
Half-cystine	ND[c]	0.4

[a] Pettersson *et al.* (1968).
[b] Dorsett and Ginsberg (1975).
[c] Not detected.

192,000–207,000 (Sundquist *et al.*, 1973) and that of the type 5 fiber is 178,000–183,000 (Dorsett and Ginsberg, 1975). It is apparent that these values for molecular weights of the fiber do not correlate with the sedimentation coefficients obtained (Levine and Ginsberg, 1967; Pettersson *et al.*, 1968; Wadell *et al.*, 1969). Thus if the fiber is assumed to sedi-, ment as a prolate ellipsoid of 180,000 daltons, with an axial ratio of 8, the calculated sedimentation coefficient should be 8.3 S. The 5.8–6.2 S sedimentation coefficient measured for the fiber (Levine and Ginsberg, 1967; Pettersson *et al.*, 1968; Wadell *et al.*, 1969; Dorsett and Ginsberg, 1975) most likely results in part from the concentration dependence observed (Dorsett and Ginsberg, 1975) and in part from the fact that the fiber is not a true prolate ellipsoid and therefore does not behave according to the theoretical treatment employed (Yphantis, 1964).

These data are at variance with earlier studies which reported that type 2 and 5 fibers have molecular weights of 60,000–80,000 (Köhler, 1965; Pettersson *et al.*, 1968). The marked underestimates of the earlier investigations probably resulted in the main from the methods employed: (1) Valentine and Pereira (1965) calculated a molecular weight of 70,000 for the fiber of type 5 adenovirus by estimating the volume of the molecule from electron micrographs; this method could have been affected by shrinkage or distortion of the fiber during fixation and staining. (2) Two analytical ultracentrifugation investigations, which reported the molecular weight of the native fiber molecule to be 70,000–80,000, determined the diffusion constant of the protein in order to calculate the molecular weight (Köhler, 1965; Pettersson *et al.*, 1968); these determinations have a greater dependence on protein concentration and are subject to greater error than equilibrium ultracentrifugation techniques.

Electrophoresis of purified fiber proteins in SDS-denaturing gels showed a single size class of polypeptides, suggesting that the polypeptides per fiber are identical (Pettersson *et al.*, 1968; Maizel *et al.*, 1968; Dorsett and Ginsberg, 1975). Tryptic peptide analysis of highly purified fiber protein, however, revealed more than 70 peptides, whereas approximately 35 peptides would be predicted, according to the arginine and lysine residues per polypeptide of 61,000 daltons (Table 2), if the three polypeptides chains were identical (Dorsett and Ginsberg, 1975). Two additional pieces of evidence imply that the three polypeptide chains may not be identical: (1) Ishibashi and Maizel (1974*b*) found that the fiber is a glycoprotein and that there are only two molecules of *N*-acetylglucosamine per fiber, and (2) Dorsett and Ginsberg (1975) showed that when the fiber protein is denatured with 10 M urea and the polypeptides are separated in denaturing gels (which contain 9 M urea, Brij 35, and dithiothreitol) on the basis of electrical charge rather than size, two protein bands are observed.

The physical and chemical data summarized suggest that the fiber consists of three polypeptide chains of similar sizes but of two species having unique amino acid sequences. Possibly the shaft of the fiber is made of two identical polypeptides, which are glycoproteins, and the terminal knob is a distinct unglycosylated polypeptide. The limited region of the genome (i.e., 2.4Kb) in which the fiber message is encoded (Lewis *et al.*, 1975) makes this model unlikely unless the two mRNAs with common 3' ends arising from this region (Nevins and Darnell, 1978) are read in different frames and translated into different proteins.

7.4. Immunological Characteristics of the Penton and Its Subunits

The penton displays antigenic reactions that reflect the summation of its component parts, i.e., base (vertex capsomer) and fiber. Hence antiserum from rabbits immunized with purified penton reacts with intact penton, penton base, and fiber (Pettersson and Höglund, 1969; Wadell and Norrby, 1969). The penton base contains a weak antigen common to all adenoviruses, the so-called β antigen (Wilcox and Ginsberg, 1961; Norrby, 1969a). In addition, of ten serotypes immunologically characterized, all penton bases carry intersubgroup and intrasubgroup antigenic determinants, except those of type 12, but none displays type-specific reactivity (Wadell and Norrby, 1969). Inter- and intrasubgroup antibodies also aggregate pentons and hence enhance hemagglutination (Norrby, 1966b, 1969a). Antibodies to purified pentons or to penton base neutralize the toxinlike activity of vertex capsomers from viruses of the same type or subgroup (Pettersson and Höglund, 1969).

Fibers possess a type-specific antigen, termed the "γ antigen," which appears to be associated with the knoblike distal portion of the projection (Pereira and de Figueredo, 1962; Pettersson et al., 1968). Antibodies to this type-specific antigen prevent attachment to RBC receptors, measured by hemagglutination inhibition, and attachment to susceptible host cells (Rosen, 1960; Philipson et al., 1968). Type-specific fiber antibodies also agglutinate viral particles and reduce viral infectivity. According to the length of the fiber, the immunological reactivity varies: the fibers from viruses belonging to subgroup I, the shortest fibers, contain only type-specific reactivity; fibers of subgroup II, which are of intermediate length, carry not only type-specific antigens but also intrasubgroup antigens, which also cross-react with subgroup III viral fibers; the longest fibers, those of subgroup III viruses, have type-specific and intersubgroup antigenic determinants shared with subgroup II fibers as well as an antigenic reactivity shared by type 1, 2, 5, and 6 viruses as intrasubgroup determinants (Pereira and de Figueredo, 1962; Norrby, 1968a; Wadell and Norrby, 1969). The vertex capsomer appears somehow to mask the intrasubgroup determinants (δ antigen) since heterotypic (intrasubgroup) fiber antibodies cannot enhance hemagglutination with intact pentons but they markedly increase the agglutination of RBC with free fibers (Pettersson and Höglund, 1969).

7.5. Biological Functions of the Penton and Its Subunits

The penton fiber (Levine and Ginsberg, 1967; Philipson et al., 1968) is the only capsid protein that efficiently combines with cell membranes, and accordingly it effects the virion's initial stage of infection, i.e., viral attachment. Either native pentons or free fibers can combine with host cell receptors (Levine and Ginsberg, 1967; Philipson, 1967), and indeed free fibers can competitively interfere with the virion-cell association (Philipson *et al.*, 1968). Just as fibers, either as a penton component or dissociated from the penton base, can combine with susceptible host cells, they can also effect hemagglutination via similar attachment (Pereira and de Figueredo, 1962; Valentine and Pereira, 1965; Norrby, 1968*a*). The interaction of adenoviruses with erythrocytes via their vertex projections offers a relatively easy, quantitative *in vitro* model to investigate the initial reactions of virus with its host cell.

Since Rosen (1958) initially described adenovirus-mediated hemagglutination, it has been demonstrated that all human adenoviruses can induce agglutination of particular species of red blood cells (Rosen, 1969; Rosen *et al.*, 1961, 1962; Bauer and Wigand, 1963; Schmidt *et al.*, 1965). Adenoviruses have even been grouped according to which erythrocytes the virions can agglutinate (Table 3). Because virions have 12 vertex units, each able to combine with RBCs, the viral particle can join with several cells and therefore produce a pattern of complete agglutination. Subgroups I and II hemagglutinate rhesus monkey and rat RBCs, respectively, whereas subgroup III and IV viruses agglutinate rat and human O RBCs (Table 3). Free pentons and dissociated fibers also are capable of effecting hemagglutination, but since the soluble proteins are univalent, only dimers or higher aggregates of pentons and fibers can clump RBCs. Pentons of some adenoviruses (e.g., types 3, 7, 11, 15) naturally form organized icosahedral structures containing 12 pentons ("dodecons") apparently associated around some central protein; they also produce patterns of complete hemagglutination (Norrby, 1966*a*, 1968*b*; Gelderblom *et al.*, 1967). The fibers and pentons of other viral types may remain as monomers or form only dimers, and hence only weak or partial hemagglutination is produced. Because the fiber protein, however, possesses intrasubgroup antigenic determinants (the δ antigen), heterotypic antibodies to the δ antigen (which cannot inhibit hemagglutination) aggregate pentons and fibers so that two or more fibers can combine with RBC producing demonstrable hemagglutination, a reaction termed "hemagglutination enhancement" (Pereira and de Figueredo, 1962; Norrby, 1968*a*; Wadell, 1970).

Pentons possess the unique feature of producing early cytopathic effects on susceptible cells in monolayer cultures (Pereira, 1958; Everett and Ginsberg, 1958; Rowe *et al.*, 1958). Within 3–6 hr after addition of

TABLE 3

Classification of Adenoviruses According to Hemagglutination Characteristics[a]

Adenovirus subgroup	RBC species agglutinated	Pattern of hemagglutination	Viral types	Additional characteristics subdividing viruses
I	Monkey	Complete	3, 7, 14, 21	Agglutinate different monkey RBCs with varying efficiency
			11, 16	Grivet and rhesus RBC
			20, 25, 28	Weak agglutination of monkey RBCs; agglutinate mouse RBCs to higher titer
II	Rat	Complete	8, 9, 10, 19	Also agglutinate mouse, human, and guinea pig RBCs
			13, 15, 16, 27	Also agglutinate mouse and human RBCs
			17, 22, 23, 24	Also agglutinate mouse RBCs
			29, 30	Agglutinate only rat RBCs
III	Rat and human	Incomplete[b]	1, 2, 5, 6	Dimers of pentons and fibers agglutinate RBCs
		Complete	4	Pentons form dodecons (like subgroup I)
IV	Rat and human	Incomplete	12, 18, 31	Weak agglutination by dimers of fibers

[a] Modified from Wadell (1970).
[b] Complete hemagglutination occurs when heterologous antibody from same hemagglutination subgroup is added to reaction mixture.

a relatively high concentration of pentons or penton bases (Pereira, 1958; Everett and Ginsberg, 1958; Rowe *et al.*, 1958; Wilcox and Ginsberg, 1961) long before the appearance of progeny virus in a productive infection, cells become rounded and clump, and many cells detach from the surface. This toxinlike action, however, does not kill the affected cells and the host cells' macromolecular synthesis is unaffected (Pereira, 1958). Moreover, removal of pentons reverses the cytopathic effect (Pereira, 1958; Rowe *et al.*, 1958). Low concentrations of trypsin (10–25 μg/ml) readily destroy the cytopathic activity of the penton and penton base (Pereira, 1958; Everett and Ginsberg, 1958), although the proteolysis does not change the protein's immunological properties (Pettersson and Höglund, 1969; Wadell and Norrby, 1969). Increased concentrations of trypsin result in degradation of the penton base and loss of immunological as well as cytopathic activities (Pettersson and Höglund, 1969).

Endonuclease activities, both double-strand- (Burlingham *et al.*, 1971) and single-strand- (Marusyk *et al.*, 1975) specific, have been reported to be associated with pentons derived from virions or the excess pool, but recent data indicate that the endonuclease can be dissociated from the penton and that the associated endonuclease is probably a host enzyme (W. Doerfler, personal communication).

Free fibers, although unable to produce a cytopathic effect like pentons, in fact establish a more profound biochemical change in sus- ceptible cells. Purified fibers can enter cells to which they attach and within 20 hr block synthesis of host DNA, RNA, and proteins (Levine and Ginsberg, 1967). The affected cells cannot divide, nor can they sup- port replication of viruses such as adenoviruses, vaccinia virus, or poliovirus (Pereira, 1960; Levine and Ginsberg, 1967). The intracellular mechanism of the fiber-inhibitory effect is still obscure, but *in vitro* the fiber protein binds cooperatively to DNA and blocks the activities of both DNA-dependent DNA polymerase and DNA-dependent RNA polymerase (Levine and Ginsberg, 1967). Whether fibers, which accu- mulate in considerable abundance late in infection, have a similar intracellular effect to terminate viral and host macromolecular syn- thesis is still uncertain.

8. OTHER CAPSID PROTEINS

As mentioned earlier (Fig. 1), the virion contains a minimum of nine unique proteins, and as many as 14 have been noted (Maizel *et al.*, 1968*a*; Anderson *et al.*, 1973; Everitt *et al.*, 1973; Ishibashi and Maizel, 1974*a*). The uncertainty of the precise number follows from the facts that some proteins are present in very low concentration, that only a few have been chemically analyzed and demonstrated to be unique, and that some may appear only as proteolytic cleavage products from major proteins. Indeed, it was initially suggested that the virion contains only five primary proteins (hexon, penton base, fiber, and two core proteins) (Russell and Skehel, 1972) and that the other components are degrada- tion products from accidental proteolytic cleavages (Pereira and Skehel, 1971). The following evidence, however, implies that this hypothesis is unlikely. Controlled degradation of virions (Everitt *et al.*, 1973, 1975; Everitt and Philipson, 1974), has consistently yielded proteins IIIa, VI, VIII, and IX in reproducible quantities sufficient to permit their

chemical and immunological characterizations as well as their topological presence in the capsid. The primary studies of these "minor"
capsid proteins have been made with type 2 virus, but SDS-polyacrylamide gel analyses have also revealed similar species in the type 3 (Prage
et al., 1972), type 5 (Kauffman and Ginsberg, 1976), and type 7 and 12
(Maizel *et al.*, 1968*b*) adenoviruses.

Polypeptide IIIa, which has a molecular weight of about 66,000
(Fig. 1) is released along with pentons when purified virions are
dialyzed against low ionic strength buffers (Everitt *et al.*, 1973). Iodination of intact virions using lactoperoxidase as a catalyst (Marchalonis
et al., 1971), which should label only the tyrosine residues of surface
proteins, did not iodinate the IIIa polypeptide (Everitt *et al.*, 1973).
Chemical cross-linking with tartryl diazide (Lutter *et al.*, 1974),
however, formed a complex of IIIa with the penton proteins (III and
IV) and protein VII (the major core protein), suggesting that protein
IIIa occupies a position near the vertex of the virion and close to the
core (Everitt *et al.*, 1975). It seems paradoxical that antisera produced
with purified protein IIIa efficiently precipitated intact virions, a reaction expected for proteins at the virion's surface (Everitt *et al.*, 1975).
The inability of IIIa to be iodinated, however, may be due to the
absence of free tyrosine residues at the protein's surface when assembled into virions. Further definitive evidence that protein IIIa is a
primary gene product follows from the facts that the mRNA has been
isolated, that its probable site of transcription has been identified by
specific hybridization, and that it has been translated *in vitro* into a
product similar in size to protein IIIa (Lewis *et al.*, 1975).

Protein VI in an undenatured form has an apparent molecular
weight of 50,000 when measured by gel exclusion chromatography
(Everitt and Philipson, 1974). On SDS-polyacrylamide gel electrophoresis, however, polypeptide VI migrates with a molecular weight of
24,000 (Anderson *et al.*, 1973; Everitt *et al.*, 1973; Ishibashi and
Maizel, 1974*a*), suggesting that the protein exists as a dimer in the
intact virion. According to pulse chase kinetics and tryptic peptide
analysis, the 24,000-dalton polypeptide VI is derived by proteolytic
cleavage (Anderson *et al.*, 1973; Ishibashi and Maizel, 1974*a*; Öberg *et
al.*, 1975) of a 27,000-dalton precursor polypeptide, variously called
"pVI" (Anderson *et al.*, 1974) or "V_a" (Ishibashi and Maizel, 1974*a*).
Amino acid analyses (Table 4) revealed that protein VI, purified from
virions, is notably rich in glycine (26%) and serine (22%) (Everitt and
Philipson, 1974).

Polypeptide VIII has a molecular weight of 13,000 and appears to be a posttranslation proteolytic cleavage product, like polypeptide VI. pVIII, which has a molecular weight of 26,000, has been presented as the putative precursor for protein VIII (Anderson *et al.*, 1973; Ishibashi and Maizel, 1974*a*; Öberg *et al.*, 1975), but comparative tryptic peptide maps of pVIII and protein VIII showed marked differences (Edvardsson *et al.*, 1976). The amino acid composition of protein VIII (Table 4) reveals a high content of glycine and serine residues (20% of each), similar to protein VI (Everitt and Philipson, 1974). However, antisera prepared against purified proteins VI and VIII do not cross-react (Everitt and Philipson, 1974; Öberg *et al.*, 1975), implying that they are not immunologically related and hence that they are unique viral gene products. Moreover, the mRNA for pVI is encoded at a site about 25 map units from the pVIII gene (Fig. 4).

Polypeptide IX is a primary translation product of about 11,000 daltons (Anderson *et al.*, 1973; Ishibashi and Maizel, 1974*a*), and is

TABLE 4

Amino Acid Composition of Core Protein VII and Minor Capsid Proteins

	Moles per 100 moles amino acid				
	VII				
Amino acid	Type 2[a]	Type 3[a]	VI[b]	VIII[b]	IX[b]
Lysine	3.8	3.7	1.6	1.8	1.8
Histidine	2.2	1.8	2.5	2.4	0.6
Arginine	20.6	23.2	6.3	5.5	6.3
Aspartic acid	7.2	7.2	5.4	7.0	9.3
Threonine	6.9	8.5	3.7	4.8	7.9
Serine	6.9	5.4	22.4	20.0	17.3
Glutamic acid	3.7	2.4	13.5	13.1	8.4
Proline	7.3	7.4	1.5	5.1	6.1
Glycine	8.3	8.0	25.8	20.0	8.7
Alanine	18.0	19.4	8.0	9.1	14.4
Valine	8.5	7.4	3.0	3.0	5.7
Methionine	Traces	ND[c]	0.4	0.5	0.3
Isoleucine	2.0	2.5	1.5	2.3	1.8
Leucine	2.4	2.2	2.2	2.7	8.5
Tyrosine	1.4	0.8	0.7	1.3	1.3
Phenylalanine	ND	ND	0.8	0.7	3.8
Tryptophan	0.7	NT[d]	ND	ND	ND
Half-cystine	NT	NT	ND	ND	ND

[a] Prage and Pettersson (1971) and Laver (1970).
[b] Everett and Philipson (1974).
[c] Not done.
[d] None detected.

produced in excess in infected cells (B. Oosterom and J. V. Maizel, unpublished data). In contrast to the other virion structural proteins, IX is synthesized prior to DNA replication, beginning about 4 hr after infection and therefore may be considered to be a "delayed early" protein serving a unique structural function (Persson *et al.*, 1978). Polypeptides X–XII are the smallest virion proteins, with molecular weights of 5000–6000 (Anderson *et al.*, 1973; Everitt *et al.*, 1973), and appear to arise by posttranslational cleavage of unknown larger proteins, since they are detected in extracts of infected cells and virions only during a chase period after a short pulse label (Anderson *et al.*, 1973). Since there are only a few copies of polypeptides X–XII per virion and their chemical composition is unknown, their structural and physiological significance are still unclear. They may represent cleavage products generated from larger proteins during virion assembly (Ishibashi and Maizel, 1974*a*) or aberrant proteolytic degradation products (Pereira and Skehel, 1971).

Controlled sequential disruption of virions (Prage *et al.*, 1970; Everett *et al.*, 1973) combined with enzymatic iodination, chemical cross linking, and immunological techniques permits assignment of the topography of proteins VI, VIII, and IX in the viral capsid (Everitt *et al.*, 1973, 1975). Proteins VI appears in association with all hexons, the so-called peripentonal and face hexons, regardless of the extraction method employed (Fig. 2). Degradation of virions yields 2 moles of polypeptide VI per mole of hexon capsomers (Everitt *et al.*, 1973). Since the lactoperoxidase procedure does not iodinate protein VI in intact virions, and antiserum against protein VI is unable to precipitate virions, this protein appears to be associated with the inner surface, i.e., the base of the hexon (Everitt *et al.*, 1975). This internal location of protein VI probably accounts for its frequent isolation with core fractions of disrupted virions (Maizel *et al.*, 1968*b*).

The face hexons of the capsid, which are arranged in groups of nine, are in approximation to proteins VIII and IX in addition to protein VI (Fig. 2). Proteins VIII and IX, however, do not appear to be associated with the hexons adjacent to pentons (Everitt *et al.*, 1973). Protein VI is dissociable from the groups of nine hexon complex (termed "nonomers") by 0.15 M NaCl, while polypeptide IX remains bound to hexons at this electrolyte concentration. In contrast, polypeptide IX is dissociated from hexons in salt-free gradients. Protein VIII appears to be internally associated with hexons since it is not iodinated by surface reactants, and specific protein VIII antibodies do not precipitate virions (Everitt *et al.*, 1975). In contrast, antiserum to protein IX precipitates virions to a small extent, suggesting that it has some surface reactive groups (Everitt *et al.*, 1975).

9. THE CORE

Several selective procedures for virion degradation yield a DNA-protein structure termed the "core." Viral cores, containing the viral genome and up to 20% of the virion protein, can be prepared by dialysis at pH 10.5 (Wilcox and Ginsberg, 1963*a*; Lawrence and Ginsberg, 1967); repeated freezing and thawing (Prage *et al.*, 1970); heating to 56°C in the presence of sodium deoxycholate (Russell *et al.*, 1967*b*, 1971); and treatment with acetone (Laver *et al.*, 1968), 5 M urea (Maizel *et al.*, 1968*b*), 10% pyridine (Prage *et al.*, 1970; Everitt *et al.*, 1973), or sarcosyl (Brown *et al.*, 1975). Although these core preparations differ in the species and molar amounts of proteins present, the common feature is the presence of a particle which contains intact viral DNA complexed with protein, but in which the DNA is nevertheless nuclease-sensitive. The restriction endonuclease *Eco*R1 cleaves the type 2 virus DNA in sarcosyl cores into six specific fragments which can be resolved if the cores are treated with pronase; without proteolytic digestion, however, the terminal DNA fragments, A and C, are complexed with a 55,000-dalton protein which is covalently linked to the 5′ terminus of each strand (Brown *et al.*, 1975; Rekosh *et al.*, 1977).

Cores prepared by any of the methods listed consistently contain DNA tightly bound to protein VII, a highly basic polypeptide of approximately 17,000 daltons (Maizel *et al.*, 1968*a*; Prage *et al.*, 1968; Anderson *et al.*, 1973). The basic charge of this polypeptide is primarily derived from its amino acid composition (Table 4), which is notable for its content of 21–23% arginine, about 20% alanine, one tryptophan residue per polypeptide, and an N-terminal alanine (Laver *et al.*, 1967; Laver, 1970; Prage and Pettersson, 1971). Thus, although protein VII resembles the arginine-rich histone, the relatively small number of lysine residues (i.e., about 4%) and the presence of tryptophan (Laver, 1970; Prage and Pettersson, 1971) distinguish protein VII from the eukaryotic cell histones. Immunologically, protein VII purified from type 2 and 3 adenoviruses contains both common and unique antigenic determinants (Prage and Pettersson, 1971). The protein is exclusively an internal component of the virion, however, and when the virion is intact protein VII is not available to antibody or to iodination by lactoperoxidase (Everitt *et al.*, 1975). Each virion contains 1100–1350 copies of protein VII, which can cover about 60% of the phosphate backbone of the viral DNA (Prage and Pettersson, 1971; Everitt *et al.*, 1975). The virion polypeptide VII is derived by posttranslational cleavage from a slightly larger precursor protein (pVII) of 19,000 daltons (Anderson *et al.*, 1973; Ishibashi and Maizel, 1974*a*).

Little is known of the structure and chemical composition of the second core protein, protein V, except that it has a molecular weight of 45,000, as measured by polyacrylamide gel electrophoresis, and is only moderately rich in arginine, 11.9% (Laver, 1970). There are only about 180 molecules of protein V per virion (Maizel *et al.*, 1968*b*; Everitt *et al.*, 1973), and these appear to be relatively superficial core components and easily removed from the DNA-protein VII complex (Brown *et al.*, 1975). In chemical cross-linking studies, using the protein cross-linker tartryl diazide, some of the protein V molecules are linked to penton, hexon, and protein IIIa, suggesting that although the core protein V molecules are located internally, at least some are situated in close approximation (within 0.6 nm) to the capsid vertices (Everitt *et al.*, 1975). Freeze-cleaved preparations strengthen the evidence that protein V is a superficial core protein since one fracture plane appears to pass between the outer capsid of the virion and polypeptide V, and a second fracture plane is probably located between polypeptide V and the remainder of the viral core (Brown *et al.*, 1975).

10. AN OVERVIEW

The adenovirus-infected cell is an effective factory for synthesizing viral DNA and proteins, which may assemble into as many as 10^5–10^6 virions in each infected cell. The major viral proteins and the viral DNA, however, are made in even greater abundance, and only about 10% of each is assembled into virions (Ginsberg and Dixon, 1961; Green, 1962; Wilcox and Ginsberg, 1963*b*). As a consequence of the high production and inefficient utilization, large nuclear DNA-protein aggregates form and characteristic inclusion bodies appear (Boyer *et al.*, 1957). It is not clear whether the excessive accumulation of viral DNA and protein results from or is a cause of the inefficient assembly of virions. The major adenovirus capsid proteins are particularly unique among viral proteins; they are soluble in aqueous solutions, and they can be purified in their native state. These valuable characteristics and the proteins' profusion have led to their extensive structural, biological, and immunological characterization.

The number of virion proteins, however, is somewhat perplexing. It does not seem economical of genetic information to provide a minimum of 11 virion proteins merely to protect the virion DNA and provide a package for its transport. Nor does it seem necessary to supply so many unique proteins to form an icosahedron suitable for attachment to host cells. The species of proteins associated with hexons and pentons may, however, be required to furnish stability to an icosahedral shell 70–80 nm in diameter, in contrast to simpler and smaller icosahedral viruses, such as picornaviruses or papovaviruses. A proposed model of the virion (Fig. 2) presents the suggested topology of its subunits and signifies the architectural relationships of the so-called "minor proteins" to the major components. Thus proteins VIII and IX may provide stability to the face hexons arranged in groups of nine (nonomers). And protein IIIa may serve as essential links between the penton base and its five neighboring peripentonal hexons. Protein VI in turn may provide an additional internal structure stabilizing the capsid as well as providing bridges to bind the capsid to the DNA-protein core.

The kinetics of assembly of viral proteins into empty capsids and virions and the posttranslational proteolytic processing of several proteins suggest that the "minor proteins" may play a critical role in morphogenesis of the stable virion. A variety of experiments using pulse-chase techniques (Sundquist *et al.*, 1973*a*; Ishibashi and Maizel, 1974*a*) yielded evidence implying that assembly consists of sequential reactions initiated with the formation of empty shells into which the viral DNA is inserted to produce "young virions" (Ishibashi and Maizel, 1974*a*). Using a temperature-sensitive mutant of type 5 adenovirus to synchronize the critical reactions, it has been possible to demonstrate that the assembly of the viral DNA in the empty capsid begins with entry of the left end of the genome (Cheng, 1978) (Fig. 4). Proteolytic cleavage of the precursor polypeptides pVI, pVII, and pVIII (Anderson *et al.*, 1973; Ishibashi and Maizel, 1974*a*) then appears to complete the assembly of mature virions. This procession of events suggests that the "minor" proteins have several functions:

1. pVI and pVIII may together act as a protein inner shell for formation of the empty capsid, similar to the gene 8 "scaffolding protein" of *Salmonella* phage P22 (King and Casjens, 1974; Casjens and King, 1974; see also Chapter 9 of this volume). When pVI and pVIII are cleaved during the final stage of morphogenesis, the products, proteins VI and VIII, may stabilize the capsid and couple it to the viral core. Protein IX may further assist in assembly of the capsid, since it is present in the

putative precursor empty shells (Sundquist *et al.*, 1973*a*; Ishibashi and Maizel, 1974*a*).

2. pVII, the precursor to the arginine-rich core protein, has been noted in empty capsids and young virions (Ishibashi and Maizel, 1974*a*), and initially it may serve to fold the entering DNA. The processing of pVII to protein VII may then establish a firm noncovalent association with the DNA phosphate backbone.

3. Protein V, which is superficial to protein VII and less firmly bound to the DNA, may promote the DNA's entrance into the shell and assist its folding; in addition, protein V may provide an attachment of the core to proteins VI, IIIa, and II through noncovalent bonds (Everitt *et al.*, 1975) (Fig. 2).

These hypotheses are not dependent on the still unproved proposal that the empty capsid is the precursor to the virion. If the components of the outer protein coat should assemble around the DNA, these proposed functions could still be ascribed to the less prominent proteins. Future investigations should furnish the missing data that will permit a final understanding of regulation of synthesis, fine structure, and morphogenesis of these virions.

11. REFERENCES

Anderson, C. W., Baum, S. G., and Gesteland, R. F., 1973, Processing of adenovirus 2-induced proteins, *J. Virol.* **12**:241.

Anderson, C. W., Lewis, J. B., Atkins, J. F., and Gesteland, R. F., 1974, Cell-free synthesis of adenovirus 2 proteins programmed by fractionated messenger RNA: A comparison of polypeptide products and messenger RNA lengths, *Proc. Natl. Acad. Sci. USA* **71**:2756.

Bauer, H., and Wigand, R., 1963, Eigenschaften der Adenovirus-Hämaggltuinine, *Z. Hyg. Infekt.-Kr.* **149**:96.

Bello, L. J., and Ginsberg, H. S., 1969, Relationship between deoxyribonucleic acid-like ribonucleic acid synthesis and inhibition of host protein synthesis in type 5 adenovirus-infected KB cells, *J. Virol.* **3**:106.

Bencze, W. L., and Schmid, K., 1957, Determination of tyrosine and tryptophan in proteins, *Anal. Chem.* **29**:1193.

Biserte, G., Samalille, J., Dautrevaux, M., Boulanger, P., Sautïère, P., Ringel, J., and Warocquier, R., 1966, Composition en acides aminés de l'atingène de structure A de l'adenovirus 5, *C. R. Acad. Sci.* **263**:1648.

Boulanger, P. A., and Warocquier, R., 1971, Improved method for virus structural polypeptide analysis on dissociating acrylamide gel, *Appl. Microbiol.* **22**:760.

Boulanger, P. A., Flamencourt, P., and Biserte, G., 1969, Isolation and comparative chemical study of structure proteins of the adenovirus 2 and 5: Hexon and fiber antigens, *Eur. J. Biochem.* **10**:116.

Boyer, G. S., Leuchtenberger, C., and Ginsberg, H. S., 1957, Cytological and cytochemical studies of HeLa cells infected with adenoviruses, *J. Exp. Med.* **105**:195.

Brown, D. T., Westphal, M., Burlingham, B. T., Winterhoff, U., and Doerfler, W., 1975, Structure and composition of the adenovirus type 2 core, *J. Virol.* **16**:366.

Burlingham, B., Doerfler, W., Pettersson, U., and Philipson, L., 1971, Adenovirus endonuclease association with the penton of adenovirus type 2, *J. Mol. Biol.* **60**:45.

Carter, T. H., and Ginsberg, H. S., 1976, Viral transcription in KB cells infected by temperature-sensitive "early" mutants of adenovirus type 5, *J. Virol.* **18**:156.

Casjens, S., and King, J., 1974, P22 morphogenesis. I. Catalytic scaffolding protein in capsid assembly, *J. Supramol. Struct.* **2**:202.

Caspar, D. L. D., and Klug, A., 1962, Physcial principles in the construction of regular viruses, *Cold Spring Harbor Symp. Quant. Biol.* **27**:1.

Cheng, C., 1978, Characterization of a type 5 adenovirus temperature-sensitive fiber mutant and its functional role, Ph.D. thesis, Columbia University.

Cornick, G., Sigler, P. B., and Ginsberg, H. S., 1971, Characterization of crystals of adenovirus type 5 hexon, *J. Mol. Biol.* **57**:397.

Cornick, G., Sigler, P. B., and Ginsberg, H. S., 1973, Mass of protein in the asymmetric unit of hexon crystals—New method, *J. Mol. Biol.* **73**:533.

Cox, H. R., Scheer, J. V. D., Aisdon, S., and Boland, E., 1947, The purification and concentration of influenza virus by means of alcohol precipitation, *J. Immunol.* **56**:149.

Crick, F. H. C., and Watson, J. D., 1956, The structure of small viruses, *Nature (London)* **177**:473.

Crowther, R. A., and Franklin, R. M., 1972, The structure of the groups of nine hexons from adenoviruses, *J. Mol. Biol.* **68**:181.

Davis, B. J., 1964, Disc electrophoresis. II. Method and application to human serum proteins, *Ann. N.Y. Acad. Sci.* **121**:404.

Dorsett, P. H., and Ginsberg, H. S., 1975, Characterization of the type 5 adenovirus fiber proteins, *J. Virol.* **15**:208.

Edvardsson, B., Everitt, E., Jörnvall, H., Prage, L., and Philipson, L., 1976, Intermediates in adenovirus assembly, *J. Virol.* **19**:533.

Ellens, D. J., Sussenbach, J. S., and Jansz, H. S., 1974, Studies on the mechanism of repliction of adenovirus DNA. III. Electron microscopy of replicating DNA, *Virology* **61**:427.

Enders, J. F., Bell, J. A., Dingle, J. H., Francis, T., Jr., Hilleman, M. R., Huebner, R. J., and Payne, A. M. M., 1956, Adenoviruses: Group name proposed for new respiratory tract viruses, *Science* **124**:119.

Ensinger, M. J., and Ginsberg, H. S., 1972, Selection and preliminary characterization of temperature-sensitive mutants of type 5 adenovirus, *J. Virol.* **10**:328.

Eron, L., Callahan, R., and Westphal, H., 1974, Cell free synthesis of adenovirus coat proteins, *J. Biol. Chem.* **249**:6331.

Everett, S. F., and Ginsberg, H. S., 1958, A toxinlike material separable from type 5 adenovirus particles, *Virology* **6**:770.

Everitt, E., and Philipson, L., 1974, Structural proteins of adenoviruses. XI. Purification of three low molecular weight virion proteins of adenovirus type 2 and their synthesis during productive infection, *Virology* **62**:253.

Everitt, E., Sundquist, B., and Philipson, L., 1971, Mechanism of arginine requirement for adenovirus synthesis. I. Synthesis of structural proteins, *J. Virol.* **8**:742.

Everitt, E., Sundquist, B., Pettersson, U., and Philipson, L., 1973, Structural proteins of adenoviruses. X. Isolation and topography of low-molecular-weight antigens from the virion of adenovirus type 2, *Virology* **52**:130.

Everitt, E., Lutter, L., and Philipson, L., 1975, Structural proteins of adenoviruses. XII. Location and neighbor relationships among proteins of adenovirion type 2 as revealed by enzymatic iodination, immunoprecipitation and chemical cross-linking, *Virology* **67**:197.

Fink, W. W., Mann, K. G., and Tanford, C., 1969, The estimation of polypeptide chain molecular weights by gel filtration in 6 M guanidine hydrochloride *J. Biol. Chem.* **244**:4989.

Flanagan, J. F., and Ginsberg, H. S., 1962, Synthesis of virus-specific polymers in adenovirus-infected cells: Effect of 5-fluorodeoxyuridine, *J. Exp. Med.* **116**:141.

Franklin, R. M., Pettersson, U., Åkervall, K., Standberg, B., and Philipson, L., 1971, Structural proteins of adenovirus. V. Size and structure of the adenovirus type 2 hexon, *J. Mol. Biol.* **57**:383.

Friedman, M. P., Lyons, M. J., and Ginsberg, H. S., 1970, Biochemical consequences of type 2 adenovirus and simian virus 40 double infection of African green monkey kidney cells, *J. Virol.* **5**:586.

Garon, C. F., Berry, K. W., Hierholzer, J. C., and Rose, J. A., 1973, Mapping of base sequence heterologies between genomes from different adenovirus serotypes, *Virology* **54**:414.

Gelderblom, H., Bauer, H., Frank, H., and Wigand, R., 1967, The structure of group II adenoviruses, *J. Gen. Virol.* **1**:553.

Gilead, Z., and Ginsberg, H. S., 1965, Characterization of a tumorlike antigen in type 12 and type 18 adenovirus infected cells, *J. Bacteriol.* **90**:120.

Ginsberg, H. S., 1957, Biological and physical properties of the adenovirus, *Ann. N.Y. Acad. Sci.* **67**:383.

Ginsberg, H. S., 1971, Structure and synthesis of adenovirus capsid proteins, in: *Nucleic Acid-Protein Interactions: Nucleic Acid Synthesis in Viral Infection* (D. W. Ribbons, J. F. Woessner, and J. Schultz, eds.), pp. 419–434, North-Holland, Amsterdam.

Ginsberg, H. S., and Dixon, M. K., 1961, Nucleic acid synthesis in types 4 and 5 adenovirus-infected HeLa cells, *J. Exp. Med.* **113**:283.

Ginsberg, H. S., and Young, C. S. H., 1977. Genetics of adenoviruses, in: *Comprehensive Virology*, Vol. 9 (H. Fraenkel-Conrat and R. R. Wagner, eds.), p. 27, Plenum Press, New York.

Ginsberg, H. S., Pereira, H. G., Valentine, R. C., and Wilcox, W. C., 1966, A proposed terminology for the adenovirus antigens and virion morphological subunits, *Virology* **28**:782.

Ginsberg, H. S., Bello, L. J., and Levine, A. J., 1967, Control of biosynthesis of host macromolecules in cells infected with adenoviruses, in: *The Molecular Biology of Viruses* (J. S. Colter, and W. Paranchych, eds.), pp. 547–572, Academic Press, New York.

Ginsberg, H. S., Ensinger, M. J., Kauffman, R. S., Mayer, A. J., and Lundholm, U., 1974, Cell transformation: A study of regulation with types 5 and 12 adenovirus temperature-sensitive mutants, *Cold Spring Harbor Symp. Quant. Biol.* **39**:419.

Green, M., 1962, Studies on the biosynthesis of viral DNA. IV. Isolation, purification and chemical analysis of adenovirus, *Cold Spring Harbor Symp. Quant. Biol.* **27**:219.

Green, M., and Piña, M., 1963, Biochemical studies on the adenovirus multiplication. IV. Isolation, purification and chemical analysis of adenovirus, *Virology* **20**:199.

Green, M., Piña, M., Kemes, R. C., Wensick, P. C., MacHattie, L. A., and Thomas, C. A., Jr., 1967, Adenovirus DNA. I. Molecular weight and conformation, *Proc. Natl. Acad. Sci. USA* **57**:1302.

Green, M., Parsons, J. T., Piña, M., Fujinaga, K., Caffier, H., and Landgraf-Leurs, I., 1970, Transcription of adenovirus genes in productively infected and in transformed cells, *Cold Spring Harbor Symp. Quant. Biol.* **35**:803.

Grütter, M., and Franklin, R. M., 1974, Studies on the molecular weight of the adenovirus type 2 hexon and its subunits, *J. Mol. Biol.* **89**:163.

Hilleman, M. R., and Wenner, J. R., 1954, Recovery of new agent from patients with acute respiratory illness, *Proc. Soc. Exp. Biol. Med.* **85**:183.

Horne, R. W., 1962, The comparative structure of adenoviruses, *Ann. N.Y. Acad. Sci.* **101**:475.

Horne, R. W., and Wildy, P., 1963, Virus structure revealed by negative staining, *Adv. Virus Res.* **10**:101.

Horowitz, M. S., Scharff, M. D., and Maizel, I. V., 1969, Synthesis and assembly of adenovirus 2. I. Polypeptide synthesis, assembly of capsomers and morphogenesis of the virion, *Virology* **39**:682.

Horowitz, M. S., Maizel, J. V., and Scharff, M. D., 1970, Molecular weight of adenovirus type 2 hexon polypeptide, *J. Virol.* **6**:569.

Horuna, J., Yaasi, H., Kono, R., and Watanabe, I., 1961, Separation of adenovirus by chromatography on DEAE-cellulose, *Virology* **13**:264.

Huebner, R. J., Rowe, W. P., and Chanock, R. M., 1958, Newly recognized respiratory tract viruses, *Annu. Rev. Microbiol.* **12**:49.

Huebner, R. J., Casey, M. J., Chanock, R. M., and Scheel, K., 1965, Tumors induced in hamsters by a strain of adenovirus type 3: Sharing of tumor antigens and "neoantigens" with those produced by adenovirus type 7 tumors, *Proc. Natl. Acad. Sci USA* **54**:381.

Ishibashi, M., and Maizel, J. V., Jr., 1974a, The polypeptides of adenovirus. V. Young virions, structural intermediates between top components and aged virions, *Virology* **57**:409.

Ishibashi, M., and Maizel, J. V., Jr., 1974b, The polypeptides of adenovirus VI. Early and late glycopolypeptides, *Virology* **58**:345.

Jörnvall, H., Oblsson, H., and Philipson, L., 1974, An acetylated N-terminus of adenovirus type 2 hexon protein, *Biochem. Biophys. Res. Commun.* **56**:304.

Jörnvall, H., Pettersson, U., and Philipson, L., 1975, Structural studies of adenovirus type 2 hexon protein, *Eur. J. Biochem.* **48**:179.

Kauffman, R. S., 1976, Characterization of a temperature-sensitive hexon transport mutant of type 5 adenovirus, Ph.D. thesis, University of Pennsylvania.

Kauffman, R. S., and Ginsberg, H. S., 1976, Characterization of a temperature-sensitive, hexon transport mutant of type 5 adenovirus, *J. Virol.* **19**:643.

Kiehn, E. D., and Holland, J. J., 1970, Synthesis and cleavage of enterovirus polypeptides in mammalian cells, *J. Virol.* **5**:358.

King, J., and Casjens, S., 1974, Catalytic head assembling proteins in virus morphogenesis, *Nature (London)* **251**:112.

Kjellen, L., and Pereira, H. G., 1968, Role of adenovirus antigens in the induction of virus neutralizing antibodies, *J. Gen. Virol.* **2**:177.

Klemperer, H. G., and Pereira, H. G., 1959, Study of adenovirus antigens fractionated by chromatography mDEAE-cellulose, *Virology* **9**:536.

Koczot, F. J., Carter, B. J., Garon, C. F., and Rose, J. A., 1973, Self-complementarity of terminal sequences within plus or minus strands of adenovirus-associated virus DNA, *Proc. Natl. Acad. Sci. USA* **70**:215.

Köhler, K., 1965, Reinigung und Charakteresierung zweier Protein des Adenovirus Type 2, *Z. Naturforsch.* **20b**:747.

Lacy, S., Sr., and Green, M., 1964, Biochemical studies on adenovirus multiplication. VII. Homology between DNA's of tumorigenic and nontumorigenic human adenoviruses, *Proc. Natl. Acad. Sci. USA* **52**:1053.

Lacy, S., Sr., and Green, M., 1965, Adenovirus multiplication: Genetic relatedness of tumorigenic human adenovirus type 7, 12, 18, *Science* **150**:1296.

Lacy, S., Sr., and Green, M., 1967, The mechanism of viral carcinogenesis by DNA mammalian viruses: DNA-DNA homology relationship among the "weakly" oncogenic human adenoviruses, *J. Gen. Virol.* **1**:413.

Laver, W. G., 1970, Isolation of an arginine-rich protein from particles of adenovirus type 2, *Virology* **41**:488.

Laver, W. G., Suviano, R. J., and Green, M., 1967, Adenovirus proteins. II. N-terminal amino acid analysis, *J. Virol.* **1**:723.

Laver, W. G., Pereira, H. G., Russell, W. C., and Valentine, B. C., 1968, Isolation of an internal component from adenovirus type 5, *J. Mol. Biol.* **37**:379.

Laver, W. G., Wrigley, N. G., and Pereira, H. G., 1969, Removal of pentons from particles of adenovirus type 2, *Virology* **39**:599.

Lawrence, W. C., and Ginsberg, H. S., 1967, Intracellular uncoating of type 5 adenovirus deoxyribonucleic acid, *J. Virol.* **1**:851.

Levine, A. J., and Ginsberg, H. S., 1967, Mechanism by which fiber antigen inhibits multiplication of type 5 adenovirus, *J. Virol.* **1**:747.

Lewis, J. B., Atkins, J. F., Anderson, C. W., Baum, P. R., and Gesteland, R. F., 1975, Mapping of late adenovirus genes by cell-free translation of RNA selected by hybridization to specific DNA fragments, *Proc. Natl. Acad. Sci. USA* **72**:1344.

Lewis, J. B., Atkins, P. R., Baum, P. R., Salem, B., and Gesteland, R. F., 1976, Location and identification of the genes for adenovirus type 2 early polypeptides, *Cell* **7**:141.

Loening, V. E., 1967, The fractionation of high molecular weight ribonucleic acid by polyacrylamide-gel electrophoresis, *Biochem. J.* **102**:251.

Lucas, J. J., and Ginsberg, H. S., 1971, Synthesis of virus-specific ribonucleic acid in KB cells infected with type 2 adenovirus, *J. Virol.* **8**:203.

Luciw, P., and Ginsberg, H. S., 1979, Variations in phenotypic expressions of type 5 adenovirus temperature-sensitive hexon mutants, submitted for publication.

Lutter, L. C., Ortonderl, F., and Fasold, H., 1974, The use of a new series of cleavable protein-cross-linkers on the *Escherichia coli* ribosome, *FEBS Lett.* **48**:288.

Maizel, J. V., Jr., 1966, Acrylamide gel electrophorograms by mechanical fractionation: Radioactive adenovirus proteins, *Science* **151**:988.

Maizel, J. V., Jr., White, D. O., and Scharff, M. D., 1968*a*, The polypeptides of adenovirus. I. Evidence for multiple protein components in the virion and a comparison of types 2, 7A and 12, *Virology* **36**:115.

Maizel, J. V., Jr., White, D. O., and Scharff, M. D., 1968*b*, The polypeptides of adenovirus. II. Soluble proteins, cores, top components and the structure of the virion, *Virology* **36**:126.

Marchalonis, J. J., Cone, R. E., and Santer, V., 1971, Enzymatic iodination, a probe for accessible surface proteins of normal and neoplastic lymphocytes, *Biochem. J.* **124:**921.

Marusyk, R. G., Morgan, A. R., and Wadell, G., 1975, Association of endonuclease activity with serotypes belonging to the three subgroups of human adenoviruses, *J. Virol.* **16:**456.

Mautner, V., and Pereira, H. G., 1971, Crystallization of a second adenovirus protein (the fiber), *Nature (London)* **230:**456.

Mautner, V., Williams, J., Sambrook, J., Sharp, P., and Grodzicker, T., 1975, The location of genes coding for hexon and fiber proteins in adenovirus DNA, *Cell* **5:**93.

Macintyre, W. M., Pereira, H. G., and Russell, W. C., 1969, Crystallographic data for the hexon of adenovirus type 5, *Nature (London)* **222:**1165.

McAllister, R. M., Nicholson, M. O., Reed, G., Kern, J., Gilden, R. V., and Huebner, R. J., 1969, Transformation of rodent cells by adenovirus 19 and other group D adenoviruses, *J. Natl. Cancer Inst.* **43:**917.

McConaby, P. J., and Dixon, F. J., 1966, A method of trace iodination of proteins for immunologic studies, *Int. Arch. Allergy Appl. Immunol.* **29:**185.

Moore, S., Spockman, D. H., and Stein, W. H., 1958, Chromatography of amino acids on sulfonated polystyrene resins—An improved system, *Anal. Chem.* **30:**1185.

Nermut, M. V., 1975, Fine structure of adenovirus type 5. I. Virus capsid, *Virology* **65:**480.

Neurath, A. R., Rubin, B. A., and Stasny, J. T., 1968, Cleavage by formamide of intercapsomer bonds in adenovirus type 4 and 7 virions and hemagglutinins, *J. Virol.* **2:**1086.

Nevins, J. R., and Darnell, J. E., 1978, Groups of adenovirus type 2 mRNAs derived from a large primary transcript: Probable nuclear origin and possible common 3' ends, *J. Virol.* **25:**811.

Norrby, E., 1966a, The relationship between the soluble antigens and the virions of adenovirus type 3. I. Morphological characteristics, *Virology* **28:**236.

Norrby, E., 1966b, The relationship between the soluble antigens and the virion of type 3. II. Identification and characterization of an incomplete hemagglutinin, *Virology* **30:**608.

Norrby, E., 1968a, Biological significance of structural adenovirus components, *Curr. Top. Microbiol. Immunol.* **43:**1.

Norrby, E., 1968b, Comparison of soluble components of adenovirus types 3 and 11, *J. Gen. Virol.* **2:**135.

Norrby, E., 1969a, The structural and functional diversity of adenovirus capsid components, *J. Gen. Virol.* **5:**221.

Norrby, E., 1969b, The relationship between the soluble antigens and the virion of adenovirus type 3. IV. Immunological complexity of soluble components, *Virology* **37:**565.

Norrby, E., 1969c, Capsid mosaics of intermediate strains of human adenoviruses, *J. Virol.* **4:**657.

Norrby, E., and Skaaret, P., 1967, The relationship between soluble antigens and the virion of adenovirus type 3. III. Immunological identification of fiber antigen and isolated vertex capsomer antigen, *Virology* **32:**498.

Norrby, E., and Wadell, G., 1969, Immunological relationships between hexons of certain human adenoviruses, *J. Virol.* **4:**663.

Norrby, E., Marusyk, H., and Hammorskjöld, M. L., 1969a, The relationship between the soluble antigens and the virion of adenovirus type 3. V. Identification of antigen specificities available at the surface of virions, *Virology* **38**:477.

Norrby, E., Wadell, G., and Marusyk, H., 1969*b*, Fiber-associated incomplete and complete hemagglutinins of adenovirus type 6, *Arch. Ges. Virusforsch.* **28**:239.

Öberg, B., Saborio, J., Persson, T., Everitt, E., and Philipson, L., 1975, Identification of the *in vitro* translation products of adenovirus mRNA by immunoprecipitation, *J. Virol.* **15**:199.

Pereira, H. G., 1958, A protein factor responsible for the early cytopathic effect of adenoviruses, *Virology* **6**:601.

Pereira, H. G., 1960, A virus inhibitor produced in HeLa cells infected with adenovirus, *Virology* **11**:590.

Pereira, H. G., and de Figueredo, M. V. T., 1962, Mechanism of hemagglutination by adenovirus types 1, 2, 4, 5, and 6, *Virology* **18**:1.

Pereira, H. G., and Laver, W. G., 1970, Comparison of adenovirus types 2 and 5 hexon by immunological and biochemical techniques, *J. Gen. Virol.* **9**:163.

Pereira, H. G., and Skehel, J. J., 1971, Spontaneous and tryptic degradation of virus particles and structural components of adenovirus, *J. Gen. Virol.* **12**:13.

Pereira, H. G., and Wrigly, N. G., 1974, *In vitro* reconstitution, hexon banding and handedness of incomplete adenovirus capsid, *J. Mol. Virol.* **85**:617.

Pereira, H. G., Huebner, R. J., Ginsberg, H. S., and Van der Veen, J., 1963, A short description of the adenovirus group, *Virology* **20**:613.

Pereira, H. G., Valentine, R. C., and Russell, W. C., 1968, Crystallization of an adenovirus protein, *Nature (London)* **219**:946.

Persson, H., Pettersson, U., and Matthews, M. B., 1978, Synthesis of a structural adenovirus polypeptide in the absence of viral DNA replication, *Virology* **90**:67.

Pettersson, U., 1970, Structural proteins of adenoviruses, Ph.D. thesis, Uppsala University, Uppsala, Sweden.

Pettersson, U., 1971, Structural proteins of adenoviruses. VI. On the antigenic determinants of the hexon, *Virology* **43**:123.

Pettersson, U., 1973, Some unusual properties of replicating adenovirus type 2 DNA, *J. Mol. Biol.* **81**:521.

Pettersson, U., and Höglund, S., 1969, Structural proteins of adenoviruses. III. Purification and characterization of the adenovirus type 2 pentons antigen, *Virology* **39**:90.

Pettersson, U., Philipson, L., and Höglund, S., 1967, Structural proteins of adenoviruses. I. Purification and characterization of the adenovirus type 2 hexon antigen, *Virology* **33**:575.

Pettersson, U., Philipson, L., and Höglund, S., 1968, Structural proteins of adenoviruses. II. Purification and characterization of adenovirus type 2 fiber antigens, *Virology* **35**:204.

Philipson, L., 1960, Separation on DEAE-cellulose of components associated with adenovirus reproduction, *Virology* **10**:459.

Philipson, L., 1967, Attachment and eclipse of adenovirus, *J. Virol.* **1**:868.

Philipson, L., and Lindberg, U., 1974, Reproduction of adenoviruses, in: *Comprehensive Virology*, Vol. 3 (H. Fraenkel-Conrat and R. R. Wagner, eds.), pp. 143–228, Plenum Press, New York.

Philipson, L., and Pettersson, U., 1973, Structure and function of virion proteins of adenovirus, in: *Oncogenic Adenoviruses: Progress in Experimental Tumor Research*, Vol. 18, p. 1, Karger, Basel.

Philipson, L., Lonberg-Holm, K., and Pettersson, U., 1968, Virus receptor interaction in an adenovirus systems, *J. Virol.* **2**:1064.

Piña, M., and Green, M., 1965, Biochemical studies on adenovirus multiplication. IX. Chemical and base composition analysis of 28 human adenoviruses, *Proc. Natl. Acad. Sci. USA* **54**:547.

Piña, M., and Green, M., 1968, Base composition of the DNA of oncogenic simian adenovirus SA7 and homology with human adenovirus DNAs, *Virology* **36**:321.

Prage, L., and Pettersson, U., 1971, Structural proteins of adenoviruses. VII. Purification and properties of an arginine-rich core protein from adenovirus type 2 and type 3, *Virology* **45**:364.

Prage, L., Pettersson, U., and Philipson, L., 1968, Internal basic proteins in adenovirus, *Virology* **36**:508.

Prage, L., Pettersson, U.,Höglund, S., Lonberg-Holm, K., and Philipson, L., 1970, Structural proteins of adenoviruses. IV. Sequential degradation of adenovirus type 2 virion, *Virology* **42**:341.

Prage, L., Höglund, S., and Philipson, L., 1972, Structural proteins of adenoviruses. VIII. Characterization of incomplete particles of adenovirus type 3, *Virology* **49**:745.

Rekosh, D. M. K., Russell, W. C., Bellet, A. J. D., and Robinson, A. J. 1977, Identification of a protein linked to the ends of adenovirus DNA, *Cell* **11**:283.

Robinson, A. J., Younghusband, H. B., and Bellet, A. J. D., 1973, A circular DNA-protein complex from adenoviruses, *Virology* **56**:54.

Rosen, L., 1958, Hemagglutination of adenoviruses, *Virology* **5**:574.

Rosen, L., 1960, A hemagglutination-inhibition technique for typing adenoviruses, *Am. J. Hyg.* **71**:120.

Rosen, L., Baron, S., and Bell, J. A., 1961, Four newly recognized adenoviruses, *Proc. Soc. Exp. Biol.* **108**:474.

Rosen, L., Havis, J. F., and Bell, J. A., 1962, Further observation on typing adenovirus and a description of two possible additional serotypes, *Proc. Soc. Exp. Biol.* **110**:710.

Rowe, W. P., Huebner, R. J., Gilmore, L. K., Parrott, R. H.. and Ward, T. G., 1953, Isolation of a cytopathogenic agent from human adenoids undergoing spontaneous degeneration in tissue culture, *Proc. Soc. Exp. Biol. Med.* **84**:570.

Rowe, W. P., Hartley, J. W., Roizmann, B., and Levey, H. B., 1958, Characterization of a factor formed in the course of adenovirus infection of tissue cultures causing detachment of cells from glass, *J. Exp. Med.* **108**:713.

Rueckert, R. R., Dunker, A. K., and Stoltzfus, C. M., 1969, The structure of mouse-Elberfeld virus: A model, *Proc. Natl. Acad. Sci. USA* **62**:912.

Russell, W. C., and Skehel, J. J., 1972, The polypeptides of adenovirus-infected cells, *J. Gen. Virol.* **15**:45.

Russell, W. C., Hayashi, K., Sanderson, P. J., Pereira, H. G., 1967a, Adenovirus antigens—A study of their properties and sequential development in infection, *J. Gen. Virol.* **1**:495.

Russell, W. C., Valentine, R. C., and Pereira, H. G., 1967b, The effect of heat on the anatomy of adenovirus, *J. Gen. Virol.* **1**:509.

Russell, W. C., McIntosch, K., and Skehel, J. J., 1971, The preparation and properties of adenovirus cores, *J. Gen. Virol.* **11**:35.

Russell, W. C., Skehel, J. J., Machado, R., and Pereira, H. G., 1972, Phosphorylated polypeptides in adenovirus-infected cells, *Virology* **50**:931.

Schlesinger, R. W., and Strohl, W. A., 1962, Natural and experimental adenovirus infections of cell cultures derived from human adenoids and tonsils, *Bacteriol. Proc.* **71**:146.

Schmidt, N. J., King, C. J., and Lennette, E. H., 1965, Hemagglutination and hemag-glutination-inhibition with adenovirus type 12, *Proc. Soc. Exp. Biol.* **118**:208.

Shapiro, A. L., Vinuela, E., and Maizel, J. V., Jr., 1967, Molecular weight estimation of polypeptide chains by electrophoresis in SDS-polyacrylamide gels, *Biochem. Biophys. Res. Commun.* **28**:815.

Shortridge, K. F., and Biddle, F., 1970, The proteins of adenovirus type 5 (assembly, differences in hexon), *Arch. Ges. Virusforsch.* **29**:1.

Smith, K. O., Geble, W. D., and Trousdale, M. D., 1965a, Architecture of the adenovirus capsid, *J. Bacteriol.* **90**:254.

Smith, K. O., Trousdale, M., and Geble, W., 1965b, Adenovirus antibody agglutination reaction, *J. Immunol.* **95**:810.

Stinski, M. F., and Ginsberg, H. S., 1975, Hexon peptides of type 2, 3, and 5 adenovirus and their relationship to hexon structure, *J. Virol.* **15**:898.

Sundquist, B., Everitt, E., Philipson, L., and Höglund, S., 1973a, Assembly of adenoviruses, *J. Virol.* **11**:449.

Sundquist, B., Pettersson, U., and Philipson, L., 1973b, Structural proteins of adenoviruses. IX. Molecular weight and subunit composition of adenovirus type 2 fiber, *Virology* **51**:252.

Sussenbach, J. S., van der Vleit, P. C., Ellens, D. J., and Jansz, H. S., 1972, Linear intermediates in the replication of adenovirus DNA, *Nature (London) New Biol.* **239**:47.

Tejg-Jensen, B., Furugrin, B., Kindquist, I., and Philipson, L., 1972, A small angle X-ray study of adenovirus type 2 hexon, *Monastsh. Chem.* **103**:1730.

Thomas, D. C., and Green, M., 1966, Biochemical studies on adenovirus multiplication. XI. Evidence of a cytoplasmic site for the synthesis of viral coded proteins, *Proc. Natl. Acad. Sci. USA* **56**:243.

Thomas, D. C., and Green, M., 1969, Biochemical studies on adenovirus multiplication. XV. Transcription of the adenovirus type 2 genome during productive infection, *Virology* **39**:205.

Valentine, R. C., and Pereira, H. G., 1965, Antigens and structure of the adenovirus, *J. Mol. Biol.* **13**:13.

van der Eb, A. J., Kestern, L. W., and von Bruggen, E. F. J., 1969, Structural properties of adenovirus DNA's *Biochim. Biophys. Acta* **182**:530.

van der Vliet, P. C., and Levine, A. J., 1973, DNA-binding proteins specific for cells infected by adenovirus, *Nature (London) New Biol.* **246**:170.

van der Vliet, P. C., Levine, A. J., Ensinger, M. J., and Ginsberg, H. S., 1975, Thermolabile DNA binding proteins from cells infected with a temperature-sensitive mutant of adenovirus defective in viral DNA sensitive, *J. Virol.* **15**:348.

Velicer, L., and Ginsberg, H. S., 1968, Cytoplasmic synthesis of type 5 adenovirus capsid proteins, *Proc. Natl. Acad. Sci. USA* **61**:1264.

Velicer, L. F., and Ginsberg, H. S., 1970, Synthesis, transport, and morphogenesis of type 5 adenovirus capsid proteins, *J. Virol.* **5**:338.

Wadell, G., 1970, Structural and biological properties of capsid components of human adenovirus, Ph.D. thesis, Karolinska Institute, Stockholm.

Wadell, G., and Norrby, E., 1969, Immunological and other biological characteristics of pentons of human adenoviruses, *J. Virol.* **4**:671.

Wadell, G., Norrby, E., and Skaaret, P., 1969, The soluble hemagglutinins of adenoviruses belonging to Rosen's subgroup III. I. The rapidly sedimenting hemagglutinin, *Arch. Ges. Virusforsch.* **26**:32.

Wasmuth, E. H., and Tytell, A. A., 1966, Physical studies with adenovirus hexon antigens, *Life Sci.* **6**:1063.

Wilcox, W. C., and Ginsberg, H. S., 1961, Purification and immunological characterization of types 4 and 5 adenoviruses soluble antigens, *Proc. Natl. Acad. Sci. USA* **47**:512.

Wilcox, W. C., and Ginsberg, H. S., 1963a, Structure of type 5 adenovirus. I. Antigen relationship of virus structural proteins to virus specific soluble antigens from infected cells, *J. Exp. Med.* **118**:295.

Wilcox, W. C., and Ginsberg, H. S., 1963b, Protein synthesis in type 5 adenovirus-infected cells. Effect of *p*-fluorophenylalanine on synthesis of protein, nucleic acids, and infectious virus, *Virology* **20**:269.

Wilcox, W. C., and Ginsberg, H. S., 1963c, Production of specific neutralizing antibody with soluble antigens of type 5 adenovirus, *Proc. Soc. Exp. Biol. Med.* **114**:37.

Wilcox, W. C., Ginbsberg, H. S., and Anderson, T. F., 1963, Structure of type 5 adenovirus. II. Fine structure of virus subunits, Morphological relationship of structural subunits to virus-specific soluble antigens from infected cells, *J. Exp. Med.* **118**:307.

Wilhelm, J. M., and Ginsberg, H. S., 1972, Synthesis *in vitro* of type 5 adenovirus capsid proteins, *J. Virol.* **9**:973.

Williams, J. F., Young, C. S. H., and Austin, P. E., 1974, Genetic analysis of human adenovirus type 5 in permissive and non-permissive cells, *Cold Spring Harbor Symp. Quant. Biol.* **39**:427.

Winters, W. D., Brownstone, A., and Pereira, H. G., 1970, Separation of adenovirus penton base antigen by preparative gel electrophoresis, *J. Gen. Virol.* **9**:105.

Wolfson, J., and Dressler, D., 1972, Adenovirus-2 DNA contains an inverted terminal repetition, *Proc. Natl. Acad. Sci USA* **69**:3054.

Yphantis, D. A., 1964, Equilibrium untracentrifugation of dilute solutions, *Biochemistry* **3**:297.

CHAPTER 7

The Adenovirus-SV40 Hybrid Viruses

Cephas T. Patch and Arthur S. Levine

Section on Infectious Disease
Pediatric Oncology Branch
National Cancer Institute
National Institutes of Health
Bethesda, Maryland 20014

and

Andrew M. Lewis, Jr.

Laboratory of Viral Diseases
National Institute of Allergy and Infectious Diseases
National Institutes of Health
Bethesda, Maryland 20014

1. INTRODUCTION

The adenovirus–simian virus 40 (Ad-SV40) hybrid viruses are stable viral recombinants which form in monkey kidney cells (MKC) coinfected with the simian papovavirus SV40 and a number of human adenovirus serotypes. The genomes of these viruses are composed mainly of Ad DNA (integrated with varying amounts of SV40 DNA) and are enclosed in capsids whose morphological and immunological properties are indistinguishable from those of the parent nonhybrid adenovirus. Studies of the Ad-SV40 hybrid viruses have made important contributions to a number of areas of molecular virology;

previous reviews of these studies include those by Rapp (1973) and Lewis (1977).

Ironically the study of Ad-SV40 hybrid viruses began before the discovery of SV40 itself. Hartley *et al.* (1956) "adapted" seven adenovirus serotypes (Ad1–Ad7) to replicate in rhesus MKC. The MKC-adapted adenoviruses were used for vaccine production. After the identification of SV40 as a common contaminant of rhesus MKC (Sweet and Hilleman, 1960) it was found that the human Ad strains adapted to grow in MKC all contained infectious SV40. O'Conor *et al.* (1963) showed that human Ad12 infection in SV40-free MKC was abortive but that large quantities of Ad12 particles could be detected when the same cells were coinfected with Ad12 and SV40. The function of SV40 in promoting Ad replication in MKC is called "enhancement." It has been a fundamental postulate in the study of the Ad-SV40 hybrid viruses that the SV40 DNA integrated in the hybrid genomes of those viruses capable of propagating in MKC must contain the SV40 enhancing function. However, a few hybrid viruses have been recognized that appear to have undergone further genetic modification, resulting in the loss of the ability to propagate in MKC while retaining integrated SV40 DNA.

The first of the MKC-adapted Ad strains to be studied extensively was Ad7LL; it was soon recognized that this strain contained Ad-encapsidated SV40 genetic information (Huebner *et al.*, 1964). Subsequently numerous Ad-SV40 hybrid viruses have been identified and studied. While these viruses have different properties with respect to both Ad and SV40 functions, they all have SV40 DNA integrated within the Ad genomes.

There are two general classes of Ad-SV40 hybrid viruses: defective and nondefective. When recombination occurs between Ad and SV40 DNAs, parts of one or both genomes may be deleted. In many cases the DNA deleted from the Ad genome plays an essential role in replication; its loss leaves the virus defective or incapable of replication unless the missing functions are provided by coinfection with a "helper" virus. If, however, DNA is deleted from a nonessential part of the Ad genome, the recombinant is nondefective and capable of independent replication. The genomes of some defective hybrid viruses contain one or more complete SV40 genomes. During infection with one of these viruses an intact SV40 genome may be excised from the hybrid DNA and undergo independent replication, giving rise to infectious SV40.

Thus the hybrid genomes are recombinants of Ad and SV40 DNAs that are composed predominantly of Ad DNA (necessary for packaging in Ad capsids), and at least that portion of the SV40 genome that provides the SV40 enhancing function (necessary for propagation in MKC). (See Section 6.1 for one exception.) The Ad portion of the hybrid genome is always incomplete although not always defective, while the SV40 portion ranges from small fragments to multiple copies of the entire SV40 genome.

The Ad-SV40 hybrid viruses are of interest since they are examples of artificially selected recombinants formed from two different classes of animal viruses. The effect of the recombination, which provides the means of selection, is to extend the host range of human adenovirus to include monkey cells. Moreover, some of these hybrid viruses are capable of propagating and expressing SV40 functions in human cells, which are only semipermissive for the highly oncogenic SV40.

The Ad-SV40 hybrid viruses have been useful in elucidating the relationship between structure and function of both Ad and SV40. Some of the defective hybrid viruses, those that give rise to infectious SV40, may provide models for the process by which small viral genomes are integrated with (and excised from) the DNAs of larger host chromosomes. The nondefective hybrids, which may be regarded as deletion mutants of SV40, have been valuable in the study of the gene products of the oncogenic region of the SV40 genome.

2. SV40 AND THE ADENOVIRUSES

Although this chapter is mainly concerned with the Ad-SV40 hybrid viruses, understanding of the properties of the parent nonhybrid viruses is essential to understanding the properties of the hybrid viruses themselves. Accordingly, this chapter will begin with a brief description of SV40, the adenoviruses, and their interactions with each other.

2.1. SV40

SV40 is a simian papovavirus first isolated from rhesus and cynomolgus monkey kidney tissue by Sweet and Hilleman (1960). SV40 produces no cytopathogenic effects in cultured rhesus monkey (*Macaca mulatta*) tissue; however, it propagates and causes extensive cytopathogenicity in cultured African green monkey (*Ceropithecus aethiops*) tissue. The pathogenicity of SV40 in its natural host is uncertain; however, SV40 has recently been isolated from degenerative lesions found in rhesus monkey brains, which resemble lesions seen in progressive multifocal leukoencephalopathy in humans (Holmberg *et al.*, 1977).

SV40 propagates efficiently in primary African green monkey kidney (AGMK) cells as well as in established lines of AGMK cells such as Vero, BSC-1, and CV-1, but human cells are only semipermissive for this virus. SV40 is highly oncogenic for hamsters (*Mesocricetus auratus*) and mastomys (*Rattus natalensis*) and can transform cells from a number of species, including human and simian, in tissue culture. The particle size of SV40 virions is about 17×10^6 daltons. The SV40 genome is a circular duplex DNA molecule with a superhelical configuration and has a molecular weight of about 3.2×10^6. A nucleotide sequence map of the entire SV40 genome (5226 nucleotide pairs) has recently been published (Reddy *et al.*, 1978; Fiers *et al.*, 1978). Other properties of SV40 are summarized in Table 1. The study of SV40 is one of the most active areas in molecular virology, and these studies have been discussed in a number of excellent reviews (Tooze, 1973; Salzman and Khoury, 1974; Levine, 1976; Kelly and Nathans, 1977; Sambrook, 1978).

2.2. The Adenoviruses

The adenoviruses are a large group of viruses that cause respiratory disease in a wide variety of natural hosts including humans and simians. Thirty-three serotypes of human adenoviruses have been identified (Beladi, 1972). In addition to sharing common antigenic determinants, the human adenoviruses are closely related in size and morphology.

In general the adenoviruses are species specific, in that they replicate efficiently only in cells derived from their natural hosts. The human serotypes grow well in human cells such as human embryonic kidney (HEK) cells and in established lines of human cells such as HeLa, KB, and WI38. However, primary monkey cells and established monkey cell lines such as CV-1 and BSC-1 are only semipermissive for human adenoviruses. For unknown reasons Vero, another continuous line of MKC, is permissive for human Ad propagation (Henry *et al.*, 1971; Eron *et al.*, 1975).

The human adenoviruses have been arranged into three groups according to their oncogenic potential in newborn hamsters: Ad12,

TABLE 1

Some Properties of SV40 and Several Adenoviruses and of Their DNAs

Virus[a]	Response of various cell types to viral challenge in vitro[b] lytic infection/transformation [$\log_{10}$(virions/pfu)/$\log_{10}$(pfu/ffu)]					Susceptibility of various animals to tumor induction[c] (% tumor incidence)			Properties of viral DNA[d]		
	Human	Monkey	Hamster	Mouse	Rat	Hamster	Mouse	Mastomys (Rattus natalensis)	Density (g/cm³)	G+C (%)	Length (µm)
SV40	SP/5	2–2.3/T	NP/7.2	NP/3	NP/T	25–100	NO	75–83	1.701	41	1.65
SV40(L)				NP/5.3		53					
SV40(S)				NP/3.7		60					
SV40(M)				NP/3.0		25					
Ad2	1.5/NT	SP/NT	SP/7.5	NP	NP/7.6	NO	NO	NO	1.716	57	12.6
Ad7	1.6/NT	SP/NT	NP/7.6	NP	NP/6.9	4–8			1.713	54	11.8
Ad12	2.5/?	SP/NT	NP/6.6	NP/T	NP/6.0	55–94	31–70	30	1.708	49	11.0

[a] SV40(L), SV40(S), and SV40(M) are large-plaque, small-plaque, and minute-plaque strains of SV40, respectively.

[b] The numerator indicates permissivity to lytic infection (SP, semipermissive; NP, nonpermissive). The numbers are the amount of virus ($\log_{10}$ number of virion particles) required to initiate a plaque (pfu) in permissive cells. The denominator indicates whether cells are transformed (T) or not transformed (NT). Where quantitative transformation data are available, they are presented as $\log_{10}$ of the number of pfu required to initiate a focus of transformed cells (ffu). References for SV40 data are Todaro et al. (1966), Black et al. (1964), A. M. Lewis, Jr. (unpublished), Black (1968), and Todaro and Takemoto (1969). References for Ad data are Green et al. (1967a), A. M. Lewis, Jr. (unpublished), and Casto (1973). Ad12 has been reported to transform human diploid cells in vitro (Sultanian and Freeman, 1966; Todaro and Aaronson, 1968); however, the significance of these results is uncertain.

[c] The data indicate the percentage of inoculated animals that develop tumors at the site of inoculation (NO, nononcogenic). References for SV40 data are Eddy et al. (1962), Girardi et al. (1962), Rabson et al. (1962), and Takemoto et al. (1966). References for Ad data are Gross (1970) and Huebner et al. (1963).

[d] The references for these data are Crawford and Black (1964), Piña and Green (1965), and Green et al. (1967b). The molecular weight of DNA is approximately $1.92 \times 10^6/\mu m$.

Ad18, and Ad31 are considered to be highly oncogenic; Ad3, Ad7, Ad11, Ad14, Ad16, and Ad21 are considered to be weakly oncogenic; the remaining Ad serotypes are nononcogenic in animals but may transform cells in tissue culture (Huebner, 1967). The particle size of Ad virions is about 175×10^6 daltons. The genomes of all the adenoviruses are linear duplex DNA molecules having molecular weights in the range $20–25 \times 10^6$. Other properties of some of the human adenoviruses are summarized in Table 1. Like SV40, the adenoviruses have been extensively studied, and several reviews of the biology and biochemistry of these viruses have been published (Tooze, 1973; Philipson and Lindberg, 1974; Levine, 1976; Flint, 1977; Wold et al., 1978; see also the preceding chapter in this volume).

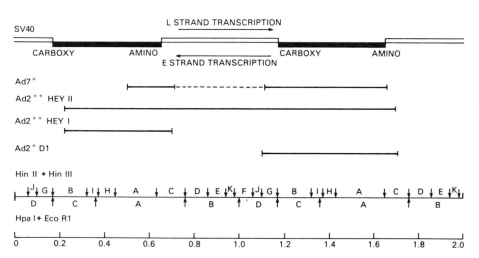

Fig. 1. Two SV40 genomes in tandem array with the origin at the *Eco*R1 cleavage site: early templates (━━) and late templates (▭) (Khoury et al., 1974, 1975). The arrows (→) indicate the direction of RNA transcription. The template regions for the amino end and the carboxy end of the early SV40 proteins are indicated. In the middle of A and B are shown the SV40 segments of several Ad-SV40 hybrid viruses: SV40 DNA (├———┤), deletions of SV40 DNA (---), and a segment of Ad DNA integrated within the SV40 segment of Ad2⁺ND₁dp2 (⏐···⏐). At the bottom of A are shown endonuclease cleavage sites (↓) for *Hin*II + *Hin*III (upper) (Danna et al., 1973) and *Eco*R1 + *Hpa*I (lower) (Sambrook et al., 1975).

A: The SV40 DNA integrated in Ad7⁺ (Kelly, 1975), Ad2⁺⁺HEY (Kelly et al., 1974), and Ad2⁺D1 (Hassell et al., 1978). The SV40 genome is depicted with the origin on the left and the early template (E strand) oriented down. The SV40 E strand is integrated in the "l" strand of Ad2⁺⁺HEY and Ad2⁺⁺D1 (Fig. 2). The strand orientation of Ad7⁺ is unknown (Section 4.3).

2.3. SV40 and Adenovirus Transcription during Lytic Infection

The lytic cycle of both SV40 and the adenoviruses occurs in two phases. The period between virus adsorption and the onset of viral DNA synthesis is called the "early phase." The "late phase" continues from the initiation of viral DNA synthesis through virus maturation.

During the early phase of SV40 and Ad infection only the early templates of the viral genomes (Figs. 1 and 2) are transcribed into mRNA. Late in infection the rate of RNA synthesis is greatly increased, and both strands of viral DNA (both SV40 and Ad) appear to be completely transcribed. The newly transcribed viral RNA which accumulates in the nucleus contains sequences transcribed from non-template DNA as well as from the early and late structural genes (Figs. 1 and 2). However, before translocation of the structural gene mRNAs into the cytoplasm for translation into polypeptides, processing occurs during which nontemplate RNA is removed, polyadenylic acid [poly(A)] sequences are attached to the 3′ ends, and the 5′ ends are "capped" with an undecanucleotide (Lavi and Shatkin, 1975; Klessig, 1977*b*). Evidence indicates that portions of the cytoplasmic mRNAs

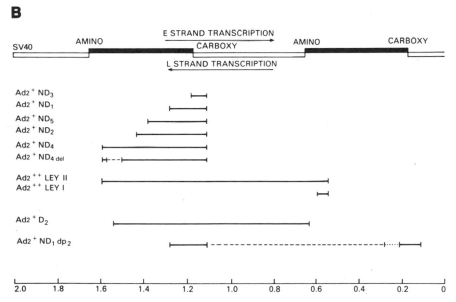

B: The SV40 DNA integrated in the nondefective Ad2-SV40 hybrid viruses (Kelly and Lewis, 1973), Ad2++LEY (Kelly *et al.*, 1974), Ad2+D2 (Hassell *et al.*, 1978), and Ad2+ND₁dp2 (Fey *et al.*, 1979). The SV40 genome is depicted with the origin on the right and with the early template (E strand) oriented up. In these hybrid genomes the SV40 E strand is integrated in the hybrid "r" strand (Fig. 2).

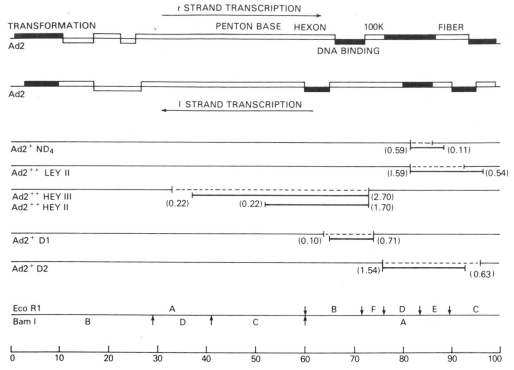

Fig. 2. Two transcription template maps of the Ad2 genome: upper (Pettersson *et al.*, 1976) and lower (Sharp *et al.*, 1974). The origins of both maps are at the G+C-rich end of the Ad2 molecule. In both maps the "r" strand (rightward transcription) templates are shown above the median and the "l" strand (leftward transcription) templates are shown below the median (Flint, 1977): early templates (████) and late templates (▭). The arrows (→) indicate the direction of RNA transcription. The genes for several Ad2 proteins are indicated (Flint, 1977). In the middle are shown the genomes of several Ad-SV40 hybrid viruses: Ad DNA (├───┤), deletions of Ad DNA (---), and integrated SV40 DNA (├───┤). The numbers in parentheses indicate the coordinates of the integrated SV40 segments (Fig. 1). The references for the hybrid genome structures are: Ad2+ND₄, Kelly and Lewis (1973); Ad2++HEY and Ad2++LEY, Kelly *et al.* (1974); and Ad2+D1 and Ad2+D2, Hassell *et al.* (1978). At the bottom are shown endonuclease cleavage sites (↓) for *Eco*R1 (upper) (Mulder *et al.*, 1973) and *Bam*1 (lower) (Sambrook *et al.*, 1975).

(the leader sequences on the 5′ ends) do not encode information directly translatable into functional polypeptides (Sambrook, 1977).

2.3.1. SV40 Transcription

The early phase of productive SV40 infection continues for 16–20 hr after virus adsorption. During this period the virus penetrates to the nucleus where uncoating occurs at 1–4 hr post infection (PI) (Hummeler *et al.*, 1970), and the early (E) strand of the viral genome is transcribed and translated (Fig. 1). At least two early SV40 proteins have been identified: a large protein having a molecular weight of 90,000–100,000 (90–100K) and a small protein having a molecular weight of 17–20K (Prives *et al.*, 1977). The large early SV40 protein is essential for both viral propagation and transformation. The function of the smaller protein has not yet been established, although there is evidence that it may play a role in SV40 transformation (Crawford *et al.*, 1978). Both early SV40 proteins are immunoprecipitable with serum from hamsters bearing SV40 tumors. The early SV40 protein(s) function to initiate both viral and host DNA synthesis but are not required for chain elongation (Martin *et al.*, 1974).

The late phase of SV40 infection begins at about 20 hr PI with the onset of viral DNA synthesis and continues through virus maturation. During the late phase the late (L) strand of the SV40 genome is transcribed and the viral capsid proteins are synthesized; transcription of the E strand as well as the L strand continues in the late phase.

2.3.2. Adenovirus Transcription

In adenovirus-infected cells the transcription pattern is more complex and events move more rapidly than in SV40-infected cells. During the early phase, four noncontiguous templates (two on each strand) are transcribed and five or six polypeptides accumulate (Lewis *et al.*, 1976) (Fig. 2). At about 8 hr PI viral DNA synthesis begins; the late templates are transcribed into mRNA, and viral capsid proteins are synthesized. RNA transcription is maximal at 18 hr and synthesis of most RNA sequences increases during the late phase. Virus replication continues for about 24–48 hr PI.

2.4. Viral Transcription in Cells Transformed by SV40 or the Adenoviruses

In cells transformed by SV40 the entire early viral template (Fig. 1) is transcribed and translated into SV40 proteins which are required for initiation and maintenance of transformation; there is little or no transcription of the late viral templates, although these are usually present in the integrated viral DNA.

Viral transcription in several rat cell lines transformed by Ad2 also appears to be limited to the early templates of the integrated viral genomes, although the late templates may be present in the integrated viral DNA (Flint and Sharp, 1976). Moreover, it has been demonstrated that rat cells can be transformed in tissue culture by endonuclease cleavage fragments of Ad2 and Ad5 DNA which comprise only the left ends, i.e., 5–7% of the viral genomes (Graham *et al.*, 1974*a,b*) (Fig. 2). Thus it appears that expression of the early gene on the left end of the Ad genome (Fig. 2) is necessary and sufficient for transformation by some and perhaps all adenoviruses.

2.5. Interactions between SV40 and the Adenoviruses during Lytic Infection

Human Ad will not propagate efficiently in primary MKC unless the cells are coinfected with an enhancing or helper monkey virus such as SV40. The simian adenoviruses SV7 and SV15 also enhance human Ad replication in MKC, but neither herpes simplex nor measles virus, which are human viruses capable of replication in MKC, enhances human Ad replication in MKC (Feldman *et al.*, 1966; Naegle and Rapp, 1967; Altstein and Dodonova, 1968). Enhancement of Ad replication by SV40 has been studied extensively and will be discussed in more detail below (Sections 3–3.4).

O'Conor *et al.* (1963) observed that when MKC were dually infected with SV40 and Ad12 the number of cells containing Ad particles increased compared to cells infected with Ad12 alone. In this study it was also observed that the number of cells containing SV40 particles decreased compared to cells infected with SV40 alone. These observations indicated not only that SV40 enhanced Ad propagation in dually infected MKC but also that Ad12 inhibited SV40 propagation in the same cells.

One of the early functions of SV40 is the induction of host DNA synthesis. In contrast, host DNA synthesis in Ad-infected cells is inhibited. The mechanism by which Ad inhibits host DNA synthesis is not entirely clear. Levine and Ginsberg (1967, 1968) showed that two late Ad5 capsid proteins, fiber and hexon, inhibit DNA polymerase from KB cells and that fiber but not hexon inhibits replication of Ad5 in the same cells. However, temperature-sensitive mutants of Ad5 inhibit host DNA synthesis at nonpermissive temperatures, although they induce no detectable capsid proteins under these conditions (Wilkie *et al.*, 1973). Friedman *et al.* (1970) showed that synthesis of SV40 DNA was reduced but not completely inhibited by coinfection with Ad2 in AGMK cells; the effectiveness of inhibition increased with increasing multiplicity of Ad infection. More recently it has been demonstrated that superinfection with Ad2 completely inhibits super-helical SV40 DNA synthesis in SV40-infected BSC-1 cells (Van Roy and Fiers, 1978; C. Patch and P. Howley, unpublished). In these experiments SV40 DNA synthesis was not affected before the onset of Ad2 DNA synthesis. However, SV40 DNA synthesis was significantly reduced at 17 hr after superinfection with Ad2 and undetectable in alkaline sucrose gradients at 21 hr.

3. SV40 ENHANCEMENT OF ADENOVIRUS REPLICATION IN MONKEY CELLS

Human adenoviruses propagate poorly in MKC; the yield of virus progeny in SV40-free MKC is only 0.1% of that obtained from human cells (O'Conor *et al.*, 1963, 1965; Rabson *et al.*, 1964; Beardmore *et al.*, 1965; Malmgren *et al.*, 1966). However, when MKC are coinfected with SV40 and Ad, the yield of Ad is comparable to that obtained from human cells (Fig. 3). Initial studies of abortive infection of MKC by Ad

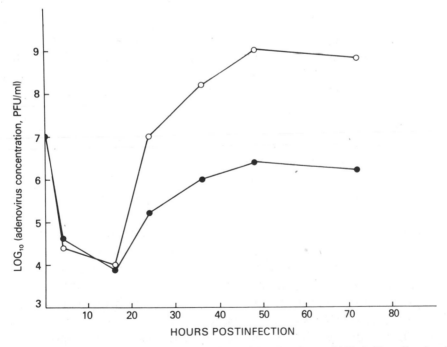

Fig. 3. Growth curves for unenhanced (●) and SV40-enhanced (○) Ad2 replication in AGMK cells; the multiplicity of infection for both Ad2 and SV40 was 30 pfu/ml. The data for Fig. 3 were taken from Friedman *et al.* (1970).

indicated that the cells undergo changes typical of Ad-infected human cells: virus particles are adsorbed and penetrate into the cells; infected cells exhibit typical Ad cytopathic effects; Ad T antigens form in most cells; but virus particles are detected in less than 1% of the infected cells (Rabson *et al.*, 1964; Beardmore *et al.*, 1965).

3.1. Adenovirus DNA and RNA Synthesis in Unenhanced and SV40-Enhanced MKC

Reich *et al.* (1966) showed that Ad7 DNA synthesis in unenhanced infection was at least 50% of that in SV40-enhanced infection. Similar results have been reported by Rapp *et al* (1966), Friedman *et al.* (1970), and Hashimoto *et al.* (1973). Since a 50% reduction in DNA synthesis would not account for a thousandfold reduction in viral propagation, these workers concluded that the block in Ad replication is manifested subsequent to viral DNA replication.

Baum *et al.* (1968) found that about half as much Ad7 RNA accumulated in MKC infected with Ad7 alone as was found in cells coinfected with SV40. Fox and Baum (1972) and Lucas and Ginsberg (1972) used hybridization competition to compare RNA prepared from enhanced and unenhanced Ad-infected MKC. These studies indicated that late in infection the Ad RNAs found in unenhanced and SV40-enhanced MKC are qualitatively indistinguishable, indicating that the enhancing effect of SV40 functions at a posttranscriptional stage.

3.2. Adenovirus Protein Synthesis in Unenhanced and SV40-Enhanced MKC

One of the initial observations in the study of abortive infection of Ad in MKC was the absence of detectable capsid antigens late in infection (O'Conor *et al.*, 1963). Baum *et al.* (1972) compared electropherograms of proteins extracted from enhanced and unenhanced Ad2-infected MKC and showed that capsid protein synthesis was deficient in unenhanced cells. Using immunoprecipitation, Lucas and Ginsberg (1972) demonstrated that the amount of Ad2 capsid protein synthesized in unenhanced MKC was only 10% of that found in SV40-enhanced cells. Thus while Ad DNA and RNA synthesis is nearly normal in unenhanced cells, late protein synthesis is greatly reduced. Henry *et al.* (1971) showed that not only is capsid protein synthesis reduced in unenhanced cells but also transport of capsid protein from the cytoplasm (where synthesis occurs) into the nucleus (where virus assembly takes place) is reduced. Fox and Baum (1974) showed that while late Ad7 mRNA is synthesized, polyadenylated, and transported to the cytoplasm in unenhanced cells, this RNA is defective in the formation of polyribosomes. Nakajima *et al.* (1974) found that an extract (high salt) of SV40-transformed MKC promoted the binding of Ad2 mRNA to ribosomes from nonpermissive cells. However, the authors note that the binding factor could be of host origin since Ad2 infection proceeds normally when unenhanced MKC are infected at high multiplicity. The observation that host restriction of Ad replication in MKC is abrogated by infection at high multiplicity has been reported by other workers (Friedman *et al.*, 1970; Eron *et al.*, 1975). Hashimoto *et al.* (1973) compared Ad replication in MKC transformed by SV40 (which express early SV40 functions) with Ad replication in untransformed MKC. By examining electropherograms of proteins synthesized in transformed (enhanced) and untransformed (unenhanced) MKC, they found that the Ad capsid proteins hexon, penton, and fiber were missing in unenhanced cells. They also showed that unenhanced cells were deficient in polyribosomes corresponding to mRNAs greater than 20 S (including the 24 S hexon mRNA), which are readily detected in enhanced cells. These authors concluded that while all Ad mRNAs are present in unenhanced cells, some (those encoding capsid proteins) do not form protein synthesizing complexes. Eron *et al.* (1975) compared electropherograms of *in vitro* (cell-free) synthesized proteins using mRNAs from unenhanced and SV40-enhanced MKC and found no difference between the mRNAs in their ability to direct the synthesis of Ad capsid proteins. On the other hand, Klessig and Anderson (1975) also using protein electrophoresis, compared *in vivo* protein synthesis in enhanced and unenhanced cells as well as *in vitro* translation of the corresponding mRNAs; they found that unenhanced late protein synthesis was defective in both systems. Although most late proteins were synthesized in unenhanced cells, fiber and 11.5K protein were not detected and several others were synthesized in significantly reduced amounts.

Klessig and Anderson (1975) studied viral RNA synthesis in enhanced and unenhanced cells using fragments of Ad2 DNA prepared by *Eco*R1 restriction endonuclease cleavage (Fig. 2). They found that while all Ad2 DNA fragments could be saturated with both enhanced and unenhanced cytoplasmic RNA the *Eco*R1 fragment, which contains the template for fiber protein (Fig. 2) (Mautner *et al.*, 1975), required 7 times more unenhanced RNA to achieve saturation than was required when using enhanced RNA. They concluded that the block to Ad replication in MKC is at least partially due to RNA metabolism and suggest that unenhanced RNA is degraded by a ribosome-associated nuclease (Nakajima *et al.*, 1974).

3.3. Enhancement: An Early SV40 Function

Compared to simultaneous coinfection, the rate of enhancement of Ad2 replication by SV40 in MKC is increased if the cells are preinfected with SV40 16 hr prior to Ad2 infection (Friedman *et al.*, 1970). Cycloheximide (an inhibitor of protein synthesis), added during the preinfection period, had the effect of nullifying the preinfection stimulus; FUdR added during the preinfection period was without effect. These results indicated that SV40 enhancement of Ad2 replication required early SV40 protein synthesis.

Apart from the work of Friedman *et al.* (1970) and the observation that SV40-transformed MKC (which express only early SV40 functions) are permissive for Ad infection, the best direct evidence that enhancement is an early SV40 function comes from studies with the Ad-SV40 hybrid viruses, which will be considered in detail in Section 12.2, and from studies with temperature-sensitive (*ts*) SV40 mutants.

Kimura (1974) observed that while several late SV40 *ts* mutants enhanced Ad replication at nonpermissive temperatures, one mutant, defective in the early SV40 region, did not. This mutant not only lacked the SV40 enhancing function but also failed to transform rat cells or initiate SV40 DNA synthesis in MKC at nonpermissive temperatures. On the other hand, Jerkofsky and Rapp (1973) and Jerkofsky (1975) studied a number of early and late *ts* mutants described by Martin *et al.* (1974) and found that only SV40 *tsD* mutants, which apparently fail to uncoat, did not enhance. The early *tsA* mutants of this series, which induce SV40 T antigen but fail to initiate transformation or viral DNA synthesis, all enhanced Ad propagation in MKC at nonpermissive temperatures.

3.4. Summary of SV40 Enhancement of Adenovirus Replication in MKC

The weight of evidence indicates that the primary restriction to Ad replication in MKC is due to the inability of certain late mRNAs to form functional polyribosomes capable of protein synthesis. Klessig and Anderson (1975) suggest that if mRNAs fail to enter protein-synthesizing complexes quickly enough they are vulnerable to nuclease degradation. Without nuclease degradation, mRNAs might enter protein-synthesizing complexes more slowly in unenhanced cells, but still direct capsid protein synthesis. Noting that Vero cells (a continuous line of MKC) are both deficient in interferon production (Desmyter et al., 1968) and permissive for Ad production, Klessig and Anderson (1975) suggest that the nuclease may be induced by interferon. The antiviral action of interferon, like the block in Ad progapation in unenhanced MKC, is directed against translation of viral mRNA (Friedman et al., 1972; Yakobson et al., 1977). However, synthesis of SV40 tumor antigen (Tag), which provides the enhancing function, is much more sensitive to human interferon (in pretreated cells) than is Ad Tag synthesis (Oxman et al., 1967; Oxman and Levin, 1971).

Although there are objections to the notion that interferon is responsible for host restriction of Ad replication in MKC, the fact that Vero cells are permissive for Ad does indicate that the block is sensitive to differences between cell types of the same host species. It has been demonstrated that pretreatment of primary MKC with IUdR permits efficient Ad replication, indicating that host restriction mechanisms are not necessarily virus-specific (Jerkofsky and Rapp, 1975; Staal and Rowe, 1975). It is possible that both Vero permissiveness and IUdR enhancement are due to cryptic viruses, such as the recently reported HD virus present in some Vero lines (Waldeck and Sauer, 1977), although the HD virus has not been shown to enhance Ad propgation. The efficiency of Ad propagation in MKC increases with the multiplicity of infection (MOI) (Friedman et al., 1970). Eron et al. (1975), using Ad2-infected MKC, showed that when the MOI was increased from 5 to 75 the rate of hexon synthesis increased fortyfold to nearly the same level as in SV40-enhanced infection. Finally, variants of Ad2 that replicate with equal efficiency in human and monkey cells have been isolated (Klessig, 1977a; A. M. Lewis, Jr., unpublished).

Nakajima and Oda (1975) showed that SV40 enhancement of Ad translation is mediated by alteration of ribosomes. Segawa et al. (1977) suggest that phosphorylation of ribosome-associated factors, which are essential for initiation of protein synthesis, may play a role in the selection of mRNAs for translation. Such a mechanism might be sensitive to differences in both viral and host functions.

Although the available data do not permit a complete understanding of the role of early SV40 proteins in unblocking late Ad translation in MKC, the fact remains that early SV40 function(s) act to extend the host range of human Ad to include monkey cells. When the appropriate region of the early SV40 genome is incorporated into Ad DNA by recombination, the recombinants are capable of supporting Ad replication in MKC in the absence of infectious SV40.

3.5.   SV40 Complementation of Adenovirus 5 Temperature-Sensitive Mutants

The temperature-sensitive mutant Ad5 *ts125* has a defective DNA binding protein and viral DNA synthesis is blocked at nonpermissive temperatures. Ad5 *ts125* is complemented by SV40 in MKC at nonpermissive temperatures, indicating that the early SV40 protein(s) can promote Ad DNA synthesis as well as provide the enhancing function (Levine *et al.*, 1974). Williams *et al.* (1974) have reported that other Ad5 *ts* mutants which are defective in hexon transport are also complemented in MKC by SV40. Thus it would appear that SV40 gene products can replace Ad gene products in a number of early viral functions essential for Ad propagation in MKC.

4.   DISCOVERY OF THE ADENOVIRUS 7–SV40 HYBRID VIRUS

The first Ad-SV40 hybrid virus to be recognized was an Ad7-SV40 hybrid virus (Huebner *et al.*, 1964). Ad7 strain LL was one of the original seven human Ad serotypes adapted to propagate in MKC (Hartley *et al.*, 1956). This virus had been carried in rhesus MKC for 22 consecutive passages when it was found to be contaminated with SV40. After two passages in AGMK in the presence of anti-SV40 rabbit serum, the virus was shown to be free of infectious SV40. Although it continued to grow well in MKC it remained free of SV40 through several passages without anti-SV40 serum. In the twenty-eighth passage, a large pool of this SV40-free, MKC-adapted Ad7LL was prepared and designated E46 (Huebner *et al.*, 1964).

Ad7 is weakly oncogenic and induces tumors in hamsters. Huebner *et al.* (1964) showed that hamsters bearing tumors induced by Ad7-SV40 developed antibodies against SV40 Tag. Moreover, they noted that tumor induction by Ad7-SV40 was completely inhibited by anti-Ad7 serum but not by anti-SV40 serum, indicating that the tumorigenic action of Ad7-SV40 was mediated by virions with Ad7 capsids (Section 13.1). Rowe and Baum (1964) and Rapp *et al.* (1964) showed that Ad7-SV40 could induce SV40 Tag in both monkey and human cells in tissue culture. The kinetics of SV40 Tag formation in Ad7-SV40-infected MKC are about the same as in SV40-infected MKC; however, SV40 Tag induction was inhibited by anti-Ad7 serum but not by anti-SV40 serum. These authors concluded that SV40 genetic information was encapsidated in Ad7 virions. The SV40 Tag induced by Ad7-SV40, like that induced by SV40, is usually localized in cell nuclei; however, variants of this hybrid induce cytoplasmic Tag (Butel *et al.*, 1969). In addition to Tag, SV40 tumor-specific transplantation antigen (TSTag), another early SV40 antigen, is induced by Ad7-SV40 (Rapp *et al.*, 1966*b*).

4.1. The Adenovirus 7–SV40 Population: A Mixture of Nonhybrid Adenovirus 7 and Defective Adenovirus 7–SV40 Hybrid Virus

Rowe and Baum (1964) found that high dilutions of E46 in HEK cells yielded an Ad7 virus population that did not induce SV40 Tag in HEK and grew poorly in MKC. In contrast, high dilutions of E46 in MKC always induced SV40 Tag. They concluded that the E46 viral population, which they designated "E46$^+$" (the plus sign indicates the presence of SV40 genetic information), was composed of two subpopulations. One subpopulation contained SV40 genetic material enclosed in Ad7 capsids and the second subpopulation, designated E46$^-$, was free of detectable SV40 genetic information. In this chapter the Ad7-SV40 hybrid virus population (including the E46$^+$ pool) will be designated "Ad7$^+$" to be consistent with the designations for other hybrid virus populations (Table 2). Rowe and Baum (1965) attempted to plaque-purify the hybrid virion in Ad7$^+$. Although they failed to isolate a pure (single-component) population of Ad7-SV40 hybrid virus, they were able to show that the hybrid virus component in the Ad7$^+$ population was defective and required nonhybrid Ad7 for replication.

In a plaque assay it is assumed that a single nondefective virus particle is capable of initiating a focus of infection or plaque (Dulbecco, 1952). On the other hand, two viruses which are individually defective for a given host may complement each other to produce a plaque only if a single cell is infected by at least one of each kind of virus (Boeyé *et al.*, 1966). Thus, for a series of dilutions in a plaque assay, the concentration(s) of the viral component(s) is proportional to the dilution. The relationship between the number of plaques (P) obtained at a

TABLE 2

Plaque Formation and SV40 Antigen Induction by the Adenovirus–SV40 Hybrid Viruses

Ad-SV40 hybrid virus[a]	Concentration dependence of plaque formation in monkey cells[b]		Induction of SV40 antigens in monkey cells[c]			
	Ad plaques	SV40 plaques	Tag	Uag	TSTag	Vag
Ad1[++]	2	+	+			
Ad2[++]	2	1	+			+
Ad2[++]HEY	2	1	+	+	+	+
Ad2[++]LEY	2	+	+	+	+	−
Ad2[+]ND$_1$	1	−	−	+	+	−
Ad2[+]ND$_1$dp2	1	−	−	?		−
Ad2[+]ND$_2$	1	−	−	+	+	−
Ad2[+]ND$_3$	1	−	−	−	−	−
Ad2[+]ND$_4$	1	−	+	+	+	−
Ad2[+]ND$_5$	1	−	−	−	−	−
Ad2[+]D1	2	−	+			
Ad2[+]D2	2	−	+			
Ad3[+]	+	−	+			
Ad4[++]	+	+	+			
Ad5[++]	2	1	+			
Ad7[+]	2	−	+		+	−
Ad12[++]	2	1	+			

[a] The double plus symbol ([++]) indicates that the hybrid virus population induces infectious SV40 in MKC. The single plus symbol ([+]) indicates that the hybrid virus population induces SV40 antigens but does not induce infectious SV40. Some defective Ad-SV40 hybrid virus populations having the same designation have different origins [e.g., Ad12[++] (Schell) and Ad12[++] (Lewis), Section 6]. Since these hybrids may have different properties, original sources should be consulted when comparing one hybrid population with another.

[b] All hybrid virus populations induce Ad plaques in human cells with a first-order concentration dependence; however, Ad plaque formation in monkey cells may be first order (1) or second order (2) (Section 4.1). Some hybrid virus populations induce SV40 plaques in MKC (+) and some do not (−).

[c] All hybrid virus populations induce Ad Tag and Vag; however, hybrid virus populations may (+) or may not (−) induce SV40 antigens. References for all data are in the text.

particular dilution (D) may be expressed as $P/P_{max} = (D_{min}/D)^{-n}$, where P_{max} is the maximum number of plaques obtained at the minimum dilution (D_{min}). The exponent n is the number of viral components that must interact to initiate a focus of infection. For non-defective viruses (e.g., SV40 in MKC or Ad2 in HEK) the value of n is 1. However, for Ad7[+] in MKC the value of n was found to be approximately 2 (Rowe and Baum, 1965; Boeyé et al., 1966) (Table 3 and Fig. 4). This result indicated that plaque formation by the Ad7[+] population in MKC required the interaction of two viral components. It was known that nonhybrid Ad7 was defective in MKC and it therefore followed that the Ad7-SV40 hybrid in the Ad7$^+$ population was defective for Ad function. However, the two viral components in Ad7$^+$ complemented each other in MKC, leading to propagation of both. On the other hand, induction of SV40 Tag by Ad7$^+$ in HEK or MKC showed a one-component dilution dependence, indicating that expression of SV40 genetic information required only that a single cell be infected by an Ad7-SV40 hybrid virus (Rowe and Baum, 1966). Some of the biological properties of Ad7$^+$ and the other Ad-SV40 hybrid viruses are shown in Table 2.

4.2. The Physical Structure of the Adenovirus 7–SV40 Hybrid Genome

Since the Ad7-SV40 hybrid virus is defective, it could not be isolated in pure culture. Attempts were made to separate Ad7-SV40 hybrid virions from nonhybrid Ad7 by physical means, but these were all unsuccessful (Rowe et al., 1965). However, Baum et al. (1970) were able to demonstrate that the Ad7-SV40 hybrid has a slightly lower density than nonhybrid Ad7 in isopycnic CsCl gradients.

When the experiments of Rowe et al. (1965) were being conducted, it had not been established that the SV40 DNA and the Ad7 DNA in the Ad7-SV40 hybrid were covalently linked; other types of combination between the two DNAs could not be excluded. Baum et al. (1966) prepared DNAs from Ad7$^+$ and a mixture of nonhybrid Ad7 and SV40. The DNAs were banded in isopyknic alkaline CsCl gradients

TABLE 3

Concentration Dependence of Adenovirus 7
Plaque Formation in MKC by the Ad7$^+$
Population[a]

Relative dilution (D)	Number of plaques (P)	D_{min}/D	P/P_{max}
1	347	1	1
1/2	113	2	0.32
1/4	41	4	0.12
1/8	15	8	0.043
1/16	3	16	0.01

[a] The concentration dependence of plaque formation is discussed in Section 4.1. These data are presented graphically in Fig. 4 (Rowe and Baum, 1965).

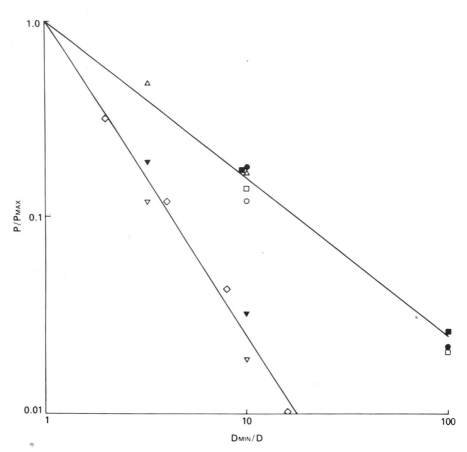

Fig. 4.   Concentration dependence of adenovirus and SV40 plaque formation in HEK and MKC. Ad7$^+$ (Table 3, ◇); Ad2^{++}HEY [Table 5, A (○), B (▽), C (□), and D (△)]; Ad2^{++}LEY [Table 5, A (●), B (▼), and C (■)]. The concentration dependence of plaque formation is discussed in Section 4.1.

and the gradients were fractionated. Each fraction was hybridized with radioactive cRNA complementary to either SV40 or Ad7. The experiment showed that while the Ad7 and SV40 DNAs [which have different densities (Table 1)] were well separated in the mixed gradient, Ad and SV40 DNAs cobanded in the Ad7$^+$ gradient. This result demonstrated unambiguously that the SV40 DNA in Ad7$^+$ was covalently integrated with Ad7 DNA.

4.3.   Heteroduplex Mapping of the Adenovirus 7–SV40 Hybrid Genome

The physical structures of the viral genomes of a number of Ad-SV40 hybrid viruses have been investigated by a variety of techniques.

The most useful technique employed in these studies has been that of heteroduplex mapping (Davis and Davidson, 1968). This technique is used to determine the extent of homology between two different DNA molecules and involves forming DNA-DNA hybrids (heteroduplexes), photographing them in an electron microscope, and measuring the regions of homology (double-stranded DNA) and heterology (single-stranded DNA) (see Fig. 9). Heteroduplex mapping provides a measure of homology and heterology which is accurate to about 50 nucleotide pairs. Kelly and Rose (1971) formed heteroduplex molecules between the hybrid and nonhybrid DNAs of Ad7[+]. They noted that about 21% of the Ad7[+] population was hybrid virus and the remainder was nonhybrid Ad7. Photographs of the molecules revealed that they contained two strands of DNA nonhomologous at a single site 5% from one end of the molecule. The two strands of single-stranded DNA were 11 and 16 Ad7 units in length [following the convention of Flint (1977) the length of the nonhybrid Ad genome is 100 units]. Baum *et al.* (1970) had shown that the Ad7-SV40 hybrid virions in Ad7[+] had a lower density than the nonhybrid virions and therefore contained less DNA. Accordingly, it was concluded that the hybrid molecules had a deletion of 16 units of Ad7 DNA and an insertion at the same site of 11 Ad7 units of SV40 DNA. One SV40 unit is defined here as the length of the SV40 genome. The length of the SV40 genome is 14.7% of the length of the Ad7 genome (Kelly and Rose, 1971); thus 1 SV40 unit is 14.7 Ad7 units and the length of the SV40 segment in Ad7-SV40, 11 Ad7 units, is 0.76 SV40 unit.

Lebowitz *et al.* (1974), by hybridizing Ad7[+] DNA to RNA transcripts of SV40 DNA fragments (obtained by endonuclease cleavage), were able to show that the SV40 DNA segment in Ad7[+] extended from about 0.12 to 0.72 SV40 unit using the *Eco*R1 restriction endonuclease cleavage site as the origin (Fig. 1A). This segment comprised 60% of the SV40 genome and included the entire early SV40 transcription region. The discrepancy between the size of the SV40 segment in Ad7[+] as determined by heteroduplex mapping (76%) and DNA fragment mapping (60%) was resolved by heteroduplex mapping of triple DNA-DNA hybrids formed between hybrid and nonhybrid Ad7[+] DNA and specific segments of SV40 DNA prepared by restriction endonuclease cleavage (Kelly, 1975). Examination of the triple heteroduplex molecules showed that the SV40 moiety in Ad7-SV40 was composed of two tandem segments of SV40 DNA; one extended from 0.50 to 0.71 SV40 unit and the other from 0.11 to 0.66 SV40 unit. Thus the region from 0.50 to 0.66 SV40 unit (16% of the SV40 genome) was repeated twice (Fig. 1A). The location of the integration site within the

Ad7-SV40 genome has not been determined beyond the fact that it lies 5% from one end of the hybrid molecule.

4.4. SV40 RNA Transcription in Cells Infected with Ad7[+]

Using hybridization competition, Oda and Dulbecco (1968) found that the RNA that accumulates late in Ad7[+]-infected cells competes effectively with 40% of the RNA that accumulates late in SV40 infection and with 90% of the RNA that accumulates early in SV40 infection. Since the hybridization competition pattern of Ad7[+] RNA was almost identical to that of SV40 early RNA, Oda and Dulbecco (1968) concluded that the entire early region of the SV40 genome and none of the late region was expressed in Ad7[+]-infected cells. More recently Lebowitz and Khoury (1975) hybridized RNA from cells productively infected with Ad7[+] to fragments of SV40 DNA prepared by cleavage with the restriction endonucleases *Hin*II and *Hin*III (Fig. 1A). Ad7[+] RNA hybridized only with fragments derived from the early region of the SV40 genome. Moreover, the SV40 RNA in Ad7[+]-infected cells is transcribed only from the E strand of the integrated SV40 genome.

4.5. Summary of Structure and Function of the Adenovirus 7–SV40 Hybrid Virus

The Ad7-SV40 hybrid virus in Ad7[+] is defective for both Ad7 and SV40. It contains the entire early region of the SV40 genome. Cells lytically infected with Ad7[+] accumulate RNA transcribed from the E strand of the SV40 genome which is translated into SV40 Tag and TSTag.

5. DNA-DNA RECOMBINATION IN THE ADENOVIRUSES AND THE ADENOVIRUS-SV40 HYBRID VIRUSES

The mechanism(s) of DNA-DNA recombination is not precisely understood; however, it is generally believed that the extent of homology between two heterologous DNA molecules is an important determinant with respect to the rate at which they recombine. Most DNA-DNA recombinations go undetected; it is only when the recombinant has a selective advantage over its progenitors that its formation becomes manifest.

There is extensive homology among the DNAs of the various human Ad serotypes (Green *et al.*, 1970; Garon *et al.*, 1973). Intergroup homology ranges from 10% between the highly oncogenic Ad viruses and the nononcogenic Ad viruses to 30% between the highly oncogenic Ad viruses and the weakly oncogenic Ad viruses; intragroup homology ranges from 70% to 95% in all three Ad virus groups. The genetic topography of the various Ad genomes is very similar (Sharp *et al.*, 1974; Pettersson *et al.*, 1976; Ortin *et al.*, 1976; Tibbetts, 1977; Flint, 1977). Accordingly, in cells coinfected with Ad of different serotypes, stable DNA-DNA recombinations occur between the two genomes (Section 10). Moreover, naturally occurring recombinants between Ad serotypes of the same hemagglutinating subgroups have been isolated (Norrby, 1968; Hierholzer, 1973).

There is no detectable homology between SV40 and the adenoviruses at high temperatures; however, unstable hybrids may form at low temperatures in formamide (P. Howley, personal communication). Accordingly, recombinations between SV40 and the adenoviruses are rare. A single passage of Ad2 with SV40 yielded no detectable hybrid viruses (Rowe, 1965), but continuous passage of SV40 with many adenoviruses usually leads to Ad-SV40 recombinations from which stable Ad-SV40 hybrid viruses may be selected in MKC. The hybrid genomes may be defective for Ad function and require helper virus for propagation, but they enhance propagation of nonhybrid Ad in MKC so that the effect of the recombination is to extend the host range of human Ad virus to monkey cells.

Zain and Roberts (1978) have identified the sequence of nucleotides at one integration site of $Ad2^+ND_1$ (map position 86, Fig. 11) and the nucleotide sequences in the corresponding regions of the Ad2 and SV40 genomes. They note that there is very little homology between Ad2 and SV40 in this region; only two nucleotide pairs adjacent to the site of recombination and several others nearby are identical. The authors conclude that the mechanism that led to recombination at this site must have involved factors other than DNA-DNA homology.

Altstein *et al.* (1968) showed that hybrid viruses capable of propagating in MKC were formed during coinfection with Ad2 and the simian adenovirus SA7, suggesting that hybrid virus formation may be a general phenomenon requiring only that the restricted virus acquire sufficient genetic information (by recombination) from the donor virus to overcome the restriction to propagation in a selecting cell type. Defective hybrid virus populations such as $Ad7^+$ are genetically unstable during low-multiplicity passage in cells permissive for nonhybrid Ad. Under these conditions the enhancing function confers no selective advantage and the hybrid virus population reverts to nonhybrid Ad (Rowe and Baum, 1964).

5.1.   A Hypothetical Model for the Formation of the Adenovirus 7–SV40 Hybrid Genome

A hypothetical model is presented in Fig. 5 to illustrate how recombinations between the DNAs of Ad7 and SV40 could have led to the formation of the Ad7-SV40 hybrid genome (Fig. 1A). Kelly and Rose (1971) suggested that initially a recombinant formed between intact molecules of Ad7 and SV40 DNAs. The hybrid molecule would be about 15% larger (for each integrated SV40 genome) than the nonhybrid Ad7 molecule. The resulting hybrid molecule would probably be too large for the Ad capsid (the largest Ad-SV40 hybrid molecule that has been characterized, $Ad2^{++}LEY$ II, is less than 5% larger than nonhybrid Ad2), and consequently would be nonviable unless it were reduced in size by further recombination during the same infectious cycle. The "viable intermediate" depicted in Fig. 5 could probably replicate through several infectious cycles. Since Ad7-SV40 contains DNA segments from noncontiguous regions of the SV40 genome it is probable that the hybrid intermediate underwent a second recombination with SV40 DNA followed by a deletion recombination to yield the final hybrid genome. The precise structures of hybrid intermediates are unknown, and there are many possibilities other than those depicted in Fig. 5; only the structure of the final form of Ad7-SV40 has been determined (Kelly, 1975).

5.2.   Transcapsidation

When MKC are coinfected with $Ad7^{+}$ and other Ad serotypes (Ad1, Ad2, Ad3, Ad4, Ad5, Ad6, and Ad12), the enhancing property of the Ad7-SV40 hybrid virus is transferred to the coinfecting serotype; this phenomenon is called "transcapsidation" (Rowe, 1965; Rapp et al., 1965, 1968). Rowe (1965) passaged $Ad7^{+}$ with Ad2 in MKC and selected for Ad2 transcapsidants by treating the progeny virus with anti-Ad7 serum. The remaining viral progeny contained the SV40-enhancing function of $Ad7^{+}$ enclosed in Ad2 capsids. The transcapsidated hybrid virus, although defective like the the parent Ad7-SV40,

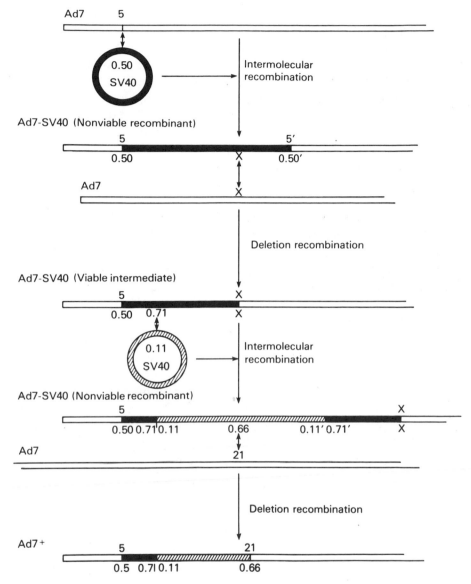

Fig. 5. How recombinations between Ad7 DNA (⊏⊐) and SV40 DNA
(▬ and ▨) could lead to the hybrid genome in Ad7⁺. The numbers (0–100) above
the hybrid molecules indicate Ad7 map positions, and the numbers 0–1.0 below the
hybrid molecules indicate SV40 map positions. When a single site is divided by recombination, one coordinate is primed. The double-pointed vertical arrows (↕) indicate the
recombination sites on the parental DNA molecules, and the vertical arrows (↓) indicate the recombination product. Map positions for a hypothetical viable intermediate
hybrid are indicated (X). The SV40 integration site is arbitrarily depicted at the left end
of the hybrid molecule.

nevertheless remained stable, without reverting to the Ad7 serotype, through repeated passage in MKC (Rapp *et al.*, 1965). However, the transcapsidated virus population continued to induce Ad7 Tag (Rowe and Pugh, 1966). One interpretation of these findings is that the defective Ad7-SV40 hybrid genomes replicate with the aid of Ad2 and are packaged in Ad2 capsids to yield a population of nonhybrid Ad2, with sufficient Ad7-SV40 hybrid genomes (enclosed in Ad2 capsids) to permit propagation in MKC. Another interpretation is that Ad7-SV40 hybrid genomes recombine with Ad2 genomes to yield a population of nonhybrid Ad2 and defective Ad2-Ad7-SV40 hybrid genomes.

6. ADENOVIRUS-SV40 HYBRID VIRUSES THAT YIELD INFECTIOUS SV40

Easton and Hiatt (1965) passaged MKC-adapted Ad4 five times in HEK and once in AGMK in the presence of anti-SV40 serum. Despite these attempts to remove contaminating SV40, this Ad4-SV40 hybrid virus population produced infectious SV40 when the anti-SV40 serum was removed. They observed that the heat lability (50°C) of infectious SV40 in $Ad4^{++}$ was almost the same as that of Ad4, although Ad4 was far more heat labile than plaque-purified nonhybrid SV40 derived from the $Ad4^{++}$ population [the double plus sign in the designations for hybrid viruses indicates that the hybrid virus induces infectious SV40 as well as SV40 antigens (Table 2)]. They next showed that production of infectious SV40 could be inhibited by adding anti-Ad4 serum to the inoculum but not by adding anti-SV40 serum, and concluded that infectious SV40 was being produced by Ad4 encapsidated virions.

Lewis *et al.* (1966*a*) studied the MKC-adapted strains of Ad1, Ad2, Ad3, Ad4, and Ad5. These viruses were all passaged 4–10 times with anti-SV40 serum. Subsequent passage without antiserum revealed that three of the viruses ($Ad2^{++}$, $Ad4^{++}$, and $Ad5^{++}$) retained the capacity to produce infectious SV40 in MKC. In this study, SV40 was not detected in $Ad1^{++}$ and $Ad3^{+}$, but it was later discovered that $Ad1^{++}$ did produce infectious SV40 in low yields (A. M. Lewis, Jr., unpublished); however, $Ad3^{+}$, like $Ad7^{+}$, remained SV40 free through many passages in MKC (Table 2). All five viruses induced SV40 Tag in HEK cells which could be inhibited by the homologous Ad antisera but not by anti-SV40 serum.

Subsequently, MKC were coinfected with SV40 and Ad12 in an attempt to hybridize this highly oncogenic Ad serotype with SV40

(Schell *et al.*, 1966; A. M. Lewis, Jr., unpublished). As anticipated, a hybrid virus was derived from these mixed infections that could propagate in MKC and induce infectious SV40. A. M. Lewis, Jr. (unpublished) showed that Ad plaque formation by both Ad12[++] and Ad5[++] followed a second-order concentration dependence in MKC, establishing the fact that the hybrid virions of Ad12[++] and Ad5[++] were defective in Ad function(s).

6.1. An Ad5[++] Hybrid Virus Population

The genomes of most Ad-SV40 hybrid viruses are comprised mainly of Ad DNA; however, a unique exception to this rule has recently been reported. The structures of the genomes of an Ad5-SV40 hybrid population [isolated from Ad5 "adapted" to replication in rhesus MKC by Hartley *et al.* (1956)] has been determined by heteroduplex mapping and restriction endonuclease cleavage (Y. Glutzman and J. Sambrook, personal communication). This viral population is comprised of a family of hybrids which differ from each other by one copy of SV40. The structure of the largest adenovirus 5–SV40 hybrid is shown in the following map:

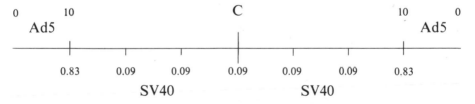

The center of this molecule (C) divides it into two identical halves, which are joined together as inverted repeats. Each half of the hybrid DNA molecule contains 2.7 SV40 genomes, organized as a tandem head-to-tail repeat, and the 10% of the adenovirus 5 genome located between map positions 0 and 10.

6.2. The Adenovirus 2–SV40 Hybrid Virus Population Ad2[++]

Lewis *et al.* (1966*b*) studied plaque induction by the SV40-yielding Ad2[++] population. They showed that Ad and SV40 plaques in MKC could be distinguished by their morphology and their kinetics of formation; Ad plaques appeared in 7 days while SV40 plaques required 12 days. Combining these criteria with the appropriate use of Ad and

TABLE 4
Influence of Ad2 and SV40 Antisera on Plaque Formation by Ad2^{++} in Monkey Cells

Antiserum added to[a]		Ad2 plaques[b]		SV40 plaques[b]	
Inoculum	Overlayer	Virus titer $\log_{10}$ (pfu/ml)	Concentration dependence	Virus titer $\log_{10}$ (pfu/ml)	Concentration dependence
NRS		6.25–6.83	2	7.57–7.72	1
Anti-SV40		6.09	2	7.32	1
Anti-Ad2		<3.5		<3.5	
	Anti-SV40	6.78	2	<3.5	
	Anti-Ad2	<3.5		7.58	1

[a] Anti-SV40 serum, anti-Ad2 serum, or nonimmune rabbit serum (NRS) was added to either the inoculum or the agar overlayer as indicated.
[b] The Ad2 titer in Ad2^{++} was $10^{8.7}$ as determined by plaque formation in HEK. The concentration dependence of plaque formation in MKC was either first order (1) or second order (2) (Section 4.1). The data were taken from Lewis et al. (1966b).

SV40 antisera, assays were devised which permitted quantitative characterization of the various components in the Ad2^{++} population (i.e., Ad2-SV40 hybrid, nonhybrid Ad2, and SV40). These studies showed that Ad2 plaque formation is inhibited only by anti-Ad2 serum whether added to the inoculum (inhibiting plaque initiation) or added to the agar overlayer (inhibiting plaque growth) (Table 4). The formation of SV40 plaques was also inhibited by adding anti-Ad2 serum to the inoculum, but anti-SV40 serum inhibited SV40 plaque formation only when it was added to the agar overlayer. In every case the concentration dependence of Ad2 plaque formation indicated that the hybrid virions were defective for Ad function while SV40 plaque formation indicated that plaque initiation required infection only by a single hybrid virion. The titer of nonhybrid Ad2 in the Ad2^{++} population ($10^{8.7}$ pfu/ml) was determined in HEK. The titer of nonhybrid SV40 was found to be $10^{3.2}$ pfu/ml in MKC when Ad2^{++} was heated at 56°C for 10 min (hybrid and nonhybrid Ad2 are inactivated under these conditions but SV40 viability remains relatively unaffected). The concentration of the Ad-SV40 hybrid virions was determined from the number of SV40 plaques formed in MKC when anti-Ad2 serum was added to the overlayer; this was found to be $10^{7.6}$ pfu/ml or 10% of the nonhybrid Ad2 titer (Table 4).

6.3. Plaque Isolation from the Ad2^{++} Population

Ad2 plaques were isolated from the Ad2^{++} population in MKC (Lewis et al., 1969; Lewis and Rowe, 1970). The progeny from these plaque isolates, which must necessarily contain Ad-SV40 hybrid viruses, were studied by plaque analysis as described above (Section 6.1). Two of the virus pools, designated Ad2^{++}HEY (high-efficiency yielder) and Ad2^{++}LEY (low-efficiency yielder), derived from plaques 1208 and 1567, respectively (Fig. 6), were similar to the parent Ad2^{++} in that they yielded SV40 in MKC and formed Ad2 plaques in MKC with a second-order concentration dependence (Table 5 and Fig. 4). However, a third pool, designated "B55," derived from plaque 1562 (Fig. 6), yielded Ad plaques in MKC with a one-component

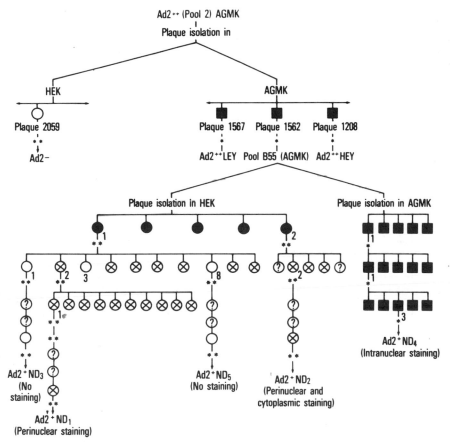

Fig. 6.   Outline of the tissue culture procedures used in the isolation of Ad2-SV40 hybrids and Ad2$^-$ from the Ad2^{++} hybrid population. □, AGMK plaque; ○, HEK plaque, with the results of testing the progeny of the plaque for SV40 antigen induction by IF indicated as follows: ○, no detectable antigen; ■,●, intranuclear antigen; ⊗, perinuclear or perinuclear and cytoplasmic antigen; ⑦, unsatisfactory test or progency were not tested; *, undiluted passage in AGMK; **, undiluted passage in HEK to establish pools. The defective Ad2^{++}HEY and Ad2^{++}LEY variants and Ad2$^-$ are included to show their relationship to the nondefective B55 pool. From Lewis (1977).

TABLE 5
Virus Composition of the Ad2++HEY and Ad2++LEY Hybrid Virus Populations

Virus assay[a]	Dilution (D) [$\log_{10}(1/D)$]	Ad2++HEY				Ad2++LEY			
		Plaques (P) (pfu/ml)	Virus titer [$\log_{10}$(pfu/ml)]	D_{min}/D	P/P_{max}	Plaques (P) (pfu/ml)	Virus titer [$\log_{10}$(pfu/ml)]	D_{min}/D	P/P_{max}
A. Ad2 in HEK	5					297	7.47	1	1
	6	134	8.12	1	1	55	7.74	10	0.18
	7	17	8.23	10	0.12	5	7.70	100	0.017
B. Ad2-SV40 as Ad2 plaques in MKC	3.5	593	6.30	1	1	492	5.69	1	1
	4	73	5.86	3.2	0.12	93	5.49	3.2	0.19
	4.5	11	5.57	10	0.019	16	5.20	10	0.032
C. Ad2-SV40 as Ad2 plaques in MKC	4	319	6.50	1	1	496	6.70	1	1
	5	46	6.66	10	0.14	87	6.94	10	0.18
	6	5	6.70	100	0.016	13	7.11	100	0.026
D. Ad2-SV40 as SV40 plaques in MKC	5	384	7.58	1	1		(2.3)		
	5.5	186	7.75	3.2	0.48				
	6	64	7.80	10	0.17				

[a] The Ad2++HEY and Ad2++LEY populations were assayed for plaque formation by inoculating cell monolayers with various dilutions (D) of virus and scoring the dishes for the number of plaques formed (P) (Lewis and Rowe, 1970). The virus titer is given by the ratio P/D, and the quantities D_{min}/D and P/P_{max} were plotted (Fig. 4) to determine the concentration dependence of plaque formation (Section 4.1). The assay conditions were as follows: (A) The concentration of nonhybrid Ad2 was determined by plaquing in HEK. (B) Ad2-SV40 hybrid virus concentrations were determined in MKC. Anti-SV40 serum was added to both the inoculum and the agar overlayer to suppress SV40 plaque formation. This assay yields Ad2 plaques with a second-order concentration dependence, indicating that the Ad2-SV40 hybrids in both Ad2++HEY and Ad2++LEY are defective in Ad2 function. (C) Ad2-SV40 hybrid virus concentrations were determined in MKC preinfected with Ad2. Anti-SV40 serum was added to both the inoculum and to the agar overlayer to suppress SV40 plaque formation. This assay yields Ad2 plaques with a first-order concentration dependence. (D) Ad2-SV40 hybrid concentrations were determined in MKC. Anti-SV40 serum was added to the inoculum to eliminate nonhybrid SV40, and anti-Ad2 serum was added to the agar overlayer to suppress Ad2 plaque formation. This assay yields SV40 plaques with a first-order concentration dependence. The Ad2-SV40 titer in Ad2++LEY (parentheses) was determined at a lower dilution than indicated.

dependence, indicating that the Ad2-SV40 hybrid virus derived from plaque 1562 was nondefective for Ad function. Although B55 induced SV40 Tag, it did not yield SV40 plaques in MKC, indicating that the hybrid virus was defective in SV40 functions. All five nondefective Ad2-SV40 hybrid viruses, discussed in Section 8, were derived from the B55 pool.

7. BIOLOGICAL PROPERTIES OF Ad2^{++}HEY AND Ad2^{++}LEY

Although Ad2^{++}HEY and Ad2^{++}LEY, like the parent Ad2^{++}, were defective for Ad function and yielded SV40 plaques in MKC, they differed in one important respect. Ad2^{++}HEY yielded 10^5 more SV40 plaques in MKC than did Ad2^{++}LEY (Table 5). Similarly, the concentration of nonhybrid SV40 was about a thousandfold higher in Ad2^{++}HEY. Analysis of plaque isolates of the two variants showed that they were genetically stable (Lewis and Rowe, 1970).

All of the known early SV40 antigens, Tag, Uag, and TSTag (Section 8), are induced by both Ad2^{++}HEY and Ad2^{++}LEY (Lewis and Rowe, 1970; Siegel et al., 1975; Tevethia and Lewis, 1976). However, only Ad2^{++}HEY induces detectable amounts of SV40 Vag (Table 2). It should be noted that Ad2^{++}LEY does not induce detectable TSTag when assayed in hamsters. TSTag is readily detected by this assay when hamsters are immunized with either SV40 or Ad2^{++}HEY (Lewis and Rowe, 1970; Siegel et al., 1975). However, Ad2^{++}LEY does induce TSTag when assayed in mice (Tevethia and Lewis, 1975). It is not understood why Ad2^{++}LEY-induced TSTag can be detected in mice but not in hamsters since both species are equally responsive to TSTag induction by SV40. Similar differences have been observed in assays for SV40 TSTag induction by Ad2$^+$ND$_1$ (Section 11.1).

The results of plaque assays of Ad2^{++}HEY and Ad2^{++}LEY are shown in Table 5 and Fig. 4. Ad2 plaque induction by both viruses follows a first-order concentration dependence in HEK, yielding titers of $10^{8.3}$ pfu/ml and $10^{7.7}$ pfu/ml, respectively. It should be noted that the calculated titers increase slightly with increasing dilution; concomitantly the slopes of the plotted data are somewhat less than the expected integral values (Fig. 4). This is due to the inherent difficulty in accurately scoring dishes with a large number of plaques. Ad2 plaque induction by both variants follows a second-order dilution dependence in MKC (Table 5B and Fig. 4); however, the concentration dependence shifts to first order when the MKC monolayer is preinfected with Ad2

(Table 5C and Fig. 4). Since the Ad2 plaques formed in the first-order assay result only from infection with Ad2-SV40 hybrids, the assay indicates that the concentration of hybrid virus in the two virus pools is about the same. In contrast, when the SV40 plaques induced by the two variants in MKC are scored, the titer of hybrid virus in Ad2^{++}HEY is about $10^{7.7}$ pfu/ml while the apparent titer of hybrid virus in Ad2^{++}LEY is only $10^{2.3}$ pfu/ml (Table 5D and Fig. 4). The titers of the genetically stable Ad2-SV40 hybrid components in the two populations are about 10% of that of the nonhybrid Ad2 component. Thus both variants initiate foci of SV40 infection; however, the Ad2^{++}LEY population does so with a much lower frequency than does Ad2^{++}HEY.

As indicated in Table 5, high-multiplicity infection of MKC by Ad2^{++}HEY yields nonhybrid SV40 titers of 10^4 pfu/ml; however, low multiplicity infection yields nonhybrid SV40 titers of 10^6–10^7 pfu/ml. If nonhybrid SV40 is removed from the inoculum by anti-SV40 serum, virus propagation occurs only in individual monkey cells infected with hybrid virus. In high-multiplicity infections, Ad2 and Ad2-SV40 hybrid replication predominates since most cells infected by hybrid virus will be coinfected with nonhybrid Ad2. Ad2 not only replicates faster than SV40 but also inhibits SV40 DNA synthesis (Section 2.5). During low-multiplicity infection, dual infection is rare, and there is a high probability that SV40 replication will be initiated in cells singly infected with an Ad2^{++}HEY hybrid virion. Consequently, during low-multiplicity Ad2^{++}HEY infection greater quantities of nonhybrid SV40 are produced than in high-multiplicity infection.

7.1. The Physical Structures of the Hybrid Viral Genomes in Ad2^{++}HEY and Ad2^{++}LEY

Wiese *et al.* (1970) attempted to separate the Ad2-SV40 hybrid virions from the nonhybrid Ad2 virions in both Ad2^{++}HEY and Ad2^{++}LEY populations using isopycnic CsCl gradients. Analysis of the gradient fractions by plaque formation in MKC revealed no significant difference in the density of the hybrid and nonhybrid components of Ad2^{++}LEY but showed that the hybrid virions in Ad2^{++}HEY were 0.004 g/cm^3 less dense than the nonhybrid component. This difference in density permitted a hundredfold enrichment of the Ad2^{++}HEY hybrid virus. The enriched hybrid virions from Ad2^{++}HEY were plaqued on MKC preinfected with Ad2 (for helper function) to yield Ad2 plaques, and on MKC without Ad2 to yield SV40 plaques. The result of this experiment showed that the ability of the enriched hybrid virus to yield SV40 or Ad2 plaques was about the same, supporting the notion that both kinds of plaques are initiated by a single virion species (i.e., the Ad2-SV40 hybrid virions).

Crumpacker *et al.* (1970) demonstrated that the SV40 DNA in the hybrid virions in Ad2^{++}HEY, like that in Ad7$^+$ (Section 4.2), is covalently linked to Ad2 DNA by showing that the two DNAs cobanded in alkaline CsCl.

7.2. Heteroduplex Mapping of the Hybrid Viral Genomes in Ad2^{++}HEY and Ad2^{++}LEY

The arrangement of the SV40 DNA in Ad2^{++}HEY and Ad2^{++}LEY was studied by heteroduplex mapping (Kelly *et al.*, 1974). After melting and reannealing, the DNAs of both populations formed heteroduplex molecules with single-stranded loops. Measurements of the single strands in the Ad2^{++}HEY heteroduplex molecules revealed that the length of one strand was the same in all molecules (40 Ad2 units) while the other strands could be grouped into three size classes. About two-thirds of the heteroduplex molecules contained single-stranded segments of 21 Ad2 units, one-third had segments of 35 Ad2 units, and a small number had segments of 6 Ad2 units. It had been previously established that the hybrid viruses in Ad2^{++}HEY were less dense than nonhybrid Ad2 (Wiese *et al.*, 1970); it therefore followed that the largest single-stranded segment represented a deletion of 40 units of Ad2 DNA in all hybrid molecules, while the smaller segment represented insertions at the same site of variable amounts of SV40 DNA. The Ad2^{++}HEY III molecule contains 2.39 genome equivalents (or 2.39 units) of SV40 DNA (1 SV40 unit equals 14.4 Ad2 units). Ad2^{++}HEY II, which contains 1.43 units of SV40 DNA, can be derived from Ad2^{++}HEY III by removing approximately one SV40 genome from the integrated SV40 segment (Figs. 2 and 7). Similarly Ad2^{++}HEY I, which has only 0.43 unit of SV40 DNA, can be derived from Ad2^{++}HEY III by removing two genomes of SV40 DNA from the integrated SV40 segment (Fig. 2). The length of the Ad2 deletion is the same in all three classes of Ad2^{++}HEY.

The organization of the SV40 DNA in the Ad2^{++}HEY molecules with respect to the SV40 genome (Figs. 1A and 2) was determined by examining triple heteroduplex molecules formed between the hybrid and nonhybrid DNAs of Ad2^{++}HEY and linear SV40 DNA fragments prepared by endonuclease cleavage (*Eco*R1 plus *Hpa*I) of superhelical SV40 DNA (Kelly *et al.*, 1974). These studies showed that the left end

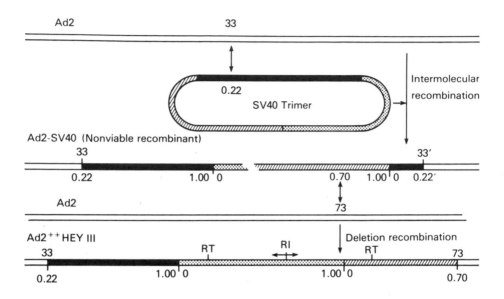

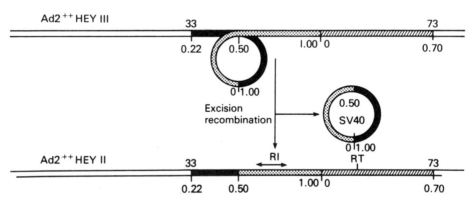

Fig. 7.   How Ad2++HEY III might have formed by an initial recombination between Ad2 DNA (⊏⊐) and an SV40 trimer (▬, ▭, and ▨). The numbers 0–100 above the hybrid molecules indicate Ad2 map positions, and the numbers 0–1.0 below the hybrid molecules indicate SV40 map positions. When a single site is divided by recombination, one coordinate is primed. The double-pointed vertical arrows (↕) indicate the recombination sites on the parental DNA molecules, and the vertical arrows (↓) indicate the recombination product. The lower part of the figure illustrates how Ad2++HEY III could undergo an intramolecular recombination within the integrated SV40 DNA to give rise to Ad2++HEY II and free SV40. The SV40 DNA replication initiation (RI) and replication termination (RT) sites are indicated on the Ad2++HEY III and Ad2++HEY II molecules; the small horizontal arrows indicate the directions of replication from the replication initiation site.

of the SV40 segment in Ad2^{++}HEY mapped at 0.22 on the SV40 genome while the right end was located at map position 0.70 (Fig. 1A).

The location of the Ad deletion in Ad2^{++}HEY was observed to be 33 Ad2 units from one end of the molecule and 27 Ad2 units from the other. By examining partially melted heteroduplex molecules it was determined that the deletion was 33 Ad2 units from the G+C-rich end of the molecule as shown in Fig. 2.

Study of heteroduplex molecules of Ad2^{++}LEY revealed that each hybrid molecule contained a deletion of 11% of the Ad2 genome near one end of the molecule (Fig. 2). Almost all molecules had an insertion of 1.05 units of SV40 DNA (Ad2^{++}LEY II) while a few had only 0.03 unit of SV40 DNA (Ad2^{++}LEY I, Figs. 1B and 2). Again examination of triple heteroduplex molecules with fragments of DNA of known structure revealed the precise oganization of the integrated SV40 DNA.

The study of triple heteroduplex molecules of both Ad2^{++}HEY and Ad2^{++}LEY using linear SV40 DNA molecules (*Eco*R1) showed that the SV40 DNA in the hybrid molecules was arranged in a tandem array of the type ABCDAB (Figs. 1A and 2). The finding that Ad2^{++}HEY contained tandem arrays of multiple copies of the SV40 genome while Ad2^{++}LEY contained only slightly more than a single copy suggested a model which could account for the different amounts of infectious SV40 yielded by the two hybrid virus populations (Kelly *et al.*, 1974). In Ad2^{++}HEY there are many more ways (and hence a greater probability) of excising an intact SV40 genome from the hybrid molecule than there are in Ad2^{++}LEY (Fig. 2). Thus the model suggests that in cells productively infected with the Ad2^{++}HEY hybrid there is a high probability that a complete SV40 genome will be excised from the hybrid molecule and undergo independent replication.

A hypothetical model is shown in Fig. 7 to illustrate how Ad2^{++}HEY III might have formed from an initial recombination between Ad2 and an SV40 trimer (Martin *et al.*, 1976), followed by a deletion recombination with Ad2. Ad2^{++}HEY II and Ad2^{++}HEY I could form from Ad2^{++}HEY III by excision of intact SV40 genomes. Alternatively, Ad2^{++}HEY I, formed from Ad2 and SV40 monomers, might have been the initial stable recombinant; Ad2^{++}HEY II and Ad2^{++}HEY III might have formed from Ad2^{++}HEY I by successive recombinations with SV40 monomers.

Figure 7 also illustrates the fact that there are many ways that an SV40 genome can be excised from Ad2^{++}HEY II and Ad2^{++}HEY III while Fig. 10 shows that there are very few ways that an SV40 genome can be excised from Ad2^{++}LEY II. Sambrook *et al.* (1974) and Botchan (unpublished) have suggested that integrated viral SV40 DNA could replicate *in situ* to yield infectious virus if the integrated DNA contained the replication initiation site (RI, Fig. 7) as well as sufficient DNA to permit complete replication in both directions to the replication termini (RT, Fig. 7). This could be the case for Ad2++HEY III but not for Ad2++HEY II or Ad2++LEY II. Replication *in situ* would probably be more efficient than recombination excision and might easily account for the difference between Ad2++HEY and Ad2++LEY in the amount of free SV40 in the two virus populations. Elucidation of the mechanism of SV40 induction in the Ad2++HEY and Ad2++LEY populations could provide insight into the mechanism of virus "rescue" from transformed cells (Section 13).

It was noted in the heteroduplex studies that about 10% of the DNA molecules in both the Ad2++HEY and Ad2++LEY populations were hybrid molecules. The biological data in Table 5 suggest that about 10% of the virions in the Ad2++HEY hybrid population induce SV40 plaques in MKC. Thus both the physical and biological data are in good agreement with respect to the amounts of hybrid molecules in the Ad2++HEY population. Moreover, the fact that these data do agree indicates that the probability of a freely replicating SV40 genome being excised from the Ad2++HEY hybrid molecule in a singly infected MKC must be very nearly 1.

7.3. SV40 Transcription in Cells Infected with Ad2++HEY and Ad2++LEY

Transcription of the SV40 DNA in Ad2++HEY and Ad2++LEY during lytic infection was studied by competition hybridization (Siegel *et al.*, 1975). These studies showed that RNA prepared from Ad2++HEY-infected MKC contained all of the sequences present, both early and late, in SV40-infected MKC. However, the concentration of SV40 RNA sequences in Ad2++HEY-infected cells was only 50% of that in SV40-infected cells. RNA prepared from Ad2++LEY-infected cells was almost as effective in competing with early SV40 RNA as was RNA from Ad2++HEY-infected cells. In contrast, Ad2++LEY RNA was much less effective than Ad2++HEY RNA in competing with late SV40 RNA. These observations correlate well with the known features of SV40 transcription; while early RNA (which provides the enhancing function) may be transcribed from nonreplicating SV40 DNA, the replicating form of the viral genome is required for late SV40 RNA synthesis. Since Ad2++LEY yields very little infectious SV40 (i.e., very little replicating SV40) it follows that the early SV40 region in Ad2^{++}LEY is transcribed mainly from integrated DNA. Thus transcription of the SV40 DNA integrated in the Ad-SV40 hybrids may be analogous to transcription of viral DNA integrated in the chromosomes of transformed cells (Section 2.4).

Although high-multiplicity infection of MKC with Ad2^{++}HEY yields relatively little infectious SV40 (Section 7), *de novo* superhelical SV40 DNA can be demonstrated under such conditions. Siegel *et al.* (1975) purified DNA from Hirt extracts (Hirt, 1967) of MKC infected for 36 hr with either Ad2^{++}HEY or Ad2^{++}LEY. The DNAs were sedimented through alkaline sucrose gradients. The gradients were fractionated and the fractions were hybridized with radioactive SV40 cRNA. Analysis of the hybridized fractions obtained from the Ad2^{++}HEY gradient revealed SV40-specific DNA in two peaks, one at the 53 S region (superhelical DNA) and another in the 16–18 S region (relaxed circular–linear DNA). No SV40 peaks were detected in the Ad2^{++}LEY gradient.

7.4. Adenovirus 2–SV40 Hybrid Viruses Derived from the Ad2^{++}HEY Population

Two additional Ad2-SV40 hybrid viruses (Ad2$^+$D1 and Ad2$^+$D2) have been derived from the Ad2^{++}HEY population (Hassell *et al.*, 1978). As the designation indicates, neither Ad2$^+$D1 nor Ad2$^+$D2 induces infectious SV40. Both viruses induce plaques in MKC with a second-order concentration dependence, indicating that both hybrids are defective for Ad function and require helper virus for propagation.

The DNAs of Ad2$^+$D1 and Ad2$^+$D2 have been studied by heteroduplex mapping and by restriction endonuclease cleavage; the structures thus derived are shown in Figs. 1 and 2 (Hassell *et al.*, 1978). In Ad2$^+$D1-infected MKC, SV40 RNA accumulates in the cytoplasm both before and after the onset of viral DNA replication. This RNA is transcribed exclusively from the early template of the integrated SV40 DNA. Since the entire early region is contained in the integrated SV40 DNA (Fig. 1A), and since the Ad2 promoter near the integration site is deleted (Fig. 2), it is likely that SV40 transcription in Ad2$^+$D1-infected cells is regulated by SV40 promoters.

In Ad2$^+$D2-infected MKC, SV40 RNA accumulates in the cytoplasm only late in infection. This RNA is transcribed mainly from the early SV40 template, although a small amount of late SV40 RNA is detected. The early SV40 promoter is deleted from Ad2$^+$D2 (Fig. 1B); however, the integrated SV40 DNA is located downstream from a late Ad2 promoter (Fig. 2). It thus seems likely that SV40 transcription in Ad2$^+$D2 is regulated by Ad2 promoters.

Both Ad2$^+$D1 and Ad2$^+$D2 induce proteins that are precipitable with serum from hamsters bearing SV40 tumors (Hassell *et al.*, 1978). Ad2$^+$D1 induces a 96K SV40 protein which may be identical to the 90–100K early SV40 protein. On the other hand, Ad2$^+$D2 induces a 115K SV40 protein which may contain Ad2 peptides on its amino end. This 115K protein is synthesized in large quantities, suggesting that its synthesis may be regulated by late Ad2 promoters. Although this protein lacks the N-terminal portion of the early SV40 protein (Fig. 1B), it nevertheless binds to SV40 DNA (Tjian, 1978) and stimulates host DNA synthesis (Tjian *et al.*, 1978).

It is not known how Ad2$^+$D1 and Ad2$^+$D2 could have arisen from Ad2^{++}HEY, but Hassell *et al.* (1978) suggest that Ad2$^+$D1 resulted from a recombination between Ad2 and an Ad2-SV40 hybrid, while Ad2$^+$D2 probably resulted from a recombination between Ad2 and free SV40 in the Ad2^{++}HEY population.

8.   ISOLATION OF THE NONDEFECTIVE ADENOVIRUS 2–SV40 HYBRID VIRUSES

The progeny of one of the plaques (no. 1562, Fig. 6) isolated from the Ad2^{++} population was nondefective and replicated with equal efficiency in MKC and HEK (Lewis *et al.*, 1969). The B55 pool derived from plaque 1562 induced SV40 Tag but did not induce SV40 plaques or SV40 Vag in MKC. The B55 pool was subjected to further plaque analysis in both MKC and HEK (Fig. 6). From this analysis three nondefective Ad2-SV40 hybrid variants were derived that induced SV40 antigens (Lewis *et al.*, 1969, 1973; Lewis and Rowe, 1971). Two of these variants were derived from HEK passage and were designated "Ad2$^+$ND$_1$" and "Ad2$^+$ND$_2$"; one variant was derived from passage in MKC and was designated "Ad2$^+$ND$_4$." It has subsequently been shown that, by the criterion of heteroduplex mapping, Ad2$^+$ND$_4$ and the parent B55 are indistinguishable (A. M. Lewis, Jr., and T. Kelly, unpublished).

The SV40 antigen induced by Ad2$^+$ND$_1$, unlike SV40 Tag, reacted with some but not all sera from hamsters bearing SV40-induced tumors. Moreover, the Ad2$^+$ND$_1$ antigen was stable under conditions (heating at 50°C for 30 min) that destroy Tag. It was evident that the

Ad2$^+$ND$_1$-induced SV40 antigen (designated "Uag") was a previously unrecognized SV40 antigen (Lewis and Rowe, 1971). It was subsequently shown that Uag is induced in MKC infected by SV40 in the presence of inhibitors of viral DNA synthesis, indicating that it is an early SV40 antigen. Anti-Uag serum can be prepared in monkeys immunized with Ad2$^+$ND$_1$-infected AGMK cells; this serum stains SV40 infected cells much like anti-Tag serum (Lewis and Rowe, 1971). Further studies (Lewis *et al.*, 1973) demonstrated that Uag can be induced by Ad2$^+$ND$_2$, Ad2$^+$ND$_4$, and B55 as well as Ad2$^+$ND$_1$ and SV40, although the staining morphology differs from one virus to another (Fig. 6). In addition to Uag induction, the nondefective Ad2-SV40 hybrid viruses were characterized with respect to induction of Tag and TSTag, the two other known early SV40 antigens. While Ad2$^+$ND$_1$ induced neither Tag nor TSTag, Ad2$^+$ND$_2$ induced TSTag and Ad2$^+$ND$_4$ induced both. Thus Ad2$^+$ND$_1$, Ad2$^+$ND$_2$, and Ad2$^+$ND$_4$ contained SV40 genetic information capable of inducing one (Uag), two (Uag and TSTag), or three (Uag, TSTag, and Tag) early SV40 antigens, respectively (Lewis *et al.*, 1973).

In the initial isolation of Ad2$^+$ND$_1$ and Ad2$^+$ND$_2$ from HEK, it was noted that three of the ten plaques isolated from the second dilution passage of B55 in HEK induced no SV40 antigens (Fig. 6). However, radioactive RNA prepared from cells infected with viral progeny derived from each of these plaques hybridized with SV40 DNA, indicating that all three contained SV40 genetic information. Two of the three plaques, subjected to further plaque purification, retained the capacity to induce SV40 RNA and were designated Ad2$^+$ND$_3$ and Ad2$^+$ND$_5$ (Lewis *et al.*, 1973). Thus, from the initial isolate (B55 pool), five stable nondefective variants were obtained which contained SV40 DNA but differed from each other in the extent of expression of SV40 genetic information.

It was apparent that the five nondefective Ad2-SV40 hybrid viruses could be useful in elucidating the genetic structure and function of both SV40 and Ad2; thus these viruses have been subjected to intensive study.

8.1. Early SV40 RNA in Cells Infected with the Nondefective Adenovirus 2–SV40 Hybrid Viruses

Using competition hybridization between RNAs prepared from cells lytically infected with Ad2$^+$ND$_1$ or SV40, Oxman *et al.* (1971) showed that Ad2$^+$ND$_1$ lytic RNA competed with about 15% of late lytic SV40 RNA and about 40% of early SV40 RNA. These experiments indicated that the segment of SV40 DNA in $Ad2^+ND_1$ included a substantial portion of the early region of the SV40 genome (Fig. 1B). Similarly, Levine *et al.* (1973) showed that the SV40 RNA expressed during lytic infection by all five nondefective Ad2-SV40 hybrid viruses competed with each other to varying extents (Fig. 8). Moreover, RNA prepared from cells infected with $Ad2^+ND_4$ competed with 90% of the viral RNA expressed early in SV40 infection. The results of the competition hybridization experiments together with the data on SV40 antigen induction led to the conclusion that the SV40 DNA in the nondefective Ad2-SV40 hybrid viruses consisted of overlapping segments of the early region of the SV40 genome.

8.2. The Physical Structures of the Nondefective Adenovirus 2–SV40 Hybrid Genomes

The SV40 DNA in all five nondefective hybrids was demonstrated to be covalently linked to Ad2 DNA (Levin *et al.*, 1971; Henry *et al.*, 1973). The DNAs were first subjected to either isopycnic banding in alkaline CsC1 or sedimentation through alkaline sucrose gradients. The

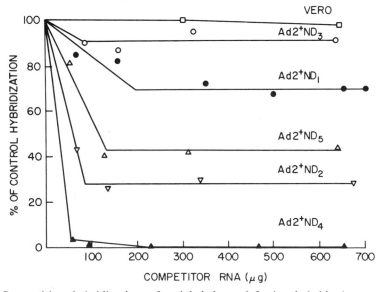

Fig. 8. Competition hybridization of unlabeled nondefective hybrid virus-specific RNAs with radioactive [³H]-$Ad2^+ND_4$ RNA. Competition hybridization experiments were performed with a saturating amount of [³H]-RNA and 0.1 μg of [¹⁴C]-SV40 DNA filters. From A. S. Levine *et al.* (1973).

gradients were fractionated and each fraction was challenged with radioactive Ad2 or SV40 cRNA. The results showed that the SV40 DNA in each hybrid was always associated with Ad2 DNA. DNAs from the hybrid viruses were indistinguishable from nonhybrid Ad2 DNA by the criteria of density, melting point, sedimentation coefficient, and molecular length as measured in the electron microscope (Crumpacker *et al.*, 1971; Henry *et al.*, 1973). The SV40 DNA content of each hybrid was estimated by reconstruction experiments. In these experiments, the amount of SV40 cRNA hybridized by known quantities of each hybrid DNA was compared with the amount of the same SV40 cRNA hybridized by known quantities of SV40 DNA. The results of these reconstruction experiments indicated that the five nondefective Ad2-SV40 hybrid DNAs contained different amount of SV40 DNA ranging from 0.02 SV40 unit in $Ad2^+ND_3$ to 0.35 SV40 unit in $Ad2^+ND_4$ (Levin *et al.*, 1971; Henry *et al.*, 1973). Although the sizes of the SV40 segments determined by hybridization are smaller than the sizes determined by heteroduplex mapping (Fig. 1B), these experiments did show correctly the relative sizes of the SV40 DNA segments in the various hybrids.

The physical structure of the nondefective Ad2-SV40 hybrid viral genomes was studied by heteroduplex mapping (Kelly and Lewis, 1973). Examination of the heteroduplex molecules formed between Ad2 DNA and DNA prepared from each of the hybrid viruses revealed that each hybrid genome had deletions of 4–7% of the Ad2 genome and contained insertions of variable amounts of SV40 DNA at the same site (Figs. 1B, 2, and 11). The site of the Ad2 deletion was the same (14% from one end) in each of the five hybrid DNAs. Moreover, DNA-DNA hybrids formed between the DNAs of the five hybrid viruses with each other demonstrated that the deletion of Ad2 DNA was located near the same end of each hybrid molecule, and the integrated SV40 segments were homologous with each other. Thus the heteroduplex mapping studies were completely consistent with the competition hybridization studies in showing that the genomes of the hybrid viruses contained overlapping segments of the SV40 genome.

Partial denaturation of DNA-DNA hybrids formed between Ad2 DNA and $Ad2^+ND_3$ DNA revealed that the deletions of Ad2 DNA were from the A+T-rich end of the molecule (Kelly *et al.*, 1974). Thus the hybrid DNAs contained deletions of varying amounts of Ad2 DNA and one end of the deletion was always at 86 Ad units from the origin of the Ad2 molecule (Figs. 2 and 11).

Triple heteroduplex molecules formed with DNAs of Ad2, $Ad2^+ND_1$, and linear SV40 DNA (derived by *Eco*R1 endonuclease cleavage of superhelical SV40 DNA) showed that the SV40 segment in Ad2$^+$ND$_1$ was colinear with 17.2% of SV40 DNA. The two segments of single-stranded SV40 DNA extending from the triple heteroduplex were 0.11 and 0.73 SV40 unit in length (Morrow and Berg, 1972). Similarly, triple heteroduplex molecules formed with Ad2, Ad2$^+$ND$_4$, and linear (EcoR1) SV40 DNAs showed that the SV40 segment in Ad2$^+$ND$_4$ was colinear with 47.3% of SV40 DNA. Again, one of the single-stranded SV40 segments extending from the triple heteroduplex molecule was 0.11 SV40 units in length while the other was 0.40 unit (Morrow et al., 1973). In the triple heteroduplexes of both Ad2$^+$ND$_1$ and Ad2$^+$ND$_4$, the 0.11-unit length of single-stranded SV40 DNA was located 14% from one end of the heteroduplex molecules.

The measurements of the triple heteroduplex molecules of Ad2$^+$ND$_4$ indicated that the integrated SV40 segment comprised the SV40 DNA region mapping either from 0.11 to 0.59 or from 0.41 to 0.89 on the SV40 genome (Fig. 1B). It was known from both the biological data and the SV40 RNA transcription studies that Ad2$^+$ND$_4$ contained most of the early region of SV40; it therefore followed that the SV40 segment integrated in Ad2$^+$ND$_4$ extended from 0.11 SV40 unit to 0.59 SV40 unit.

It should be noted that examination of the triple heteroduplex molecules of Ad2$^+$ND$_4$ (Morrow et al., 1973) revealed that about one-half of the Ad2$^+$ND$_4$ molecules contained deletions from the SV40 segment between map positions 0.50 and 0.57; this variant was designated "Ad2$^+$ND$_4$ del" (Fig. 1B).

Recent heteroduplex mapping studies of Ad2$^+$ND$_4$ propagated in human cells indicate that the genomes of the hybrid virus population are heterogeneous with respect to the integrated SV40 DNA (Westphal et al., 1979). These findings together with those of Morrow et al. (1973) show that a large proportion of the Ad2$^+$ND$_4$ genomes contain DNA deletions in the region between SV40 map positions 0.50 and 0.60 (Fig. 1B). Moreover, the studies of Westphal et al. (1979) indicate that the left end of the integrated SV40 DNA maps near 0.62, or 0.03 SV40 unit to the left of the position reported by Kelly and Lewis (1973) (Fig. 1B). This difference could be significant in view of the discussion in Section 13.4.

Lebowitz et al. (1974) hybridized RNA transcripts of restriction endonuclease (HinII plus HinIII) cleavage fragments of SV40 DNA to the DNAs of the five nondefective Ad2-SV40 hybrid viruses. The results of these experiments led to maps of the SV40 segments in the hybrid viruses which were in good agreement with those obtained by heteroduplex mapping.

It was now clear that the five nondefective hybrid viruses contained overlapping segments of SV40 DNA which extended from a common point in each segment (0.11 SV40 unit from the *Eco*R1 cleavage site, Fig. 11) for varying lengths through the early region of the SV40 genome. Moreover, the common point in the SV40 segment was located 14% from the end of the A+T-rich region in each hybrid molecule. Thus it was possible to relate the various early SV40 antigens to a physical map of the SV40 genome (Fig. 11) (Kelly and Lewis, 1973; Morrow *et al.*, 1973; Lebowitz *et al.*, 1974).

The separated complementary strands of each nondefective hybrid DNA were immobilized on nitrocellulose filters and challenged with early and late lytic SV40 RNA as well as SV40 cRNA asymmetrically transcribed from superhelical SV40 DNA with *E. coli* RNA polymerase (Patch *et al.*, 1972, 1974). The results of these experiments indicated that only the "r" strands (Fig. 11) of the hybrid DNAs were homologous with SV40 early RNA or SV40 cRNA, while late SV40 RNA was homologous with both strands. These findings demonstrated that the early SV40 template strand (E strand) is integrated in the r strand of Ad2 DNA (Figs. 1B and 2); in addition, the results demonstrated that the SV40 segment in the hybrid DNAs contained both early and late SV40 templates, and therefore contained a transcription initiator or terminator. The template map of SV40 shown in Fig. 1 indicates that the terminator region for both early and late SV40 mRNAs (at map position 0.17) is located in the SV40 DNA segments contained within the nondefective hybrid DNAs.

Gel electrophoresis of Ad2 DNA cleaved by the restriction endonuclease *Eco*R1 shows that the Ad2 DNA is cut at five sites, yielding six DNA fragments of varying lengths (Fig. 2). A similar analysis of Ad2$^+$ND$_1$ DNA revealed that the *Eco*R1 cleavage site located at map position 83.6 (Figs. 2 and 11) was deleted (Mulder *et al.*, 1974). Thus *Eco*R1 cleavage of the nondefective Ad2-SV40 hybrid DNAs yields four fragments that are identical to Ad2 DNA fragments A, B, C, and F and a fifth fragment composed of parts of Ad2 fragments D and E plus the integrated SV40 DNA (Figs. 2 and 11).

8.3. The Origin of the Nondefective Adenovirus 2–SV40 Hybrid Viruses

Kelly *et al.* (1974) prepared heteroduplex molecules by hybridizing DNAs from Ad2$^+$ND$_4$ and Ad2^{++}LEY and found that the two hybrid molecules were colinear over much of the region of recombination

(Figs. 9 and 11). This result established the fact that the recombination region in Ad2^{++}LEY, like that in Ad2$^+$ND$_4$, was in the A+T-rich region (right end) of the Ad2 molecule (Figs. 2 and 11). Moreover, it suggested a model (Fig. 10) for the origin of Ad2$^+$ND$_4$ and the other nondefective hybrid viruses (Kelly *et al.*, 1974). The structures of the integration sites in the genomes of Ad2^{++}LEY and the five nondefective hybrid viruses are depicted in Fig. 11. As can be seen, an intermolecular recombination between Ad2^{++}LEY DNA and non-hybrid Ad2 DNA at map position 86 would lead to the structure observed for Ad2$^+$ND$_4$ (Figs. 10 and 11). This hypothetical recombination would delete about half of the SV40 DNA in Ad2^{++}LEY, but more importantly it would replace the essential portion of the Ad2 genome (missing from Ad2^{++}LEY), yielding a hybrid molecule that

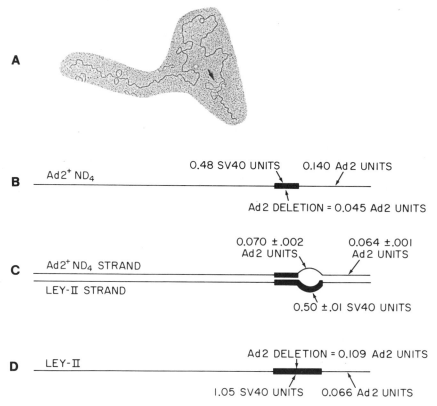

Fig. 9. Ad2$^+$ND$_4$/LEY II heteroduplex. A: Micrograph at 20,000× magnification. The arrow indicates the substitution loop. B: Dimensions of the Ad2$^+$ND$_4$ DNA molecule (Kelly and Lewis, 1973; Morrow *et al.*, 1973). C: Dimensions of Ad2$^+$ND$_4$/LEY II heteroduplexes. D: Dimensions of the LEY II DNA molecule. From Kelly *et al.* (1974).

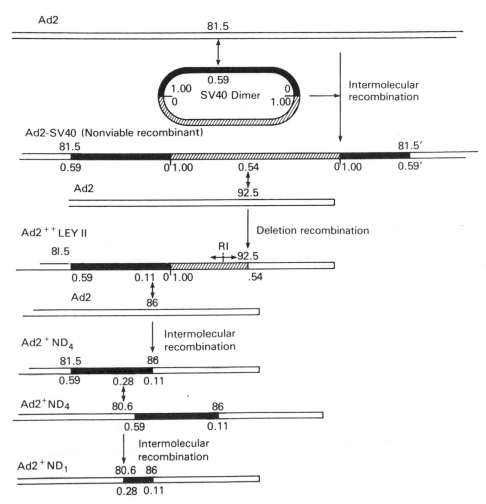

Fig. 10. How Ad2^{++}LEY II might have formed by an initial recombination between Ad2 DNA (▭) and an SV40 dimer (▬ and ▨). The numbers 0–100 above the hybrid molecules indicate Ad2 map positions, and the numbers 0–1.0 below the hybrid molecules indicate SV40 map positions. When a single site is divided by recombination, one coordinate is primed. The double-pointed vertical arrows (↕) indicate the recombination sites on the parental DNA molecules, and the vertical arrows (↓) indicate the recombination product. The middle part of the figure illustrates how Ad2^{+}ND$_{4}$ could have formed by recombination between Ad2^{++}LEY II and Ad2 DNAs. The bottom part of the figure illustrates how Ad2^{+}ND$_{1}$ could have formed by recombination between two Ad2^{+}ND$_{4}$ molecules. The SV40 DNA replication initiation site (RI) is indicated on the Ad2^{++}LEY molecule.

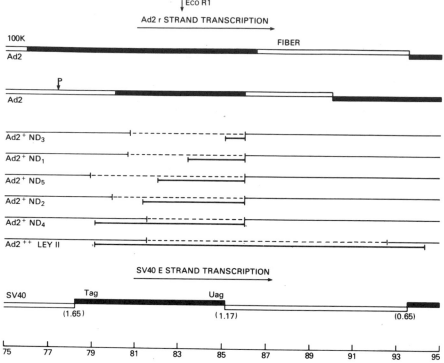

Fig. 11.   Enlargement of the two Ad2 transcription template maps (depicted in Fig. 2) between map positions 75 and 95: early templates (━━) and late templates (▭). The genes for Ad2 100K and fiber proteins are indicated. The position of a proposed new Ad2 promotor located in Ad2⁺⁺LEY and the nondefective Ad2-SV40 hybrids is indicated (P) (Flint *et al.*, 1975). The bottom part of the figure shows tandem SV40 genomes in register with the SV40 segments in the hybrid genomes: early templates (━━) and late templates (▭). The numbers in parentheses indicate the coordinates in SV40 units. The locations of the SV40 Tag and Uag determinates are indicated. The horizontal arrows indicate the direction of Ad2 r strand and SV40 E strand transcription. In the middle of the figure are shown the genomes of Ad2⁺⁺LEY and the five nondefective Ad2-SV40 hybrid viruses; Ad2 DNA (├──┤), deletions of Ad2 DNA (---), and SV40 DNA (├──┤). See Figs. 1 and 2 for references. The *Eco*R1 cleavage site at map position 83.6 (↓) is indicated.

was no longer defective. The genome of the original nondefective isolate, B55, is indistinguishable from that of Ad2⁺ND₄ by the criterion of heteroduplex mapping (A. M. Lewis, Jr., and T. Kelly, unpublished). It is also possible that both Ad2⁺⁺LEY and B55 (or Ad2⁺ND₄) arose from a common precursor different from both. In either case the nondefective recombinant would have a selective advantage since it could replicate both in MKC and HEK without helper virus. When the B55 hybrid, which contains more Ad2 and SV40 DNA than any of the other hybrids, was subsequently passed in HEK, further recombination (Fig. 10) could have led to the formation of other hybrid viruses; any recombinants that remained nondefective for Ad2 functions would propagate in HEK.

8.4. SV40 RNA Transcription during Lytic Infection with Nondefective Adenovirus 2–SV40 Hybrid Viruses

As indicated in Section 7.1, the SV40-specific RNA that accumulates in cells lytically infected with the nondefective hybrid viruses competes effectively with early SV40 RNA. Khoury *et al.* (1973) prepared RNA from MKC infected with each of the five nondefective hybrid viruses and hybridized it with separated strands of SV40 DNA. They showed that only the early SV40 strand hybridized. This result indicated that only the early strand of the SV40 DNA integrated in the Ad2-SV40 hybrid viruses is expressed during lytic infection. Moreover, the early strand of the integrated SV40 segment appeared to be completely transcribed, including the antilate template region between map positions 0.11 and 0.17 (Fig. 1B).

Flint *et al.* (1975; unpublished) infected KB cells with all five of the nondefective Ad2-SV40 hybrid viruses and hybridized RNA accumulating early in the cytoplasm with separated strands of fragments of SV40 DNA prepared by cleavage of superhelical SV40 DNA with the restriction endonucleases *Eco*R1 and *Hpa*I (Fig. 1A). In each case the transcription pattern is consistent with the notion that the SV40 sequences are transcribed from the 5' end of the integrated SV40 early strand to the terminator site at 0.17 (Fig. 1B). Although Flint *et al.* did not detect SV40 RNA sequences from the region 0.17–0.11 SV40 unit (Fig. 1B), it should be noted that they used early cytoplasmic RNA, while Khoury *et al.* (1973) employed late whole cell RNA.

The current view of SV40 mRNA synthesis and processing is that both the E strand and the L strand are transcribed in their entirety (Section 2.3). After transcription the mRNAs are processed to yield functional mRNAs which are transported to the cytoplasm for translation into early and late SV40 proteins. It would be of interest to learn how the processing enzymes recognize the ends of the functional mRNAs. Dhar *et al.* (1974*a,b*, 1975) employed DNA from $Ad2^+ND_1$ and $Ad2^+ND_3$ (both separated strands and double-stranded DNA) to select, by hybridization, early and late SV40 mRNA sequences; the RNAs were then subjected to nucleotide sequencing analysis. These studies have led to nucleotide sequence maps of the 3′ ends of both early and late SV40 mRNAs which show similarities to analogous regions of other mammalian mRNAs. These workers speculate that such regions of homology, which presumably function as processing controls, might provide convenient sites for recombination between viral and mammalian DNA (Dhar *et al.*, 1975). Similar studies of SV40 cRNA synthesis indicate that there are five initiation sites for *E. coli* RNA polymerase within the SV40 segment of $Ad2^+ND_4$ and one site within the SV40 segment of $Ad2^+ND_1$ (Lebowitz *et al.*, 1977).

8.5. Adenovirus 2 Transcription during Lytic Infection with Nondefective Adenovirus 2–SV40 Hybrid Viruses

The initial studies of transcription in cells infected with the nondefective Ad2-SV40 hybrid viruses were limited to examination of SV40 RNA. Subsequently, the same radioactive (late whole cell RNA) preparations were used to challenge separated strands of Ad2 DNA immobilized on nitrocellulose filters (Y. Wewerka and C. Patch, unpublished). The results of these experiments indicated that Ad2 transcription in cells infected by hybrid viruses was indistinguishable from transcription in cells infected by nonhybrid Ad2. More recently, Flint *et al.* (1975) hybridized separated strands of *Eco*R1 fragments of Ad2 DNA (Fig. 2) with cytoplasmic RNA accumulating early (8 hr) in KB cells infected by Ad2, $Ad2^+ND_1$, or $Ad2^+ND_3$. They found that transcription of Ad2 regions of the nondefective hybrid virus DNA differed slightly from transcription of nonhybrid Ad2 DNA. Cells infected with the nondefective viruses failed, of course, to accumulate RNA from the early r-strand template deleted from the hybrid genomes; however, they did accumulate RNA transcripts from a small Ad2 r-strand region (1000 nucleotides long) which is contiguous with the 3′ end of the integrated SV40 DNA (Fig. 11). These Ad2 RNA sequences are not present in early cytoplasmic RNA prepared from cells infected with nonhybrid Ad2, but are found in the cytoplasm late in Ad2 infection. Recently J. Flint (unpublished) has examined early cytoplasmic RNA prepared from KB cells infected with $Ad2^+ND_2$, $Ad2^+ND_4$, or $Ad2^+ND_5$ and the results indicate that transcription of Ad2 RNA from these viruses follows the same pattern as that of $Ad2^+ND_1$ and $Ad2^+ND_3$. Moreover, $Ad2^{++}LEY$, which may be the progenitor of $Ad2^+ND_4$ (Section 8.3), also induces the same late Ad2 RNA sequences as do the nondefective hybrids early in infection (J. Flint, unpublished). These results indicate that the Ad2 and SV40 RNA that accumulates in the cytoplasm early in infection by the nondefective hybrid viruses and Ad2^{++}LEY appears to contain sequences that extend from map position 77.6 (Fig. 11) through the integrated SV40 segment, ending at the SV40 terminator at Ad map position 85.1 (Fig. 11). It is not clear why some RNA sequences that appear to accumulate in the cytoplasm only late in Ad2 infection should be found in early cytoplasmic RNA prepared from cells infected with Ad2^{++}LEY and all of the nondefective hybrid viruses. It is possible that an early Ad2 promoter (Fig. 11) that functions in the hybrid genome is either not present or repressed in the nonhybrid Ad2 genome. Ad2 RNA transcription is complex (Flint and Sharp, 1976) and the nonessential early Ad2 protein which is encoded between map positions 80 and 86, a region that is largely deleted from hybrid genomes (Fig. 11), may play a role in regulation of expression of other Ad2 cistrons. Also, mutations occurring concomitantly during recombination with SV40 could act as new promoters. Furthermore, it is possible that the transcriptional anomaly results from a processing defect. The Ad2 RNA sequences at the 5' ends of mRNAs which accumulate early in hybrid virus infection may be protected from processing enzymes by the presence of SV40 sequences at the 3' ends of the mRNAs (Flint *et al.*, 1975).

It should be noted that the early Ad2 promoter shown at map position 80 on the transcription map of Sharp *et al.* (1974) appears at position 76 on the map of Pettersson *et al.* (1976) (Figs. 2 and 11). This difference could be due to differences in virus strains and might account for the apparent transcriptional anomaly observed by Flint *et al.* (1975). However, with this possibility in mind J. Flint (unpublished) mapped RNA prepared from Ad2$^-$ infected cells and found that the Ad2$^-$ transcription map was essentially the same as the map of Sharp *et al.* (1974) (Figs. 2 and 11). Since it is likely that Ad2$^-$ is the parent nonhybrid Ad2 for all five nondefective Ad2-SV40 hybrids (Fig. 6), it is unlikely that the transcriptional anomaly observed for the hybrid viruses can be entirely due to differences in virus stocks.

The results of Flint *et al.* (1975) suggest that mRNAs accumulating in cells infected with nondefective Ad2-SV40 hybrid viruses may be composed of Ad2 RNA covalently linked to SV40 RNA. Oxman *et al.* (1974) showed that SV40 expression in cells infected with Ad2$^+$ND$_4$ was resistant to interferon. Since interferon inhibits SV40 expression (but not Ad2 expression) in the same cells, this finding implied that SV40 expression in Ad2$^+$ND$_4$-infected cells was regulated by Ad2 promoters. More directly, Oxman *et al.* (1974) demonstrated that 27% of the RNA prepared from Ad2$^+$ND$_4$-infected cells and hybridized to Ad2 DNA could be eluted and rehybridized to SV40 DNA, suggesting that the Ad2 and SV40 RNA sequences were covalently linked. More recently, Dunn and Hassell (1977) and Dunn et al. (1978) have demonstrated that the SV40 RNA that accumulates in cells infected with Ad2$^+$ND$_1$ or Ad2$^+$ND$_1$dp2 is covalently linked to Ad2-specific RNA sequences. Moreover, the Ad2 sequences in the SV40-containing RNA species appear to include leader sequences transcribed from regions distant from the SV40 integration site as well as from Ad2 regions adjacent to the integrated SV40 DNA.

8.6. SV40 Protein Synthesis in Cells Lytically Infected with the Nondefective Adenovirus 2–SV40 Hybrid Viruses

Cell protein synthesis, like cell DNA synthesis, is stimulated by SV40 infection; as a consequence, it is difficult to resolve *de novo* viral proteins from host proteins early in SV40 infection. In contrast, host protein synthesis in cells infected with Ad2 or the Ad2-SV40 hybrid viruses is abrogated, and late in infection protein synthesis is mainly viral. Thus studies of protein synthesis in cells productively infected with the Ad2-SV40 hybrid viruses have proved useful in characterizing early SV40 proteins.

Lopez-Revilla and Walter (1973) detected a protein in gel electropherograms of lysates of Ad2$^+$ND$_1$-infected HeLa cells that was not detectable in Ad2-infected cells. This protein has a molecular weight of 28,000–30,000 (28K–30K) as estimated by electrophoretic mobility (Lopez-Revilla and Walter, 1973; Grodzicker et al., 1976; Mann et al., 1977). Using similar techniques, proteins have been detected in Ad2$^+$ND$_2$-, Ad2$^+$ND$_4$-, and Ad2$^+$ND$_5$-infected HeLa cells which are not found in either Ad2- or Ad2$^+$ND$_3$-infected cells (Table 6) (Walter and Martin, 1975; Anderson et al., 1976). Deppert and Walter (1976) demonstrated that the two new proteins induced by Ad2$^+$ND$_2$ (42K and 56K) were both precipitable with serum from hamsters bearing SV40 tumors, indicating that at least the antigenic determinants of these proteins, which are expressed in SV40-induced hamster tumors, are also encoded by Ad2$^+$ND$_2$ DNA. Using pulse chase experiments, Deppert and Walter (1976) showed that the 42K and 56K proteins induced in HeLa cells by Ad2$^+$ND$_2$ were unstable in the cytoplasm but stable in both the nucleus and plasma membrane of infected cells. This suggested that the nucleus and the plasma membrane were the functional sites of these two proteins. Recently, Deppert (1978) has found that the nuclear-associated SV40 proteins induced by Ad2$^+$ND$_1$ and Ad2$^+$ND$_2$ are principally contained in the nuclear matrix. Nuclear matrices are derived from nuclei by high salt treatment; they are composed principally of protein (87%) and are largely devoid of membranous material as determined by electron microscopy (Hodge *et al.*, 1977). Most of the SV40 proteins induced by Ad2$^+$ND$_4$ are also associated with the nuclear matrix; however, the 72K, 74K, and 95K proteins are partially lost from the nuclear fraction when the nuclear membrane is dissociated (Deppert, 1978).

Jay *et al.* (1977) have also studied the 42K and 56 K SV40 proteins induced in KB cells by Ad2$^+$ND$_2$. These workers found that about two-thirds of the 56K protein and one-third of the 42K protein were localized in the plasma membrane fraction of Ad2$^+$ND$_2$-infected KB cells at 24 hr PI, and the remainder of both proteins was found in the cytoplasm; in contrast to Ad2$^+$ND$_2$-infected HeLa cells (Deppert and Walter, 1976), neither protein was detected in the nucleus. Jay *et al.* (1977) found that much of the cytoplasmic 42K and 56K protein synthesized in Ad2$^+$ND$_2$-infected KB cells was tightly bound to 40 S ribosomes. Moreover, unbound cytoplasmic 42K and 56K protein was shown to bind to purified 40 S ribosomes *in vitro*, the 42K protein binding quantitatively. These observations suggest that one or more SV40 early proteins may function at the level of translation and relate to SV40's Ad-enhancing role (Section 11.2).

Jay *et al.* (1978*a*) have demonstrated that Ad2$^+$ND$_1$ induces two proteins (28K and 30K) in infected KB cells which can be immunoprecipitated by serum from hamsters bearing SV40 tumors. Both proteins are exclusively associated with the plasma membrane and the outer nuclear membrane. The 30K protein, which appears to be a precursor of the 28K protein, is primarily associated with the outer nuclear membrane. The stable 28K protein, which is rapidly formed from the 30K protein by peptide cleavage, is mainly (80%) found in the plasma membrane fraction. The localization of the stable 28K Ad2$^+$ND$_1$ protein on the plasma membrane agrees well with the localization of Uag in the plasma membrane of SV40-transformed cells (Lin *et al.*, 1977).

Ad2$^+$ND$_5$, which induces none of the early SV40 antigens, does induce a 42K protein in infected HeLa cells (Walter and Martin, 1975). However, this protein is unstable in both the nucleus and plasma membrane as well as in the cytoplasm and cannot be precipitated with serum from SV40 tumor-bearing hamsters. The 42K protein induced by Ad2$^+$ND$_5$ is neither functionally nor antigenically active and is presumably the translation product of a partially nonsense mRNA.

Eight proteins ranging in size from 28K to a 95K doublet (Table 6) have been identified in Ad2$^+$ND$_4$-infected HeLa cells; all of these proteins are immunoprecipitable with serum from hamsters bearing SV40 tumors except the small 28K protein (Deppert *et al.*, 1977). The authors suggest that the failure to precipitate the 28K proteins in Ad2$^+$ND$_1$- and Ad2$^+$ND$_4$-infected cells is due to a low titer of antibodies for that protein. Recently Jay *et al.* (1978*a*) precipitated the 28K protein induced by Ad2$^+$ND$_1$ using the serum from T$^+$U$^+$ tumor-bearing hamsters (Lewis and Rowe, 1971). With the exception of the 42K protein, all of the proteins induced by Ad2$^+$ND$_4$ were stable in the nucleus and plasma membrane; the 56K and the 95K doublet as well as the 42K protein were unstable in the cytoplasm (Table 6).

Mann *et al.* (1977) have prepared trypsin digests of methionine-labeled proteins induced by the nondefective Ad2-SV40 hybrid viruses and subjected these digests to two-dimensional peptide separation by electrophoresis and chromatography. Analysis of the resulting peptide patterns indicates that all of the proteins induced by the Ad2-SV40 hybrid viruses have common amino acid sequences at their C termini which are translated from the 3' end of the mRNA(s) (Fig. 11). In addition, this analysis suggests that most of the tryptic peptides derived from the smaller proteins are contained within the larger proteins. The methionine-labeled peptide pattern of the largest SV40 protein induced by Ad2$^+$ND$_4$ (95K) is identical to that derived from SV40 Tag (both lytic and transformed Tag). Mann *et al.* (1977) suggest that the identity between the 95K protein induced by Ad2$^+$ND$_4$ and SV40 Tag provides definitive evidence that SV40 Tag is entirely encoded in SV40 DNA and contains no host encoded peptide sequences.

Most of the SV40 proteins induced *in vivo* by the nondefective Ad2-SV40 hybrid viruses can be synthesized *in vitro* using cell-free protein-synthesizing systems together with RNA purified from cells infected with the various hybrid viruses (Anderson *et al.*, 1976; Grodzicker *et al.*, 1976; Mann *et al.*, 1977). Moreover, the same SV40 proteins can be synthesized *in vitro* using RNA preselected on SV40 DNA, a process that removes all RNAs that do not contain SV40 sequences. In addition, to SV40 proteins, SV40-selected RNAs direct *in vitro* synthesis of non-SV40 proteins whose properties indicate that they are encoded in the Ad2 genome. This finding implies that some RNA species direct the synthesis of both Ad2 and SV40 proteins and indicates that the RNA templates for these proteins are covalently linked. It should be noted that these putative Ad2 proteins are the only proteins synthesized by RNA prepared from cells infected with Ad2$^+$ND$_3$ and preselected on SV40 DNA (Mann *et al.*, 1977). Two of these puta-

TABLE 6

Early SV40 Proteins Induced by Nondefective Ad2-SV40 Hybrid Viruses: Antigenic and Functional Properties

	Virus						
	SV40	Ad2+ND$_1$	Ad2+ND$_1$dp2	Ad2+ND$_2$	Ad2+ND$_3$	Ad2+ND$_4$	Ad2+ND$_5$
Amount of early SV40 template (SV40 units)	0.48	0.12	0.04	0.26	0.01	0.42	0.22
Early SV40 proteins induced (molecular weight × 10^{-3})							
17–20	+						
23							+
28–30		+	+			+	
42				+		+	
56				+		+	
60						+	
64						+	
72						+	
74						+	
95–100	+					+	
Early SV40 antigens induced							
Uag	+	+	?	+	−	+	−
TSTag	+	+		+	−	+	−
Tag	+	−	−	−	−	+	−
Early SV40 functions expressed							
Enhancement of Ad2 replication	+	+	+	+	−	+	−
Initiation of host DNA synthesis	+					−	
Initiation of SV40 DNA synthesis	+					−	
Induction of SV40-like transformation	+	−		−	−	−	−
Induction of SV40-like tumors	+	−		−	−	+	−

tive Ad2 proteins appear to be similar to the Ad2 100K and the Ad2 fiber protein (Grodzicker *et al.*, 1976; Mann *et al.*, 1977); the DNA templates for these proteins lie on either side of the integrated SV40 DNA (Figs. 2 and 11). This finding, together with the observation that late Ad2 RNA sequences are induced early in infection with the nondefective Ad2-SV40 hybrid viruses (Flint *et al.*, 1975), suggests that some RNA polymerases can initiate transcription at a promoter located on the r strand of Ad2 DNA (Fig. 11) and proceed into the integrated SV40 DNA. Most of the transcripts appear to terminate at the SV40 terminator (Fig. 11) early in infection (Flint *et al.*, 1975; unpublished). However, it would appear that at least some of the SV40 transcripts (perhaps initiated late in infection) contain Ad2 sequences on their 3' ends as well.

Some of the hybrid mRNAs apparently contain the appropriate information required to regulate the initiation and termination of translation of various portions of the mRNAs into specific Ad2 or SV40 proteins. None of the proteins studied appears to contain both Ad2 and SV40 peptide sequences within the same molecule (Mann *et al.*, 1977). The smaller SV40 proteins induced by Ad2$^+$ND$_2$ and Ad2$^+$ND$_4$ contain some of the same peptide sequences as the larger proteins. However, it is not known whether this is a consequence of multiple initiation sites for transcription (or translation) or a consequence of mRNA (or polypeptide) processing. However, the fact that the synthesis of both Ad2 and SV40 proteins is directed by mRNAs that have been selected on SV40 DNA suggests that the mRNAs themselves are Ad2-SV40 hybrid mRNAs.

Westphal *et al.* (1979) examined SV40-specific mRNA accumulating in Ad2$^+$ND$_4$-infected HeLa cells by annealing the RNA to SV40, Ad2, or Ad2$^+$ND$_4$ DNA. Most of the DNA-RNA heteroduplex molecules appeared to have non-SV40 RNA at both ends [the RNA on the 3' end presumably includes poly(A) sequences]. Thus the SV40-specific mRNAs induced by Ad2$^+$ND$_4$, like those induced by Ad2$^+$ND$_1$ and Ad2$^+$ND$_1$dp2, are hybrid mRNAs containing Ad2 leader sequences as well as RNA sequences which encode information for both Ad2 and SV40 proteins (Section 8.5).

Westphal *et al.* (1979) observed two classes of SV40 mRNA sequences: The most abundant class (62%) appeared to be a continuous transcript between SV40 map positions 0.16 and 0.46. However, the observed coordinates of the individual heteroduplex molecules varied widely, indicating that this class of mRNAs was a heterogeneous population. The second class of SV40 mRNAs mapped between 0.14 and

0.62, and the coordinates of the ends were much less variable than those of the first class. This latter class of mRNA appears to be transcribed from noncontiguous segments of the SV40 DNA; however, the amount of SV40 RNA deleted is variable. The mRNA which contained the smallest deletion (between SV40 map positions 0.52 and 0.60) resembled the early SV40 mRNA observed by Berk and Sharp (1978) in SV40-infected MKC (Section 13.4). Other mRNAs contained larger deletions of SV40 sequences. Additional evidence indicates that the synthesis of each SV40-specific protein induced by $Ad2^+ND_2$ and $Ad2^+ND_4$ is directed by a specific mRNA, suggesting that these proteins result from processing of the hybrid mRNAs (Lawrence *et al.*, 1979). Westphal *et al.* (1979) and Lawrence *et al.* (1979) suggest that the largest SV40 mRNA (i.e., containing the smallest deletion and closely resembling an SV40-induced mRNA) encodes the information for synthesis of the 90–100K early SV40 protein, while the smaller mRNAs (which are much more abundant) direct the synthesis of smaller SV40 proteins.

Westphal *et al.* (1979) suggest that since the SV40 sequences integrated in $Ad2^+ND_4$ contain translation stop signals near SV40 map position 0.54 (Section 13.4), and since the SV40-specific mRNAs are hybrid mRNAs, it is possible that these stop signals may interfere with efficient synthesis of Ad2 fiber protein encoded downstream from the integrated SV40 DNA. In monkey cells an efficient mechanism (RNA splicing) exists for bypassing these stop signals at the level of transcription. If human cells are deficient in this mechanism, selection pressure in such cells would favor propagation of variants of $Ad2^+ND_4$ from which the SV40 translation stop signals have been deleted. Thus $Ad2^+ND_4$, propagated in human cells, contains a high proportion (80%) of deletion variants (Section 8.2) while B55, propagated in MKC, has remained undeleted. This concept is further supported by the fact that all of the other nondefective Ad2-SV40 hybrids were derived by passage of B55 in human cells (Section 8, Fig. 6).

9. HOST RANGE MUTANTS OF $Ad2^+ND_1$

Grodzicker *et al.* (1974, 1976) have derived host range (*hr*) mutants of $Ad2^+ND_1$ which, like nonhybrid Ad2, propagate well in human cells but yield a hundred- to a thousandfold less virus in MKC. Monkey kidney cells infected with *hr* mutants of $Ad2^+ND_1$ are deficient in the synthesis of SV40 Uag and Ad2 capsid proteins.

The DNAs of *hr* mutants of Ad2⁺ND₁ are indistinguishable from that of nonmutant Ad2⁺ND₁ by the criteria of heteroduplex mapping with Ad2 DNA and the fragment patterns produced by electrophoresis of endonuclease cleavage products. The physical similarity between mutant and nonmutant DNAs suggests that the *hr* mutants of Ad2⁺ND₁ arise from point mutations in the SV40 segment of the viral genomes. The *hr* mutants of Ad2⁺ND₁ do not induce the 28–30K SV40 protein induced by Ad2⁺ND₁ in either human or monkey cells. Moreover, unlike nonmutant Ad2⁺ND₁, cell-free translation of mRNAs, selected from cells infected with *hr* Ad2⁺ND₁ by hybridization with SV40 DNA, fails to yield the 28–30K SV40 protein. However, these mRNAs do direct the synthesis of several new proteins that are smaller than 30K as well as several Ad2 proteins (including the 100K and fiber proteins) whose templates are located on either side of the integrated SV40 DNA (Fig. 11).

The *hr* mutants of Ad2⁺ND₁ fall into two general classes (Grodzicker *et al.*, 1976). Class 1 *hr* mutants are similar to Ad2 in that they yield a thousandfold fewer plaques when assayed in MKC than in human cells. H71, a class 1 *hr* mutant, induces no detectable SV40 Uag in either MKC or human cells; however, it does induce a 10K protein that is not present in either Ad2- or Ad2⁺ND₁-infected cells. Class 2 *hr* mutants are leaky, and the virus yield in MKC is only a hundredfold less than in human cells. H39, a class 2 *hr* mutant, induces SV40 Uag in infected cells; however, the kinetics of induction are slower than in Ad2⁺ND₁-infected cells.

Recent evidence indicates that some of the *hr* mutants of Ad2⁺ND₁ are amber or ochre mutants in which codons that are read as instructions for particular amino acids in the nonmutant genome have mutated to stop signals. These mutations can be suppressed by providing the appropriate yeast tRNA in cell-free translation systems (R. Gesteland, N. Wills, J. Lewis, and T. Grodzicker, manuscript in preparation).

10. REVERTANTS OF HOST RANGE MUTANTS OF Ad2⁺ND₁

Revertants of the *hr* mutants of Ad2⁺ND₁ have been obtained. These revertants appear spontaneously and are selected by their ability to propagate in MKC. The DNAs of the revertants have been examined by heteroduplex mapping and endonuclease cleavage; they appear to be of three types (Sambrook *et al.*, unpublished). The DNAs of one type are indistinguishable from those of the parent $Ad2^+ND_1$ and apparently result from the reversion of a point mutation to the wild-type (WT) nucleotide sequence. The second type of revertant has deletions of portions of the integrated SV40 DNA. This type of revertant could result from intermolecular recombinations between the SV40 segments of two *hr* $Ad2^+ND_1$ molecules in such a way as to delete the ochre or amber mutation which blocks translation of the mRNA. The third type of revertant has an apparent rearrangement of DNA near the region of the integrated SV40 DNA. $Ad2^+ND_1dp2$ (Fig. 1B), which is a revertant of the ochre *hr* mutant H71, is an example of this type (E. Lukanidin, unpublished), and may have resulted from an intermolecular recombination between a point within the SV40 segment of one *hr* mutant and a point in the Ad fiber gene of another *hr* mutant. The revertant molecule would contain the original SV40 segment with its *hr* mutation and a smaller piece of SV40 DNA free of mutations; the two pieces of SV40 DNA would be separated by a small portion (290 base pairs) of the Ad2 fiber gene. $Ad2^+ND_1dp2$ propagates well in MKC and induces a 23K protein which apparently provides the SV40 enhancing function. Unlike in the parent $Ad2^+ND_1$, expression of SV40 genetic information in cells infected with $Ad2^+ND_1dp2$ appears late in infection and the 23K protein is synthesized in much larger quantities than is the 28–30K protein of $Ad2^+ND_1$. Peptide analysis of the 23K protein indicates that the genetic information for only about 55 amino acids is encoded in the SV40 genome; the remainder of this protein (67%) appears to be encoded in the contiguous segment of the Ad2 fiber gene which apparently regulates expression of the 23K protein (Fey *et al.*, 1979). Since this virus is capable of propagating in MKC it follows that the enhancing function of the early SV40 protein requires no more than the 55 amino acids on the C terminus of the SV40 protein. The 23K protein of $Ad2^+ND_1dp2$ is not immunoprecipitable by serum from hamsters bearing SV40 tumors and may lack the Uag determinant of the early SV40 protein (T. Grodzicker, personal communication); however, the 23K protein can be precipitated by anti-Ad2 fiber serum.

11. TEMPERATURE-SENSITIVE MUTANTS OF $Ad2^+ND_1$

Temperature-sensitive (*ts*) mutants of $Ad2^+ND_1$ have been derived that have *ts* defects in the Ad portion of the genome (Williams *et al.*, 1975). Recombinations between the *ts* mutants of $Ad2^+ND_1$ and *ts* mutants of Ad5 have been used to map the defects in the latter (Williams *et al.*, 1975). The frequency with which WT recombinants form from two defective viruses is assumed to be proportional to the distance between the defects on the viral genomes. Similarly, a determination of the proportion of WT recombinants (obtained in a particular cross) that can propagate in MKC provides a measure of the location of the mutation with respect to the integrated SV40 DNA.

The *Eco*R1 restriction endonuclease fragment patterns of Ad2$^+$ND$_1$ and Ad5 DNAs are different (Mulder *et al.*, 1974). Since the genomes of the nondefective recombinants formed between Ad2$^+$ND$_1$ and Ad5 are necessarily composed of DNA from both viruses, it is possible to determine the approximate location of the recombination site by comparing restriction endonuclease fragment patterns of the recombinant DNA with those of the parent viruses (Sambrook *et al.*, 1975). It is of interest to note that only the recombinants selected on MKC contain the *Eco*R1 fragment C' (Mulder *et al.*, 1974), which in turn contains the integrated SV40 DNA (Fig. 2). It is also of interest to note that Williams *et al.* (1970) observed that some nondefective recombinants formed between Ad2$^+$ND$_1$ and Ad5 could be neutralized by both anti-Ad2 and anti-Ad5 sera, indicating that the capsid antigens of the recombinant virions were composed of proteins of both viruses. Temperature-sensitive mutants of Ad2$^+$ND$_1$ have been used to determine the location of the templates for Ad hexon and fiber antigens on the Ad genome (Mautner *et al.*, 1975).

12. EARLY SV40 ANTIGENS AND FUNCTIONS EXPRESSED BY THE NONDEFECTIVE ADENOVIRUS 2–SV40 HYBRID VIRUSES

In cells permissive for SV40 infection, the early SV40 gene products induce viral and host DNA synthesis and enhance Ad propagation in cells coinfected with Ad (Martin *et al.*, 1974). In cells nonpermissive or semipermissive for SV40 infection, the early SV40 gene products may function to induce and maintain cell transformation (Section 13) (Martin *et al.*, 1974). In both permissive and nonpermissive infection, two early intranuclear SV40 antigens (Tag and Uag) can be detected either by immunofluorescent staining or by complement fixation, and a third early antigen, TSTag, can be demonstrated by the ability of SV40-immunized animals to reject tumor induction by SV40.

12.1. Early SV40 Antigens

Robb (1977) has shown that proteins having molecular weights of 84K, 89K, and 94K, which are induced in cells permissively or non-permissively infected with SV40, can be precipitated by both anti-SV40 Tag serum (from tumor-bearing hamsters) and anti-SV40 Uag serum [from monkeys immunized with $Ad2^+ND_1$-infected MKC (Lewis and Rowe, 1971)]. This finding indicates that both antigenic sites are located on the same molecular species. Anderson et al. (1977a,b) have studied the properties of cells transformed by SV40 tsA mutants and have concluded that Tag and TSTag are functionally related. This evidence suggests that all three of the early SV40 antigens are associated with a single early protein (or with derivatives of this protein), which has a molecular weight of 90K–100K. This protein may have different antigenic and functional sites which mediate early SV40 functions.

Studies with the nondefective Ad2-SV40 hybrid viruses have revealed the relative relationship of the templates for Tag, Uag, and TSTag on the physical map of the SV40 genome (Fig. 11) (Kelly and Lewis, 1973). The Tag determinant is probably located near the amino end of the 90–100K early SV40 protein (Fig. 1B) since $Ad2^+ND_4$, but none of the other nondefective hybrid viruses (which contain less SV40 DNA) induces SV40 Tag. The Uag determinant must be localized on the C terminus of the early SV40 protein since it is induced by $Ad2^+ND_1$, which contains only this portion of the early SV40 genome. The third early SV40 antigen, TSTag, is located near the C terminus of the early SV40 protein, perhaps between Uag and Tag. $Ad2^+ND_2$, but not $Ad2^+ND_1$, induces TSTag in immunized hamsters (Lewis and Rowe, 1973). However, Jay et al. (1978b) have shown that TSTag is induced in mice immunized with large amounts (2×10^9 pfu) of $Ad2^+ND_1$. Moreover, virus-free cell fractions (containing the 28K protein) of $Ad2^+ND_1$-infected cells can be used to immunize mice against tumor induction by SV40-transformed cells (Jay et al., 1978b). The reason for this discrepancy remains unclear but may indicate that the mouse system is more sensitive to TSTag than is the hamster system (Section 6.2) (Tevethia and Lewis, 1976). Alternatively, there may be several different protein species having TSTag activity which differ in their antigenicity in different animals.

Studies with the nondefective Ad2-SV40 hybrid viruses have shown that expression of early SV40 antigenic determinants does not require that the 90–100K early SV40 protein be intact. Uag and TSTag are expressed on proteins no more than one-third to one-half the size of the early SV40 protein. It is also evident from these studies that functional sites of the 90–100K early SV40 protein may act independently. Moreover, SV40 *tsA* mutants, which do not express most early SV40 functions, nevertheless enhance Ad replication in MKC at nonpermissive temperatures (Martin *et al.*, 1974; Jerkofsky and Rapp, 1975).

12.2. SV40 Enhancement of Adenovirus Replication in Monkey Kidney Cells

Although the mechanism of SV40 enhancement of Ad propagation in MKC is not yet understood, the nondefective Ad2-SV40 hybrid viruses have been useful in the study of this early SV40 function. Only the C terminus of the early 90–100K SV40 protein appears to be required for the enhancement function, since Ad2$^+$ND$_1$ (which contains only about 25% of the early SV40 genome encoding the C terminus of the early SV40 protein) is capable of enhancing Ad propagation in MKC. Moreover, a 23K protein induced by Ad2$^+$ND$_1$dp2, which contains only 55 SV40-encoded amino acids, provides the enhancing function (Fey *et al.*, 1979).

As discussed in Section 3.5, the block to Ad propagation in MKC appears to be due to the failure of certain late Ad2 mRNAs to form functional polyribosomes which are capable of protein synthesis. Jay *et al.* (1977) showed that the 42K and 56K proteins induced by Ad2$^+$ND$_2$ (which enhances Ad2 replication in MKC) bind strongly to 40 S ribosomes. Studies with the host range mutants of Ad2$^+$ND$_1$ indicate that the failure of these mutants to induce a 30K SV40 protein is closely correlated with the failure to induce SV40 Uag and the inability of these viruses to propagate in MKC. Together these results suggest that SV40 enhancement of Ad2 propagation in MKC is mediated by SV40 proteins that carry the Uag site. [The Uag determinant may not be an absolute requirement since the 23K protein of Ad2$^+$ND$_1$dp2 apparently lacks Uag activity (Section 10).] These SV40 proteins may bind to ribosomes and permit late Ad2 mRNAs to form functional polyribosomes and be efficiently translated into Ad capsid proteins.

Jay *et al.* (1978*a*) have demonstrated that a stable 28K protein induced by Ad2$^+$ND$_1$ is primarily associated with the plasma membrane fraction of infected cells, while its apparent precursor, an unstable 30K protein, is mainly associated with the outer nuclear membrane. Although the plasma membrane fraction studied by Jay *et al.* (1978*a*) includes a rough endoplasmic reticulum and therefore may be involved in viral protein synthesis, these authors also suggest that SV40 enhancement of Ad2 propagation may be mediated by transport of viral mRNA from the nucleus to the cytoplasm. Deppert (1978) has concluded that most of the proteins induced by the nondefective Ad2-SV40 hybrid viruses are associated with the nuclear matrix (Section 8.6). He suggests that the association of these proteins with the nucleus may imply that SV40 enhancement of Ad replication involves processing and/or transport of Ad mRNA.

12.3. Host DNA Synthesis

Host cell DNA synthesis is stimulated during productive infection with SV40 (Gershon et al., 1966). In contrast, host cell DNA synthesis is inhibited during productive infection by Ad, both in HEK and in SV40-enhanced MKC (Ginsberg et al., 1967). Since initiation of cellular DNA synthesis is an early SV40 function, it was of interest to determine whether or not host DNA synthesis was stimulated by infection with Ad2$^+$ND$_4$. Accordingly, Schnipper et al. (1973) examined cellular DNA synthesis in MKC and hamster cells infected with Ad2$^+$ND$_4$. These workers found that, like Ad2, Ad2$^+$ND$_4$ inhibits cellular DNA synthesis in MKC. In contrast, both viruses stimulate host DNA synthesis in semipermissive hamster cells. Thus Schnipper et al. (1973) found no detectable differences between Ad2 and Ad2$^+$ND$_4$ with respect to influence on host DNA synthesis.

13. CELL TRANSFORMATION AND TUMOR INDUCTION BY SV40 AND THE ADENOVIRUSES

SV40 will induce tumors in hamsters and mastomys in vivo and transform the cells of a variety of mammalian species in vitro. Many of the human adenoviruses (Ad) induce tumors in hamsters and all transform hamster cells in tissue culture (Table 1). Several comprehensive reviews on SV40 and Ad oncogenicity have been published (Black, 1968; Gross, 1970; Butel et al., 1972; Rapp, 1973; Tooze, 1973).

When newborn hamsters are inoculated with various strains of SV40, 25–100% of the animals develop tumors at the site of injection (subcutaneous, intracerebral, intraperitoneal, or intrathoracic) within 3–12 months (Eddy et al., 1962; Girardi et al., 1962; Rabson et al., 1962; Takemoto et al., 1966) (Table 1). The incidence of tumor induction as well as the latent period before tumor development appears to depend on the amount of virus inoculated. The oncogenicity of SV40 in older hamsters is much less than in newborn animals (Girardi *et al.*, 1963; Allison *et al.*, 1967).

SV40 transforms a number of permissive, semipermissive, and nonpermissive cell types in tissue culture. Hamster cells transformed by SV40 *in vitro* develop into tumors when injected into hamsters; with some cell lines, fewer than 100 transformed cells will induce tumors in half the animals injected (Rapp and Melnick, 1966). Similarly, SV40 tumor cells taken from one hamster can be transplanted in other animals.

SV40 does not induce tumors in newborn mice; however, when nonpermissive mouse 3T3 cells are infected in tissue culture at high multiplicity (e.g., 1000 pfu/cell), as many as 50% of the cells become transformed (Todaro and Green, 1966). Mouse embryo cells (BALB/c) newly transformed by SV40 do not induce tumors in immunoin-competent mice; however, after prolonged passage in tissue culture SV40-transformed mouse cells will induce tumors in newborn mice (Tevethia and McMillan, 1974). Both hamsters and mice can be immunized against SV40 tumor induction with either SV40 or Ad-SV40 hybrid viruses that induce SV40 TSTag (Table 2).

The highly oncogenic adenoviruses (Table 1), when injected into newborn hamsters, will induce tumors in 55–94% of the animals within 2–3 months after injection (Gross, 1970). Fewer animals develop tumors when inoculated with the weakly oncogenic adenoviruses, and the latent period is longer (4–18 months). Although tumor induction differs between the highly oncogenic and weakly oncogenic adenoviruses, the tumors, once induced, are morphologically similar (Tooze, 1973). Hamster cells transformed *in vitro* by the adenoviruses will produce tumors when inoculated into newborn hamsters.

Studies with Ad2-transformed rat cells indicate a correlation between the oncogenicity of the transformed cells in immunosuppressed rats and the multiplicity of infecting virus used to effect transformation (Harwood and Gallimore, 1975). This finding suggests that the onco-genicity of transformed cells may depend on the number of viral genomes that become integrated in the cellular chromosomes. It is possible that oncogenicity is conferred on transformed cells by viral integration at particular loci and that the more viral genomes integrated the higher the probability of integration at one of these loci.

Although transformation by either SV40 or the adenoviruses is relatively inefficient compared to lytic infection (Table 1), viral dilution assays exhibit a first-order concentration dependence, indicating that cell transformation is effected by single virions. Cell transformation is induced *in vitro* by DNA purified from either SV40 or Ad, although transformation efficiency is much less than with intact virus (Graham *et al.*, 1974*b*). Moreover, fragments of SV40 or Ad DNA that contain the oncogenic regions of these viruses (SV40 early region or the left end of the Ad genome, Figs. 1 and 2) will transform cells *in vitro* (Graham *et al.*, 1974*b*; Yano *et al.*, 1977).

Viral transformation is usually accompanied by loss of contact inhibition, which limits cell density in untransformed cells by inhibition of cell division and motility. Loss of contact inhibition together with changes in cell morphology often leads to the marked changes in colony morphology associated with transformation. Individual cells transformed by SV40 are usually larger than untransformed cells and are more polygonal in shape, having enlarged nuclei with prominent nucleoli. Cells transformed by Ad can readily be distinguished from untransformed or SV40-transformed cells; they are more uniform, smaller, and rounder, with little cytoplasm (Black, 1968).

Most transformed cells are aneuploid or polyploid and exhibit altered chromosomal morphology. Cells transformed by SV40 frequently exhibit chromosomal breaks and translocations. Changes in the chromosomal morphology of Ad-transformed cells are much less pronounced than those of SV40-transformed cells (Black, 1968).

In addition to loss of contact inhibition and cytomorphological changes, transformed cells usually differ from untransformed cells in their growth requirements. Unlike most untransformed cells, transformed cells will grow in medium containing very low concentrations of serum or in semisolid agar (0.33%) and frequently even in suspension culture. Since the rate of propagation of transformed cells is greater than that of untransformed cells and since their growth requirements are less fastidious, transformed cells usually overgrow and eliminate untransformed cells from mixed populations of transformed and untransformed cells (Black, 1968).

Cells semipermissive for SV40, and transformed by nondefective SV40, may yield low levels of infectious virus. Transformed cells that are either semipermissive or nonpermissive may yield infectious SV40 when fused with permissive cells (Gerber, 1966). The mechanism(s) of virus "rescue" whereby integrated viral genomes become freely replicating viral genomes is not understood. However, it is possible that the mechanism of virus rescue from transformed cells is similar to that of SV40 induction by the Ad2^{++}HEY and Ad2^{++}LEY populations (Section 7.2).

The precise sequence of molecular events that leads to the transformed state is not known. However, all cells transformed by

SV40 or Ad contain viral DNA integrated in cellular chromosomes. The integrated viral DNA found in stably transformed cells may be composed of fragments of one or more viral genomes or multiple copies of the complete viral genome. In these transformed cells the early regions of integrated SV40 and Ad are always transcribed and translated into early viral antigens (Section 2.4). Studies with temperature-sensitive mutants of SV40 indicate that the entire early region must function to induce and maintain SV40-transformed cells in their neoplastic state (Martin and Chou, 1975; Tegtmeyer, 1975; Brugge and Butel, 1975; Osborn and Weber, 1975). Since cells transformed with temperature-sensitive mutants of SV40 cannot be tested in their mammalian hosts at permissive and nonpermissive temperatures, the influence of these mutations on the tumor-inducing potential of these transformed cells cannot be determined. SV40 proteins induced by the nondefective Ad2-SV40 hybrid viruses are frequently found associated with the nuclear and cytoplasmic membranes (Section 8.6). Since these proteins are all encoded in the early region of the SV40 genome, this finding suggests that the transformed state may result from perturbations of normal membrane functions due to the presence of the viral proteins *per se* or due to preemptive early viral functions.

13.1.   Cell Transformation and Tumor Induction by Ad7$^+$

The first Ad-SV40 hybrid virus to be studied extensively was Ad7$^+$, which was derived from the weakly oncogenic Ad7 (Section 4). Huebner *et al.* (1964) demonstrated that the defective Ad7$^+$ hybrid, which was free of infectious SV40, induced tumors in 75% of newborn hamsters 2–4 months after inoculation. The observed latent period for tumor induction by Ad7$^+$ was shorter than that of either SV40 or Ad7. The histomorphology of tumors induced by Ad7$^+$ generally resembled that of SV40-induced tumors; however, the tumors frequently contained regions of small uniform cells characteristic of Ad-induced tumors. The sera of animals bearing Ad7$^+$-induced tumors usually contained antibodies against SV40 Tag. Antibodies against Ad7 Tag were found only in animals bearing tumors with Ad or mixed Ad and SV40 morphology (Rapp, 1973).

Black and Todaro (1965) transformed hamster cells *in vitro* with Ad7$^+$. Transformation was inhibited with anti-Ad7 serum but not with anti-SV40 serum. Cells transformed by Ad7$^+$ accumulate SV40 Tag, and the cytomorphological characteristics of Ad7$^+$-transformed cells are similar to those of SV40-transformed cells (Black and White, 1967).

Transformation by Ad7$^+$, unlike Ad7$^+$ lytic infection in MKC, exhibits a first-order dilution dependence, indicating that neither Ad-like nor SV40-like transformation requires helper function (Duff and Rapp, 1970). Hamster cells transformed by Ad7$^+$ induce tumors when inoculated into newborn hamsters; the histomorphology of most of these tumors is similar to that of tumors induced by SV40 (Igel and Black, 1967).

The Ad7$^+$ hybrid virus population is composed of both nonhybrid Ad7 (80%) and Ad7-SV40 hybrid virus (20%); thus transformation and tumor induction could be induced by hybrid virus, nonhybrid Ad7, or both. However, most of the tumors induced by Ad7$^+$ express SV40 genetic information and are morphologically similar to SV40 tumors. Thus it would appear that the oncogenic potential of Ad7$^+$ is mediated mainly by the SV40 genetic material contained in the hybrid virus despite the fact that it comprises only a small part of the total genetic information in the Ad7$^+$ population.

It is not clear why the defective Ad7-SV40 hybrid virus should induce tumors more efficiently than either Ad7 or SV40. However, it is likely that the tumorigenicity of any virus is determined by a variety of factors such as the ability of the virus to penetrate the host defenses and infect cells at the site of inoculation, the probability that an infected cell will become transformed, the frequency with which transformed cells become incipient tumors and the number of cell generations required for this to occur, and the likelihood that an incipient tumor will be rejected by its host. The tumor incidence and the latent period for tumor development in any virus–host system are probably determined by a combination of these and other factors. Thus it is possible that a hybrid virus, which has various oncogenic features of both parent viruses, could be more oncogenic than either of its parents.

13.2. Oncogenicity of Transcapsidated Adenovirus 7–SV40 Hybrid Viruses

The SV40 genetic material in Ad7$^+$ is readily transferred to capsids of other Ad serotypes (Section 5.2). Black *et al.* (1969) transcapsidated the SV40 component of Ad7$^+$ to the highly oncogenic Ad12 and the nononcogenic Ad2. The transcapsidated viruses, designated Ad12^{+t7} and Ad2^{+t7}, were used to transform hamster cells *in vitro*. The transformed cells were cloned and the clonal lines were used to induce tumors in hamsters. Cytomorphological analysis of the cloned transformed cell lines indicated that both Ad12^{+t7}- and Ad2^{+t7}-transformed cells consisted of three different cell phenotypes. Some resembled cells transformed by SV40, others resembled cells transformed by Ad, and a third intermediate type had features of both SV40- and Ad-transformed cells. Histomorphological analysis of tumors induced by the various clones indicated that clones having SV40 or Ad cytomorphology usually induced tumors with SV40 or Ad histomorphology, respectively. However, the histomorphology of tumors induced by clones with intermediate cytomorphology more often resembled that of Ad tumors.

Levin *et al.* (1969) extracted radioactive RNA from the transformed clones characterized by Black *et al.* (1969) and hybridized it with DNA from SV40, Ad7, Ad2, and Ad12. In general, cells with SV40 cytomorphology accumulated SV40 and Ad7 RNA, while those with Ad cytomorphology accumulated either Ad2 or Ad12 RNA. Clones with intermediate morphology usually accumulated SV40, Ad7, and either Ad2 or Ad12 RNA. Thus there was a correlation between the transformed cell morphological phenotype and the expression of integrated viral genomes.

Butel *et al.* (1972) demonstrated that the latent period for tumor induction in newborn hamsters by Ad12^{+t7} was only 1–2 months, much shorter than for either SV40 or Ad12. The tumors accumulated both SV40 and Ad12 Tag, indicating that both viral genomes were expressed in the transformed cells.

The *in vivo* oncogenic potential of other transcapsidants derived from Ad7$^+$ was studied by Rapp *et al.* (1968). Transcapsidation of Ad1, Ad2, Ad5, and Ad6 changed these nononcogenic Ad serotypes into viruses that induced tumors in hamsters. The oncogenicity of the weakly oncogenic Ad3 was enhanced, while that of Ad14, Ad16, and Ad21 remained unchanged. Although the oncogenicity of transcapsidated viruses was variable, all induced SV40 TSTag and animals immunized with these viruses rejected tumor induction by SV40.

Thus studies of transformation and tumor induction by Ad7$^+$ and its transcapsidated derivatives show that the oncogenic potential of some Ad serotypes is significantly enhanced by the presence of SV40 genetic material in the infecting viral population. Transformed cell and tumor morphology varies from that characteristic of SV40 to that characteristic of Ad with intermediate morphological types as well. The latent period of tumor induction by these Ad-SV40 recombinants is frequently shorter than the latent period of tumor induction by either SV40 or Ad alone.

13.3. Cell Transformation and Tumor Induction by Defective Adenovirus-SV40 Hybrid Viruses That Yield Infectious SV40

Schell *et al.* (1966) created an Ad12-SV40 hybrid virus by coinfecting MKC with SV40 and Ad12 (Section 6). The hybrid virus population, which we have designated "Ad12^{++}", induced tumors in hamsters as efficiently as Ad12 and SV40; however, the latent period of tumor induction was significantly reduced (27 days, as compared with 42 days for nonhybrid Ad12 and 117 days for nonhybrid SV40). Tumor induction by Ad12^{++} was inhibited with anti-Ad12 serum but not with anti-SV40 serum. The tumors induced by Ad12^{++} accumulated both Ad12 and SV40 Tags.

Fifteen to forty percent of newborn Syrian hamsters injected subcutaneously with the Ad-SV40 hybrid virus population Ad1^{++}, Ad2^{++}, or Ad5^{++} developed tumors in 3–10 months (A. M. Lewis, Jr., unpublished). Although all three hybrid virus populations induce infectious SV40 (Table 2), the incidence of tumor development was not reduced by mixing the inoculum with SV40-neutralizing antibodies. Hamsters carrying transplants of the tumors induced by Ad1^{++} and Ad2^{++} develop antibodies to both SV40 and Ad Tag. Black *et al.* (1967) and Gilden *et al.* (1968) used sera from these animals to define the subgroup C Ad Tag.

Black and White (1967) transformed hamster cells with Ad2^{++}, Ad3^{+}, and Ad12^{++} hybrid populations. Cell lines designated "Ad2^{++}HK1" and "Ad2^{++}HK2," established from Ad2^{++}-transformed cultures, contained serologically detectable SV40 Tag but not Ad2 Tag and appeared morphologically similar to SV40 transformed hamster cells. Despite the absence of detectable Ad2 Tag in Ad2^{++}-transformed lines, hamsters carrying tumors induced by these cells developed antibodies to both Ad2 and SV40 Tag.

Igel and Black (1967) examined hamster tumors induced by hamster cells transformed by Ad2^{++}, Ad3^{+}, Ad7^{+}, and Ad12^{++}. Histomorphologically these tumors were pleomorphic fibrosarcomas. Although they appeared to be similar to tumors induced by SV40-transformed hamster cells, they contained carcinomatous components and occasional "nests of cells" resembling those seen in Ad-induced tumors.

Black *et al.* (1967) showed that hamsters carrying tumors induced by Ad1^{++} or by hamster cells transformed by Ad2^{++} developed antibodies to both Ad and SV40 Tag. Eleven of 23 sera from animals bearing Ad2^{++}-transformed cell-induced tumors (and immune ascites fluids prepared from four different animals by immunization with virus-free Ad2^{++} tumor extracts) reacted only with FUdR-sensitive (i.e., late) Ad2 antigens when tested by immunofluorescence (IF). None of these sera contained detectable Ad2-neutralizing antibody, and it is possible that the IF staining patterns were due to the early Ad DNA binding protein which undergoes an altered morphological pattern in cells treated with FUdR (Sugawara *et al.*, 1977). Twenty-five percent of the sera from hamsters carrying Ad1^{++} and Ad2^{++} tumors reacted (by IF) with early antigens in Ad3- and Ad7-infected cells, while none of the sera tested reacted with cells infected by Ad4, Ad8, or Ad12. Cloned lines of Ad1^{++}- and Ad2^{++}-transformed cells produced tumors when injected into hamsters. Animals carrying tumors induced by these clones developed antibodies to Ad2 T ag. The authors concluded from these results that the nononcogenic Ad1 and Ad2 genomes were integrated into the chromosomes of hamster cells transformed by Ad1^{++} and Ad2^{++} hybrid populations and that the T ag of Ad1 and Ad2 were closely related to each other but distinct from the T ag induced by the human adenovirus A and B subgroups. These conclusions were verified by Gilden *et al.* (1968) in their characterization of the subgroup specificity of group C Ad T ag by complement fixation.

Thus transformation and tumor induction by defective Ad-SV40 hybrid virus populations that contain infectious SV40 are like those of Ad7$^+$, which contains the early region of SV40 but does not induce free SV40. Moreover, the fact that anti-SV40 serum has no influence on the oncogenicity of Ad1^{++}, Ad2^{++}, or Ad5^{++} indicates that the oncogenicity of these viruses is mediated mainly by the hybrid virus component of the virus population.

13.4. Cell Transformation and Tumor Induction by Adenovirus 2 and the Nondefective Adenovirus 2–SV40 Hybrid Viruses

The usefulness of the nondefective Ad2-SV40 hybrid viruses in associating segments of the early SV40 genome with induction of the three early SV40 antigens has been discussed in Section 12. Since the early region of the SV40 genome is evidently responsible for the oncogenicity of SV40, the presence of the appropriate segment of SV40 DNA in the genome of one of the nondefective Ad2-SV40 hybrid viruses might alter its oncogenicity compared to that of nonhybrid Ad2.

SV40 oncogenicity appears to be mediated by early SV40 protein(s) (Section 2.3.1). Both the large (90–100K) and the small (17–20K) early SV40 proteins appear to be translated from 19 S mRNAs encoded in the SV40 genome between map positions 0.65 and 0.17 (Fig. 1). However, the mRNA for the 17–20K protein appears to contain multiple translation stop signals (in all three reading frames) near map position 0.54 (Reddy *et al.*, 1978). The mRNA for the 90–100K protein appears to contain a deletion (including the stop signals) between map positions 0.59 and 0.54 (Berk and Sharp, 1978). Both early SV40 proteins have identical N termini (Paucha *et al.*, 1978), indicating that translation of both mRNAs begins at the same point on the 5' end of the mRNAs. Translation of one mRNA stops near 0.54, giving rise to the 17–20K protein, while the other mRNA (from which the stop signal has been deleted) is translated in its entirety, giving rise to the 90–100K protein (Berk and Sharp, 1978). If both early SV40 proteins have the same N termini encoded near 0.65, then the 90–100K SV40 protein induced by $Ad2^+ND_4$, whose N terminus is encoded near 0.59, cannot be identical to the 90–100K early protein induced by SV40 (Fig. 1 and Table 6). Moreover, the 17–20K early protein induced by SV40 has not been demonstrated in $Ad2^+ND_4$-infected cells. Thus the precise structural relationship between the SV40 proteins induced by $Ad2^+ND_4$ and the large and small early proteins induced by SV40 remains unclear. However, it is not known whether the small early SV40 protein is required for tumor induction by SV40, and the absolute requirement for this protein in cell transformation has not been established (Sleigh *et al.*, 1978). Thus study of the oncogenic potential of the nondefective Ad2-SV40 hybrid viruses could provide insight into the molecular mechanism(s) of SV40 oncogenicity.

Lewis *et al.* (1974a) found that nonhybrid Ad2 and each of the nondefective hybrids would transform hamster kidney cells in tissue culture. All transformed cell lines contained Ad2 Tag and Ad2 RNA. However, only cells transformed by $Ad2^+ND_2$, $Ad2^+ND_4$, and B55 [which is indistinguishable from $Ad2^+ND_4$ (Section 8)] contained early SV40 antigens and detectable amounts of SV40 RNA. Cell lines established from these cultures induced tumors when injected into hamsters. The morphology of the hybrid-transformed colonies and histopathology of tumors induced by hybrid-transformed cells were indistinguishable from those of Ad2-transformed colonies and Ad2-transformed cell-induced tumors. These results implied that transformation of hamster cells was governed by the Ad portion of the hybrid viral genomes.

Breeden *et al.* (1976) and Patch *et al.* (1979) found that cellular DNA prepared from all of the transformed hamster lines characterized by Lewis *et al.* (1974a) contained Ad2 DNA. The amount of integrated viral DNA varied from fragments (39%) to multiple copies of the complete viral genome. In addition, these workers prepared RNAs from all of the transformed cell lines and hybridized them with separated strands of radioactive Ad2 or SV40 DNA. They found that both Ad2 DNA strands were transcribed more extensively in cells transformed by hybrid viruses than in cells transformed by nonhybrid Ad2 (Fig. 2). Ad2 "l"-strand transcription was much more extensive in cells transformed by hybrid viruses, exceeding even that observed in cells lytically infected with Ad2. SV40 RNA was detected in two cell lines transformed by $Ad2^+ND_2$ and $Ad2^+ND_4$; in both lines the entire E strand of the integrated SV40 DNA was transcribed while cellular RNA showed no homology with the SV40 L strand.

Thus, while genetic expression in cells transformed by either Ad2 or the nondefective hybrid viruses is quite different, all of the transformed cells are morphologically indistinguishable. While a variety of factors (i.e., integration site and host promoters) might influence genetic expression, it would appear that the transformed cell phenotype of cells stably transformed by the nondefective hybrid viruses is governed by the Ad2 transforming function.

Since hamster cells transformed by Ad2-SV40 hybrid viruses are morphologically indistinguishable from hamster cells transformed by nonhybrid Ad2, the next question to be studied was whether any of the SV40 DNA segments in the nondefective hybrids alter the efficiency with which these viruses transform cells. To answer this question, the transforming efficiencies of Ad2 and the three nondefective hybrids that induce early SV40 antigens (Table 6) were compared in hamster and rat embryo cells (A. M. Lewis, Jr., unpublished). Using Ad2 inactivated by exposure to ultraviolet light (UV) to retard virus-induced cytopathology, assays were developed which related the dose of Ad2 virions to the number of transformed foci developing in infected hamster and rat embryo cells (Lewis *et al.*, 1974*b*; unpublished). In these assays the number of foci was proportional to the virus dose at the dilutions assayed; therefore, the transforming efficiency of Ad2 could be determined and compared with the transforming efficiency of the nondefective hybrids.

Initial studies comparing transforming efficiencies of UV inactivated Ad2, $Ad2^+ND_2$, $Ad2^+ND_4$, and B55 (grown in different lots of AGMK or HEK cells) indicated that $Ad2^+ND_4$ and B55 transformed hamster cells somewhat more efficiently than did Ad2 or $Ad2^+ND_2$ [10^6 pfu/ffu (plaque-forming units per focus of transformed cells) as compared with 10^7 pfu/ffu]. However, when all virus stocks were grown in the same lot of Vero cells, inactivated by UV, and tested for transforming efficiency in rat embryo cells, the observed differences were even less. Thus, in these assays, the SV40 DNA segments in the nondefective hybrids did not appear to render the recombinants significantly more efficient than Ad2 in transforming cells (A. M. Lewis, Jr., unpublished).

A third approach to the question of the influence of the SV40 DNA segment within the nondefective hybrids on the oncogenicity of the Ad2 genome involved injecting virus into large numbers of newborn hamsters. In a single experiment hamsters injected with Ad2 and four of the five nondefective hybrids failed to develop tumors during observation periods ranging from 199 to 643 days (Lewis *et al.*, 1974*b*).

In a fourth study, newborn hamsters were injected with either Ad2 or nondefective hybrids (after UV inactivation) and observed for 500–540 days. These results showed that the tumor incidence (number of hamsters with tumors/number of hamsters surviving) for UV-inactivated $Ad2^+ND_4$ and B55 was 12% and 3% respectively (Lewis and Cook, 1979). In another experiment, the incidence of tumors in injected animals was reduced from 3/13 (23%) to 1/31 (3%) when the UV-inactivated $Ad2^+ND_4$ was pretreated with anti-Ad2 serum. On the other hand, no virus-specific tumors developed in hamsters injected with UV-inactivated Ad2 or Ad^+ND_2. The tumors induced by $Ad2^+ND_4$ and B55 contained both Ad2 and SV40 Tag. Tumor-bearing animals developed antibodies against both Ad and SV40 antigens. Histopathologically the tumors appeared to be either SV40 type fibrosarcomas; small cell, undifferentiated Ad-type tumors; or a mixture of both. Cell lines were established from the tumors induced by UV-inactivated $Ad2^+ND_4$. The rate of reassociation between tumor cell DNA from two of these lines and radioactive Ad2 DNA indicated that cells from both $Ad2^+ND_4$ tumor lines contained Ad2 DNA (Lewis and Cook, 1979).

It would appear from these experiments that UV-inactivated $Ad2^+ND_4$ induced SV40-like as well as Ad-like tumors in hamsters while UV-inactivated Ad2 or $Ad2^+ND_2$ did not. The incidence of tumors induced by UV-inactivated $Ad2^+ND_4$ is less than that observed with infectious SV40 in the same host (Table 1). The low incidence of tumor induction by $Ad2^+ND_4$ may be a consequence of damage to the oncogenic region of the SV40 genome by UV irradiation, of Ad2 TSTag function, or of other unknown factors.

Thus the segment of SV40 DNA in $Ad2^+ND_4$, which contains most but not all of the early SV40 region (Figs. 1B and 11), is sufficient to induce SV40-like tumors *in vivo*. Since $Ad2^+ND_2$ does not induce tumors, it follows that all or part of the segment of SV40 DNA between 0.43 and 0.59 (Figs. 1B and 11) is essential for SV40 oncogenicity. This finding confirms and extends the results of Martin and Chou (1975), Tegtmeyer (1975), Brugge and Butel (1975), and Osborn and Weber (1975), which imply that the entire early region in SV40 temperature-sensitive mutants must function to induce and maintain the phenotype of the SV40-transformed cell. However, all of these data leave unanswered the question of whether the Tag determinant of the early SV40 protein(s) (encoded between 0.43 and 0.59) is sufficient to induce carcinogenesis, or whether other antigenic determinants (Uag and TSTag) (encoded between 0.17 and 0.43) are also required.

14. REFERENCES

Allison, A. C., Chesterman, F. C., and Baron, S., 1967, Induction of tumors in adult hamsters with SV40, *J. Natl. Cancer Inst.* **38**:567.

Altstein, A. D., and Dodonova, N. N., 1968, Interaction between human and simian adenoviruses in simian cells: Complementation, phenotypic mixing and formation of monkey cell "adapted" virions, *Virology* **35**:248.

Altstein, A. D., Dodonova, N. N., Vassilyeva, N. N., and Tsetlin, E. M., 1968, Hybrid of monkey and human adenoviruses, *J. Virol.* **2**:488.

Anderson, C. W., Lewis, J. B., Baum, D. R., and Gesteland, R. F., 1976, Simian virus 40-specific polypeptides in $Ad2^+ND_1$- and $Ad2^+ND_4$-infected cells, *J. Virol.* **18**:685.

Anderson, J. L., Chang, C., Mora, P., and Martin, R. G., 1977*a*, Expression and thermal stability of SV40 tumor specific transplantation antigen and tumor antigen in wild type and *tsA* mutant-transformed cells, *J. Virol.* **21**:459.

Anderson, J. L., Martin, R. G., Chang, C., Mora, P., and Livingston, D., 1977*b*, Nuclear preparations of SV40-transformed cells contain tumor specific transplantation antigen activity, *Virology* **76**:420.

Baum, S. G., Reich, P. R., Hybner, C. J., Rowe, W. P., and Weissman, S. M., 1966, Biophysical evidence for linkage of adenovirus and SV40 DNA's in adenovirus 7–SV40 hybrid particles, *Proc. Natl. Acad. Sci. USA* **56**:1509.

Baum, S. G., Wiese, W. H., and Reich, P. R., 1968, Studies on the mechanism of enhancement of adenovirus 7 infection in African green monkey cells by simian virus 40: Formation of adenovirus-specific RNA, *Virology* **34**:373.

Baum, S. G., Wiese, W. H., and Rowe, W. P., 1970, Density differences between hybrid and nonhybrid particles in two adenovirus–simian virus 40 hybrid populations, *J. Virol.* **5**:353.

Baum, S. G., Horwitz, M. S., and Maizel, J. V., Jr., 1972, Studies of the mechanism of enhancement of human adenovirus infection in monkey cells by simian virus 40, *J. Virol.* **10**:211.

Beardmore, W. B., Havlick, M. J., Serafini, A., and McLean, I. W., Jr., 1965, Interrelationship of adenovirus (type 4) and papovavirus (SV-40) in monkey kidney cell cultures, *J. Immunol.* **95**:422.

Beladi, I., 1972, Adenoviruses, in: *Strains of Human Viruses* (M. Majer and S. Plotkin, eds.), pp. 1–19, Karger, New York.

Berk, A., and Sharp, P., 1978, Spliced early mRNAs of SV40 *Proc. Natl. Acad. Sci. USA* **75**:1274.

Black, P., 1968, The oncogenic DNA viruses: A review of *in vitro* transformation studies, *Annu. Rev. Microbiol.* **22**:391.

Black, P. H., and Todaro, G. J., 1965, *In vitro* transformation of hamster and human cells with the adeno 7–SV40 hybrid virus, *Proc. Natl. Acad. Sci. USA* **54**:374.

Black, P. H., and White, B. J., 1967, *In vitro* transformation by the adenovirus-SV40 hybrid viruses. II. Characteristics of the transformation of hamster cells by the adeno 2-, adeno 3- and adeno 12-SV40 viruses, *J. Exp. Med.* **125**:629.

Black, P., Crawford, E., and Crawford, L., 1964, The purification of SV40, *Virology* **24**:381.

Black, P. H., Lewis, A. M., Jr., Blacklow, N. R., Austin, J. B., and Rowe, W. P., 1967, The presence of adenovirus-specific antigens in hamster cells rendered neoplastic by adenovirus 1–SV40 and adenovirus 2–SV40 hybrid viruses, *Proc. Natl. Acad. Sci. USA* **57**:1324.

Black, P. H., Berman, L. D., and Dixon, C. B., 1969, *In vitro* transformation by the adenovirus-SV40 hybrid viruses. IV. Properties of clones isolated from cell lines transformed by adenovirus 2–simian virus 40 and adenovirus 12–simian virus 40 transcapsidant hybrid viruses, *J. Virol.* **4**:694.

Boeyé, A., Melnick, J. L., and Rapp, F., 1966, SV40-adenovirus "hybrids": Presence of two genotypes and the requirement of their complementation for viral replication, *Virology* **28**:56.

Breeden, J. H., Wewerka-Lutz, Y., Schnipper, L. E., Hauser, J., Patch, C. T., Lewis, A. M., Jr., and Levine, A. S., 1976, The content and expression of integrated viral DNA in hamster cells transformed by the nondefective adenovirus 2–simian virus 40 hybrid viruses, *J. Virol.* **20**:555.

Brugge, J. S., and Butel, J. S., 1975, Role of simian virus 40 gene A function in maintenance of transformation, *J. Virol.* **15**:619.

Butel, J. S., Guentzel, M. J., and Rapp, F., 1969, Variants of defective simian papovavirus 40 (PARA) characterized by cytoplasmic localization of simian papovavirus 40 tumor antigen, *J. Virol.* **4**:632.

Butel, J. S., Tevethia, S. S., and Melnick, J. L., 1972, Oncogenicity and cell transformation by papovavirus SV40: The role of the viral genome, *Adv. Cancer Res.* **15**:1.

Casto, B. C., 1973, Biologic parameters of adenovirus transformation; oncogenic adenoviruses, *Progr. Exp. Tumor Res.* **18**:166.

Crawford, L. V., and Black, P. H., 1964, The nucleic acid of simian virus 40, *Virology* **24**:388.

Crawford, L., Cole, C., Smith, A., Paucha, E., Tegtmeyer, P., Rundell, K. and Berg, P., 1978, Organization and expression of early genes of SV40, *Proc. Natl. Acad. Sci. USA* **75**:117.

Crumpacker, C. S., Levin, M. J., Wiese, W. H., Lewis, A. M., Jr., and Rowe, W. P., 1970, Adenovirus type 2–simian virus 40 hybrid population: Evidence for a hybrid deoxyribonucleic acid molecule and the absence of adenovirus-encapsidated circular simian virus 40 deoxyribonucleic acid, *J. Virol.* **6**:788.

Crumpacker, C. S., Henry, P. H., Kakefuda, T., Rowe, W. P., Levin, M. J., and Lewis, A. M., Jr., 1971, Studies of nondefective adenovirus 2–simian virus 40 hybrid viruses. III. Base composition, molecular weight, and conformation of the Ad2⁺ND₁ genome, *J. Virol.* **7**:352.

Danna, K. J., Sack, G. H., Jr., and Nathans, D., 1973, Studies of simian virus 40 DNA. VII. A cleavage map of the SV40 genome, *J. Mol. Biol.* **78**:363.

Davis, R., and Davidson, N., 1968, Electron microscopic visualization of deleted mutations, *Proc. Natl. Acad. Sci. USA* **60**:243.

Deppert, W., 1978, SV40-specific proteins associated with the nuclear matrix isolated from Ad2-SV40 hybrid virus-infected HeLa cells carry SV40 U-antigen determinants, *J. Virol.* **26**:165.

Deppert, W., and Walter, G., 1976, Simian virus 40 (SV40) tumor-specific proteins in nucleus and plasma membrane of HeLa cells infected by adenovirus 2–SV40 hybrid virus Ad2⁺ND₂, *Proc. Natl. Acad. Sci. USA* **73**:2505.

Deppert, W., Walter, G., and Linke, H., 1977, SV40 tumor specific proteins: Subcellular distribution and metabolic stability in HeLa cells infected with nondefective adenovirus 2–SV40 hybrid viruses, *J. Virol.* **21**:1170–1186.

Desmyter, J., Melnick, J. L., and Rawls, W. E., 1968, Defectiveness of interferon production and of rubella virus interference in a line of African green monkey kidney cells (Vero), *J. Virol.* **2**:955.

Dhar, R., Zain, S., Weissman, S. M., Pan, J., and Subramanian, K., 1974*a*, Nucleotide sequences of RNA transcribed in infected cells and by *Escherichia coli* RNA polymerase from a segment of simian virus 40 DNA, *Proc. Natl. Acad. Sci. USA* **71**:371.

Dhar, R., Weissman, S. M., Zain, B. S., Pan, J., and Lewis, A. M., Jr., 1974*b*, The nucleotide sequence preceding an RNA polymerase initiation site on SV40 DNA. Part 2. The sequence of the early strand transcript, *Nucleic Acids Res.* **1**:595.

Dhar, R., Subramanian, K. N., Zain, B. S., Levine, A. S., Patch, C., and Weissman, S. M., 1975, Sequences in SV40 DNA corresponding to the "ends" of cytoplasmic mRNA, in: *Colloque: In Vitro Transcription and Translation of Viral Genomes* (A. L. Haenni and G. Beaud, eds.), pp. 25–31, Institut National de la Santé et de la Recherche Medicale, Paris.

Duff, R., and Rapp, F., 1970, Quantitative characteristics of the transformation of hamster cells by PARA (defective simian virus 40)–adenovirus 7, *J. Virol.* **5**:568.

Dulbecco, R., 1952, Production of plaques in monolayer tissue cultures by single particles of an animal virus, *Proc. Natl. Acad. Sci. USA* **38**:747.

Dunn, A., and Hassell, J., 1977, A novel method to map transcripts: Evidence for homology between an adenovirus mRNA and discrete multiple regions of the viral genome, *Cell* **12**:23.

Dunn, A. R., Mathews, M. B., Chow, L. T., and Sambrook, J., 1978, A supplementary adenoviral leader sequence and its role in messenger translation, *Cell* **15**:511.

Easton, J. M., and Hiatt, C. W., 1965, Possible incorporation of SV40 genome within capsid proteins of adenovirus 4, *Proc. Natl. Acad. Sci. USA* **54**:1100.

Eddy, B. E., Borman, G. S., Grubbs, G. E., and Young, R. D., 1962, Identification of the oncogenic substance in rhesus monkey kidney cell cultures as SV40, *Virology* **17**:65.

Eron, L., Westphal, H., and Khoury, G., 1975, Post-transcriptional restriction of human adenovirus expression in monkey cells, *J. Virol.* **15**:1256.

Feldman, L. A., Butel, J. S., and Rapp, F., 1966, Interaction of a simian papovavirus and adenoviruses. I. Induction of adenovirus tumor antigen during abortive infection of simian cells, *J. Bacteriol.* **91**:813.

Fey, G., Lewis, J. B., Grodzicker, T., and Bothwell, A., 1979, Characterization of a fused protein specified by the Ad2-SV40 hybrid Ad2+ND₁dp2, *J. Virol.* **30**:201.

Fiers, W., Contreras, R., Haegeman, G., Rogiers, R., van de Voorde, A., van Heuverswyn, H., van Herreweghe, J., Volkaert, G., and Ysebaert, M., 1978, Complete nucleotide sequence of SV40, *Nature (London)* **273**:113.

Flint, J., 1977, The topography and transcription of the adenovirus genome, *Cell* **10**:153.

Flint, S. J., and Sharp, P. A., 1976, Adenovirus transcription. V. Quantitation of viral RNA sequences in adenovirus 2 infected and transformed cells, *J. Mol. Biol.* **106**:749.

Flint, S. J., Werwerka-Lutz, Y., Levine, A. S., Sambrook, J., and Sharp, P. A., 1975, Adenovirus transcription. II. RNA sequences complementary to SV40 and adenovirus 2 DNA in Ad2+ND₁ and Ad2+ND₃ infected cells, *J. Virol.* **16**:662.

Fox, R. I., and Baum, S. G., 1972, Synthesis of viral ribonucleic acid during restricted adenovirus infection, *J. Virol.* **10**:220.

Fox, R. I., and Baum, S. G., 1974, Posttranscriptional block to adenovirus replication in nonpermissive monkey cells, *Virology* **60**:45.

Friedman, M. P., Lyons, M. J., and Ginsberg, H. S., 1970, Biochemical consequences of type 2 adenovirus and simian virus 40 double infections of African green monkey kidney cells, *J. Virol.* **5**:586.

Friedman, R., Metz, D., Esteman, R., Tovell, D., Ball, L., and Kerr, I., 1972, Mechanism of interferon action: Inhibition of viral mRNA translation in L-cell extracts, *J. Virol.* **10**:1184.

Garon, C. F., Berry, K. W., Hierholzer, J. C., and Rose, J. A., 1973, Mapping of base sequence heterologies between genomes from different adenovirus serotypes, *Virology* **54**:414.

Gerber, P., 1966, Studies on the transfer of subviral infectivity from SV40-induced hamster tumor cells to indicator cells, *Virolgy* **28**:501.

Gershon, D. P., Sacks, L., and Winocour, E., 1966, The induction of cellular DNA synthesis by simian virus 40 in contact-inhibited and x-irradiated cells, *Proc. Natl. Acad. Sci. USA* **56**:918.

Gilden, R. V., Kern, J., Freeman, A. E., Martin, C. E., McAllister, R. C., Turner, H. C., and Huebner, R. J., 1968, T and tumour antigens of adenovirus group C-infected and transformed cells, *Nature (London)* **219**:517.

Ginsberg, H. S., Bello, L. J., and Levine, A. J., 1967, Control of biosynthesis of host macromolecules in cells infected with adenovirus, in: *The Molecular Biology of Viruses* (J. S. Colter and W. Paranchych, eds.), pp. 547–572, Academic Press, New York.

Girardi, A. J., Sweet, B. H., Slotnick, V. B., and Hilleman, M. R., 1962, Development of tumors in hamsters inoculated in neonatal period with vacuolating virus, SV40, *Proc. Soc. Exp. Biol.* **109**:649.

Girardi, A., Sweet, B., and Hilleman, M., 1963, Factors influencing tumor induction in hamsters by vacuolating virus, SV40, *Proc. Soc. Exp. Biol. Med.* **112**:662.

Graham, F., van der Eb, A., and Heijneker, H., 1974a, Size and location of the transforming region in human Ad5 DNA, *Nature (London)* **251**:687.

Graham, F., Abrahams, P., Mulder, C., Heijneker, H., Warnaar, S., de Vries, F., Fiers, W., and van der Eb, A., 1974*b*, *Cold Spring Harbor Symp. Quant. Biol.* **39**:637.

Green, M., Piña, M., and Kimes, R. C., 1967*a*, Biochemical studies on adenovirus multiplication. XII. Plaquing efficiencies of purified human adenoviruses, *Virology* **31**:562.

Green, M., Piña, M., Kimes, R., Wensink, P., MacHattie, L., and Thomas, C. A., Jr., 1967*b*, Adenovirus DNA. I. Molecular weight and conformation, *Proc. Natl. Acad. Sci. USA* **57**:1302.

Green, M., Parson, J. T., Piña, M., Fujinaga, K., Caffier, H., and Landgraf-Leurs, I., 1970, Transcription of adenovirus genes in productively infected and in transformed cells, *Cold Spring Harbor Symp. Quant. Biol.* **35**:803.

Grodzicker, T., Anderson, C., Sharp, P. A., and Sambrook, J., 1974, Conditional lethal mutants of adenovirus 2–simian virus 40 hybrids. I. Host range mutants of Ad2$^+$ND$_1$, *J. Virol.* **13**:1237.

Grodzicker, T., Lewis, J., and Anderson, C., 1976, Conditional lethal mutants of Ad2-SV40 hybrids. II. Ad2$^+$ND$_1$ host-range mutants that synthesize fragments of the Ad2$^+$ND$_1$ 30K protein, *J. Virol.* **19**:559.

Gross, L., 1970, *Oncogenic Viruses*, 2nd ed., Pergamon Press, New York.

Hartley, J. W., Huebner, R. J., and Rowe, W. P., 1956, Serial propagation of adenoviruses (APC) in monkey kidney tissue cultures, *Proc. Soc. Exp. Biol.* **92**:667.

Harwood, L. M. J., and Gallimore, P. H., 1975, A study of the oncogenicity of adenovirus type 2 transformed rat embryo cells, *Int. J. Cancer* **16**:498.

Hashimoto, K., Nakajima, K., Oda, K., and Shimojo, H., 1973, Complementation of translational defect for growth of human adenovirus type 2 in simian cells by a simian virus 40-induced factor, *J. Mol. Biol.* **81**:207.

Hassell, J., Lukanidin, E., Fey, G., and Sambrook, J., 1978, The structure and expression of two defective Ad2-SV40 hybrids, *J. Mol. Biol.* **120**:209.

Henry, C. J., Slifkin, M., and Merkow, L., 1971, Mechanism of host cell restriction in African green monkey kidney cells abortively infected with human adenovirus type 2, *Nature (London) New Biol.* **233**:39.

Henry, P. H., Schnipper, L. E., Samaha, R. J., Crumpacker, C. S., Lewis, A. M., Jr., and Levine, A. S., 1973, Studies of nondefective adenovirus 2–simian virus 40 hybrid viruses. VI. Characterization of the DNA from five nondefective hybrid viruses, *J. Virol.* **11**:665.

Hierholzer, J. C., 1973, Further subgrouping of adenoviruses by differential hemagglutination, *J. Infect. Dis.* **128**:541.

Hirt, B., 1967, Selective extraction of polyoma DNA from infected mouse cell cultures, *J. Mol. Biol.* **26**:365.

Hodge, L. D., Mancini, P., Davis, F. M., and Heywood, P., 1977, Nuclear matrix of HeLa S$_3$ cells: Polypeptide composition during adenovirus infection and in phases of the cell cycle, *J. Cell Biol.* **72**:194.

Holmberg, C. A., Gribble, D. H., Takemoto, K. K., Howley, P. M., Espana, C., and Osburn, B. I., 1977, Isolation of SV40 from rhesus monkeys (*Macaca mulatta*) with spontaneous progressive multifocal leukoencephalopathy, *J. Infect. Dis.* **136**:593.

Huebner, R. J., 1967, Adenovirus-directed tumor and T antigens, in: *The Gustav Stern Symposium: Perspectives in Virology V. Virus-Directed Host Response* (M. Pollard, ed.), pp. 147–166, Academic Press, New York.

Huebner, R., Rowe, W., Turner, H., and Lane, W., 1963, Specific adenovirus comple-
ment-fixing antigens in virus-free hamster and rat tumors, *Proc. Natl. Acad. Sci.
USA* **50**:379.

Huebner, R. J., Chanock, R. M., Rubin, B. A., and Casey, M. J., 1964, Induction by
adenovirus type 7 of tumors in hamsters having the antigenic characteristics of
SV40 virus, *Proc. Natl. Acad. Sci. USA* **52**:1333.

Hummeler, K., Tomassini, N., and Sokol, F., 1970, Morphological aspects of the
uptake of simian virus 40 by permissive cells, *J. Virol.* **6**:87.

Igel, H. J., and Black, P. H., 1967, *In vitro* transformation by the adenovirus-SV40
hybrid viruses. III. Morphology of tumors induced with transformed cells, *J. Exp.
Med.* **125**:647.

Jay, G., Jay, F. T., Friedman, R. M., and Levine, A. S., 1977, Simian virus 40-specific
ribosome-binding proteins induced by a nondefective adenovirus 2–simian virus 40
hybrid, *J. Virol.* **23**:692.

Jay, G., Jay, F., Friedman, R., and Levine, A. S., 1978*a*, Biosynthesis immunological
specificity and intracellular distribution of the SV40-specific protein induced by the
nondefective hybrid Ad2$^+$ND$_1$, *J. Virol.* **26**:411.

Jay, G., Jay, F., Chang, C., Friedman, R., and Levine, A. S., 1978*b*, Tumor-specific
transplantation antigen: Use of the Ad2$^+$ND$_1$ hybrid virus to identify the protein
responsible for SV40 tumor rejection and its genetic origin, *Proc. Natl. Acad. Sci.
USA* **75**:3055.

Jerkofsky, M., 1975, Enhancement of the replication of human adenovirus in simian
cells by a series of temperature-sensitive mutants of SV40, *Virology* **65**:579.

Jerkofsky, M., and Rapp, F., 1973, Host cell DNA synthesis as a possible factor in the
enhancement of replication of human adenoviruses in simian cells by SV40,
Virology **51**:466.

Jerkofsky, M., and Rapp, F., 1975, Stimulation of adenovirus replication in simian
cells in the absence of a helper virus by pretreatment of the cells with iododeoxyu-
ridine, *J. Virol.* **15**:253.

Kelly, T. J., Jr., 1975, Structure of the DNA of the adenovirus 7–simian virus 40
hybrid, E46$^+$, by electron microscopy, *J. Virol.* **15**:1267.

Kelly, T. J., Jr., and Lewis, A. M., Jr., 1973, Use of nondefective adenovirus–simian
virus 40 hybrids for mapping the simian virus 40 genome, *J. Virol.* **12**:643.

Kelly, T. J., Jr., and Nathans, D., 1977, The genome of simian virus 40, *Adv. Virus
Res.* **21**:85.

Kelly, T. J., Jr., and Rose, J. A., 1971, Simian virus 40 integration site in an adenovirus
7–simian virus 40 hybrid DNA molecule, *Proc. Natl. Acad. Sci. USA* **68**:1037.

Kelly, T. J., Jr., Lewis, A. M., Jr., Levine, A. S., and Siegel, S., 1974, Structure of two
adenovirus–simian virus 40 hybrids which contain the entire SV40 genome, *J. Mol.
Biol.* **89**:113.

Khoury, G., Lewis, A. M., Jr., Oxman, M. N., and Levine, A. S., 1973, Strand orientation of SV40 transcription in cells infected by nondefective adenovirus 2–SV40
hybrid viruses, *Nature (London) New Biol.* **246**:202.

Khoury, G., Howley, P., Brown, M., and Martin, M., 1974, The detection and quantitation of SV40 nucleic acid sequences using single-stranded SV40 DNA probes,
Cold Spring Harbor Symp. Quant. Biol. **39**:147.

Khoury, G., Howley, P., Nathans, D., and Martin, M., 1975, Posttranscriptional selection of simian virus 40-specific RNA, *J. Virol.* **15**:433.

Kimura, G., 1974, Genetic evidence for SV40 gene function in enhancement of replication of human adenovirus in simian cells, *Nature (London)* **248**:590.

Klessig, D., 1977*a*, Isolation of a variant of Ad2 that multiplies efficiently in monkey cells, *J. Virol.* **21**:1243.

Klessig, D., 1977*b*, Two adenovirus mRNAs have a common 5′ terminal leader sequence encoded at least 10 kb upstream from their main coding regions, *Cell* **12**:9.

Klessig, D. F., and Anderson, C. W., 1975, Block to multiplication of adenovirus serotype 2 in monkey cells, *J. Virol.* **16**:1650.

Lavi, S., and Shatkin, A., 1975, Methylated SV40-specific RNA from nuclei and cytoplasm of infected BSC-1 cells, *Proc. Natl. Acad. Sci. USA* **72**:2012.

Lawrence, C., Hunter, T., and Walter, G., 1979, Characterization of the SV40 specific mRNAs isolated from HeLa cells infected with the nondefective Ad2-SV40 hybrid viruses Ad2$^+$ND$_2$ and Ad2$^+$ND$_4$, *J. Mol. Biol.* (submitted for publication).

Lebowitz, P., and Khoury, G., 1975, Simian virus 40 DNA segment of the adenovirus 7–simian virus 40 hybrid, E46$^+$, and its transcription during permissive infection of monkey kidney cells, *J. Virol.* **15**:1214.

Lebowitz, P., Kelly, T. J., Jr., Nathans, D., Lee, T. N. H., and Lewis, A. M., Jr., 1974, A colinear map relating the simian virus 40 (SV40) DNA segments of six adenovirus-SV40 hybrids to the DNA fragments produced by restriction endonuclease cleavage of SV40 DNA, *Proc. Natl. Acad. Sci. USA* **71**:441.

Lebowitz, P., Stern, R., Ghosh, P., and Weissman, S., 1977, Specificity of initiation of transcription of SV40 DNA I by *Escherichia coli* RNA polymerase: Identification and localization of five sites for initiation with [γ^{32}P]ATP, *J. Virol.* **22**:430.

Levin, M. J., Black, P. H., Coghill, S. L., Dixon, C. B., and Henry, P. H., 1969, *In vitro* transformation by the adenovirus–simian virus 40 hybrid viruses. V. Virus-specific ribonucleic acid in cell lines transformed by the adenovirus 2–simian virus 40 and adenovirus 12–simian virus 40 transcapsidant hybrid viruses, *J. Virol.* **4**:704.

Levin, M. J., Crumpacker, C. S., Lewis, A. M., Jr., Oxman, M. N., Henry, P. H., and Rowe, W. P., 1971, Studies of nondefective adenovirus 2–simian virus 40 hybrid viruses. II. Relationship of adenovirus 2 deoxyribonucleic acid and simian virus 40 deoxyribonucleic acid in the Ad2$^+$ND$_1$ genome, *J. Virol.* **7**:343.

Levine, A. J., 1976, SV40 and adenovirus early functions involved in DNA replication and transformation, *Biochim. Biophys. Acta* **458**:213.

Levine, A. J., and Ginsberg, H. S., 1967, Mechanism by which fiber antigen inhibits multiplication of type 5 adenovirus, *J. Virol.* **1**:747.

Levine, A. J., and Ginsberg, H. S., 1968, Role of adenovirus structural proteins in the cessation of host-cell biosynthetic functions, *J. Virol.* **2**:430.

Levine, A. J., van der Vliet, P. C., Rosenwirth, B., Rabek, J., Frenkel, G., and Ensinger, M., 1974, Adenovirus-infected, cell-specific DNA-binding proteins, *Cold Spring Harbor Symp. Quant. Biol.* **39**:559.

Levine, A. S., Levin, M. J., Oxman, M. N., and Lewis, A. M., Jr., 1973, Studies of nondefective adenovirus 2–simian virus-40 hybrid viruses. VII. Characterization of the simian virus 40 RNA species induced by five nondefective hybrid viruses, *J. Virol.* **11**:672.

Lewis, A. M., Jr., 1977, Defective and nondefective Ad2-SV40 hybrids, *Progr. Med. Virol.* **23**:96.

Lewis, A. M., Jr., and Cook, J. L., 1979, Studies of nondefective Ad2-SV40 hybrids. XI. The association of tumor induction by ultraviolet light inactivated Ad2-SV40 recombinants with a specific segment of SV40 DNA, *J. Natl. Cancer Inst.* (in press).

Lewis, A. M., Jr., and Rowe, W. P., 1970, Isolation of two plaque variants from the adenovirus type 2–simian virus 40 hybrid population which differ in their efficiency in yielding simian virus 40, *J. Virol.* **5**:413.

Lewis, A. M., Jr., and Rowe, W. P., 1971, Studies on nondefective adenovirus–simian virus 40 hybrid viruses. I. A newly characterized simian virus 40 antigen induced by the Ad2$^+$ND$_1$ virus, *J. Virol.* **7**:189.

Lewis, A. M., Jr., and Rowe, W. P., 1973, Studies of nondefective adenovirus 2–simian virus 40 hybrid viruses. VIII. Association of simian virus 40 transplantation antigen with a specific region of the early viral genome, *J. Virol.* **12**:836.

Lewis, A. M., Jr., Baum, S. G., Prigge, K. O., and Rowe, W. P., 1966a, Occurrence of adenovirus-SV40 hybrids among monkey kidney cell adapted strains of adenovirus, *Proc. Soc. Exp. Biol.* **122**:214.

Lewis, A. M., Jr., Prigge, K. O., and Rowe, W. P., 1966b, Studies of adenovirus-SV40 hybrid viruses. IV. An adenovirus type 2 strain carrying the infectious SV40 genome, *Proc. Natl. Acad. Sci. USA* **55**:526.

Lewis, A. M., Jr., Levin, M. J., Wiese, W. H., Crumpacker, C. S., and Henry, P. H., 1969, A nondefective (competent) adenovirus-SV40 hybrid isolated from the Ad2-SV40 hybrid population, *Proc. Natl. Acad. Sci. USA* **63**:1128.

Lewis, A. M., Jr., Levine, A. S., Crumpacker, C. S., Levin, M. J., Samaha, R. J., and Henry, P. H., 1973, Studies of nondefective adenovirus 2–simian virus 40 hybrid viruses. V. Isolation of additional hybrids which differ in their simian virus 40-specific biological properties, *J. Virol.* **11**:655.

Lewis, A. M., Jr., Rabson, A. S., and Levine, A. S., 1974a, Studies of nondefective adenovirus 2–simian virus 40 hybrid viruses. X. Transformation of hamster kidney cells by adenovirus 2 and the nondefective hybrid viruses, *J. Virol.* **13**:1291.

Lewis, A. M., Jr., Breeden, J. H., Wewerka, Y. L., Schnipper, L. E., and Levine, A. S., 1974b, Studies of hamster cells transformed by adenovirus 2 and the nondefective Ad2-SV40 hybrids, *Cold Spring Harbor Symp. Quant. Biol.* **39**:651.

Lewis, J. B., Atkins, J. F., Baum, P. R., Solem, R., Gesteland, R. F., and Anderson, C. W., 1976, Location and identification of the genes for adenovirus type 2 early polypeptides, *Cell* **7**:141.

Lin, P. S., Schmidt-Ullrich, R., and Wallach, D. F. H., 1977, Transformation by simian virus 40 induces virus-specific, related antigens in the surface membrane and nuclear envelope, *Proc. Natl. Acad. Sci. USA* **74**:2495.

Lopez-Revilla, R., and Walter, G., 1973, Polypeptide specific for cells with adenovirus 2-SV40 hybrid Ad2ND$_1$, *Nature (London) New Biol.* **244**:165.

Lucas, J. J., and Ginsberg, H. S., 1972, Transcription and transport of virus-specific ribonucleic acids in African green monkey kidney cells abortively infected with type 2 adenovirus, *J. Virol.* **10**:1109.

Malmgren, R. A., Rabson, A. S., Carney, P. G., and Paul, F. J., 1966, Immunofluorescence of green monkey kidney cells infected with adenovirus 12 and with adenovirus 12 plus simian virus 40, *J. Bacteriol.* **91**:262.

Mann, K., Hunter, T., Walter, G., and Linke, H., 1977, Evidence for simian virus 40 (SV40) coding of SV40 T-antigen and the SV40-specific proteins in HeLa cells infected with nondefective adenovirus type 2-SV40 hybrid viruses, *J. Virol.* **24**:151.

Martin, M. A., Howley, P. M., Byrne, J. C., and Garon, C. F., 1976, Characterization of supercoiled oligomeric SV40 DNA made in productively infected cells, *Virology* **71**:28.

Martin, R. G., and Chou, J. Y., 1975, Simian virus 40 functions required for the establishment and maintenance of malignant transformation, *J. Virol.* **15**:599.

Martin, R. G., Chou, J. Y., Avila, J., and Saral, R., 1974, The semiautonomous replicon: A molecular model for the oncogenicity of SV40, *Cold Spring Harbor Symp. Quant. Biol.* **39**:17.

Mautner, V., Williams, J., Sambrook, J., Sharp, P., and Grodzicker, T., 1975, The location of the genes coding for hexon and fiber proteins in adenovirus DNA, *Cell* **5**:93.

Morrow, J. F., and Berg, P., 1972, Cleavage of simian virus 40 DNA at a unique site by a bacterial restriction enzyme, *Proc. Natl. Acad. Sci. USA* **69**:3365.

Morrow, J. F., Berg, P., Kelly, T. J., Jr., and Lewis, A. M., Jr., 1973, Mapping of simian virus 40 early functions on the viral chromosome, *J. Virol.* **12**:653.

Mulder, C., Sharp, P. A., Delius, H., and Pettersson, U., 1974, Specific fragmentation of DNA of adenovirus serotypes 3, 5, 7, and 12, and adenosimian virus 40 hybrid virus Ad2$^+$ND$_1$ by restriction endonuclease R·*Eco*RI, *J. Virol.* **14**:68.

Naegele, R. F., and Rapp, F., 1967, Enhancement of the replication of human adenoviruses in simian cells by simian adenovirus SV15, *J. Virol.* **1**:838.

Nakajima, K., and Oda, K., 1975, The alteration of ribosomes for mRNA selection concerned with adenovirus growth in SV40-infected simian cells, *Virology* **67**:85.

Nakajima, K., Ishitsuka, H., and Oda, K., 1974, An SV40-induced initiation factor for protein synthesis concerned with the regulation of permismiseness, *Nature (London)* **252**:649.

Norrby, E., 1968, Comparative studies on soluble components of Ad9 and Ad15 and the intermediate strain 9-15, *J. Virol.* **2**:1200.

O'Conor, G. T., Rabson, A. S., Berezesky, I. K., and Paul, F. J., 1963, Mixed infection with simian virus 40 and adenovirus 12, *J. Natl. Cancer Inst.* **31**:903.

O'Conor, G. T., Rabson, A. S., Malmgren, R. A., Berezesky, I. K., and Paul, F. J., 1965, Morphologic observations of green monkey kidney cells after single and double infection with adenovirus 12 and simian virus 40, *J. Natl. Cancer Inst.* **34**:679.

Oda, K., and Dulbecco, R., 1968, Regulation of transcription of the SV40 DNA in productively infected and in transformed cells, *Proc. Natl. Acad. Sci. USA* **60**:525.

Ortin, J., Schneidtmann, K. H., Greenberg, R., Westphal, H., and Doerfler, W., 1976, Transcription of the genome of adenovirus type 12. III. Maps of stable RNA from productively infected human cells and abortively infected and transformed hamster cells, *J. Virol.* **20**:355.

Osborn, M., and Weber, K., 1975, Simian virus 40 gene A function and maintenance of transformation, *J. Virol.* **15**:636.

Oxman, M., and Levin, M., 1971, Interferon and transcription of early virus-specific RNA in cells infected with SV40, *Proc. Natl. Acad. Sci. USA* **68**:299.

Oxman, M. N., Baron, S., Black, P. H., Takemoto, K. K., Habel, K., and Rowe, W. P., 1967, The effect of interferon SV40 T antigen production in SV40 transformed cells, *Virology* **32**:122.

Oxman, M. N., Levine, A. S., Crumpacker, C. S., Levin, M. J., Henry, P. H., and Lewis, A. M., Jr., 1971, Studies of nondefective adenovirus 2–simian virus 40 hybrid viruses. IV. Characterization of the simian virus 40 ribonucleic acid species induced by wild-type simian virus 40 and by the nondefective hybrid virus, Ad2$^+$ND$_1$, *J. Virol.* **8**:215.

Oxman, M. N., Levin, M. J., and Lewis, A. M., Jr., 1974, Control of simian virus 40 gene expression in adenovirus–simian virus 40 hybrid viruses: Synthesis of hybrid adenovirus 2–simian virus 40 RNA molecules in cells infected with a nondefective adenovirus 2–simian virus 40 hybrid virus, *J. Virol.* **13**:322.

Patch, C. T., Lewis, A. M., Jr., and Levine, A. S., 1972, Evidence for a transcription-control region of simian virus 40 in the adenovirus 2–simian virus 40 hybrid, Ad2$^+$ND$_1$, *Proc. Natl. Acad. Sci. USA* **69**:3375.

Patch, C. T., Lewis, A. M., Jr., and Levine, A. S., 1974, Studies of nondefective adenovirus 2–simian virus 40 hybrid viruses. IX. Template topography in the early region of simian virus 40, *J. Virol.* **13**:677.

Patch, C. T., Hauser, J., Lewis, A. M., Jr., and Levine, A. S., 1979, A method for determining the extent and copy number of overlapping and nonoverlapping segments of integrated viral genomes, *J. Virol.* **31**:575.

Paucha, E., Mellor, A., Harvey, R., Smith, A. E., Hewick, R. M., and Waterfield, M. D., 1978, Large and small tumor antigens from SV40 have identical termini mapping at 0.65 map units, *Proc. Natl. Acad. Sci. USA* **75**:2165.

Pettersson, U., Tibbetts, C., and Philipson, L., 1976, Hybridization maps of early and late messenger RNA sequences on the adenovirus type 2 genome, *J. Mol. Biol.* **101**:479.

Philipson, L., and Lindberg, U., 1974, Reproduction of adenoviruses, in: *Comprehensive Virology*, Vol. 3 (H. Fraenkel-Conrat and R. R. Wagner, eds.), pp. 143–175, Plenum Press, New York.

Piña, M., and Green, M., 1965, Biochemical studies on adenovirus multiplication. IX. Chemical and base composition analysis of 28 human adenoviruses, *Proc. Natl. Acad. Sci. USA* **54**:547.

Prives, C., Gilboa, E., Revel, M., and Winocour, E., 1977, Cell-free translation of simian virus 40 early messenger RNA coding for viral T-antigen, *Proc. Natl. Acad. Sci. USA* **74**:457.

Rabson, A. S., and Kirschstein, R. L., 1962, Induction of malignancy *in vitro* in newborn hamster kidney tissue infected with simian vacuolating virus (SV40), *Proc. Soc. Exp. Biol.* **111**:323.

Rabson, A. S., O'Conor, G. T., Berezesky, I. K., and Paul, F. J., 1964, Enhancement of adenovirus growth in African green monkey kidney cell cultures by SV40, *Proc. Soc. Exp. Biol.* **116**:187.

Rapp, F., 1973, The para-adenoviruses: Oncogenic adenoviruses, *Progr. Exp. Tumor Res.* **18**:104.

Rapp, F., and Melnick, J. L., 1966, Papovavirus SV40, adenovirus and their hybrids: Transformation, complementation and transcapsidation, *Progr. Med. Virol.* **8**:349.

Rapp, F., Melnick, J. L., Butel, J. S., and Kitahara, T., 1964, The incorporation of SV40 genetic material into adenovirus 7 as measured by intranuclear synthesis of SV40 tumor antigen, *Proc. Natl. Acad. Sci. USA* **52**:1348.

Rapp, F., Butel, J. S., and Melnick, J. L., 1965, SV40-adenovirus "hybrid" populations: Transfer of SV40 determinants from one type of adenovirus to another, *Proc. Natl. Acad. Sci. USA* **54**:717.

Rapp, F., Butel, J. S., Tevethia, S. S., Katz, M., and Melnick, J. L., 1966*a*, Antigenic analysis of tumors and sera from animals inoculated with PARA-adenovirus populations, *J. Immunol.* **97**:833.

Rapp, F., Feldman, L. A., and Mandel, M., 1966*b*, Synthesis of virus deoxyribonucleic acid during abortive infection of simian cells by human adenoviruses, *J. Bacteriol.* **92**:931.

Rapp, F., Jerkofsky, M., Melnick, J. L., and Levy, B., 1968, Variation in the oncogenic potential of human adenoviruses carrying a defective SV40 genome (PARA), *J. Exp. Med.* **127**:77.

Reddy, V. B., Thimmappaya, B., Dhar, R., Subramanian, K., Zain, B., Pan, J., Ghosh, M., Celma, M., and Weissman, S. M., 1978, The genome of SV40, *Science* **200**:494.

Reich, P. R., Baum, S. G., Rose, J. A., Rowe, W. P., and Weissman, S. M., 1966, Nucleic acid homology studies of adenovirus type 7–SV40 interactions, *Proc. Natl. Acad. Sci. USA* **55**:336.

Robb, J., 1977, Identification of SV40 tumor and U antigens, *Proc. Natl. Acad. Sci. USA* **74**:447.

Rowe, W. P., 1965, Studies of adenovirus-SV40 hybrid viruses. III. Transfer of SV40 gene between adenovirus types, *Proc. Natl. Acad. Sci. USA* **54**:711.

Rowe, W. P., and Baum, S. G., 1964, Evidence for a possible genetic hybrid between adenovirus type 7 and SV40 viruses, *Proc. Natl. Acad. Sci. USA* **52**:1340.

Rowe, W. P., and Baum, S. G., 1965, Studies of adenovirus SV40 hybrid viruses. II. Defectiveness of the hybrid particles, *J. Exp. Med.* **122**:955.

Rowe, W. P., and Pugh, W. E., 1966, Studies of adenovirus-SV40 hybrid viruses. V. Evidence for linkage between adenovirus and SV40 genetic materials, *Proc. Natl. Acad. Sci. USA* **55**:1126.

Rowe, W., Baum, S., Pugh, W., and Hoggan, M. D., 1965, Studies of Ad-SV40 hybrid viruses. I. Assay system and further evidence for hybridization, *J. Exp. Med.* **122**:943.

Salzman, N. P., and Khoury, G., 1974, Reproduction of papovaviruses, in: *Comprehensive Virology*, Vol. 3 (H. Fraenkel-Conrat and R. Wagner, eds.), pp. 63–141, Plenum Press, New York.

Sambrook, J., 1977, Adenovirus amazes at Cold Spring Harbor, *Nature (London)* **268**:101.

Sambrook, J., 1978, The molecular biology of the papovaviruses, in: *The Molecular Biology of Animal Viruses*, Vol. 2 (D. P. Nayak, ed.), pp. 589–672, Marcel Dekker, New York.

Sambrook, J., Sugden, B., Keller, W., and Sharp, P. A., 1973, Transcription of simian virus 40. III. Mapping of "early" and "late" species of RNA, *Proc. Natl. Acad. Sci. USA* **70**:3711.

Sambrook, J., Botchan, M., Gallimore, P., Ozanne, B., Pettersson, U., Williams, J. F., and Sharp, P. A., 1974, Viral DNA sequences in cells transformed by simian virus 40, adenovirus type 2 and adenovirus type 5, *Cold Spring Harbor Symp. Quant. Biol.* **39**:615.

Sambrook, J., Williams, J. F., Sharp, P. A., and Grodzicker, T., 1975, Physical mapping of temperature-sensitive mutations of adenoviruses, *J. Mol. Biol.* **97**:369.

Schell, K., Lane, W. T., Casey, M. J., and Huebner, R. J., 1966, Potentiation of oncogenicity of adenovirus type 12 grown in African green monkey kidney cell cultures preinfected with SV40 virus: Persistence of both T antigens in the tumors and evidence for possible hybridization, *Proc. Natl. Acad. Sci. USA* **55**:81.

Schnipper, L. E., Lewis, A. M., Jr., and Levine, A. S., 1973, Induction of cellular DNA synthesis by the nondefective adenovirus 2–simian virus 40 hybrid viruses, *J. Virol.* **12**:940.

Segawa, K., Yamaguchi, N., and Oda, K., 1977, Simian virus 40 gene A regulates the association between a highly phosphorylated protein and chromatin and ribosomes in SV40-transformed cells, *J. Virol.* **22**:679.

Sharp, P. A., Gallimore, P. H., and Flint, S. J., 1974, Mapping of adenovirus 2 RNA sequences in lytically infected cells and transformed cell lines, *Cold Spring Harbor Symp. Quant. Biol.* **39**:457.

Siegel, S. E., Patch, C. T., Lewis, A. M., Jr., and Levine, A. S., 1975, Simian virus 40 DNA replication, transcription, and antigen induction during infection with two adenovirus 2–SV40 hybrids that contain the entire SV40 genome, *J. Virol.* **16**:43.

Sleigh, M. J., Topp, W. C., Hanich, R., and Sambrook, J., 1978, Mutants of SV40 with an altered small t protein are reduced in their ability to transform cells, *Cell* **14**:79.

Staal, S., and Rowe, W., 1975, Enhancement of adenovirus infection in WI-38 and AGMK cells by pretreatment of cells with 5-iododeoxyuridine, *Virology* **64**:513.

Sugawara, K., Gilead, Z., Wold, W., and Green, M., 1977, Immunofluorescence study of the Ad2 single stranded DNA binding protein in infected and transformed cells, *J. Virol.* **22**:527.

Sultanian, I., and Freeman, G., 1966, Enhanced growth of human embryonic cells infected with Ad12, *Science* **154**:665.

Sweet, B. H., and Hilleman, M. R., 1960, The vacuolating virus, SV40, *Proc. Soc. Exp. Biol.* **105**:420.

Takemoto, K. K., Kirschstein, R. L., and Habel, K., 1966, Mutants of simian virus 40 differing in plaque size, oncogenicity and heat sensitivity, *J. Bacteriol.* **92**:990.

Tegtmeyer, P., 1975, Function of simian virus 40 gene A in transforming infection, *J. Virol.* **15**:613.

Tevethia, S. S., and Lewis, A. M., Jr., 1976, Two adenovirus type 2–simian virus 40 hybrid populations which contain the entire SV40 genome differ in their ability to induce SV40 transplantation immunity in hamsters but not in mice, *J. Virol.* **20**:539.

Tevethia, S. S., and McMillan, V. L., 1974, Acquisition of malignant properties by SV40-transformed mouse cells: Relationship to type-C viral antigen expression, *Intervirology* **3**:269.

Tibbetts, C., 1977, Physical organization of subgroup B human adenovirus genomes, *J. Virol.* **24**:564.

Tjian, R., 1978, The binding site on SV40 DNA for a T antigen related protein, *Cell* **13**:165.

Tjian, R., Fey, G., and Graessmann, A., 1978, Biological activity of purified SV40 antigen proteins, *Proc. Natl. Acad. Sci. USA* **75**:1279.

Todaro, G., and Aaronson, S., 1968, Human cell strains susceptible to focus formation by human adenovirus type 12, *Proc. Natl. Acad. Sci. USA* **61**:1272.

Todaro, G., and Green, H., 1966, High frequency of SV40 transformation of mouse cell line 3T3, *Virology* **28**:756.

Todaro, G., and Takemoto, K., 1969, "Rescued" SV40: Increased transformation efficiency in mouse and human cells, *Proc. Natl. Acad. Sci. USA* **62**:1031.

Todaro, G., Green, H., and Swift, M., 1966, Susceptibility of human diploid fibroblast strains to transformation by SV40, *Science* **153**:1252.

Tooze, J., 1973, *The Molecular Biology of Tumor Viruses*, Cold Spring Harbor Laboratory, Cold Spring Harbor, N.Y.

Van Roy, F., and Fiers, W., 1978, Interference with SV40 DNA replication by Ad2 during mixed infection of monkey cells, *J. Virol.* **27**:275.

Waldeck, W., and Sauer, G., 1977, New oncogenic papovavirus from primate cells, *Nature (London)* **269**:171.

Walter, G., and Martin, H., 1975, Simian virus 40-specific proteins in HeLa cells infected with nondefective adenovirus 2–simian virus 40 hybrid viruses, *J. Virol.* **16**:1236.

Westphal, H., Lai, S.-P., Lawrence, C., Hunter, T., and Walter, G., 1979, Mosaic adenovirus-SV40 RNA specified by a nondefective hybrid virus, *J. Mol. Biol.* **130**:337.

Wiese, W. H., Lewis, A. M., Jr., and Rowe, W. P., 1970, Equilibrium density gradient studies on simian virus 40-yielding variants of the adenovirus type 2–simian virus 40 hybrid population, *J. Virol.* **5**:421.

Wilkie, N. M., Ustacelebi, S., and Williams, J. F., 1973, Preliminary characteristics of temperature-sensitive mutants of adenovirus type 5: Nucleic acid synthesis, *Virology* **51**:499.

Williams, J. F., Young, C. S. H., and Austin, P. E., 1974, Genetic analysis of human Ad5 in permissive and nonpermissive cells, *Cold Spring Harbor Symp. Quant. Biol.* **39**:427.

Williams, J., Grodzicker, T., Sharp, P., and Sambrook, J., 1975, Adenovirus recombination: Physical mapping of crossover events, *Cell* **4**:113.

Wold, W. S. M., Green, M., and Buttner, W., 1978, Adenoviruses, in: *The Molecular Biology of Animal Viruses*, Vol. 2 (D. P. Nayak, ed.), pp. 673–768, Marcel Dekker, New York.

Yakobson, E., Prives, C., Hartman, J., Winocour, E., and Revel, M., 1977, Inhibition of viral protein synthesis in monkey cells treated with interferon late in SV40 lytic cycle, *Cell* **12**:73.

Yano, S., Ojima, S., Fujinaga, K., Shiroki, K., and Shimojo, H., 1977, Transformation of a rat cell line by an Ad12 DNA fragment, *Virology* **82**:214.

Zain, S., and Roberts, R., 1978, Characterization and sequence analysis of a recombination site in the hybrid virus Ad2$^+$ND$_1$, *J. Mol. Biol.* **120**:13.

Bacteriophage Structure

Frederick A. Eiserling

Department of Microbiology and Molecular Biology Institute
University of California, Los Angeles
Los Angeles, California 90024

1. INTRODUCTION

1.1. Advantages of Bacteriophages for Structural Studies of Viruses

More is known about the physical and chemical properties of the bacterial viruses than of any other virus group except for several simpler plant viruses. The reasons are based on the availability of homogeneous populations of uniform particles which are relatively easy to prepare in large quantities in moderate-sized fermentors. These particles have been extensively used in studies of nucleic acid packaging, in studies of protein–protein interactions, and more recently in characterization of the intermediates in virus assembly. As a result of continued study, a great deal is known about phage structural organization, which has provided insight into such viral functions as adsorption on cell surface receptors, unfolding and penetration of nucleic acids, and the interaction of viral structural components with the host cell membrane during maturation. Understanding of some of the earliest and most obscure steps in viral morphogenesis has been advanced by the discovery, in bacteriophages, of structural "cores" or "scaffolding" proteins which interact to guide, in as yet unknown ways, the assembly of the major capsid proteins. Ingenious structural studies using immunoelectronmicroscopy, direct examination of mutationally defective particles, and selective chemical extraction of capsids have provided much new information about the localization of virion components. Most important, *in vitro* assembly systems have progressed to the point where the early intermediates in virus assembly can be formed and isolated, providing biochemical access to the shape- and size-determining steps of viral morphogenesis. From all these studies it is becoming apparent that the virion, the end result of morphogenesis, is considerably more than a passive container for nucleic acid. The virion itself undergoes a number of major structural transformations, both during assembly and on infection, which are an essential part of the program of gene expression of the virus. In principle, a viral shell can be constructed from the product of a single gene, and this is apparently so for the simplest plant viruses. However, many viruses devote more than one-third of their total genetic information to the design, production, and assembly of additional structural components. Examples of some of these essential structural interactions in virus assembly which require additional components are the displacive lattice expansions during bacteriophage capsid maturation, tail sheath contraction, hexagonal baseplate expansion and rearrangement, tail fiber retraction and extension on cell surface adsorption, internal protein entry and exit, and the coupling of DNA packaging, maturation, and replication. Some of these are discussed in Chapter 9 of this volume and others will be mentioned later.

1.2. Methods of Structure Analysis

Bacterial viruses are exceptionally favorable objects for the study of the relations between structure and assembly. One major advantage is the ease of genetic manipulation and the availability of genetic lesions, such as amber (*am*) and temperature-sensitive (*ts*) mutants, which result in the accumulation of structural components that can be isolated and purified for further structural studies. In addition, it is possible to identify the individual polypeptide species of the structural components by SDS gel electrophoresis. In favorable cases structures lacking identifiable components can be used to demonstrate directly the location of that component by comparing it with the wild-type structure as, for example, with T4 baseplate components (Crowther *et al.*, 1977). Another approach to localization of structural components is immunoelectronmicroscopy (Lake *et al.*, 1974). This had been applied earlier with success to bacteriophages by Yanagida and Ahmad-Zadeh (1970) and more recently by Müller-Salamin *et al.* (1977).

Image processing of electron micrographs has yielded valuable information on the detailed structure of bacteriophage components at the 2 nm level of resolution (DeRosier and Klug, 1972). These procedures can be applied to any repeating array of subunits with translational symmetry, rotational symmetry, or combinations of the two. Examples are tail tubes, extended and contracted sheaths, capsid surface lattices, hexagonal baseplates, and artificially ordered aggregates of virtually any viral component. The image analysis procedure involves placing an electron micrograph in a beam of coherent light and recording the optical Fourier transform or scanning the micrograph with a densitometer and converting the image into its harmonic components computationally. The periodic features of the structure can be separated from the random noise and recombined to give a clearer, filtered image. These techniques can be used to separate overlapping images which come from the two sides of a structure, and they have also been used to generate three-dimensional information about the specimen. Examples of several different viruses and other macromolecular assemblies treated by these techniques are given in a graphic review by Crowther and Klug (1975). This structure analysis has been extended to the 0.5–1 nm level by employing unstained specimens and image-averaging techniques which permit exposure of the specimen to very low doses of damaging radiation. The effects of electron beam damage have been quantified in recent years (Glaeser, 1974; Isaacson, 1977) and shown to restrict resolution in negative-contrast specimens by destroying biological macromolecules and by causing stain migration (Unwin, 1974), giving rise to false positions of the transparent biological material within the electron-dense stain. A new procedure described by Unwin and Henderson (1975) involves embedding the unstained sample in an amorphous layer of glucose, which provides some three-dimensional support. A regular array of specimens in then photographed at a dose so low that the specimen is not significantly damaged by the beam. The faint periodic information (the micrograph appears almost transparent to the eye) is extracted by computer analysis of the digitized image density and then further studied by standard image-processing methods (Crowther and Klug, 1975).

Recently Aebi et al. (1977a) have developed a promising new technique which combines immunoelectronmicroscopy and image processing of electron micrographs. They have prepared antibody fragments (Fab) from antisera directed against purified phage structural proteins and used these antibodies to label proteins on the bacteriophage T4 capsid surface. Optically filtered electron micrographs of the antibody-labeled capsids not only reveal the location of specific virus-coded proteins but also have the potential for revealing different conformational states of the protein subunits.

Selective extraction of viral structural components has also been used successfully to localize capsid proteins in T4 (Aebi *et al.*, 1977*b*). The idea is to find a mild, selective denaturant which removes the most weakly bound elements of the structure leaving behind the intact framework. Structural differences can be localized by electron microscopy and image-processing techniques, and the extracted components can be identified by SDS gel electrophoresis. Finally, it is also possible to identify structural arrangements of viral macromolecules by purifying the isolated components and assembling them *in vitro* to form various polymorphic structures, such as linear aggregates, planar sheets, helical tubes, and other regular arrays. These will reveal basic bonding properties of the structural subunits, although they are not definitive in establishing which contacts are the ones chosen by the final viral structure itself. The structures are ideal for image processing techniques.

The plan of this chapter resembles that of Chapter 9 in discussing the results of structural analysis of the major bacteriophage subassemblies, followed by a discussion of the relationship between structure and assembly.

2. STRUCTURE OF BACTERIOPHAGE HEADS AND CAPSIDS

All bacteriophage head shells analyzed in sufficient detail have been shown to be derived from the icosahedral design postulated by Caspar and Klug (1962). Some embellishments of the original principles include the discovery of minor protein components at specific locations such as at the center of a ring of six structure units or a 5-fold vertex. The original models established hierarchical structural levels of organization. The basic structure unit or protomer, equivalent to the crystallographic asymmetrical unit, can consist of a single polypeptide chain or several polypeptide chains which associate to form the fundamental structural repeat unit. To date, such protomers in large complex bacteriophage capsids have been found to be single polypeptide chains, but there is no requirement that this be so. Picornaviruses, for example, have protomers composed of several polypeptide chains (Ruekert, 1976) and this is probably also true for ϕX174 (Fujisawa and Hayashi, 1977). The clustering of protomers about axes of symmetry gives rise to morphological units visible at low resolution in the electron microscope, the capsomers. With improvements of electron microscopic techniques over the past 10 years, it is now possible, using image-processing techniques on suitable specimens, to resolve clearly the capsid structure units themselves. Thus the use of the term "capsomer" (of large complex bacteriophages) will diminish as structural analysis improves. In many cases, however, it has been shown that the capsomer is a definite subassembly of the capsid. Structural studies of the heads of the phages ϕCbK, λ, and T4 among others, have established that additional polypeptide chains are placed on or into the basic lattice design at symmetry-related locations as described later. In some cases these adjunct proteins are known to be added after the basic lattice is established by assembly of the major capsid protein, and the subunits are selectively removable by detergent treatment. Their function may be to provide additional stability to the capsid or to regulate ion passage across it. An additional feature of most large bacteriophage capsids is the provision of a specialized subunit structure at one of the icosahedral vertices, which serves as the attachment point for an adsorption structure such as the short baseplate or tail. It is likely that this structure is also the remnant of an initiation point for capsid assembly at a site on the cell membrane, explaining its unique origin and suggesting a relationship to its ultimate function in adsorption to the cell surface.

2.1. Isometric Phage and Head Structure: λ, P22, T7, and P2

The well-studied bacteriophages, λ, P22, T7, and P2 are reviewed in some detail with regard to their assembly in Chapter 9. On first inspection the phages look very different: the large complex contractile tail of P2, the narrow λ tube, and the short baseplate structure of P22 and T7. However, the heads of these phages have quite similar structural characteristics (Table 1). Each has a capsid diameter of some 55–60 nm, and the DNA masses range from 21 to about 30×10^6 daltons. The major head protein or proteins are arranged in a $T = 7$ surface lattice (possibly, in the case of P2, $T = 9$) containing 420–540 copies of the major protein. About five or six component polypeptide species are found as constituents of the capsid of each of these phages. The molecular weight of the major capsid protein is around 40,000 in each case.

The identification of the exact number of structural components of bacteriophage heads, or of any virus for that matter, is not straightforward. Heads are usually prepared using mutants defective in tail attachment, followed by chemical and physical purification. These manipulations usually cause the loss of DNA and the associated internal pro-

TABLE 1
Phage Head Structures

Phage	DNA mass (mega-daltons)	Head size (nm) EM	Head size (nm) X-ray	Probable surface lattice design	Major capsid protein genes	Approximate number of copies of major protein	Molecular weight × 10⁻³	Number of proteins in head[a]	Number of genes in head assembly	References
Isometric										
λ	32	55	64	$T = 7l$	E, D	420	38, 12	5–6	11	Hohn and Katsura (1977)
P22	27	60	61	$T = 7$	5	420	42	6	11	King et al. (1976)
T7	25	55	60	$T = 7$	10	460	38	5	7–8	Studier et al. (1972), Serwer (1976)
P2	22	60	—[b]	$T = 7$ or 9	N^c	550	44 → 36	4	6	Goldstein et al. (1974)
T5	75	65	—	$T = 12$ or 13	$D20^c$	7–800	50 → 32	≥6	—	Zweig and Cummings (1973a,b)
SP01	86	87	—	$T = 16$	—	900–1000	50 → 45	≥7	—	Parker (1979)
Elongated										
φ29	12	32 × 42	—	$T = 1$	8	100	45	3	5	Nelson et al. (1976)
T4	111	80 × 110	85	$T = 13l$	23,^{c} soc	960	56 → 46, 10	10–15	20	Wood and Revel (1976)
φCbK	120	60 × 200	—	$T = 7l$	—	1150, 2452	36, 13.5	3	—	Lake and Leonard (1974)

[a] May include connector proteins.
[b] Not known.
[c] Cleaved during assembly.

teins. The molecular weights of capsid components are sometimes very similar, and major capsid protein bands on SDS gels can obscure minor components. Viral nonstructural proteins may adhere nonspecifically. A number of protein bands identified as head or capsid components may actually be part of the connecting structure between head and tail. Depending on growth and isolation conditions, these connector proteins may form aberrant associations with either head or tail (Coombs and Eiserling, 1977).

The general organizational plan of these isometric phage heads appears to be a major structural framework constructed according to the icosahedral surface lattice properties predicted by Caspar and Klug (1962) from a fairly large 35,000- to 40,000-dalton protein. Assembly takes place via a prohead precursor in which the structural proteins are tightly packed into a thick-walled structure. Maturation is accompanied by a displacive expansion of the previously determined surface lattice, which may then incorporate a small 10,000- to 13,000-dalton protein in near-equivalent numbers to the major protein (e.g., λ, ϕCbK, and T4). The location of all the other minor proteins is not known with certainty. Possibilities include internal location with the DNA, the icosahedral vertices, and the tail attachment site, but these have not yet been generally established for the phages considered here.

2.2. λ Head Structure

Structural studies (Williams and Richards, 1974) determined the triangulation number of λ head structure to be $T = 7l$. The two major structure proteins, gpE and gpD, are clustered as hexamers–pentamers and as trimers. From studies on tubular polyheads made of gpE, or gpE plus gpD, Wurtz et al. (1976) concluded that the most likely arrangement is gpE hexamers surrounded by gpD trimers. The minor proteins gpB, gpC, and gpFII are present in from six to 15 copies/capsid (Hohn and Katsura, 1977) and the total capsid mass is 21×10^6 daltons. One of the minor proteins, gpFII, is known to lie at the connector vertex for tail attachment (Casjens, 1974; Hohn and Katsura, 1977). Drawings showing the structure of λ during assembly can be found in the review by Hohn and Katsura (1977); see Fig. 1 for a sketch of the mature phage and probable gene product locations.

2.3. P22 Head Structure

Although the head size and DNA packing arrangement have been determined for phage P22 by X-ray diffraction analysis, somewhat less

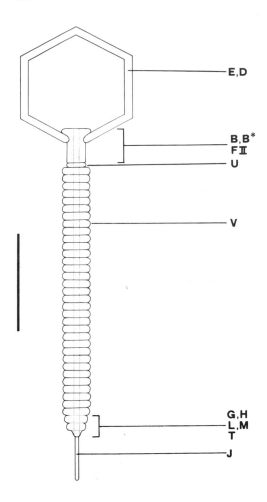

E,D

B,B*
F II
U

V

G,H
L,M
T
J

Fig. 1. Sketch of the components and gene product locations of bacteriophage λ, based on references from the text. The head contains the two major capsid proteins gpE and gpD. The detailed structure of the connector region has not yet been determined, but it contains at least three or four proteins. These gene product locations on the sketch are estimates, based on unpublished data from R. Hendrix. The bar represents 50 nm.

is known about the structure of P22 than of λ. From the known number of copies of the major head protein, gp5, the surface lattice design must be $T = 7$, although it has not yet been directly demonstrated. The locations of the minor head components are uncertain. Like that of λ the P22 prohead expands during maturation, but unlike λ there is no stoichiometric addition of a second small capsid protein. Proheads accumulate in cells infected with several DNA packaging mutants and contain the capsid protein, gp5, and a scaffolding protein, gp8, not found in mature phage. Using both electron microscopy and low-angle X-ray diffraction analysis, Earnshaw *et al.* (1976) established that proheads are made of a 51-nm-diameter outer shell about 4 nm thick, with an inner core 15 nm thick. The empty head and the mature phage have a single 61-nm-diameter shell, 4 nm thick (Fig. 2). Treatment of the proheads with SDS at room temperature removes the gp8 scaffolding protein and all the minor capsid components as well, and leaves an expanded, 4-nm-thick shell the same size as heads and capsids. Thus, in the case of phage P22, the expansion of the prohead shell is a property of the head protein itself and need not involve DNA entry or cleavage of any head proteins. The DNA inside the phage is regularly packed in concentric layers except for a region near the center, where it is likely to be disordered.

2.4.   T7 Head Structure

The size of the T7 capsid is essentially identical to that of phage P22 as determined by low-angle X-ray diffraction (Earnshaw *et al.*, 1976; Ruark *et al.*, 1978). T7 appears structurally distinct from both λ and P22 in containing a hollow cylindrical protein core, 20 nm long by 12–15 nm wide, with a 3- to 5-nm central hole (Serwer, 1976). This core is seen in whole phages which have lost their DNA as well as in certain precursor capsids and is attached to the capsid at the same point where the tail is joined. Its role in morphogenesis is unclear, but it may function in capsid initiation and/or DNA packaging. From the estimated number of copies of the major capsid protein (coded for by gene 10) the surface lattice design should be $T = 7$ (Studier, 1972). Figure 3 gives a schematic drawing with gene product locations.

2.5.   P2 Head Structure

Phage P2 and its satellite phage P4 are of interest because of the question of head size determination. The small P4 phage requires all the structural proteins of phage P2 yet somehow assembles them into a smaller head (Goldstein *et al.*, 1974). Little is known regarding the prohead structure of these phages, and genetic characterization of the proteins involved in head morphogenesis is incomplete. Estimates for the number of copies of the cleaved major head protein (gpN*) fit estimates of either $T = 7$ or $T = 9$. From the size of the genome it seems that a $T = 7$ surface lattice is more likely (Table 1). A schematic diagram of P2 and P4 is shown in the review by Goldstein *et al.* (1974).

2.6.   Structure of T5 and SP01 Heads

The large isometric phages T5 and SP01 have not been characterized in extensive detail, yet are probably representative of a

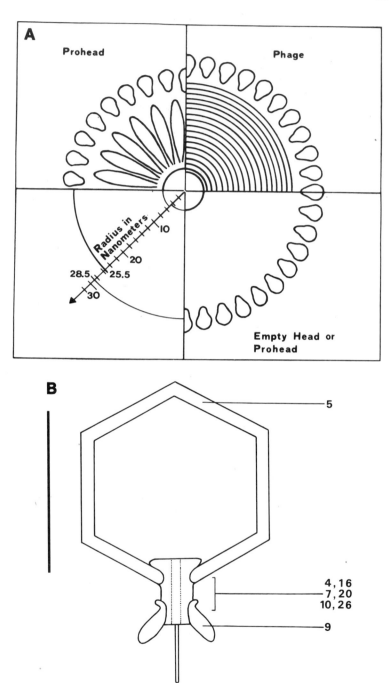

Fig. 2.   A: Drawing, modified from Earnshaw *et al.* (1976), of the dimensions of the prohead, empty head, and phage particle of phage P22 based on low-angle X-ray diffraction results. The central region is difficult to study and its structure is undetermined. At higher radii in intact phages, the DNA is highly ordered, indicated by the

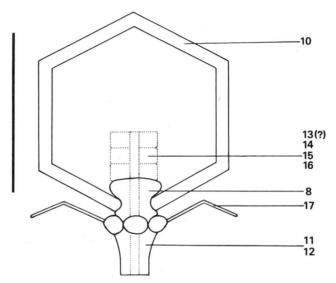

Fig. 3. Structure of bacteriophage T7, based on data given in the text. Only two of the tail fibers are shown, but end-on views of isolated tails show that there are six. The fainter structure in the center is a representation of the internal core structure described by Serwer (1976). Its division into rings is suggested but not yet established. Locations of gene products in the virion are indicated at the right. The bar represents 50 nm.

large number of phages in nature (Bradley, 1967). Zweig and Cummings (1973a,b) studied the structure of coliphage T5 heads, demonstrated more than six proteins in isolated heads, and also showed cleavage of the major head protein (Table 1). Their estimates of the number of copies of the major head protein (gpD20*) would predict surface lattice structures of $T = 12$ or 13.

Phage SP01 has been extensively studied because of interest in its transcriptional program (Rabussay and Geiduschek, 1977). Little is known about its morphogenesis, but some structural parameters have been determined (Parker, 1979) (Fig. 4). Isolated heads contain at least seven proteins. The major head protein has a mass of about 50,000 daltons when it is part of the polyheads produced by suppressible mutants in several head-defective genes. When mature phages are dissociated in SDS and the proteins are separated by gel elec-

---

concentric lines. The prohead structure contains no DNA but has an inner core structure represented by elongated objects extending from 6 to 20 nm. The prohead shell is apparently the same thickness as the mature phage shell, but is smaller, and expands on maturation. B: Sketch, compiled from cited text references and unpublished data of W. Earnshaw, of the head and tail component of phage P22. The location of the phage proteins is given where known. The bar represents 50 nm.

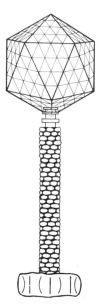

Fig. 4. Schematic drawing of bacteriophage SP01 of *Bacillus subtilis*. The head shows a suggested icosahedral surface lattice design of $T = 16$, and a complex connector structure is indicated between the head and tail. The tail subunit arrangement is that derived from analysis of electron micrographs made by Parker (1979). The baseplate structure is difficult to make out on extended tails, but clearly has 6-fold symmetry when converted to the expanded state after sheath contraction. The bar represents 50 nm.

trophoresis, the major head protein migrates at a position corresponding to a mass of about 45,000 daltons, suggesting that it is processed to a smaller form by proteolytic cleavage during maturation. Both SP01 and T5 heads (Zweig and Cummings, 1973a) contain a 19,000- to 21,000-dalton protein in fairly large quantity (5–10% of total head protein) which is missing in heads lacking DNA. This probably corresponds to the major internal protein of phage T4 (see below), which is packaged in the head along with the DNA and injected into the host cell on infection. Inspection of electron micrographs of SP01 and SP01-like phages (Hemphill and Whiteley, 1975) suggests hexamer–pentamer clustering in a $T = 16$ icosahedral surface lattice, which agrees with rough estimates of the chemically determined number of head protein subunits (Table 1).

2.7. Elongated Head Structures: ϕ29, T4, and CbK

The structure of anisometric viral capsids requires the regulation of both diameter and length during assembly. The proheads are built with the anisometric form already determined (Nelson *et al.*, 1976; Eiserling *et al.*, 1970). Initiation of a properly designed cap with the appropriate triangulation number and built-in curvature must be followed by elongation via addition of capsid subunits and additional regulatory protein components.

In the case of T4, an assembly core plays a role in both diameter selection and length determination, but the structural arrangement of neither the core proteins nor the initiation complex has yet been determined. The core is, however, highly organized, as described below.

2.8. ϕ29 Structure

The very small phage ϕ29 nonetheless has a very complex morphology (Nelson *et al.*, 1976; Hagen *et al.*, 1976), and over 60% of the genetic information of the phage is used for virion assembly and structural proteins (Pène *et al.*, 1973; Reilly *et al.*, 1977). The head consists of a 32 × 42-nm capsid equipped with protein fibers at each end, and a collar connector to the tail (Fig. 5). The dispensible fibers do not appear to project only from the 5-fold vertices, but their attachment sites are poorly defined. The head protein is present in about 100

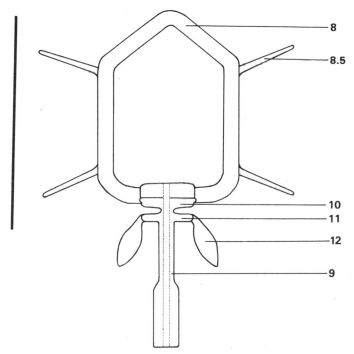

Fig. 5. Outline of the arrangment and protein composition of *Bacillus subtilis* phage ϕ29. This tiny phage has a remarkably complex structure, including an anisometric head and head fibers. The upper collar structure is involved in head shape determination, and the lower collar appendages somehow facilitate phage adsorption. Gene product locations are given at the right of the sketch. The bar represents 50 nm.

copies, suggesting that the design of the shell is an elongated $T = 1$ structure. If the gp8 subunits have pentamer–hexamer clustering, a single band of five hexamers could provide the necessary elongation. However, since electron micrographs show a smooth capsid with no obvious morphological units, it is possible that either a minor protein fills in the spaces, or the clustering is trimer or dimer, which would make the repeating unit too small to be seen easily by electron microscopy. The head is reported (Nelson *et al.*, 1976) to consist of only the fiber, head, and collar proteins, although Pène *et al.* (1973) reported a minor capsid protein co-migrating with gp8. The head shows a curious asymmetry in that the tail attachment end (with upper collar) is more flattened than the opposite end of the particle. Presumably this is due to a distortion introduced by the gp10 collar structure. In the absence of this structure, isometric rather than elongated capsids are produced. It is not completely clear whether the anisotropy is induced by gp10 adding to a shell containing the full complement of gp8 head protein or whether the isometric structure has fewer gp8 subunits, since neither direct protein composition comparison nor mature isometric phages have yet been described. An estimate has been made by Hagen *et al.* (1976), based on model building, of about 72 subunits for the isometric form, suggesting a smaller capsid.

2.9. T4 Head Structure

Phage T4 represents the extreme in structural complexity among bacterial viruses. Twenty genes are involved in head morphogenesis, and the head itself (depending on the presence of connector proteins and whether some protein bands seen on gels are truly head proteins) has from nine to 19 different polypeptide components (see Table 2). Four of these are internal proteins (Black and Ahmad-Zadeh, 1971; Stone and Cummings, 1972; Horwitz, 1974), and there are two internal peptides (Kurtz and Champe, 1977) packaged inside the head along with the DNA and released from it on infection.

The icosahedral surface lattice is $T = 13l$, elongated along a 5-fold axis (Branton and Klug, 1975; Aebi *et al.*, 1974). The precise length of the head and thus the number of protein components are not known with certainty. Branton and Klug (1975) favor one additional band of 20 capsomers ($Q = 17$) while we (Bijlenga *et al.*, 1976; Aebi, Doermann, and Eiserling, unpublished results) favor two ($Q = 21$) (Fig. 6). We have used the latter value in computing the number of copies of

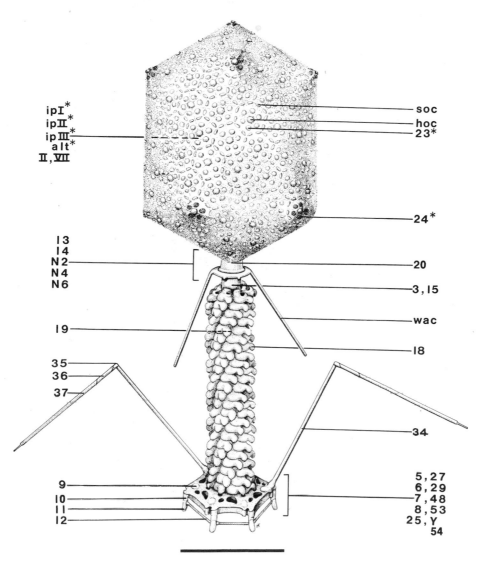

ipI*
ipII*
ipIII*
alt*
II,VII

soc
hoc
23*

24*

13
14
N2
N4
N6

20
3,15
wac
18

19

35
36
37

34

9
10
11
12

5,27
6,29
7,48
8,53
25,Y
54

Fig. 6. Structure of bacteriophage T4, based on electron microscopic structure analysis to a resolution of about 2–3 nm. Near the head are shown the locations of the known major and minor proteins. The icosahedral vertices are the location of gp24*, but it is not known precisely where they are or whether an additional subunit in fact lies on the local 5-fold axis, as depicted. The gene 20 protein is located at the connector vertex, bound in an unknown way to the neck structure. The six whiskers and collar structure appear to be made of a single protein species; only two whiskers are shown here. The gp18 sheath subunits fit into holes in the baseplate, and the short tail fibers (gp12) are shown in a stored position. The long tail fibers (only two of the six are shown) are usually bent at a constant angle of 156° when free. Their position shown here is closer to that seen on adsorption to the cell surface. The bar represents 50 nm.

TABLE 2

Structural Proteins of Bacteriophage T4

	Designation of gene product	Estimated size (kilodaltons)	Estimated number of copies per virion	Daltons per virion $\times 10^{-6}$	References[a]
Head	23[c]	46	960	44.00	Aebi et al. (1974, 1976, 1977b)
(15 proteins)[b] (73.5×10^6 daltons)	soc	10	960	9.60	Ishii and Yanagida (1977)
	hoc	40	148	5.90	Yanagida (1977)
	24[c]	45	55	2.50	Müller-Salamin et al. (1977)
	ipIII[c]	18	400	4.80	Showe and Black (1973), Hosoda and Cone (1970), Onorato et al. (1978)
	ipI[c]	9	180	1.60	Show and Black (1973), Hosoda and Cone (1970)
	20	64	15	0.96	Müller-Salamin et al. (1977)
	ipII[c]	10	90	0.90	Showe and Black (1973), Hosoda and Cone (1970)
	alt(B1)	67	10	0.67	Horvitz (1974)
	H12	29	34	0.98	Coombs and Eiserling (1977), Aebi et al. (1974)
	Peptide II	3.9	140	0.55	Kurtz and Champe (1977)
	Peptide VII	2.5	180	0.45	Kurtz and Champe (1977)
	H7	36	6	0.21	Coombs and Eiserling (1977)
	H9	34	6	0.20	Coombs and Eiserling (1977)
	H10	33	6	0.20	Coombs and Eiserling (1977)

Structure	Gene				Reference
Neck (6 proteins) (3.4 × 10⁶ daltons)	wac	53	38	2.05	Coombs and Eiserling (1977)
	13	33	18	0.59	Coombs and Eiserling (1977)
	N2	35	6	0.21	Coombs and Eiserling (1977)
	N4	32	6	0.19	Coombs and Eiserling (1977)
	N5(14)	30	6	0.18	Coombs and Eiserling (1977)
	N6	28	6	0.17	Coombs and Eiserling (1977)
Tail (4 proteins) (11.1 × 10⁶ daltons)	18	70(56)	114	10.00 (8.10)	Moody (1973)
	19	18.5	144	2.66	Moody (1973)
	15	32	6	0.19	Coombs and Eiserling (1977)
	3	29	1–6	0.17	Coombs and Eiserling (1977)
Baseplate (15 proteins) (7.5 × 10⁶ daltons)	10	88	12	0.06	Crowther et al. (1977)
	6	85	12	1.02	Crowther et al. (1977)
	12	55	18	0.99	Crowther et al. (1977)
	7	140	6	0.84	Crowther et al. (1977)
	9	34	24	0.82	Crowther et al. (1977)
	11	24	24	0.58	Crowther et al. (1977)
	29	80	6	0.48	Crowther et al. (1977)
	27	48	6	0.29	Crowther et al. (1977)
	8	46	6	0.28	Crowther et al. (1977)
	5	44	6	0.26	Crowther et al. (1977)
	48	44	6	0.26	Crowther et al. (1977)
	54	36	6	0.22	Crowther et al. (1977)
	53	23	6	0.14	Crowther et al. (1977)
	Y	22	6	0.13	Crowther et al. (1977)
	25	15	6	0.09	Crowther et al. (1977)
Tail fibers (4 proteins) (3.7 × 10⁶ daltons)	34	145	12	1.74	Wood and King (this volume)
	37	115	12	1.38	Wood and King (this volume)
	36	24	12	0.30	Wood and King (this volume)
	35	39	6	0.24	Wood and King (this volume)

[a] Molecular weights are from Wood and Revel (1976) unless otherwise noted.
[b] Head completion genes 2, 4, 50, 64, and 65 are candidates for minor structural contributions.
[c] Cleaved during assembly.

TABLE 3
Phage Tail Structures

Short hexagonal

Phage	Tube size (nm) Width	Length	Tail appendages
φ29	4–6	32.5	Lower collar: 6 copies, gp11; Lower collar appendages: 12 copies, gp12
T7	9	20	Collar: 6 copies gp11 or 12; 6 fibers gp17
P22	10	10	Collar: 18 copies gp9; single tail fiber

Tubular

	Width	Length	$M_r \times 10^{-3}$ tube protein	Number of subunits	Annular repeat (nm)	Number of annuli	Symmetry	Number of tail proteins
λ	15	135	31	192	4.0	32	6-fold	9
φCbK	13	298	58	234	3.8	78	3-fold	3–4
T5	14	180	55	270	4.0	45	—	≥7

Contractile

	Sheath size (nm) Width	Length	$M_r \times 10^{-3}$ sheath protein	Number of subunits	Annular repeat (nm)	Number of annuli	Symmetry	Hand, coarse helical groove	Ω^c
T4	19.8	98.2	70(56)[b]	144	4.1	24	6-fold	Right	−102.2
SP01	18.6	140.3	61	198–216	4.1	33–36	6-fold	Right	−97.5
G	13	455	—[a]	612–828	3.8	102–138	6-fold	Probably right	−80.0
Mu	18	100	52	198	3.0	31–33	6-fold	Right	+144

[a] Not known.   [b] Glycoprotein, uncertain M_r.   [c] Helical screw angle (Smith et al., 1976).

the head proteins given in Table 3. The surface lattice design was determined directly by freeze-fracture techniques on phage T2 (Branton and Klug, 1975) which lacks the minor proteins hoc and soc (Ishii and Yanagida, 1977; Yanagida, 1977; Aebi *et al.*, 1976; Forrest and Cummings, 1970). However, in the case of T4, these additional proteins made the structural determination very difficult until the discovery of "giant" phages, elongated much more than normal along the 5-fold axis (Doermann *et al.*, 1973; Cummings *et al.*, 1973). These giant heads permitted detailed optical diffraction analysis of the electron micrographs because of the larger number of repeats, thus a higher signal-to-noise ratio. The location of the proteins soc (*small outer capsid*) and hoc (*highly antigenic outer capsid*) was determined by Ishii and Yanagida (1977) and by Aebi *et al.* (1976) using giant T4 phage. The protein hoc lies at the center of a ring (capsomer) of gp23* while there are six copies of soc around each six-membered capsomer of gp23*. Recently the location of the other capsid components has been accomplished by Müller-Salamin *et al.* (1977). Using antibody directed against purified gp24, they showed the most likely location of gp24* to be the icosahedral vertices, excluding the tail-joining vertex. In principle, the 5-fold vertices could be made of gp23*, but they are not. Differential extraction of T4 capsids (in 7 M urea, pH 11) removes all the gp24* as seen by SDS gel electrophoresis, and gaps appear at the vertices, confirming this as the gp24* location. It is not known whether another protein such as hoc binds at the vertices, but we have indicated something like it on Fig. 6. Finally, gp20 has been localized at the tail-joining vertex, where it probably serves a role in capsid initiation during assembly.

The neck of the phage is itself a complex structure composed of at least five proteins (Coombs and Eiserling, 1977). In T4 and T6, six whiskers are attached to the lower of the two knobs protruding from the connector structure. These serve a role in long tail fiber attachment, described later (Conley and Wood, 1975). Aside from the localization of the whiskers, the *wac* gene product, the position of the neck proteins in this structure is unknown.

As described earlier for the smaller isometric phages P22 and λ, the T4 prohead expands during maturation. The early prohead lacks minor proteins, and, as for the phage λ D protein, hoc and soc are added later, after expansion of the lattice of P23 from 11.2 nm to the lattice of 12.5 nm followed by the cleavages of gp23 and gp24, producing gp23* and gp24*. Most of the T4 head proteins have now been localized in the head structure; however, some protein components have not yet been correlated with genetic lesions, for example, H 7, 9, 10,

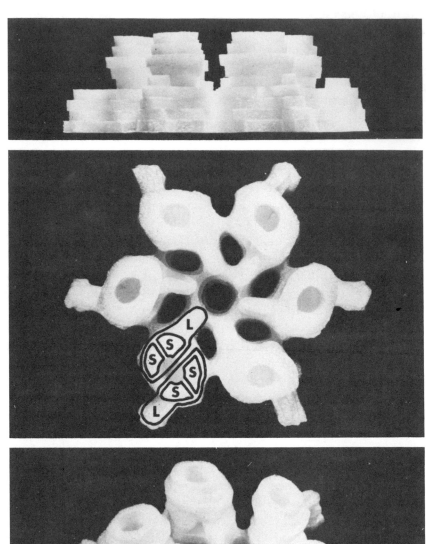

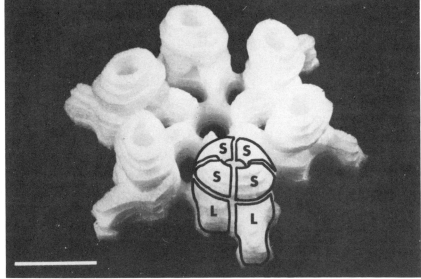

and 12, and N 2, 4, and 6 (Table 2). Since the products of five genes known to be involved with head morphogenesis (genes 2, 4, 50, 64, 65) have not yet been identified as protein bands on gels, it is likely that several of these gene products will turn out to be head internal proteins or neck proteins, or will have transient associations with the head.

The subtotal for the molecular mass of the head depends on whether the minor unidentified components and the neck are included. From Table 2 the capsid mass is 73.5×10^6 daltons, and the neck 3.4×10^6 daltons; thus the head should total 183×10^6 daltons (187 with the neck). The value of 183×10^6 agrees well with the value of 176×10^6 calculated by Benbasat and Bloomfield (1975) for purified T4 heads from hydrodynamic measurements. The same authors determined that fiberless particles are 195×10^6 daltons, thus tails are 19×10^6 daltons. Again, this is in good agreement with the value of 18.6×10^6 from summing up the protein components (Table 2).

2.10. Phage ϕCbK Head Structure

Phage ϕCbK infects *Caulobacter crescentus*, and, although virtually nothing is known about its assembly or genetics, its large head size and prominent subunit structure made it a favorable subject for structural studies by Lake and Leonard (1974). In fact, its head structure is known in more detail than for any other large phage except T4, since it has a naturally occurring, very elongated head structure. Compositional studies by Leonard *et al.* (1972) established that there are two major capsid proteins, defined as "peak 6" from SDS gels, a 36,000-dalton protein present in 1150 copies, and "peak 8," containing twice as many copies of a small (13,500-dalton) protein. Metal shadowing and negative staining established the icosahedral surface lattice as $T = 7l$. Metal shadowing also revealed that the small protein probably lies on top of the basic lattice formed by the large protein. Computer filtering confirmed this model, presented in Fig. 7, which shows several views of a model of

←

Fig. 7. Views of a three-dimensional model of the protein positions in the ϕCbK capsid according to Lake and Leonard (1974). Top: An edge-on view, perpendicular to the local 6-fold axis. Middle: A view down the 6-fold axis. The proteins are outlined in black, with the large 36,000-dalton protein marked L and the small 13,500-dalton protein marked S. Bottom: A 45° tilted view of the model. In the ϕCbK capsid, the prominent morphological units visible on electron micrographs consist of two large and four small proteins. The more common arrangement for phage capsomers consists of a grouping of six large and 12 small subunits about the local 6-fold axis, or half (L_1S_2) of each unit shown in this model. The edge view shows the considerable height of the small proteins above the surface, which are very clearly visible in metal shadowed micrographs. The bar represents 5.0 nm.

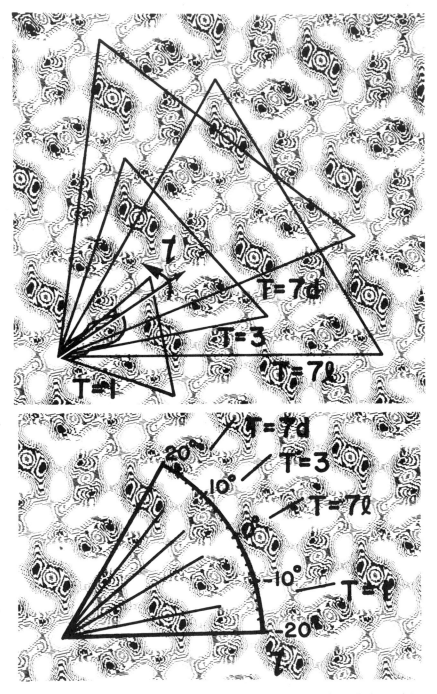

Fig. 8.   Computer-averaged image of the ϕCbK surface lattice, from Lake and Leonard (1974). Protein is dark. Top: The equilateral triangles drawn on the surface lattice
all have their corners on a local 6-fold axis, which would be transformed into a 5-fold

an "expanded" capsomer. The capsomer structure consists of six large and 12 small subunits arranged about a local 6-fold axis. Thus, unlike in T4 where soc is inserted between capsomers of gp23*, the ϕCbK small protein dimer binds to the outer surface of the capsomer formed by the large capsid protein. The small proteins are clustered in rings of four over local 2-fold axes, in contact with two large proteins below (Figs. 7 and 8). Although the data are indirect, Lake and Leonard (1974) speculate that the 5-fold vertices are composed of a different protein, as is the case for T4.

3. STRUCTURE OF PHAGE TAILS

Three morphologically distinguishable bacteriophage tail types form the basis for Bradley's (1967) groupings of types A, B, and C: contractile, noncontractile–long, and noncontractile–short. For the phages discussed in this chapter, these categories are referred to as "contractile," "tubular," and "short hexagonal" (Table 3). Phage tails probably originate from the specialized vertex used to initiate capsid assembly and are designed to attach to cell surfaces and initiate nucleic acid transfer to the host cell. All phages described here have a head-to-tail connecting structure as well, part of which can be considered as a tail component. Besides the appendages at the head end, many phage tails also have fibrous structures attached to the distal end which interact with the cell surface. A detailed collection of electron micrographs and a survey of many phage morphological types are found in the monograph by Tikhonenko (1970).

3.1. Short Hexagonal Tail Structure

Previously thought to be simple structures, the P22, T7, and ϕ29 tail structures are complex if the connector is included. In phage P22, six dimers or trimers of the gene 9 product make up a hexagonal collar

---

when forming a curved icosahedral structure (see Caspar and Klug, 1962) of different T numbers indicated on the triangles. At the common vertex of all four triangles, the outline of a single L_1S_2 unit is shown. The long axis of this protein is shown by an arrow, and the tilt angle is indicated by t. Bottom: The tilt angle, t, needed to produce a surface lattice of the appropriate design is shown. The long axis of the penton protein will point in different directions depending on the T number, and Lake and Leonard (1974) suggest that this tilt may be used to select the $T = 7l$ structure rather than the $T = 7d$ enantiomer, and thus account for the fact that a given virus produces a unique capsid design.

(or baseplate) surrounding a short tubular neck which enters the capsid; the neck is possibly made of gps 4, 7, 10, 16, 20, and 26. This connector and tail structure requires a minimum of five or six gene products for its construction, resulting in a fairly complex organelle with specificity for the recognition and hydrolysis of rhamnosyl-galactose groups in the lipopolysaccharide of the *Salmonella* outer envelope (Iwashita and Kanegasaki, 1973; Israel, 1976). Inactivating antiserum prepared against P22 specifically blocks the gp9 hexagonal collar (Israel *et al.*, 1967), and mutants lacking the collar clearly show the short tube but are unable to adsorb. A 20-nm-long fiber projects from the base of the 10-nm tube. Most of the phage structural proteins are located around the head–tail connecting region (Fig. 2B), although their positions within it are unknown.

Phage T7 is very similar to P22 in its tail structure (Fig. 3). There is an additional fiber component coded for by gene 17 (Studier, 1972; Studier, Costello, and Maizel, unpublished, 1976). The tubular part of the tail is made of the gene 11 and/or 12 proteins and is attached to the gene 8 neck protein, usually referred to as a head protein. Tails produced from heat-disrupted wild-type phage contain gp8 in addition to gps 11, 12, and 17, similar to the neck proteins in T4 produced by osmotic shock (Coombs and Eiserling, 1977). The core structure described by Serwer (1976), composed of gps 14, 15, 16, and possibly 13, is bound to gp8 on the inside of the head.

Like P22 and T7, *Bacillus subtilis* phage ϕ29 has a neck and collar arrangement surrounding a short tube (Fig. 5). Variations include 12, rather than six, tail appendages and an increase in tube diameter about halfway down; the molecular explanation for this is unknown. Proteolytic cleavage during assembly occurs for the ϕ29 appendages (Tosi *et al.*, 1975). The tail tip structure is particularly unclear, since only three copies of the gene 9 product are thought to be in the tail tube (Viñuela *et al.*, 1976; Nelson *et al.*, 1976). In ϕ29, the upper and lower collar rings of six subunits each are coded for by different genes (10 and 11), and the upper collar protein has a major role in head shape determination (Nelson *et al.*, 1976). For all three of these phages and others constructed like them, the basic design is a head–tail connector structure, to which is attached a short tube made of a stack of rings of six subunits. Attached to this are six or some multiple appendages (fibers, baseplate) involved in adsorption to the cell surface. The appendages may, in addition to recognizing specific cell surface receptors, have enzymatic activity (receptor-destroying) similar to animal viruses, such as influenza.

3.2. Tubular Tail Structure

In addition to the neck structures common to all tailed bac-teriophages, these phages λ, T5, and ϕCbK have a long flexible tube made of rings of three or six subunits terminating in a complex adsorp-tion organelle. For λ and probably the others, this organelle serves as the initiator for tail tube assembly and is the most complex part of the tail. The steps in lambda tail assembly are reviewed both by Wood and King (Chapter 9) and extensively by Hohn and Katsura (1977). The structural parameters for these phages are given in Table 3 (see also Figs. 1 and 9). Both λ and T5 show proteolytic cleavage of a tail component during assembly (Hendrix and Casjens, 1974; Zweig and Cummings, 1973a,b); however, the function of these cleavages is unknown.

An interesting variation on the standard rings of six subunits com-posing the tail tube is found in the structure of the ϕCbK tail (Leonard *et al.*, 1973). The tail of this phage has a relatively uncharacterized neck and baseplate, but the tubular portion has been analyzed in detail by optical diffraction methods, and has been found to consist of rings of three subunits with asymmetrical projections aimed toward the head, giving the entire structure a strong polarity and pronounced helical twist (Fig. 9). The tail length of 78 annuli of 3-fold symmetry is tightly controlled, estimated at 78 ± 2.2 annuli.

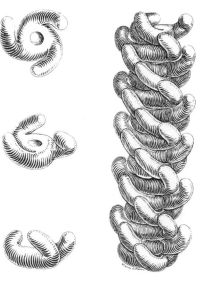

Fig. 9. Model of a portion of the ϕCbK tail structure taken from Leonard *et al.* (1973). Three views of an isolated trimer ring are shown at left, and the stacked disk structure arranged with the rotational angle seen on electron micrographs is indicated at the right. The cylindrical subunit projections point upward toward the head. This is the only phage described which has 3-fold rather than 6-fold rotational symmetry in the tail.

3.3. Contractile Tail Structure

These tails show the most complex arrangement of proteins, including an intricate baseplate with tail fibers composed of many pro- teins which change conformation during infection, resulting in sheath contraction and DNA injection. The steps in the assembly of phage T4, the paradigm for such structures, are given in Chapter 9. Detailed studies of the T4 sheath (Moody, 1973; Amos and Klug, 1975; Smith *et al.*, 1976) and the baseplate (Crowther *et al.*, 1977) have given perhaps the most complete structure analysis for any complex virus. Because of the large number of repeating units in the extended sheath and the fact that they are arranged with helical symmetry, a single electron mic- rograph simultaneously presents many different views of the equivalent subunits, which permits a three-dimensional analysis of its struc- ture (Crowther and Klug, 1975). The T4 tail sheath is composed of a single protein, gp18 (King and Mykolajewycz, 1973; Dickson, 1974). On SDS gels the protein appears to have an M_r of 70,000, but other chemical studies suggest a mass closer to 56,000 daltons (Dickson, 1974). There are 144 copies of gp18 arranged in 24 rows of six subunits each. The distal row of subunits is in contact with the baseplate proteins (Fig. 6), and the row nearest the head binds to gp3 and gp15. All subunits are in close contact with the central tube, made of gp19. The subunits in each 4.1-nm-thick hexagonal row are rotated by about 103° with respect to the one below (Smith *et al.*, 1976), giving rise to helical lines visible in electron micrographs. The stacked disk structure repeats after seven hexagonal rows, giving 42 subunits in each repeat. This represents 21 different views of the subunit in a single electron mic- rograph, since half the views are the same. The main features of the structure are six helical "tunnels" and two sets of grooves on the sur- face (Fig. 6). The deepest grooves give rise to the prominent right- handed helix seen on the surface. The gp18 subunit has protruding knobs at the tips, which are likely to fit into corresponding holes in the baseplate. Amos and Klug (1975) portray each gp18 in the extended sheath as sloping downward from inner to outer radius. We have used this feature in constructing Fig. 6, although it should be noted that there is little or no downward slope in the model presented by Smith *et al.* (1976). The sheath surrounds a central tube or core, composed of gp19. Moody (1971) determined the structural features of polytubes from phage T2 as having a 4.1-nm repeat between rings of six subunits. The spacings in electron micrographs of sheath and core are identical. Moody's data give a diameter of 9.0 nm, with a 3.0-nm hole in the center of the tube.

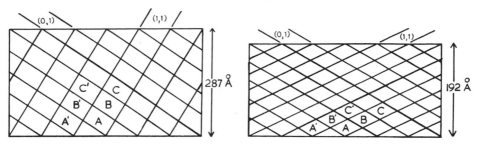

Fig. 10. Schematic drawing, from Amos and Klug (1975), of the extended and contracted tail sheath lattice of phage T4, using the terminology of Moody (1973). Left: The "long pitch helices" (1,1) give rise to the strong, right-handed helical grooves seen in Fig. 6. The lattice repeats after seven rings of six subunits. The shallower, left-handed helices are indicated by the (0,1) notation. Right: On contraction, the subunits above (B',B) move downward as the subunits (A,A') move apart. This lattice repeats after 11 rings of six subunits.

Sheath contraction has been shown by Moody (1973) to be a displacive transition from the extended to the contracted state (Fig. 10). From three-dimensional reconstructions of extended sheath and polysheath (an aberrant assembly form of gp18 in the contracted state), Amos and Klug suggest that the dramatic change in the shape of the sheath on contraction is related to relatively small changes in the overall conformational form of gp18. Both Moody (1973) and Donelli *et al.* (1972) have shown micrographs of partially contracted sheaths, the latter from a *Bacillus subtilis* phage, G. These convincingly establish the displacive nature of the sheath subunit rearrangement, and show that for T4, the gp18 conformational change occurs before sheath contraction itself is completed. The contraction process begins when signals, transmitted to the baseplate by the tail fibers, trigger a rearrangement of the baseplate. The connection of the annulus of sheath subunits at the surface of the baseplate to the central tube weakens and the gp18 subunits move apart. As the ring expands, subunits above are pulled down into the spaces created by the baseplate expansion, setting off the contraction process and driving the tail tube downward into the bacterial cell.

The key structure in the contraction process is the hexagonal baseplate. It consists of a central hub and six outer wedges, six tail spikes and six 140-nm-long fibers. There are also six short (35-nm) tail fibers bound to the spikes. During attachment to the cell surface, the baseplate undergoes expansion from a compact hexagon to a thin six-pointed star (Simon and Anderson, 1967*a,b*; Crowther *et al.*, 1977). Using a rotational filtering process to improve the signal-to-noise ratio of electron micrographs of isolated baseplates, Crowther *et al.* (1977) have determined the architecture of the hexagonal and star-shaped baseplates to about 3.0 nm resolution. Having described the complete structures (Fig. 11), they examined mutants lacking various components with the goal of localizing these components in the structure. Fortunately for this analytical approach, three of the proteins, gps 9, 11, and 12, account for a considerable fraction of the total mass of the baseplate (40%) and gps 9 and 11 are added after the hexagonal structure is completed. This permits relatively unambiguous determination of their locations, which are given in Figs. 6 and 11. Since gp9 is needed

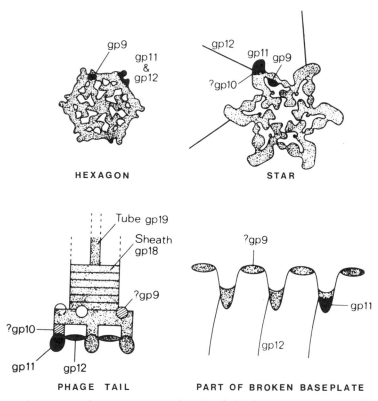

Fig. 11. Summary of the structural details of the hexagon-to-star transition in the baseplate of bacteriophage T4, taken from Crowther *et al.* (1977). Top: Anatomy of the hexagon and star and the location of the major structural proteins gp 9, 10, 11, and 12. Bottom: Schematic diagrams of side views of the extended sheath with hexagonal baseplate and of a piece of broken baseplate. The latter is thought to represent a form of the outer hexagonal rim of the baseplate, in which the gp12 short fibers are fully extended. This should be compared with the "stored" form of gp12 on the lower left, also represented in Fig. 6.

for tail fiber attachment and is found to be located near the site where the tail fibers join to the baseplate, it is reasonable to assume that gp9 may be involved in tail fiber binding although direct evidence is lacking. The gene 11 product has been shown to be the distal portion of the tail pin. If gp11 is missing, gp12 cannot bind; thus gp11 must supply the gp12 binding site. Kells and Haselkorn (1974) showed that gp12 forms the six 35-nm fibers. In wild-type phage these 35-nm fibers are not usually visibly extended from the baseplate, suggesting that they occupy a stored or folded position (Fig. 6).

Using the same analytical approach, Crowther *et al.* (1977) determined the structural changes which take place during the hexagon–star transformation. The major events in this process are the outward extension of the tail pins, the switch of gp9 from the outside of the hexagon toward the inside of the star, and the switch in the position of gp12 (Fig. 11). The hexagon is stabilized by the presence of gp12; in its absence, many isolated baseplates spontaneously convert from hexagon to star. The contraction process is probably monitored by the long tail fibers, since Yamamoto and Uchida (1975) and Arscott and Goldberg (1976) have shown that fiberless phages are more resistant to induced contraction than are phages with the normal complement of long tail fibers. Crowther *et al.* (1977) postulate that the long tail fibers, moving over the bacterial cell surface, transmit receptor-modulated binding and conformational change information to the baseplate, possibly via the gene 9 product. This step is thought to activate the baseplate, which is triggered into the hexagon–star transformation by the contact of the gp12 short tail fibers with the cell surface. This structural transformation is the key event in inducing sheath contraction.

4. DISCUSSION

4.1. Head Structure and Assembly

As mentioned earlier, bacteriophage head structure follows the rules of icosahedral surface lattice design predicted by Caspar and Klug (1962). One result of recent structural and chemical studies on phage heads is that the initiation event in head assembly must include several shape-determining steps. The logical structural site for head initiation is the part of the head where the tail attaches, referred to as the neck or connector. For all the phages described here, some such structure

exists: the core and neck proteins of T7 (gps 9, 13–16) described by
Serwer (1976) and by Studier *et al.* (unpublished, 1976), the gene
products 4, 7, 10, 16, 20, and 26 for phage P22 (Botstein *et al.*, 1973),
the four or five proteins of the λ connector (Hendrix, unpublished,
1978), the gene 10 product of φ29 (Hagen *et al.*, 1976), and the six neck
proteins of T4 (Coombs and Eiserling, 1977) plus gp20 (Müller-
Salamin *et al.*, 1977). In all cases where the data are available, the connector components have 6-fold symmetry and the structure is inserted
into the 5-fold icosahedral vertex. This symmetry mismatch has been
described earlier (Moody, 1965; Katsura and Kühl, 1974) and may have
some significance or may simply reflect the junction of two structures
of different symmetry which are mechanically joined by a constriction
at the head vertex. This seems possible, since relatively mild osmotic
shock of T4 produces tails with the connector structure still attached
(Coombs and Eiserling, 1977). Müller-Salamin *et al.* (1977) have
localized gp20 in the head at the vertex where the tail joins, yet gp20 is
not found on the expelled T4 connectors (Coombs and Eiserling, 1977);
thus it seems likely that gp20 is part of the head vertex which provides a
weak binding site to the connector structure. The role of T4 gp20 is a
key one in head assembly. In its absence, head proteins are assembled
into tubular structures without icosahedral caps, and it has been postulated that gp20 is an icosahedral cap initiator for this reason. T4 gene
20 [located at 102 Kb on the genetic map (Wood and Revel, 1976)] has
an estimated protein molecular weight of 64,000, and is present in at
least five to ten copies per phage. Hsiao and Black (1977) have shown
that a cold-sensitive mutant in gene 20 shows an unusual phenotype: it
makes empty heads with cleaved proteins which appear normal and
contain gp20. Since DNA is not packaged, this vertex protein appears
to have a second role in structure determination. Using an ingenious
method devised by Jarvik and Botstein (1975) for ordering the steps in
assembly with *ts* and *cs* mutants, Hsiao and Black showed that the gp20
vertex protein functions both early in assembly, at the icosahedral cap
stage, and later, at the time of DNA packaging.

One aspect of head structure determination which has received
little attention is the choice of direction for the skew classes of icosahedral surface lattices such as $T = 7l$ (for λ and φCbK) and $T = 13l$ for
phage T4. Mixtures of $T = 7l$ and $T = 7d$ heads are not observed, so
some positive control mechanism must exist. One suggestion, made by
Lake and Leonard (1974), utilizes the discovery that the capsid penton
vertex protein is different from the hexagonal lattice (as for phage T4
and φCbK). Figure 8 shows equilateral triangles corresponding to different triangulation numbers. Lake and Leonard show that, depending

on the triangulation number, the long axis of the specific vertex protein will point in different directions, because the 5-fold axis is inclined at an angle to the icosahedral face. A combination of intrinsic curvature of the major capsid protein plus the regulatory effect of the specialized vertices could act together to specify the size and hand of the lattice.

4.2. Tail Structure

Contractile phage tails, as pointed out by Bradley (1967), have remarkably constant structural design: an inner tubular part that is a roughly 20,000-dalton protein composed of 4.0-nm stacked disks, surrounded by a sheath with the same periodicity made of a larger, roughly 60,000-dalton protein. Bacteriophage μ is somewhat of an exception to this general rule, since it has a smaller sheath subunit, smaller annular spacing, and different coarse pitch helix sense (Admiraal and Mellema, 1976) (Table 3). The phages with non-contractile tails resemble the inner tube if the tails are short hexagonal (P22, T7) or appear to be more variable in design (Table 3) if the tails are long (λ, ϕCbK).

The regulation of the length of the bacteriophage tail is a model problem in the search for biological length-determining mechanisms. For all phage tails, the problem reduces to how the length of the central tube is determined, since it happens independently of sheath formation. All phage systems described apparently are similar: a basal structure initiates the polymerization of tail subunits which are present in large numbers but which are designed to remain unassembled within the cell. The basal structure presumably imposes a conformational change on the first bound tail subunits, which in turn exposes new binding sites. This permits the addition of more subunits, possibly in a manner similar to binding of bacterial flagellin monomer to short fragments of assembled flagella (Asakura, 1970).

Models have been discussed (Kellenberger, 1972) for length regulation, but none has yet been convincingly established. The remarkable homogeneity in length of phage tails (usually $\pm$ 1–2 disks) requires some well-defined ruler or a switching mechanism of highly cooperative sensitivity. Many phage tails contain 20–50 or more disks; thus models which propose uniform changes in the structural conformation of the growing structure at the addition of each disk seem unlikely to give such a narrow length distribution. However, such a theoretical model has been constructed (Wagenknecht and Bloomfield, 1975).

The best-studied phage tail length measuring system at present is phage λ. Studies by Katsura *et al.* (1974, 1975*a,b*, 1976) have established the pathway for tail assembly and demonstrated the requirement for an initiator structure and for a termination protein. The normal initiator, like the phage T4 baseplate, requires many (at least seven) gene products for its formation. Once properly formed, the initiator facilitates the assembly of about 200 molecules (32 disks) of the major tail protein (gene V product). In the presence of the gene U "termination" protein, tail assembly stops at the proper length and the stable structure is ready for joining to heads. The mechanism of action of the gene U product is unknown, but it appears to bind to the tail protein itself. Recent evidence (Hohn and Katsura, 1977) shows that it apparently acts by adding a single ring at the head attachment end. Even in the absence of gpU, however, the growing tail apparently stops at the normal length, caught in a "kinetic trap," although this structure is unstable and is later converted into an aberrant tail of indeterminate length, incapable of joining to heads (Katsura, 1976).

Phage T4 has a similar sequence. The initiator is the baseplate, itself composed of 15 gene products. After the addition of the gene 54 product, the baseplate can bind the tube protein. *In vitro* studies on assembly by Wagenknecht and Bloomfield (1977) show the same result as for phage λ: purified tube protein gp19 adds to baseplate to form structures near the normal length, but these two are unstable and eventually grow past the normal length. These experiments have not yet been done in the presence of the T4 gp3 terminating protein, which should stablize the structure. Further work is needed to define the mechanism of length determination, but the problem is becoming experimentally accessible.

Another related question is the polarity of assembly of the tail tube protein. Once an initiator structure is present, clearly, elongation is polar and proceeds in one direction. However, it is not known for λ or T4 whether the tail tube grows in a polar manner *in vitro*, free of the baseplate, by the structural information contained in the tube protein subunit itself. Assembly studies by Leonard *et al.* (1973) on the flexible φCbK tail protein demonstrated closed circular polymers, suggesting unregulated polymerization of the protein in both directions. No data are yet available for other phages, but this result is different from that of bacterial flagella (Asakura, 1970) where free subunits add only to a single end of a broken fragment of the flagellar filament.

5.   SUMMATION

From the recent increase in structural information on bacteriophage assembly it has become clear that an impressive number of structural transformations of the virion take place during assembly and on infection. For a single phage such as T4 these include at least eight major structural rearrangements of viral components: during head assembly (prohead lattice expansion and addition of accessory proteins, entry and exit of core proteins, entry and packaging of DNA); during tail fiber assembly (positioning of long fiber subassemblies on whiskers); and during adsorption and injection [whisker–fiber–sheath interactions during long tail fiber extension and retraction (Conley and Wood, 1975), short tail fiber extension, baseplate hexagon–star rearrangement, tail sheath contraction, tail core movement, and DNA ejection]. More of these structural transitions remain to be discovered, and many are known in outline for other phage systems. The elucidation of the molecular mechanisms of these transformations over the next few years should continue to provide further insights into the problems of viral adsorption and penetration and into the more general problems of the genesis and function of subcellular structures.

ACKNOWLEDGMENTS

My thanks to many colleagues who made unpublished data available, in particular Dwight Anderson, William Earnshaw, Roger Hendrix, Jonathan King, Michael Parker, and F. William Studier. Thanks also to Susan Sheby, Hermine Kavanaugh, and all the others in our group who helped in production of the figures. The research in our laboratory is supported by grants from the U.S. National Science Foundation and the Institute of Allergy and Infectious Diseases, NIH. Special thanks to Donald Caspar, who provided inspiration and critical insight.

6. REFERENCES

Admiraal, G., and Mellema, J. E., 1976, The structure of the contractile sheath of bacteriophage mu, *J. Ultrastruct. Res.* **56**:48.

Aebi, U., Bijlenga, R., Broek, J., Eiserling, F., Kellenberger, C., Kellenberger, E., Mesyanzhinov, V., Müller, L., Showe, M., Smith, R., and Steven, A., 1974, The transformation of τ particles into T4 heads, *J. Supramol. Struct.* **2**:253.

Aebi, U., Bijlenga, R., ten Heggeler, B., Kistler, J., Steven, A. C., and Smith, P. R., 1976, Comparison of the structural and chemical composition of giant T-even phage heads, *J. Supramol. Struct.* **5**:475.

Aebi, U., ten Heggeler, B., Onorato, L., Kistler, J., and Showe, M. K., 1977a, A new method for localizing proteins in periodic structures: Fab fragment labeling combined with image processing of electron micrographs, *Proc. Natl. Acad. Sci. USA* **74**:5514.

Aebi, U., van Driel, R., Bijlenga, R., ten Heggeler, B., van den Broek, R., Steven, A.,
    and Smith P., 1977*b*, Capsid fine structure of T-even bacteriophages: Binding and
    localization of two dispensible capsid proteins into the P23 surface lattice, *J. Mol.
    Biol.* **110**:687.
Amos, L. A., and Klug, A., 1975, Three dimensional image reconstructions of the
    contractile tail of the T4 bacteriophage, *J. Mol. Biol.* **99**:51.
Arscott, P., and Goldberg, E., 1976, Cooperative action of the T4 tail fibers and base-
    plate in triggering conformational change and in determining host range, *Virology*
    69:15.
Asakura, S., 1970, Polymerization of flagellin and polymorphism of flagella, *Adv.
    Biophys.* **1**:99.
Beckendorf, S. K., 1973, Structure of the distal half of the bacteriophage T4 tail fiber,
    J. Mol. Biol. **73**:37.
Benbasat, J. A., and Bloomfield, V., 1975, Joining of bacteriophage T4D heads and
    tails: A kinetic study by inelastic light scattering, *J. Mol. Biol.* **95**:335.
Bijlenga, R. G. L., Aebi, U., and Kellenberger, E., 1976, Properties and structure of a
    gene 24-controlled T4 giant phage, *J. Mol. Biol.* **103**:469.
Black, L. W., and Ahmad-Zadeh, C., 1971, Internal proteins of bacteriophage T4D:
    Their characterization and relation to head structure and assembly, *J. Mol. Biol.*
    57:71.
Botstein, D., Waddell, C. H., and King, J., 1973, Mechanism of head assembly and
    DNA encapsulation in *Salmonella* phage P22. I. Genes, proteins, structures, and
    DNA maturation, *J. Mol. Biol.* **80**:669.
Bradley, D. E., 1967, Ultrastructure of bacteriophages and bacteriocins, *Bacteriol. Rev.*
    31:230.
Branton, D., and Klug, A., 1975, Capsid geometry of bacteriophage T2: A freeze-etch-
    ing study, *J. Mol. Biol.* **92**:559.
Casjens, S., 1974, Bacteriophage lambda *FII* gene protein: Role in head assembly, *J.
    Mol. Biol.* **90**:1.
Caspar, D. L. D., and Klug, A., 1962, Physical principles in the construction of regular
    viruses, *Cold Spring Harbor Symp. Quant. Biol.* **27**:1.
Conley, M. P., and Wood, W. B., 1975, Bacteriophage T4 whiskers: A rudimentary
    environment-sensing device, *Proc. Natl. Acad. Sci. USA* **72**:3701.
Coombs, D. H., and Eiserling, F. A., 1977, Studies on the structure, protein composi-
    tion and assembly of the neck of bacteriophage T4, *J. Mol. Biol.* **116**:375.
Crowther, R., and Klug, A., 1975, Structural analysis of macromolecular assemblies by
    image reconstruction from electron micrographs, *Annu. Rev. Biochem.* **44**.
Crowther, R. A. Lenk, E. V., Kikuchi, Y., and King, J., 1977, Molecular reorganiza-
    tion in the hexagon to star transition of the baseplate of bacteriophage T4, *J. Mol.
    Biol.* **116**:489.
Cummings, D. J., Chapman, V. A., DeLong, S. S., and Couse, N. L., 1973, Structural
    aberrations in T-even bacteriophage. III. Induction of "lollipops" and their partial
    characterization, *Virology* **54**:245.
DeRosier, D. J., and Klug, A., 1972, Structure of the tubular variants of the head of
    bacteriophage T4 (polyheads). I. Arrangement of subunits in some classes of poly-
    heads, *J. Mol. Biol.* **65**:469.
Dickson, R. C., 1974, Protein composition of the tail and contracted sheath of bac-
    teriophage T4, *Virology* **59**:123.

Doermann, A. H., Eiserling, F. A., and Boehner, L. A., 1973, Genetic control of capsid length in bacteriophage T4. I. Isolation and preliminary description of four new mutants, *J. Virol.* **12**:374.

Donelli, G., Gugliemli, F., and Pauletti, L., 1972, Structure and physicochemical properties of bacteriophage G. 1. Arrangement of protein subunits and contraction process of tail sheath, *J. Mol. Biol.* **71**:113.

Earnshaw, W., Casjens, S., and Harrison, S. C., 1976, Assembly of the head of bacteriophage P22: X-ray diffraction from heads, proheads, and related structure, *J. Mol. Biol.* **104**:387.

Eiserling, F. A., Geiduschek, E. P., Epstein, R. H., and Metter, E. J., 1970, Capsid size and deoxyribonucleic acid length: The petite variant of bacteriophage T4, *J. Virol.* **6**:865.

Forrest, G. L., and Cummings, D. J., 1970, Head proteins from T-even bacteriophage. I. Molecular weight characterization, *J. Virol.* **5**:398.

Fujisawa, H., and Hayashi, M., 1977, Assembly of bacteriophage ϕX174: Identification of a virion capsid precursor and proposal of a model for the functions of bacteriophage gene products during morphogenesis, *J. Virol.* **24**:303.

Glaeser, R. M., 1974, Radiation damage and resolution limitations in biological specimens, in: *High Voltage Electron Microscopy* (P. R. Swann *et al.*, eds.), p. 370, Academic Press, London.

Goldstein, R., Lengyel, J., Pruss, G., Barrett, K., Calendar, R., and Six, E., 1974, Head size determination and the morphogenesis of satellite phage P4, *Curr. Top. Microbiol. Immunol.* **68**.

Hagen, E. W., Reilly, B. E., Tosi, M. E., and Anderson, D. L., 1976, Analysis of gene function of bacteriophage ϕ29 of *Bacillus subtilis*: Identification of cistrons essential for viral assembly, *J. Virol.* **19**:501.

Hemphill, H. E., and Whiteley, H. R., 1975, Bacteriophages of *Bacillus subtilis*, *Bacteriol. Rev.* **39**:257.

Hendrix, R. W., and Casjens, S., 1974, Protein cleavage in bacteriophage λ tail assembly, *Virology* **61**:156.

Hohn, T., and Katsura, I., 1977, Structure and assembly of bacteriophage lambda, *Curr. Top. Microbiol. Immunol.* **78**:69.

Horvitz, H. R., 1974, Bacteriophage T4 mutants deficient in alteration and modification of the *Escherichia coli* RNA polymerase, *J. Mol. Biol.* **90**:739.

Hosoda, J., and Cone, R., 1970, Analysis of T4 phage proteins. I. Conversion of precursor proteins into lower molecular weight peptides during normal capsid formation, *Proc. Natl. Acad. Sci. USA* **66**:1275.

Hsiao, C., and Black, L., 1977, DNA packaging and the pathway of bacteriophage T4 assembly, *Proc. Natl. Acad. Sci. USA* **74**:3652.

Isaacson, M. S., 1977, Specimen damage in the electron microscopy. in: *Principles and Techniques of Electron Microscopy*, Vol. 7: *Biological Applications* (M. A. Hayat, ed.), p. 1, Van Nostrand Reinhold, New York.

Ishii, T., and Yanagida, M., 1977, The two dispensible structural proteins (*soc* and *hoc*) of the T4 phage capsid; their purification and their binding with the defective heads in vitro, *J. Mol. Biol.* **109**:487.

Israel, J. V., Anderson, T. F., and Levine, M., 1967, *In vitro* morphogenesis of phage P22 from heads and baseplate parts, *Proc. Natl. Acad. Sci. USA* **57**:284.

Israel, V., 1976, Role of the bacteriophage P22 tail in the early stages of infection, *J. Virol.* **18**:361.

Iwashita, S., and Kanegasaki, S., 1973, Smooth specific phage adsorption: Endorhamnosidase activity of tail parts of P22, *Biochem. Biophys. Res. Commun.* **55**:403.

Jarvik, J., and Botstein, D., 1975, Conditional-lethal mutations that suppress genetic defects in morphogenesis by altering structural proteins, *Proc. Natl. Acad. Sci. USA* **72**:2738.

Katsura, I., 1976, Morphogenesis of bacteriophage lambda tail: Polymorphism in the assembly of the major tail protein, *J. Mol. Biol.* **107**:307.

Katsura, I., and Kühl, P. W., 1974, A regulator protein for the length determination of bacteriophage lambda tail, *J. Supramol. Struct.* **2**:239.

Katsura, I., and Kühl, P. W., 1975a, Morphogenesis of the tail of bacteriophage λ. II. In vitro formation and properties of phage particles with extra long tails, *Virology* **63**:238.

Katsura, I., and Kühl, P. W., 1975b, Morphogenesis of the tail of bacteriophage λ. III. Morphogenesis pathway, *J. Mol. Biol.* **91**:257.

Kellenberger, E., 1972, Assembly in biological systems, in: *The Generation of Subcellular Structure*, Proc. 1st John Innes Symp., p. 62, Elsevier, Amsterdam.

Kells, S. S., and Haselkorn, R., 1974, Bacteriophage T4 short tail fibers are the product of gene 12, *J. Mol. Biol.* **83**:473.

King, J., and Mykolajewycz, N., 1973, Bacteriophage T4 tail assembly: Proteins of the sheath, core, and baseplate, *J. Mol. Biol.* **75**:339.

King, J., Botstein, D., Casjens, S., Earnshaw, W., Harrison, S., and Lenk, E., 1976, Structure and assembly of the capsid of bacteriophage P22, *Philos. Tr. Roy. Soc. London Ser. B* **276**:37.

Kurtz, M. B., and Champe, S., 1977, Precursors of the T4 internal peptides, *J. Virol.* **22**:412.

Lake, J., and Leonard, K. R., 1974, Structure and protein distribution for the capsid of *Caulobacter crescentus* bacteriophage φCbK, *J. Mol. Biol.* **86**:499.

Lake, J. A., Pendergast, M., Kahan, L., and Nomura, M., 1974, Localization of *Escherichia coli* ribosomal proteins S4 and S14 by electron microscopy of antibody-labeled subunits, *Proc. Natl. Acad. Sci. USA* **71**:4688.

Leonard, K. R., Kleinschmidt, A. K., Agabian-Keshishian, N., Shapiro, L., and Maizel, J. V., Jr., 1972, Structural studies of the capsid of *Caulobacter crescentus* bacteriophage φCbK, *J. Mol. Biol.* **71**:201.

Leonard, K. R., Kleinschmidt, A. K., and Lake, J., 1973, *Caulobacter crescentus* bacteriophage φCbK: Structure and *in vitro* self assembly of the tail, *J. Mol. Biol.* **81**:349.

Moody, M. F., 1965, The shape of the T-even bacteriophage head, *Virology* **26**:567.

Moody, M. F., 1971, Structure of the T2 bacteriophage tail-core, and its relation to the assembly and contraction of the sheath, in: *First European Biophyics Congress, Baden, Austria* (E. Broda, A. Locker, and H. Springer-Lederer, eds.), p. 543, Weiner Medizinische Akademie, Vienna.

Moody, M. F., 1973, Sheath of bacteriophage T4. III. Contraction mechanism deduced from partially contracted sheaths, *J. Mol. Biol.* **60**:613.

Müller-Salamin, L., Onarato, L., and Showe, M., 1977, Localization of minor protein components of the head of the bacteriophage T4, *J. Virol.* **24**:121.

Nelson, R. A., Reilly, B. E., and Anderson, D. L., 1976, Morphogenesis of bacteriophage φ29 of *Bacillus subtilis*: Preliminary isolation and characterization of intermediate particles of the assembly pathway, *J. Virol.* **19**:518.

Onorato, L., Stirmer, B., and Showe, M. K., 1978, Isolation and characterization of bacteriophage T4 mutant preheads, *J. Virol.* **27**:409.

Parker, M., 1979, Ph.D. thesis, University of California, Los Angeles.

Pène, J. J., Murr, P. C. and Barrow-Carraway, J., 1973, Synthesis of bacteriophage ϕ29 proteins in *Bacillus subtilis*, *J. Virol.* **12**:61.

Rabussay, D., and Geiduschek, E. P., 1977, Regulation of gene action in the development of lytic bacteriophages, in: *Comprehensive Virology*, Vol. 8 (H. Fraenkel-Conrat and R. Wagner, eds.), p. 1, Plenum, New York.

Reilly, B. E., Nelson, R. A., and Anderson, D. L., 1977, Morphogenesis of bacteriophage ϕ29 of *Bacillus subtilis*: Mapping and functional analysis of the head fiber gene, *J. Virol.* **24**:363.

Ruark, J. E., Serwer, P., Ross, M. J., and Stroud, R. M., 1979, Structural study of bacteriophage T7 and T7 capsids, *J. Mol. Biol.* (in press).

Rueckert, R. R., 1976, On the structure and morphogenesis of picornaviruses, in: *Comprehensive Virology*, Vol. 6 (H. Fraenkel-Conrat and R. Wagner, eds.), pp. 131–213, Plenum, New York.

Serwer, P., 1976, The internal proteins of bacteriophage T7, *J. Mol. Biol.* **107**:271.

Showe, M. K., and Black, L. W., 1973, Assembly core of bacteriophage T4: An intermediate in head formation, *Nature (London) New Biol.* **242**:70.

Simon, L. D., and Anderson, T. F., 1967*a*, The infection of *Escherichia coli* by T2 and T4 bacteriophages as seen in the electron microscope. I. Attachment and penetration, *Virology* **32**:279.

Simon, L. D., and Anderson, T. F., 1967*b*, The infection of *Escherichia coli* by T2 and T4 bacteriophages as seen in the electron microscope. II. Structure and function of the baseplate, *Virology* **32**:298.

Smith, P. R., Aebi, U., Josephs, R., and Kessel, M., 1976, Studies of the structure of the T4 bacteriophage tail sheath, *J. Mol. Biol.* **106**:243.

Stone, K. W., and Cummings, D. J., 1972, Comparison of the internal proteins of the T-even bacteriophages, *J. Mol. Biol.* **64**:651.

Studier, F. W., 1972, Bacteriophage T7, *Science* **176**:367.

Tikhonenko, A. S., 1970, *Ultrastructure of Bacterial Viruses*, Plenum, New York.

Tosi, M., Reilly, B., and Anderson, D., 1975, Morphogenesis of bacteriophage ϕ29 of *Bacillus subtilis:* Cleavage and assembly of the neck appendage protein, *J. Virol.* **16**:1282.

Unwin, P. N. T., 1974, Electron microscopy of stack disk aggregate of tobacco mosaic virus protein. II. The influence of electron irradiation on the strain distribution, *J. Mol. Biol.* **87**:657.

Unwin, P. N. T., and Henderson, R., 1975, Molecular structure determination by electron microscopy of unstained crystalline specimens, *J. Mol. Biol.* **94**:425.

Viñuela, E., Camacho, A., Jimenez, F., Carrascosa, J. L., Ramirez, G., and Salas, M., 1976, Structure and assembly of phage ϕ29, *Philos. Tr. Roy. Soc. London Ser. B* **276**:29.

Wagenknecht, T., and Bloomfield, V., 1975, Equilibrium mechanisms of length regulation in linear protein aggregates, *Biopolymers* **14**:2297.

Wagenknecht, T., and Bloomfield, V., 1977, *In vitro* polymerization of bacteriophage T4D tail core subunits, *J. Mol. Biol.* **116**:347.

Williams, R. C., and Richards, K. E., 1974, Capsid structure of bacteriophage lambda, *J. Mol. Biol.* **88**:547.

Wood, W. B., and Revel, H. R., 1976, The genome of bacteriophage T4, *Bacteriol. Rev.* **40**:849.

Wurtz, M., Kistler, J., and Hohn, T., 1976, Surface structure of *in vitro* assembled bacteriophage lambda polyheads, *J. Mol. Biol.* **101**:39.

Yamamoto, M., and Uchida, H., 1975, Organization and function of the tail of bacteriophage T4. II. Structural control of tail contraction, *J. Mol. Biol.* **92**:207.

Yanagida, M., 1977, Molecular organization of the shell of the T-even bacteriophage head. II. Arrangement of subunits in the head shells of giant phages, *J. Mol. Biol.* **109**:515.

Yanagida, M., and Ahmad-Zadeh, C., 1970, Determination of gene product positions in bacteriophage T4 by specific antibody association, *J. Mol. Biol.* **51**:411.

Zweig, M., and Cummings, D. J., 1973*a*, Structural proteins of bacteriophage T5, *Virology* **51**:443.

Zweig, M., and Cummings, D. J., 1973*b*, Cleavage of head and tail proteins during T5 assembly: Selective host involvement in the cleavage of a tail protein, *J. Mol. Biol.* **80**:505.

CHAPTER 9

Genetic Control of Complex Bacteriophage Assembly

William B. Wood

Department of Molecular, Cellular,
and Developmental Biology
University of Colorado
Boulder, Colorado 80309

and

Jonathan King

Department of Biology
Massachusetts Institute of Technology
Cambridge, Massachusetts 02139

1. INTRODUCTION

1.1. Scope and Purposes of This Chapter

Assembly of complex bacterial viruses has been investigated intensively during the past decade, revealing, in rich detail, the explicit steps from the information stored in genes to the formation of three-dimensional structure. Research in this area has been motivated by curiosity about virus assembly as an important aspect of virus multiplication, as well as by the conviction that knowledge of the genetic control of viral morphogenesis would provide a foundation for approaching the more difficult problems of the assembly of organelles in higher organisms. Although basic questions remain to be answered about bacteriophage assembly, a great deal already has been learned, primarily because of the convenience of bacteriophages as genetically, biochemically, and structurally accessible experimental systems.

The results of recent research in this area have been summarized in several comprehensive reviews (Eiserling and Dickson, 1972; Casjens and King, 1975; Showe and Kellenberger, 1975; Russell and Winters, 1975; Murialdo and Becker, 1978). Here we present a more concise summary of current knowledge and use it as the basis for discussion of the questions, answers, and general principles that have emerged so far from research into bacterial virus assembly and its genetic control.

1.2. Approaches to the Problem of Phage Assembly

The functions of a virion are to protect the viral nucleic acid and to provide a means for its delivery into host cells. Unlike some eukaryotic cell viruses that are uncoated by the host, bacteriophages must build their delivery system into the virion during morphogenesis. In the complex bacteriophages, the viral nucleic acid is DNA, and the delivery system takes the form of an intricate tail structure that allows recognition and penetration of the bacterial cell wall. Thus all the complex bacteriophages consist of a head, which contains the viral DNA, and a tail, which serves as an adsorption and penetration organelle (for the comparative anatomy of bacteriophages, see chapters by Mathews, and Rabussay and Geiduschek, Volumes 7 and 8 of this series, and Eiserling, this volume).

The formation of bacteriophage head and tail structures inside the infected host cell presents a well-defined opportunity to analyze molecular events in morphogenesis. Considerable success with this analysis has been achieved by genetic dissection of the assembly process, exploiting conditionally lethal phage mutations that block phage assembly. Such mutations, introduced by Edgar and Epstein (Epstein *et al.*, 1963) for bacteriophage T4 and by Campbell (1961) for bacteriophage λ, are of two principal types: amber (*am*), also referred to as "chain termination" or "suppressor-sensitive" (*sus*), and temperature-sensitive (*ts*). During the past decade, T4, λ, P22, T7, and a few other phages have been characterized genetically to the point where most if not all of their essential genes have been identified by conditionally lethal mutations. Under nonpermissive conditions, these mutations can result in arrest of the assembly process at many different stages, generally with accumulation of structural intermediates or side products, which can be isolated and characterized conveniently.

Bacteriophage T4 has the advantage that host protein synthesis is shut down rapidly after phage infection, so that radioactive amino acids added to infected cells are incorporated only into phage-coded polypeptides. These polypeptides can be analyzed by separation according to molecular weight on polyacrylamide gels in the presence of the denaturant sodium dodecylsulfate (SDS) (Laemmli, 1970). Autoradiography of dried gels permits visualization of the labeled phage polypeptide bands without interference from the background of unlabeled host proteins (Fairbanks *et al.*, 1965; Hosoda and Levinthal, 1968). Since *am* mutations lead to premature termination of translation and thus decreased molecular weight of the defective gene product, gel bands often can be identified as products of particular genes by their disappearance from the normal band pattern as the result of *am* mutations in these genes (Laemmli, 1970; King and Laemmli, 1973; O'Farrell *et al.*, 1973; Vanderslice and Yegian, 1974).

A further tool for analyzing assembly mutants became available with the discovery that infectious phage could be produced when cell-free extracts of mutant-infected cells were mixed in appropriate combinations (Edgar and Wood, 1966). When one step in an assembly process is blocked by mutation, extracts of the infected cells often contain the remaining unassembled proteins in active form. If the structural intermediate that accumulates is also active, then addition of the missing gene product leads to infectious virus formation. By analogy to *in vivo* genetic complementation, this process is termed "*in vitro* complementation." The *in vitro* complementation test provides an assay for the biological function of phage gene products involved in assembly.

The general approach to elucidating processes of phage assembly has exploited the foregoing techniques as follows. The general function of an assembly gene is deduced from the phage structures, identified by electron microscopy, that accumulate in infected cells as the result of *am* or *ts* mutations in the gene. These structures then can be isolated and characterized with respect to their protein composition, nucleic acid composition, antigenicity, detailed morphology in the electron microscope, and *in vitro* complementation activity. If a structure is active in *in vitro* complementation, then it is possible to ascertain which gene products have acted on the structure within the cell and which have not, by determining which mutant-infected cell extracts are complemented by the isolated structure, as first described by Edgar and Lielausis (1968).

If the protein product of the mutant gene can be identified by polyacrylamide gel electrophoresis, then it is possible to determine whether the protein is a component of the mature virus and whether it is found in components or incomplete precursor structures isolated from other mutant-infected cells. The results of such experiments indicate whether or not the gene product is a structural protein and where it acts in the assembly process relative to other gene products involved in assembly of the same component.

Early physiological characterization of mutants and *in vitro* complementation experiments showed that T4 assembly is a strictly ordered process, which can be written as a sequential series of steps or assembly pathway. The pathway is branched, with independent formation of subassemblies that subsequently combine to complete the structure (reviewed in Kellenberger and Edgar, 1971; Wood, 1973; Casjens and King, 1975). Unlike many developmental processes in cellular systems, however, the order of steps in assembly is not controlled by sequential gene expression but by the properties of the interacting gene products themselves, all of which are synthesized at the same time during the latter half of the infectious cycle (Hosoda and Levinthal, 1968). Subsequent work has shown that these generalizations are true for other phages as well.

More recent investigations have focused on understanding the nature of individual steps in assembly. Different problems have been encountered in head and tail subassemblies, and quite different features have emerged from these branches of the overall pathway. Likewise, apparently different mechanisms for similar processes are found in different phages. Comparing these mechanisms for common features provides clues to the nature of steps that are not yet understood. The most intensively studied of the complex bacteriophages have been the virulent *coli* phage T4, the temperate *coli* phage λ, and the temperate *Salmonella* phage P22. Additional information has come from the investigation of other *coli* phages T7, P2 and its satellite phage P4, T5, T3, and the *Bacillus subtilis* phage φ29. In the following sections we discuss the major subassemblies in turn, summarizing the problems posed by each and comparing the information currently available for λ, P22, T4, and other phages that have yielded relevant results. In the final section we discuss the general principles that have emerged and the problems that still remain.

2. ASSEMBLY OF PHAGE HEADS

2.1. General Problems of Head Assembly

The packaging of nucleic acid inside a protein shell is common to all viral infections. This process poses two major problems: building a shell of precisely specified size and shape, and packaging within it the correct length of nucleic acid in a highly condensed state. All the complex viruses so far investigated appear to determine shell size and shape first, in the form of a prohead into which the DNA is introduced subsequently. In addition, most complex phages replicate their DNA to form long concatemers that consist of many genomes in tandem. If head assembly is mutationally blocked, the DNA remains concatemeric. Thus the packaging process involves introduction of concatemeric DNA into a prohead and cleavage of the concatemer to lengths of approximately the size of the genome.

The mechanism by which a DNA molecule many micrometers in length can be threaded into a preformed shell is difficult to imagine. Packaging presents a thermodynamic problem as well. Entry of DNA into the prohead must occur with a net decrease in free energy; however, on subsequent infection the DNA must exit spontaneously from the head, again with a decrease in free energy. One possible solution would be to drive a thermodynamically unfavorable packaging process by coupling to an energy-yielding reaction such as ATP hydrolysis, to form a quasi-stable head structure which would release DNA spontaneously when appropriately triggered. Alternatively, packaging could be a spontaneous condensation driven by thermodynamically favorable protein–nucleic acid interactions. If so, however, chemical changes must occur within the completed head to increase the energy of the packaged nucleic acid to the point where its release will be spontaneous (Laemmli and Favre, 1973; Hohn and Hohn, 1974).

Cleavage of the DNA concatemer is obligatorily coupled to the packaging process for most of the complex bacteriophages. An exception is P2, in which the packaging substrate is circular monomeric DNA (Pruss *et al.*, 1975). In some phages (e.g., T4 and other T-even phages, P22) the point of concatemer cleavage appears to be determined by the headful mechanism originally proposed by Streisinger *et al.* (1967). The amount of DNA packaged per virion in these phages is not affected by deletion mutations, which reduce the genome size. In other phages (e.g., λ, T7, T3, T5) cleavage of a concatemer occurs at a specific site, presumably recognized as a specific nucleotide sequence in the DNA. The amount of DNA per virion in these phages is decreased by deletion mutations.

Not surprisingly, head assembly is a complex process, controlled by many phage genes, and most of the problems posed above are not yet solved. Recent progress has been reviewed in detail by Murialdo and Becker (1978). In the following paragraphs we summarize currently available evidence on head assembly of phages λ, P22, T7, and T4. In considering the specific features of these systems, it is helpful to keep in mind five currently discernible general stages of the capsid assembly process. These stages can be described as follows: (1) *Initiation of capsid formation:* This process is obscure but some of the proteins involved can be identified. (2) *Capsid assembly:* Assembly of the major capsid protein into a shell always seems to require at least one additional protein that is not found in the mature phage. These scaffolding or assembly-core proteins are removed from the prohead prior to DNA packaging, either intact or with proteolysis. (3) *DNA packaging:* This process requires proteins that also are absent from the mature phage, and that function only in concert with the prohead particle. (4) *Capsid conformational change:* The entire capsid goes through a conformational alteration or lattice transition during the process of DNA packaging. (5) *Stabilization and completion:* Additional proteins act either to stabilize the structure or to complete construction of the injection apparatus.

2.2. λ Head Assembly

The λ phage head is a regular icosahedron about 55 nm in diameter with a $T = 7$ surface lattice (Casjens and Hendrix, 1974*b*; Williams and Richards, 1974). Its assembly requires the products of 11 mutationally identified phage genes, which are clustered near the left end of the genetic map as shown in Fig. 1. The completed structure contains the protein products of genes D and E (gpD and gpE) as major proteins, and gpB and gpC as minor components (Hendrix and Casjens, 1975). The protein gpFII is located at the head–tail junction and probably forms the site for tail attachment to the completed head (Casjens, 1974).

The process of λ head assembly is diagrammed in Fig. 2. The prohead forms as a shell composed of gpE, gpB, gpC, and a protein not present in the mature phage, gpNu3 (Hohn *et al.*, 1974, 1975; Ray and

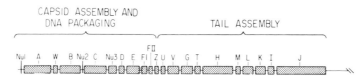

Fig. 1. Map of bacteriophage λ morphogenetic genes. Stippled bars represent minimum lengths of genes whose polypeptide products have been identified and sized by SDS-polyacrylamide gel electrophoresis. Map includes only the left arm of the vegetative λ chromosome. Map data from Parkinson (1968) with additions according to Jara and Murialdo (1975).

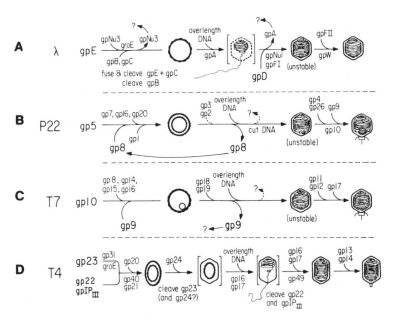

Fig. 2. Pathways of bacteriophage head morphogenesis. The four panels summarize information on the order of gene product (gp) interaction in assembly of the capsids of phages λ, P22, T7, and T4. Although these sequences are fairly well established based on analysis of mutant phenotypes and on protein composition of isolated intermediates, the mechanisms of shell assembly and DNA packaging are still poorly understood. Adapted from Casjens and King (1975), with information on T7 from Serwer (1976) and Roeder and Sadowski (1977).

Murialdo, 1975; Hendrix and Casjens, 1975). This structure, originally referred to as "petit" λ, is spherical with about three-fourths the diameter of the completed phage head. Mutants defective in gene B or gene C accumulate aberrant nonmaturable proheads (Murialdo and Ray, 1975; Zachary *et al.*, 1976). Mutants defective in gene Nu3 form aberrant tubular or spiral structures composed of the major protein gpE; therefore, gpNu3 is thought to form a core or scaffold that is involved in the specification of capsid shape (Murialdo and Siminovitch, 1972b; Ray and Murialdo, 1975).

The following steps are dependent on prohead assembly and at least one host gene, designated groE (Georgopoulos and Eisen, 1974), but they occur prior to DNA packaging; gpB is cleaved, and gpNu3 and the smaller fragment of gpB are released from the prohead structure. gpNu3 also is cleaved into fragments, but perhaps only after its release from the prohead (Ray and Murialdo, 1975). Then in a bizarre series of reactions still poorly understood, each gpC molecule becomes covalently linked to an adjacent gpE molecule. This reaction is followed by cleavage of a terminal fragment from either the C or the E portion of the fusion product. The remaining gpE molecules are not cleaved (Hendrix and Casjens, 1974a). The function of these reactions is obscure. Ray and Murialdo (1975) have suggested that gpB, gpC, and gpNu3 might combine to form an initiation complex for capsid assembly. It is not yet certain whether the gpB and gpC molecules are distributed symmetrically over the phage head or are restricted to one location, but there is some evidence that gpB is localized at the vertex to which the tail subsequently attaches (discussed in Hohn and Katsura, 1977).

Since mature λ DNA molecules have specific ends, packaging must include a cutting mechanism that recognizes a specific nucleotide sequence. Packaging and cutting occur sequentially along replicating concatemers (Wake et al., 1972; Skalka et al., 1972; Emmons, 1974; Syvanen, 1975). These steps require in addition to the prohead the products of genes A and D and those of the more recently recognized genes Nu1 and FI. Protein gpA is not in the mature virion; gpD is a major capsid protein. The gpA protein is thought to be a nuclease responsible for cutting the DNA at the appropriate point when packaging is complete. However, cutting generally will not occur in the absence of prohead or of gpD, which normally becomes incorporated as a major component on the outer surface of the capsid, present in equimolar amount with gpE (Wang and Kaiser, 1973; Kaiser et al., 1975; Becker and Gold, 1975). The functional and structural roles of gpNu1 and gpFI are not yet known. During the packaging process, the shell expands by about 20% in diameter, to the size and icosahedral shape of the completed head. This expansion can occur in the absence of gpD and can be induced artificially by urea treatment (Hohn et al., 1976).

In vitro packaging of DNA to form infectious virus first was demonstrated in extracts of λ-infected cells (Kaiser and Masuda, 1973; Hohn and Hohn, 1974; Kaiser et al., 1974), and further study of this reaction will be important in understanding the packaging mechanism. So far the reaction has been shown to require a complete prohead (Kaiser et al., 1975), either mature or concatemeric DNA (Hohn, 1975; Syvanen, 1975), gpA, gpNu1, gpFI, and the presence of ATP and spermidine in the reaction mixture (Kaiser et al., 1975).

Completion of the head requires the action of gpW in addition to gpFII, which is incorporated at one vertex to form the site for subsequent joining of the tail (Casjens, 1974). For a more comprehensive review of λ head assembly, see Hohn and Katsura (1977).

2.3. P22 Head Assembly

The head of P22 is icosahedral, with a diameter of 60 nm. Its assembly requires the products of 11 mutationally identified genes, shown on the genetic map in Fig. 3. The completed head structure contains gp5 as the major component, and at least five other proteins as minor components (King *et al.*, 1973; Botstein *et al.*, 1973; Poteete and King, 1976). The most notable feature of P22 head assembly is the involvement of a nonvirion component, gp8, as a recycling scaffolding protein in shell formation and DNA packaging (see Fig. 2B). Head assembly begins with formation of a double-shell prohead. The inner shell consists of about 250 molecules of the scaffolding protein gp8, and the outer shell consists of about 420 molecules of the coat protein gp5. During the subsequent packaging of DNA, all of the gp8 molecules are released intact into the cell cytoplasm, where they participate in further rounds of prohead formation (King and Casjens, 1974). In mutants that lack the gp5 protein, gp8 accumulates as free subunits (King and Casjens, 1974). In mutants that lack gp8 function, gp5 assembles into aberrant aggregates, indicating that the scaffolding protein is crucial for determination of head size and shape (King *et al.*, 1973; Lenk *et al.*, 1975). A simple model consistent with the data would be that scaffolding protein and coat protein molecules combine with each other to form small complexes that can polymerize efficiently into a shell of proper dimensions.

The prohead also contains four other gene products as minor components. Three of these proteins, gp16, gp20, and gp7, are not required for prohead assembly, but must be incorporated into the prohead if the final phage particles are to be infectious. In their absence, morphologically normal phages are formed, but they are unable to inject their DNA into the next host cell (Hoffman and Levine,

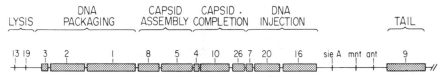

Fig. 3. Map of bacteriophage P22 morphogenetic genes. Stippled bars represent minimum lengths of genes whose polypeptide products have been identified and sized by SDS-polyacrylamide gel electrophoresis. Map includes only the left end of the P22 vegetative chromosome. The region between genes 16 and 9 contains genes that control superinfection exclusion, maintenance of lysogeny, and antirepressor. Map data from Botstein *et al.* (1972) with additions according to Poteete and King (1977).

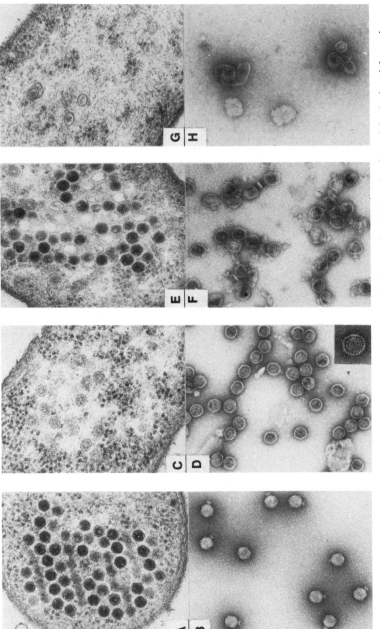

Fig. 4. Electron micrographs of P22 head structures. Upper panels show negatively stained particles isolated from the corresponding infected cells. A,B: Wild-type particles. C,D: Proheads from cells infected with gene 2-defective mutants blocked in DNA packaging. E,F: Unstable and empty capsids from gene 10-defective mutants blocked in head completion. The 10⁻ particles lose their DNA both within the cell and after lysis. G,H: Aberrant protein aggregates from cells infected with gene 8-defective mutants, which lack scaffolding protein. Photographs from the work of Lenk *et al.* (1975).

1975). The remaining minor protein, gp1, is involved in DNA packaging. In the absence of gp1, or either of two nonstructural proteins, gp2 or gp3, proheads, and uncut concatemeric DNA accumulate (Botstein *et al.*, 1973).

In P22, the DNA packaging process seems to be obligatorily coupled with the exit of the scaffolding protein. In this respect P22 differs from λ, in which gpNu3 exits from the prohead prior to the DNA packaging process. No protein cleavages have been found to occur during P22 morphogenesis, again in contrast to λ and T4.

Packaging and cutting of DNA proceed sequentially along replicating DNA concatemers as in λ infection, but the ends of mature P22 DNA molecules are not unique (Tye *et al.*, 1974). The molecules are terminally redundant, containing about 2% more DNA than a complete genome. These features suggest that the cutting mechanism is triggered when the head becomes filled and not when a specific nucleotide sequence is encountered. Since defects in genes 1, 2, and 3 lead to accumulation of proheads and uncut DNA concatemers, all three of these proteins are implicated in the packaging and cutting process. Following encapsidation of the DNA the head is unstable until three more minor proteins, gp4, gp10, and gp26, are added to the structure. These steps complete the head and prepare it for tail attachment (King *et al.*, 1973; Casjens and King, 1974; Lenk *et al.*, 1975). Electron micrographs of P22 capsid structures are shown in Fig. 4.

2.4. T7, T3, and φ29 Head Assembly

Mechanisms of head assembly and packaging in the virulent *coli* phage T7 (see Figs. 5 and 2C) appear similar to those in P22 and λ on the basis of the evidence so far available (Studier and Maizel, 1969; Roeder and Sadowski, 1977). A major protein present in proheads is lacking from complete phage, but is not cleaved during assembly. Therefore, it is a candidate for a scaffolding protein, although it does not seem to recycle (Roeder and Sadowski, 1977). T7 proheads display an additional internal structure, which may represent an initiation complex for capsid assembly (Serwer, 1976). The mechanism for cutting DNA to mature length probably resembles that of λ more than that of P22, since mature T7 DNA molecules terminate with a specific nucleotide sequence (Ritchie *et al.*, 1967). The demonstration that T7 proheads can incorporate DNA efficiently *in vitro* to form infectious virions (Kerr and Sadowski, 1974) offers promise for a direct biochemical attack on the packaging process.

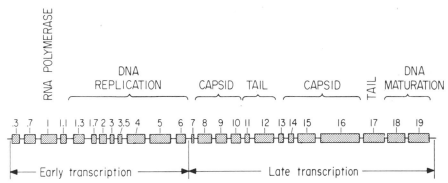

Fig. 5. Map of bacteriophage T7 genes. Stippled bars represent minimum lengths of genes whose products have been identified and sized. The product of gene 13 recently has been shown to be a head protein, essential for infectivity but not for phage assembly (Roeder and Sadowski, 1977). Map data primarily from Studier (1972); map adapted from Watson (1976).

Bacteriophage T3, morphologically similar to P22 and T7, has been extensively characterized with respect to particle assembly by Minagawa, Fujisawa, and co-workers (Matsuo-Kato and Fujisawa, 1975). Its assembly pathway is similar to that of P22 and T7, in that a prohead is formed from a coat protein and scaffolding protein, and subsequently encapsidates DNA. These events proceed without substantial proteolytic cleavages.

Bacteriophage ϕ29 of *Bacillus subtilis* is morphologically distinct from the phages discussed so far. It is smaller, with a chromosome of molecular weight about 11×10^6, whose ends are joined by a protein linker (Ortin *et al.*, 1971). The particles are not isometric and display a complex tail structure (Fig. 6). Despite these differences, the morphogenetic pathway displays the same general features seen previously. The major coat protein (Hd; gene 8 product) is assembled with the help of a scaffolding protein gp7 into a precursor prohead (Nelson *et al.*, 1976; Hagen *et al.*, 1976). Prohead assembly also requires the gene 10 product, which is thought to be located at the base of the capsid (Mendez *et al.*, 1971). The prohead is the precursor in the DNA packaging process, which requires the gene 9 and gene 16 proteins and is accompanied by the release of the scaffolding protein, which recycles (Nelson *et al.*, 1976).

2.5.   T4 Head Assembly

T4 heads are the largest and most complex of those that have been studied in detail. Unlike the heads of most phages, the T4 head is not

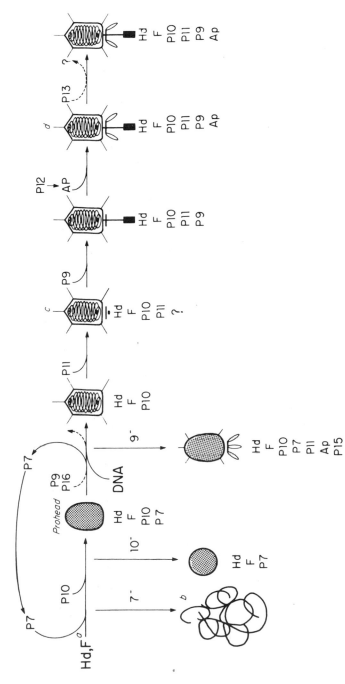

Fig. 6. Morphogenetic pathway of phage $\phi29$. Gene products are indicated as P followed by the gene number. $\phi29$ gene numbers reflect their order on the genetic map. The major coat protein (Hd) is the product of gene 8. Formation of the prohead involves a scaffolding protein coded by gene 7, which maps adjacent to the coat protein gene. Structures shown below the main pathway are aberrant side products of defective assembly. From Nelson et al. (1976).

isometric but elongated, with a diameter of about 85 nm and a length of about 110 nm, posing specific problems for shape determination. Freeze-etch electron micrographs of the closely related phage T2 show a $T = 13$ surface lattice with an extra equatorial band of hexamers that accounts for the elongation (Branton and Klug, 1975).

T4 head assembly (Fig. 2D) involves the products of at least 20 genes, which occur in two major clusters on the genetic map as shown in Fig. 7. Of these gene products, nine are known to contribute to the finished structure along with additional nonessential structural proteins (for recent reviews, see Laemmli et al., 1974; Wood and Revel, 1976). The T4 prohead, originally called the "τ particle" by Kellenberger and co-workers, is formed by aggregation of roughly equimolar amounts of the major capsid subunit gp23 and the major assembly core proteins gp22 and gpIP3 (Showe and Black, 1973). This process occurs on or near the host cell membrane (Simon, 1972) and requires the products of T4 genes 31, 20, and 40. It also requires the normal function of host E. coli genes at at least two loci: mop, also called tabB or groE (Georgopoulos and Eisen, 1974; Takahashi et al., 1975), and fatA (Simon et al., 1975).

Defects in gene 31 or in the host function result in the aggregation of the major coat protein in "lumps" along the cell membrane. This state of the coat protein is distinguished from its condition in the absence of gp20 and gp40, in which the protein aggregates into long tubes (polyheads), which although not intermediates are related to the normal capsid structure. The gene 20 and gene 40 products can be viewed as proteins involved in correct capsid initiation (Showe and Onorato, 1978); in their absence the major protein aggregates into an incorrect structure (Laemmli et al., 1970a,b).

The polyheads just described have the same diameter as the normal complete head. They contain within them a core composed of the gene 22 product (Laemmli and Quittner, 1974). In the absence of gp22, the polyheads that form have various diameters, suggesting that this protein normally plays a role in diameter selection. As demonstrated by Showe and Black (1973), gp22 together with one of the internal proteins, gpIP3, forms an assembly core, which is necessary for the proper assembly of the major capsid protein. The minor proteins gp20 and gp40 may be necessary for the proper initiation of the assembly core, which is itself a complex structure. Surprisingly, the internal protein is generally dispensable; mutants that lack it produce phage particles that are infectious except in a few host strains (Showe and Black, 1973; Black, 1974).

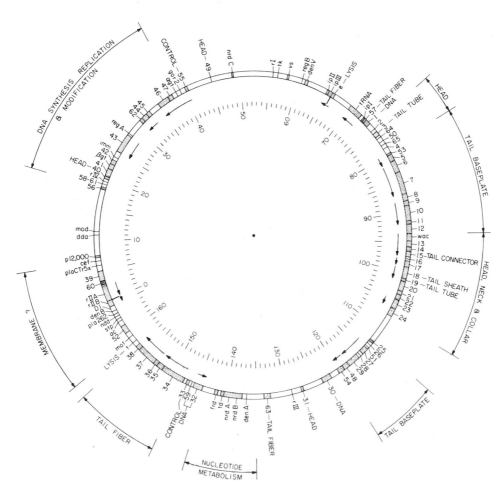

Fig. 7. Map of bacteriophage T4 genes. The circular numerical scale indicates physical distances in kilobase-pairs (kb) from an arbitrary zero point. The map circle shows the relative locations of T4 genes. Heavy radial lines inside the map circle indicate positions determined by heteroduplex mapping of deletion mutants in the electron microscope. Arrows indicate transcription direction; those that extend over more than one gene indicate cotranscription. Stippled bars on the map circle represent minimum lengths of genes whose polypeptide products have been identified and sized by SDS-polyacrylamide gel electrophoresis. The outermost circle indicates gene functions. Smaller radial labels adjacent to gene names indicate functions that differ from those of the surrounding genes in a cluster. Most of the genes that function in assembly were defined by the conditionally lethal amber and temperature-sensitive mutations isolated and characterized by Epstein *et al.* (1963). Adapted from Wood and Revel (1976).

Following prohead formation but prior to DNA packaging, the minor protein gp24 is incorporated and a major transformation occurs: all the major subunit gp23 molecules are cleaved, with release of an N-terminal fragment and a reduction of about 20% in molecular weight (Laemmli, 1970; Hosoda and Cone, 1970; Kellenberger and Kellenberger-van der Kamp, 1970; Dickson et al., 1970; Celis et al., 1973). Subsequently, all the gp24 molecules also lose a fragment, but the stage at which this cleavage occurs is not clear. The activated prohead then initiates DNA encapsidation from a replicating concatemer. This process is associated with a second major transformation of the capsid: the proteolytic cleavage of the gp22 assembly core protein to small peptides, and the cleavage of gpIP3 to a lower molecular weight form (Laemmli, 1970; Showe and Black, 1973; Laemmli et al., 1974; Tsugita et al., 1975).

The events of T4 head maturation differ considerably from those of λ and P22 in the number and apparent importance of proteolytic cleavage reactions. There is little cleavage of the outer capsid proteins in λ and none in P22. In λ, gpNu3 probably is removed intact; in P22, the scaffolding protein is removed intact and recycled; in T4, the assembly core protein is removed by proteolysis. The relationship of core removal to DNA packaging is discussed in Section 7.7.

The T4 cleavage reactions are dependent on the organizational state of the entire structure, because they do not occur in vivo if capsid assembly is prevented by mutation. However, cleavage of the unassembled proteins has been demonstrated in vitro and shown to be dependent on the product of gene 21 (Onorato and Showe, 1975; Giri et al., 1976). This protein is not found in mature phage. The primary gene 21 product undergoes a series of cleavages to yield an active protease, which appears to be associated with the prohead structure. This protease initiates most if not all of the cleavages described above, and then largely disappears from the head, possibly by autodigestion, when packaging is complete (Showe et al., 1976).

DNA packaging and cutting also requires the products of genes 16, 17, and 49 (Luftig et al., 1971). gp16 and gp17 could be analogous to gpA of λ, and to gp2 and gp3 of P22. gp49, which recently has been purified and characterized, shows DNase activity on replicating DNA concatemers and probably functions to trim branch points or other obstructions to packaging from the replicating DNA rather than to complete the packaging process (Frankel et al., 1971; Kemper and Brown, 1976; Minagawa and Ryo, 1978). Whatever the cutting mechanism for completion of packaging; it appears to be triggered by the presence of a filled head rather than by a specific nucleotide sequence, since mature T4 DNA molecules are circularly permuted in sequence and terminally redundant to the extent of about 2% (Streisinger *et al.*, 1967; MacHattie *et al.*, 1967).

Two capsid surface proteins, designated soc and hoc, have been identified recently and shown to be major components of the mature capsid, but not necessary for infectivity (Ishii and Yanagida, 1976). These proteins fill in the lattice formed by the essential head proteins and are responsible for the smooth appearance of mature T4 capsids. They may be related in function to the gene D product of bacteriophage λ in that they add to the lattice after the DNA packaging process.

Several other gene products are essential for assembly of a functional head, although their absence has no clear effect on head morphology. The products of these genes, 2, 4, 50, 64, and 65, have not been identified in gels, so their presence or absence in the phage is not established. The heads produced by mutants that lack one of these gene products show reduced cleavage of structural proteins and reduced ability to attach tails, and the complete particles that do form are noninfectious (Laemmli *et al.*, 1974). Recent experiments suggest that one of these proteins, gp2, normally is injected with the phage DNA and performs an essential function after infection (Silverstein and Goldberg, 1976*a*,*b*).

The head is completed and readied for tail attachment by the addition of two more proteins, gp13 and gp14, which form the neck structure that subsequently attaches to the tail (Coombs and Eiserling, 1977).

Head assembly in the coli phage P2 and its satellite phage P4 may be similar to that of T4, since the major P2 head subunit also undergoes cleavage during assembly (Pruss *et al.*, 1974). The head of P4, although smaller than that of P2, is assembled primarily from P2 proteins. Shore *et al.* (1978) have isolated a P4 mutant that is unable to direct the assembly of a P4-size head from these proteins. Thus P2 and P4 provide an intriguing experimental system for investigating the problem of capsid geometry determination.

3. ASSEMBLY OF PHAGE TAILS

3.1. General Problems of Tail Assembly

The tail structures of complex bacteriophages are unique to this class of viruses. Although they are essential components of the nucleic

acid delivery system, they take on widely differing forms in different
phages, ranging from the rudimentary six-subunit structure of P22 to
the intricate contractile tail of T4. All consist of a tube of 6-fold symmetry and varying length, with one or more adsorption organelles at
the distal tip which interact with and help to penetrate the bacterial surface (see Chapter 1, Volume 7).

Problems common to the various pathways of tail assembly and
attachment to the head include specification of tube length, interaction
of a 6-fold-symmetrical tube with a head vertex that has 5-fold symmetry, insertion of DNA into the tube, and, in the case of contractile
tails, assembly of a complex quasi-stable structure that will be triggered
only by interaction with the appropriate bacterial surface. In general,
tail proteins form relatively few aberrant polymorphic structures when
normal assembly is blocked by mutation, so that pathways of tail
assembly are more amenable to elucidation by the genetic approach
and are consequently better understood than the head assembly
pathways.

The assembly of the complex tails generally can be divided into
three stages: (1) initiation, involving the formation of a complex basal
structure; (2) elongation, through polymerization of the major tube
subunits onto the initiation structure; and (3) termination to form the
structure at the proximal end of the tail, which will form the joint with
the head.

The attachment of tails or tail parts of the phage head results in
the creation of a channel for the passage of DNA. It is not clear
whether this channel is opened to the head during head–tail joining, or
during the infectious process. The DNA delivery functions of phage
tails have only recently become amenable to experimental analysis
(Benz and Goldberg, 1973; Dawes and Goldberg, 1973; Yamamoto and
Uchida, 1975). This subject is discussed further in Section 4.

3.2. P22 and T7 Tail Assembly

The tail structures of phages P22 and T7 are rudimentary, consisting of one and three gene products, respectively. The P22 tail is formed
by attachment of six subunits composed of the gene 9 product to the
completed head, in a reaction that was one of the first phage assembly
steps to be studied *in vitro*. The kinetics of infectious phage production
in this reaction suggests that the six subunits are added randomly and
one at a time, and that several are necessary for infectivity (Israel *et al.*,

1967). The tail parts of P22 and other morphologically related phages are enzymatically active depolymerases of host cell capsular polysaccharides (Iwashita and Kanegasaki, 1973). This activity seems to be expressed independently of the state of assembly of the protein (Israel, 1976).

The T7 tail is slightly more complex, consisting of three proteins, gp11, gp12, and gp17. The gene 11 and 12 proteins add to completed heads to form a rudimentary baseplate with sites for the subsequent attachment of six short bent fibers composed of gp17 (Studier, 1972; Roeder and Sadowski, 1977).

3.3. λ Tail Assembly

The λ tail is deceptively simple in appearance; it consists of a long, stacked-disk tube about 150 nm in length, connected through a small basal structure to a single fiber at the distal tip, which serves as an adsorption organelle. Assembly of the tail structure, however, requires the products of 11 phage genes, which are clustered on the left arm of the vegetative phage chromosome as shown in Fig. 1. The pathway of assembly has been partially defined by characterization of the tail-related structures that accumulate as the result of mutations in these genes, using sucrose gradient sedimentation and assays of *in vitro* complementation (Kühl and Katsura, 1975; Katsura and Kühl, 1975*a,b*; Katsura, 1976; reviewed in Hohn and Katsura, 1977). Although the protein compositions of intermediates have not yet been determined, most of the steps can be carried out *in vitro* and a partial order of assembly reactions can be written (Fig. 8).

Seven of the 11 gene products required for tail formation are

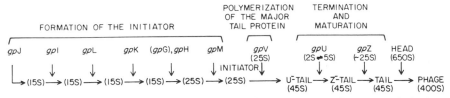

Fig. 8. Pathway of gene product interaction in λ tail assembly. Most of the intermediate structures so far have been characterized only with regard to sedimentation coefficient (in parentheses). As in T4 tail assembly, the sequence of steps appears to be fixed. Data from Kühl and Katsura (1975), Katsura and Kühl (1975*b*), and Katsura (1976). Adapted from Hohn and Katsura (1977).

present in complete phage. gpV is the major tube subunit; gpJ makes up the distal fiber, gpG, gpH, and gpL are components of the basal structure, and gpZ probably forms the terminator. The products of genes I, M, and T have not yet been identified on gels. gpK appears not to be a structural protein (Murialdo and Siminovitch, 1972a).

In the initial step of assembly, gpJ forms a 15 S structure which then is acted on sequentially by gpI, gpL, and gpK with no alteration in sedimentation coefficient. Interaction with gpG and gpH then converts the complex to a 25 S structure, which is acted on by gpM with no change in sedimentation coefficient. gpH undergoes a proteolytic cleavage with a loss of a fragment, either at this stage or subsequently (Hendrix and Casjens, 1974b). The resulting basal structure serves as an initiator for polymerization of gpV to form the tail tube, in a reaction that also requires gpU. This protein, although only a minor component of the completed tail, is a major protein of the infected cell. For efficient attachment to heads, the tail structure also must be acted on by gpZ, which normally completes the tail assembly. The role of gpT in the pathway is not yet known. Gene T-defective mutants, as well as all other tail defective mutants except those lacking gpZ or gpU functions (see following paragraph) form no tail-related structures identifiable in electron micrographs, presumably because they are unable to form the complete initiation structure (Murialdo and Siminovitch, 1972a).

An intriguing aspect of λ tail assembly is the mechanism of length determination and the function of gpU. Single mutants unable to form the complete 25 S complex form no tube structures; however, if gpU also is absent, gpV tube subunits polymerize into aberrantly long tubes. If gpU alone is absent, gpV tube subunits polymerize on the 25 S complex to form abnormally long "polytails." These structures do not attach to heads *in vivo* but can be attached *in vitro* if gpU is supplied, to form phage particles with very long tails and low infectivity. The molar amount of gpU in the completed tail is much smaller than that of gpV. Thus gpU appears to be required for proper length determination in tube polymerization and also for tail attachment to the head (Katsura and Kühl, 1974; Katsura, 1976). However, experiments with λ and φ80, which have tails of similar structure but different length, show that neither gpU nor gpV alone directly specifies the length of the tail. When nonpermissive cells are mixedly infected with φ80 and λ that carries an *am* mutation in either gene U or gene V, some phage with λ-length tails still are produced (P. Youderian, E. Lenk, and J. King, unpublished results).

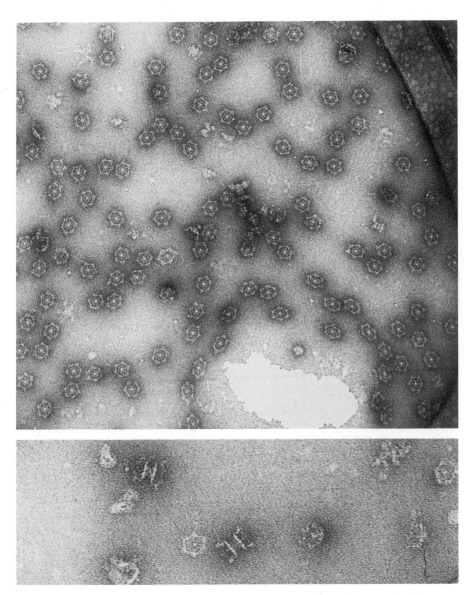

Fig. 9.   Electron micrographs of baseplates from T4 mutant-infected cells. The upper panel shows precursor baseplates isolated by sucrose gradient sedimentation from cells infected with a mutant defective in gene 19, which codes for the major tail tube subunit. Baseplates are suspended in a sheet of stain stretching across a hole in the carbon film. The side-to-side baseplate diameter is about 40 nm. The lower panel shows dimers of baseplate precursors joined by their inner faces and lying on their sides to reveal the spikes that are prominent on mature phage. These baseplates apparently dimerize because of lack of gene product 48, which is needed for initiation of tail tube polymerization (King, 1971; Berget and Warner, 1975).

3.4. T4 Tail Assembly

The tail of T4 is structurally and functionally more complex than that of λ. The tail tube, surrounded by a contractile sheath, connects to the phage head through a neck and collar region, and terminates at the distal end in an intricate hexagonal baseplate, to which are attached six long tail fibers and six short tail fibers. The tail is metastable; when triggered by attachment to the bacterial surface, the baseplate opens out into a starlike configuration and the sheath contracts irreversibly, driving the distal end of the tube through the bacterial cell wall and allowing the DNA to penetrate the cell (Simon and Anderson, 1967*a,b*). The baseplate (Fig. 9) is particularly interesting. Kozloff and co-workers have shown that baseplates include folic acid derivatives,

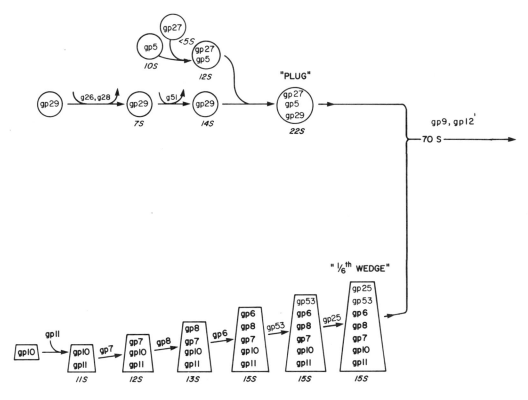

Fig. 10. Pathway of gene product interaction in T4 tail assembly. The two major structural intermediates in baseplate assembly are shown schematically as a wedge-shaped arm and a circular plug. Sedimentation coefficients are shown beneath each intermediate. Gene products (gp) listed inside each intermediate represent those proteins found in the structure. Proteins shown in boldface type are those that contribute the major portion of the mass of the completed structure. Gene numbers preceded by "g" indicate dependence of a step on function of a gene whose product has not yet been

dihydrofolate reductase (Kozloff *et al.*, 1970*a,b*), and Zn^{2+} (Kozloff and Lute, 1977), all of which might be components of the triggering reaction (Male and Kozloff, 1973).

The assembly pathway of the T4 tail has been worked out in detail by King and his collaborators, by identifying on polyacrylamide gels the products of genes essential for tail formation, and by characterizing the structures that these proteins form in various mutants, with regard to sedimentation constant, morphology in electron micrographs, *in vitro* assembly activity, and protein composition. Tail assembly requires the products of 21 T4 genes, which occur predominantly in two large clusters on the genetic map (see Fig. 1). The tail is formed primarily by self-assembly; none of the tail assembly proteins so far identified is cleaved, and all but three of them are structural components of the

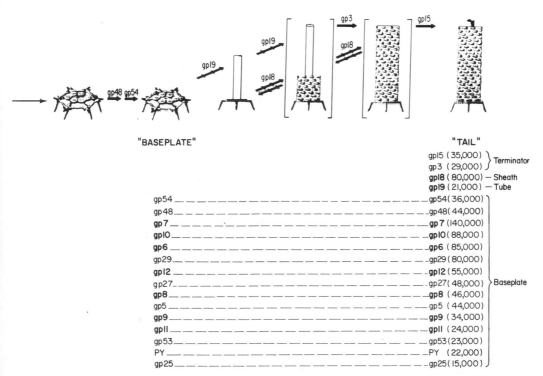

identified. The two columns at the lower right indicate the gene products present in the completed baseplate and in the completed tail, respectively. All but one of the proteins in the arm pathway are specified by one cluster of genes (53–12; see Fig. 7), and all but one of the proteins in the plug pathway are specified by a second cluster (25–54). Six of the 15 S arm complexes assemble radially around one 22 S plug complex to form a hexagonal precursor of the baseplate. From Kikuchi and King (1975*c*).

completed tail. Assembly proceeds by formation of the baseplate, followed by polymerization of tube and sheath subunits on its top surface (King, 1968). Attachment of the long tail fibers occurs only after joining of the tail to the phage head (see Section 5) (King and Wood, 1969).

The pathway of tail formation is diagrammed in Fig. 10. Formation of the baseplate proceeds via two independent subassemblies: seven gene products interact to form a wedge-shaped component that makes up a 1/6 arm of the outer hexagonal structure. In an independent series of steps, six other proteins interact to form a central plug. A plug and six of the completed arms combine to form an unstable hexagonal precursor structure, which is completed and prepared for tube and sheath initiation by addition of four other gene products. The tube, a stacked-disk helix of 24 annuli that each consist of six molecules of gp19, then initiates polymerization on the top surface, and the sheath, a larger helix of gp18 molecules in one-to-one correspondence with the tube subunits, polymerizes around it. gp3 is added to the end of the tube, where it acts as the terminator for sheath polymerization; when this process is complete, gp15 is added to stabilize the sheath and form the connector for subsequent attachment to the neck and collar (King and Mykolajewycz, 1973; Kikuchi and King, 1975a,b,c).

A striking feature of this pathway is its strictly sequential order of steps. Only three proteins are exceptions: gp9, gp11, and gp12 (which is the subunit of the short tail fibers; Kells and Haselkorn, 1974) can be added to otherwise complete tails or phage, although they normally are added early in baseplate assembly (Edgar and Lielausis, 1968). The remaining 18 gene products interact *only* in the order shown. If an early protein is missing, the remaining components remain as unassembled soluble monomers. Of these components only the sheath subunit, gp18, eventually will polymerize into long aberrant polysheath helices if no baseplate structures are present to initiate normal sheath polymerization (King, 1968). In the absence of the central plug, the arm complexes will slowly aggregate to form inactive hexagonal structures (Kikuchi and King, 1975b).

As in the λ tail assembly pathway, the mechanism of tube length determination remains a mystery. Soluble preparations of gp19 and baseplates will combine to form tubes of only the correct length, regardless of the presence or absence of gp3 and sheath protein (King, 1968). Mutants that produce longer or shorter tubes have not been found. Possible mechanisms of length determination are considered in Section 7.

3.5. Assembly of Other Phage Tails

Bacteriophage T5 tail assembly may resemble that of λ. The T5 and λ tails are morphologically similar, and T5 tail assembly involves cleavage of a high-molecular-weight minor protein. T5 tail assembly also may involve a host component (see Section 6) (Zweig and Cummings, 1973*a,b*).

The P2 tail is contractile and similar in morphology to that of T4, and its assembly also proceeds by formation of a baseplate structure followed by polymerization of tube and sheath (Lengyel *et al.*, 1974).

4. HEAD–TAIL JOINING

In all of the assembly pathways so far examined, the joining of completed heads and tails appears to be a spontaneous reaction that requires special junctions on both head and tail, but no additional gene products. Nevertheless, this process raises some intriguing and still unanswered questions. For example, how is only one vertex of the head specified as the site for tail attachment? To allow subsequent injection, the tail must attach at a vertex near one end of the packaged DNA molecule. All phages with tails have specific connector proteins on the head, presumably added to the correct vertex as a terminal step in DNA packaging. In support of this notion, the right end of packaged λ DNA remains nuclease sensitive until the probable tail connector protein gpFII is added to the head (Boklage *et al.*, 1974). However, Showe and Onorato (1978) have presented evidence for T4 that the head vertex at which capsid assembly *initiates* is also the vertex at which the tail later attaches, and that the same protein, gp20, may determine both events.

The connector also must somehow form a compatible link between the 6-fold rotational symmetry of the tail and the 5-fold rotational symmetry of an icosahedral vertex on the head. Possible solutions to this problem, common to all the complex phages, have been discussed by Moody (1965). In T4 an intricate collar with six whiskers is added to the neck region after head–tail joining (Coombs and Eiserling, 1977). The function of these structures is discussed in the following section.

Different phages may differ in whether DNA penetrates the tail at the time of attachment or only during subsequent injection. In λ there is evidence that the right end of the DNA is extended into the tail tube at the time of tail attachment (Saigo and Uchida, 1974); in T4 the tail tube of complete phage appears to be empty (J. King, unpublished observations).

Silverstein and Goldberg (1976*a,b*) have described a situation in T4 in which both injection and morphogenetic functions are affected by the absence of a protein, the gene 2 product. This protein is required for protection of newly injected DNA and may accompany the DNA into the host. Particles assemble without it, but inefficiently. These authors suggest that the initial interaction of this protein with a terminus of the DNA aids morphogenesis, for example, in the positioning of the DNA ends in the head.

5. ASSEMBLY OF PHAGE TAIL FIBERS

Long slender tail fibers (Fig. 11) attached to the six vertices of the baseplate are a unique feature of the largest bacteriophages such as T2 and T4. These adsorption organelles provide increased efficiency (Kellenberger *et al.*, 1965) and control (Conley and Wood, 1975) of phage attachment to bacterial cells with which they collide. T4 tail fiber assembly, which has been studied in detail, exhibits two distinctive features of general interest: it involves the formation of novel fibrous pro-

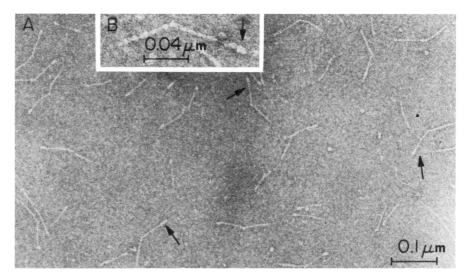

Fig. 11. Electron micrograph of negatively stained T4 tail fibers. Both completed whole fibers and their precursor half-fibers may be seen in this photograph. The thickening at one end of the whole fiber (arrows) is the site at which the tail fiber joins to the phage baseplate. The tapered tip is probably the active site for adsorption to the bacterial cell surface. Tail fibers are the target of most of the neutralizing antibody in anti-T4 sera. From Ward *et al.* (1970).

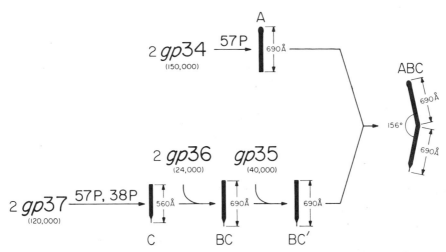

Fig. 12. Pathway of gene product interaction in T4 tail fiber assembly. Numbers preceded by "gp" represent polypeptide products of the corresponding genes. Numbers followed by "P" represent the active form (unknown) of the phage gene product. Dimensions and general appearance of structural intermediates are based on electron microscopy, and antigens A, B, and C are determined by serum blocking assay (King and Wood, 1969; Ward et al., 1970). The molecular weights of the four structural proteins are indicated in parentheses (King and Laemmli, 1971; Ward and Dickson, 1971; Dickson, 1973). The molecular weights of the two nonstructural proteins are 26,000 for gp38 (King and Laemmli, 1971) and probably 3000–7000 for gp57 (R. O. Herrmann and H. R. Revel, unpublished experiments). From Bishop and Wood (1976).

tein structures as well as participation of accessory proteins that appear to catalyze noncovalent interactions between structural components (for reviews, see Wood and Bishop, 1973; Bishop et al., 1974).

T4 tail fiber assembly and attachment to the phage are under the control of eight phage genes. Four of the corresponding proteins are structural components of the tail fiber, and the remaining four play accessory or catalytic roles, in that they are required for efficient assembly and yet are not structural elements of the finished tail fiber or any of its assembly precursors. The pathway of tail fiber assembly is shown in Fig. 12. The four structural proteins are gp34, gp35, gp36, and gp37. Their molecular weights and order of addition to the structure are shown in the figure. The complete tail fiber probably contains two molecules each of gp34, gp36, and gp37, and one molecule of gp35, through which the two half-fibers are thought to connect (Dickson, 1973). A, B, and C represent serum blocking antigens (Edgar and Lielausis, 1965) which are exhibited by the assembled forms of gp34, gp36, and gp37, respectively (King and Wood, 1969; Ward et al., 1970).

The tapered tip of the BC′ half-fiber carries the site that interacts with the cell surface to initiate infection, and the knobbed end of the A half-fiber is the site of attachment to the phage baseplate (see Fig. 11). By locating the binding sites of antibodies specific to known regions of the gp37 polypeptide chain, Beckendorf (1973) was able to show that the two molecules of this protein in the distal (BC') half-fiber are arranged in parallel, with their C termini at the distal tip, their N termini near the central kink of the fiber, and the remainder of the polypeptides distributed fairly uniformly along the length of the half-fiber. If the two polypeptides are twisted into a helix, as seems likely, it can be calculated from their molecular weights and the length of the C half-fiber that the average rise per residue along the helix axis is about 0.05 nm, considerably lower than the value of this parameter for any known protein helix. Earnshaw *et al.* (1979) have recently presented evidence that the two polypeptides are folded together in a cross-β conformation. The configuration of the two gp34 molecules in the proximal half-fiber is not so well understood, but may be similar, since mutational alterations at the N-terminal ends of the polypeptide affect attachment of tail fibers to the baseplate, whereas alterations at the C-terminal end of gp34 affect the attachment of proximal to distal half-fiber (King and Wood, 1969; Seed, Del Zoppo, Conley, and Wood, unpublished observations).

The two accessory proteins for assembly are gp38, required for dimerization of gp37 in the first step of distal half-fiber assembly, and gp57, which also is required or gp37 dimerization and in addition is required for the analogous dimerization of gp34 in proximal half-fiber assembly (Ward and Dickson, 1971; King and Laemmli, 1971). The two remaining proteins, gp63 and gp*wac*, are required for the efficient attachment of tail fibers to the phage baseplate. gp63, a soluble protein not present in the phage particle, mediates the interaction of the proximal tip of the A half-fiber with the baseplate (Wood and Henninger, 1969; Wood *et al.*, 1977). gp*wac* is the protein of the phage whiskers, 2 × 40 nm filaments that extend outward from the collar region at the base of the phage head (Coombs and Eiserling, 1977). The whiskers somehow promote tail fiber attachment by transiently interacting with distal half-fibers, perhaps serving as jigs (Terzaghi, 1971) to position them correctly for attachment (Bishop *et al.*, 1974; Wood and Conley, 1979; Terzaghi *et al.*, 1979).

Since there appear to be no covalent bonds formed or broken in the course of tail fiber assembly and attachment, the four accessory proteins somehow promote the noncovalent association of structural subunits. Therefore, their mechanisms of action are of considerable interest, both intrinsically and as possible models for other macromolecular assembly reactions in higher cells.

6. ROLE OF THE HOST CELL IN PHAGE ASSEMBLY

Complex bacteriophages, like all viruses, depend for their reproduction on interaction with the host cell at many stages of the infectious cycle, from attachment of the virion, penetration of nucleic acid, and biosynthesis of viral macromolecules, to the cell lysis which releases finished virus. The nature of these virus-host interactions has been elucidated partly by study of host cell mutations that affect viral multiplication. Recently, host mutations have been discovered that affect several steps in particle assembly, indicating that the complex bacteriophages depend on host cell components at some stages of morphogenesis.

Mutations in several bacterial genes, designated *groE*, *mop* (morphogenesis of phage), and *tabB* (T4 abortive infection) by various authors, prevent multiplication of λ, T4, and several other phages, although adsorption and injection are normal. Some of these *mop* mutants have been shown to block both λ and T4 at the stage of prohead formation (reviewed in Georgopoulos and Eisen, 1974). When *mop* host cells are infected with wild-type T4, the major capsid protein gp23 accumulates in amorphous lumps on the bacterial membrane, just as had been previously observed to occur as the result of defects in phage gene 31 (Laemmli *et al.*, 1970a). The *mop* block can be overcome by mutations in gene 31, supporting the notion that gp31 and a host component under the control of a *mop* gene must interact to allow proper organization of gp23 for prohead assembly. However, this interaction may not be highly specific, since mutations in gene 23 also can compensate for the *mop* defect (Takahashi *et al.*, 1975; Simon *et al.*, 1975). Moreover, *mop* mutations with similar effects on head assembly now have been shown to occur in at least three sites on the bacterial chromosome, and all such *mop* defects can be overcome by mutations in either gene 31 or gene 23 of T4 (Revel *et al.*, 1979). In λ, mutations in gene B or gene E, which codes for the major capsid protein, can compensate for the bacterial defect (Georgopoulos and Eisen, 1974).

The nature of these host effects is not clear. The apparent association of proheads with the bacterial membrane in electron micrographs, as well as findings that some *mop* mutants show altered morphology and impaired cell division, have led to the speculation that mop mutations affect bacterial membrane properties. Preliminary results from spin-labeling studies with one such mutant are consistent with this notion (Simon *et al.*, 1975).

Host mutations also have been reported to block T5 tail assembly (Zweig and Cummings, 1973b), T4 tail production (Simon *et al.*, 1974) and T4 tail fiber attachment (Pulitzer and Yanagida, 1971), but the natures of these blocks are not known.

7. DISCUSSION, CONCLUSIONS, AND REMAINING PROBLEMS

7.1. General Nature of Assembly Pathways

Two germinal concepts in early attempts to understand virus structure and assembly were *subassembly*, the idea that large structures are built up by successive addition of subcomponents (Crane, 1950; Crick and Watson, 1957), and *self-assembly*, the proposition that the information and energy required for correct, stable assembly of subunits are supplied by the subunits themselves (Fraenkel-Conrat and Williams, 1955; Crick and Watson, 1957). These concepts were given more precise geometric formulation in the analysis of icosahedral virus structure by Caspar and Klug (1962).

Independently of the structural consideration of simple viruses, Epstein and Edgar (Epstein *et al.*, 1963) and Campbell (1961), working with complex viruses, exploited conditionally lethal mutants to mutationally identify essential genes, including those that carry the information for viral subunits and their assembly. From subsequent studies of such mutants we have learned a great deal about the kinds of information these genes provide. The findings, reviewed in this chapter, corroborate the validity of the subassembly and self-assembly concepts. Phage subcomponents tend to be assembled independently and then subsequently joined to form complete viruses. A large fraction of the genes required for assembly code for self-assembling structural proteins. However, the concepts of subassembly and self-assembly were proposed originally as solutions to the problem of assembling small regular viruses composed of only a few kinds of subunits. The complex bacteriophages are large asymmetrical viruses composed of many different kinds of macromolecules. Attempts to understand their construction have raised new problems, as outlined in the following paragraphs, and have led to some new general insights into macromolecular assembly processes.

1. For small regular viruses it could be assumed that the free energy of subunit association strongly favored one assembly state—the complete correct structure—over all others, so that spontaneous

assembly could be explained by thermodynamic equilibria alone. Complex virus assembly requires *sequential ordering* of assembly steps. In many instances the association of one set of interacting proteins must not occur until after the association of another set in order to avoid formation of aberrant structures and waste of subunits. This control must be exerted at the gene product level rather than at the gene level, since almost all the macromolecules involved in viral assembly are synthesized simultaneously in infected cells. Sequential ordering is accomplished by kinetic controls on assembly; to understand them we must consider the relative rates of association reactions as well as their thermodynamic equilibria.

2.   In large capsid shells, not all of the subunits can have strictly equivalent environments (Caspar and Klug, 1962). To associate in *quasi-equivalent* environments, these proteins must be able to form more than one set of thermodynamically permissible bonding relationships. Consequently, such proteins and some others in phage have the potential for *polymorphic assembly*, that is, formation of more than one thermodynamically favorable structure. Prevention of polymorphic assembly so that only the correct structure forms also must be accomplished by kinetic controls.

3.   The complex viruses require special mechanisms for specifying the dimensions of structures composed of proteins that are capable of polymorphic assembly. Examples are the specification of tail length and head size and shape in long-tailed bacteriophages such as λ and T4.

4.   Complex viruses require controls on the relative levels of some structural proteins inside the cell. For example, if a structure A must acquire six molecules of a protein B in order to function in a subsequent step, and if the attachment of B molecules to A is noncooperative, then the fraction of structures completed will decrease rapidly if the A/B ratio falls below a critical value.

5.   Finally, complex viruses pose new problems in the energetics of assembly. Many of the structures that form during phage assembly are only metastable; they are capable of extensive spontaneous alteration either later in the assembly process or on subsequent interaction of complete virus with host cells. The energy for these alterations may be acquired by coupling early assembly steps to energy-yielding hydrolytic reactions, or by building metastable lattices that can be triggered to undergo cooperative lattice transitions to lower-energy conformations.

The studies reviewed here provide solutions to some of these problems, as discussed in the following sections.

7.2. Sequential Ordering

Rates of association can be controlled by structural proteins themselves to give sequential ordering. The recent work on T4 tails has shown that an extremely complex structure can be formed by self-assembly, and that a long sequence of steps can be constrained to a unique order by protein interactions alone. Interaction between the tail proteins is highly favored thermodynamically, judging from the ability of tail assembly to go to completion in extracts of infected cells with formation of an extremely stable structure. However, each of these interactions is undetectable unless the preceding step in the pathway has taken place (Kikuchi and King, 1975a,c). This observation can be explained most straightforwardly by assuming that each individual association reaction by itself has a considerable activation energy, which acts as a kinetic barrier to interaction. The normal assembly process proceeds in such a manner that some of the binding energy of each association goes toward reducing the activation energy of the succeeding step, thus increasing its rate.

Experiments with model polymer systems (e.g., Hartman *et al.*, 1974) as well as other associating proteins such as TMV coat subunits (Klug, 1972), tubulin from dissociated microtubules (Olmstead and Borisy, 1973; Erickson, 1974; Kirschner and Williams, 1974), and even subunits of oligomeric enzymes (reviewed by Paulus and Alpers, 1971) suggest that the rate-limiting step in many self-assembly reactions is subunit conformational change. Presumably in tail assembly the mechanism by which one step promotes the next is by inducing conformational changes in the binding of each subunit that eliminate the energy barrier to binding of the next subunit.

The demonstration that this mechanism can control such a long sequence of steps has important implications for organellogenesis and morphogenesis in eukaryotic cells. Subunits for an organelle may be prefabricated and stored as soluble monomers with no danger of premature aggregation, until a nucleating protein is supplied which overcomes the conformational activation energy barrier to the first step and thereby triggers a cascade of assembly reactions. Moreover, direction of growth of a polymerizing system can be controlled by positioning the nucleation site on a membrane or other structure. These considerations have particular relevance to control of microtubule assembly.

Prevention of polymorphic assembly can be explained by similar considerations. Stable aberrant assemblies such as T4 polyheads and polysheaths occur abundantly only when mutations block the formation of normal heads and tails, thereby causing accumulation of unassembled capsid and sheath proteins, respectively. In normal infections these structures appear only very late in the latent period and then accumulate rapidly, suggesting that their rates of initiation, although observable, are much slower than those of normal head and tail assembly. Preferential formation of correct structures is again, presumably, the result of kinetic control. It can be explained, for example, in sheath assembly, by assuming that the activation energy barrier to initiation of polymerization on a baseplate around the tail tube is much lower than the barrier to initiation of polysheath by association of free subunits.

7.3. Nonstructural Accessory Proteins in Assembly

Proteins that serve catalytic functions in assembly may provide additional control of rates. The study of complex phage morphogenesis has turned up a number of gene products that play accessory roles; that is, they are required for assembly, and yet they are not structural components of the finished product. These proteins are of interest because it is likely that analogous accessory functions generally may be important for biological assembly processes, and because their existence was not expected by early investigators who assumed that all viral morphogenesis, and indeed subcellular morphogenesis in general, could be explained by self-assembly.

The accessory gene products so far encountered or inferred to exist appear to be of three principal classes: (1) template or scaffolding proteins, (2) orthodox enzymes that catalyze formation or breakage of covalent bonds, and (3) a possible new class of catalysts that promote noncovalent interaction between structural subunits.

The clearest case of a scaffolding protein has been found in P22 head assembly, as described above in Section 2. However, some scaffolding, in the form of a protein "core" that is a structural participant in prohead assembly but is absent from mature virus, is a common feature of all the head assembly pathways so far studied. The mechanism of core elimination in the course of DNA packaging varies: gp22 of T4 is degraded to small peptides; gp8 of P22 exits intact and is recycled; and gpNu3 of λ is released in an unknown manner. The functions of these core proteins are not clear, but they may be required to make bond angles of interacting capsid subunits precise enough to allow successful formation of a closed shell structure (King *et al.*, 1973).

Of the orthodox enzymes in phage assembly, the most notable are those that catalyze the proteolysis of specific structural proteins following their assembly. Such cleavages seem to be a universal feature of the more complex phages; they occur in the assembly of T4, λ, and P2 heads as well as in assembly of the flexible noncontractile tails of λ and T5. The functions of these cleavages are not established, but they are probably related to the necessity that phage particles assemble spontaneously and yet form metastable structures. An analogy may be the well-known proteolytic cleavages that convert thermodynamically stable zymogens, bridged by disulfide bonds, to kinetically stable but thermodynamically unstable digestive enzymes. Similarly the cleavages in phage assembly may be required to convert a thermodynamically stable prohead or protail, formed by spontaneous aggregation of structural components, to a metastable structure capable of being triggered to release DNA upon infection.

Another group of orthodox enzymes in phage assembly are the presumed nucleases that cut the replicating DNA concatemer to mature length pieces during packaging. Some of these enzymes appear to be nonspecific as in T4 and P22, whereas others must recognize a particular nucleotide sequence as in λ and T7. Yet another kind of enzyme, perhaps a transpeptidase, is suggested by the covalent fusion of two gene products in λ head assembly, but the enzymatic basis for this unusual reaction has not yet been demonstrated.

Purification and initial characterization of an assembly-related protease and an assembly-related nuclease have been reported recently. The protease is gp21 of T4 (Onorato and Showe, 1975; Showe *et al.*, 1976). and the nuclease is gpA of λ (Becker and Gold, 1975). The activities of both of these enzymes appear to depend on their assembly state and that of their substrates. The gp21-mediated cleavage of gp22, gp23, and gp24 of T4 occurs *in vivo* only if the three structural proteins are assembled into a prohead, although this requirement can be bypassed *in vitro*. The gpA-mediated cleavage of λ DNA concatemers to genome-size molecules requires concomitant DNA packaging into a competent prohead, both *in vivo* and *in vitro*. Further investigation of these enzymes will be of considerable interest.

A final group of orthodox enzymes is associated with asssembly and function of T4 baseplates. One of the required gene products in baseplate plug formation, gp28, appears to be an enzyme that alters the length of the oligoglutamate chains of host pteroyl glutamate conjugates to provide the folate cofactor that is incorporated into the baseplate (Kozloff *et al.*, 1973). Because gp28 function also appears to activate the structural protein gp29 for further assembly (Kikuchi and King, 1975c), the incorporated folate derivatives may act as cofactors in the assembly process. Two additional phage-coded enzymes, dihydrofolate reductase and thymidylate synthetase, are structural components of the baseplate (Kozloff *et al.*, 1975*a,b*). Neither of these enzymes is necessary for baseplate assembly or subsequent phage infection, and their functions remain obscure. However, phage can be inactivated by treatment with hog kidney conjugase, an enzyme that cleaves glutamate residues from pteroyl glutamate conjugates, suggesting that the folate cofactors may be important for tail function (Kozloff *et al.*, 1970*a*).

The third class of accessory proteins, postulated to catalyze noncovalent association of structural components, could represent a new kind of enzymatic activity not previously recognized or predicted. In the past enzymes have been assumed to catalyze only reactions that involve breakage and formation of covalent bonds, but this assumption could be unwarranted. As discussed in the preceding section, conformational activation energy barriers in tail assembly must be overcome to allow subunit associations that are thermodynamically favored. If permanent binding of a subunit to a growing structure can overcome such a barrier and promote subsequent association, it is easy to imagine that transient binding to a catalytic protein, with an accompanying conformational change, could serve the same purpose. The most likely candidate for such a catalyst so far is the dimeric active form of T4 gp63, which promotes tail fiber attachment as described above in Section 5. Understanding the action and physiological role of this protein has been made more difficult by the recent unexpected finding that gp63 is responsible for the RNA ligase activity in T4-infected cells (Snopek *et al.*, 1977). Evidence available so far suggests that the protein is bifunctional and that its two activities are not mechanistically related.

Another example of such a catalyst may be provided by the lipid-containing double-stranded-RNA bacteriophage φ6. Mindich *et al.* (1976; see also Volume 12 of this series) have shown that the lipid envelopes of this virus, although derived primarily from host phospholipid, form in the center of the cell out of contact with the host cell membrane. Envelope formation is blocked by mutations in gene 12, which codes for a protein not present in mature virions. Mindich has speculated that this protein might function as a phospholipid transferase analogous to those demonstrated to catalyze transfer of phospholipids between membranes of mammalian cells (Enholm and Zilversmit, 1973; Wirtz, 1974). Such proteins are probably the best understood examples of catalysts that act by reducing energy barriers not associated with covalent bond breakage or formation.

Alternatively or in addition, accessory proteins of this class could combine transiently with structural components to prevent aberrant associations. All viruses are faced with the problem of maintaining hydrophobic structural proteins in an active form, within the hydrophobic membrane of the host cell, until assembly has taken place. Moreover, some viral proteins such as gp37 of T4 are specifically constructed to interact with receptors in the membrane that surrounds them. Conceivably, mechanisms for protection of structural proteins from hydrophobic interaction with intracellular membranes may be a general feature of viral systems. The nonstructural T4 proteins gp38 and gp57, which are required for tail fiber assembly as described in Section 5, could play either catalytic or protective roles (Bishop and Wood, 1976; Revel et al., 1976).

7.4. Specification of Dimensions

A sharply defined and longstanding problem in phage morphogenesis is the mechanism of tail length determination. In both T4 and λ the tail tubes are repeating cylindrical structures composed of a precise number of annuli. The lengths of these tubes appear to be specified by properties of the tail proteins themselves, rather than by some external template, because tubes of the correct length will form in preparations that contain no structures larger than the baseplate (King, 1971; Kikuchi and King, unpublished experiments). Two models have been proposed to account for this length determination. One is the accumulated strain model of Kellenberger (1969), which postulates that the fit of annuli into the tube structure is imperfect, causing increasing conformational strain with the addition of each annulus. Polymerization stops when the strain becomes too great to be overcome by the binding energy of association. A possible objection to this model is that the proposed gradual increase in strain would produce a distribution of lengths rather than the precise length seen, for example, in the T4 tail tube, which always consists of 24 annuli.

An alternative to the strain model is that length is determined directly by a measuring device, presumably an extended polypeptide chain, that is part of the structure (King, 1971). A familiar analogy would be the determination of the length of TMV virus rods by the viral RNA (Fraenkel-Conrat and Williams, 1955). However, the hypothetical length determiner of the tail cannot be seen in electron micrographs, and so far attempts to demonstrate its existence, for example by looking for an effect of limited proteolysis on tube length, have been ambiguous (Kikuchi and King, unpublished results).

Another problem in specification of dimensions is posed by the T4 head, which has a prolate icosahedral structure longer than it is wide;

how is the long dimension determined? Mutants of T4 have been isolated that produce both longer and shorter heads (Doermann et al., 1973; Paulson et al., 1976; Bijlenga et al., 1976), and treatment of wild-type infected cells with canavanine results in production of long-headed phage (Cummings et al., 1973). Mutations that affect head length map in genes 22, 23, and 24, indicating that the length is determined by the interaction of these gene products. The mutations in genes 22 and 24 are temperature-sensitive lethals whose effect on length is seen on growth at sublethal temperatures.

Paulson et al. (1976) have proposed a vernier model for head length determination in which the critical interaction is between the inner assembly core lattic of gp22 and the outer lattice of gp23. These lattices show different helical pitches. According to the model, the proper length would be determined by the number of helical repeats in the inner and outer lattices between the site of capsid initiation at one end of the core and the point at which the two lattices come back into phase. The gene 24 product could be involved in recognizing sites where the two lattices are aligned, and there forming vertices. The idea is consistent with the results of Bijlenga et al. (1976), who show that the ability to form particles of correct length depends on the amount of gp24 in the cell and that the gp24/gp23 ratio in completed heads decreases as head length increases. Showe and Onorato (1978) have confirmed the suggestion that gp24 is the vertex protein, and have presented evidence to support the novel idea that head length is determined kinetically by the relative rates of capsid, vertex, and core protein production.

The size problem presents itself in a slightly different manner in the case of Escherichia coli bacteriophage P2 and its satellite phage P4 (Pruss et al., 1974). Both phage capsids are isometric, but that of P4 is considerably smaller. Normally P4 coinfection results in the formation of only P4 size capsids, even though these capsids are constructed from P2 gene products. Geisselsoder et al. (1978) have obtained evidence that P4 causes formation of a smaller icosahedral shell by altering the transcriptional regulation of P2 head proteins so as to change their relative rates of synthesis. These results also are consistent with kinetic influence in the control of capsid dimensions.

The capsid of Bacillus subtilis ϕ29, like that of T4, is longer than it is wide (Fig. 6). In ϕ29 assembly it is clear that the product of gene 10, the upper collar protein, is responsible for the elongated dimension. In the absence of gp10, isometric structures are formed, as shown in Fig. 6. However, gp10 must provide some additional function besides dimension specification, since the isometric capsids do not encapsidate DNA (Hagen *et al.*, 1976). Since gp10 is a minor protein of the particle, it seems likely that its dimension-specifying properties are expressed during the initiation of ϕ29 capsid assembly.

7.5. Gene Clustering and Control of Synthetic Rates

The relative map locations of phage morphogenetic genes probably reflect some aspect of their origins or their functions. For example, the genes for the major coat and scaffolding proteins are adjacent to each other in most of the phages considered in this review. In phages whose components, such as heads and tails, are assembled independently of each other (T4, λ, T5), the relevant genes tend to be clustered separately. The map order of λ tail genes is similar to the temporal order of interaction of the corresponding proteins during λ tail assembly (Casjens and Hendrix, 1974*a*).

Such clustering could reflect the evolutionary origin of present-day assembly genes by tandem duplication and divergence of ancestral assembly genes (discussed in Wood and Revel, 1976). Alternatively or in addition, clustering could reflect the selective advantage of minimizing recombination between genes for proteins that must interact structurally, so as to decrease the probability of nonviable hybrids in interstrain matings (Stahl and Murray, 1966). At present we do not have enough comparative data for related phages to explore evolutionary relationships further. However, clustering of related genes may be functionally important for coordinate control of gene expression.

The efficiency with which structural proteins are converted to virions in the infected cell is relatively insensitive to changes in the overall rate of protein synthesis caused by changes in external conditions. However, changes in the ratios of certain phage-coded proteins, due to mutations that specifically affect their synthetic rates, can lead to greatly decreased efficiency, presumably because some assembly steps that involve addition of many subunits to a structure are non-cooperative (Floor, 1970; Bijlenga *et al.*, 1976). Normally these ratios appear to be fixed and are determined by translational rather than transcriptional rates (Ray and Pearson, 1974).

Generally, assembly pathways exhibit no feedback from substructures to either the gene product or the gene level. For example, most defects that prevent tail assembly have no effect on either head assembly or on the synthesis of head and tail proteins. One exception is the scaffolding protein gp8 in P22 head synthesis, which shows autogenous regulation at the DNA or RNA level. The free form of the protein represses further gp8 synthesis; hence in mutants that do not form proheads less gp8 is synthesized than in normal infections where at any given time a large fraction of the total gp8 protein is sequestered in the form of proheads (King *et al.*, 1978).

Although the genes that control assembly generally are not feedback regulated, cotranscription of functionally related genes may be important in maintaining intracellular levels of key proteins at optimum ratios under various physiological conditions (discussed in King and Laemmli, 1973). This consideration could provide some explanation for the extensive clustering of functionally related genes in phage genomes, and for the observed patterns of cotranscription (see Fig. 7).

7.6. Lattice Transitions

The cooperative transition of entire arrays of subunits from one conformation and lattice structure to another has become recognized as an important feature of viral function and morphogenesis. One of the first such transitions to be analyzed in detail was the contraction of the T4 tail sheath in infection (Moody, 1967, 1973). More recently, lattice transitions have been shown to occur in the morphogenesis of phage capsids. Analysis of the arrangement of subunits in phage capsids has been aided greatly by the development of optical diffraction techniques. The polyheads that accumulate in cells infected with T4 gene 20- and gene 22-defective mutants have been the major experimental material since studies by DeRosier and Klug (1972) showed that high-resolution information could be obtained from these structures.

All the phages so far studied exhibit one or more transitions in the nature of bonding between capsid subunits during head assembly. Both the mechanism and the functions of these transitions are obscure. In T4, lattice transitions (Fig. 13) are associated with the cleavages of capsid proteins (Laemmli *et al.*, 1976; Steven *et al.*, 1976); however, it is not clear whether the cleavage reactions trigger rearrangement of subunits, or vice versa. Capsid lattice transitions in λ have been analyzed by Wurtz *et al.* (1976) and Hohn *et al.* (1976).

Several subunit rearrangements appear to be associated with DNA packaging. These reactions involve the additional problem of releasing an internal protein from the structure. In phage P22 maturation, for example, all the molecules of scaffolding protein gp8, which in the prohead are stably bonded both to each other and to the major capsid protein, are released intact to the surroundings. Since the scaffolding protein is inside the prohead (Lenk *et al.*, 1975; Earnshaw *et al.*, 1976), these molecules somehow must pass out through the coat protein lattice. Another apparently general feature of such capsid transitions, demonstrated so far for phages T4, P22, and λ, is expansion of the surface lattice structure to cause an increase in the internal volume of the phage head. This volume increase conceivably could be an important feature of the mechanism for DNA packaging, discussed in the following section.

7.7.   The Problem of DNA Packaging

Packaging of DNA within a protein shell, although basic to the reproduction of all viruses, still represents the most poorly understood aspect of phage morphogenesis. Packaged DNA is highly ordered, as inferred from electron micrographs such as Fig. 14 and confirmed by

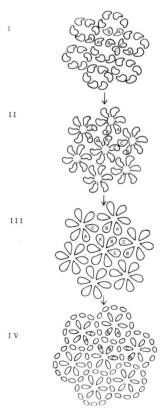

Fig. 13.   Lattice transitions in T4 capsid maturation. Schematically represented lattice structures are based on optical diffraction of electron micrographs of various aberrant T4 polyheads. Class I lattices are composed of uncleaved coat proteins. In the class II lattice the coat proteins have been cleaved, but still are anchored in the original coarse-surfaced configuration. The class III lattice appears to be related to the class II lattice by a cooperative rearrangement and expansion. In the class IV lattice the small outer capsid protein soc (Ishii and Yanagida, 1976) has assembled onto the surface, stabilizing it and giving it a finer appearance. The transitions implied by these structures are thought to occur in precursor particles during the normal assembly of infectious virus. Similar conclusions have been reached by Ishii and Yanagida (1976) and by Steven *et al.* (1976). From Laemmli *et al.* (1976).

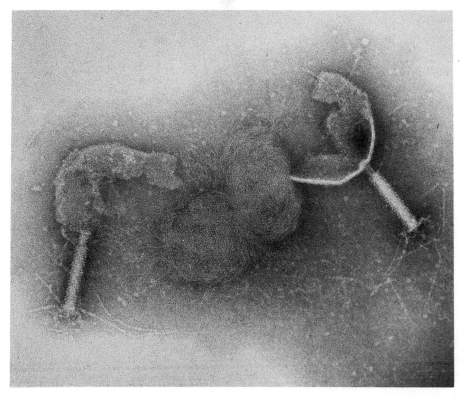

Fig. 14.   Electron micrographs of negatively stained condensed T4 chromosomes. The photograph shows two phage chromosomes from particles which are thought to have broken on the electron microscope grid, releasing their DNA in the condensed form. The DNA shows a distinct pattern suggestive of cylindrical coiling. Electron micrograph courtesy of K. Richards. Similar micrographs of P2, λ, T5, and T7 DNA are shown in Richards *et al.* (1973).

X-ray scattering experiments (W. Earnshaw and S. Harrison, personal communication). It is difficult to imagine the working details of a mechanism whereby a charged, rigid DNA molecule with a length of up to 100 times the head diameter could be threaded into and tightly wound within a preformed shell. Somehow the process must overcome the charge repulsion of the sugar–phosphate backbone and the rigidity of the DNA double helix, perhaps by local denaturation, and must compensate for the decrease in conformational entropy of the molecule as it becomes folded in an ordered coil within the head (Fig. 14). There are few clues available so far as to the source of the necessary free energy. In all the packaging processes studied, uptake of DNA seems to occur concomitantly with a lattice transition that causes expansion of the head shell from a more spherical to a more clearly icosahedral shape. In most phages, with the exception of λ (Kaiser *et al.*, 1975; Hohn *et al.*, 1975), DNA uptake appears to be accompanied by the exit of one or more proteins from the prohead, although the precise relative timing of these events is difficult to establish. In some but not all phages the packaging process includes cleavages of head proteins. *In vitro* packaging of λ DNA (Kaiser *et al.*, 1975; Becker and Gold, 1975), P22 DNA (Poteete and Botstein, 1976), and P2 DNA (R. Calendar, personal communication) requires ATP, but *in vitro* packaging of T7 DNA probably does not (Kerr and Sadowski, 1974; Wood, Conley, and Serwer, unpublished results), although the T7 experiments so far have been carried out in crude extract mixtures so that requirements for the reaction are not yet certain.

Possible sources of energy for packaging are favorable binding interactions of DNA with internal proteins of the prohead, ATP hydrolysis, and, in some phage, peptide bond hydrolysis, although a mechanism for coupling DNA movement to hydrolytic reactions is not apparent. Another source of energy was suggested by Serwer (quoted in Hohn *et al.*, 1974; Serwer, 1975) for T7 packaging and reiterated by Hohn *et al.* (1974) as a possibility for λ packaging as well. When the proheads of these phages expand in the course of DNA packaging, their internal volumes increase. If one end of a replicating DNA molecule were inside the prohead, and if the shell remained impermeable to water, then expansion of the head would create a pressure differential that could suck the DNA inside. Serwer (1976) has shown that only about half the internal volume of the T7 head is occupied by DNA, and has isolated an infectious particle with an expanded shell which could be a packaging intermediate. If it is, the volume increase from prohead to expanded-shell intermediate would be more than sufficient to cause uptake of the phage DNA. Possibly analogous examples of water-impermeable protein shells that fill because of a pressure differential created by shell expansion are the gas vacuoles by which halobacteria and some other prokaryotes regulate their buoyancy (Walsby, 1972).

A detailed model for DNA packaging has been proposed by Laemmli (1975) for phage T4. He has shown that the acidic peptides found within mature T4 are capable of collapsing purified viral DNAs into compact balls *in vitro*. The bulk of these acidic peptides is formed from the cleavage of the gp22 assembly core protein. Laemmli has suggested that one end of the DNA is attached within the prohead and that proteolysis of the assembly core proteins results in a local high concentration of acidic peptides. The resulting collapse of the DNA within the head draws in more DNA, until packaging is complete. Apparently at odds with this model is the finding that fully cleaved hollow proheads made at nonpermissive temperature by a gene 20 cold-sensitive mutant can package DNA when the infected cells are shifted to permissive temperature (Hsiao and Black, 1977).

A general problem with such models is to explain how the packaged DNA subsequently becomes capable of spontaneous injection. As pointed out in Section 2, chemical changes in the virion following DNA uptake may be required to increase the free energy of the packaged nucleic acid, that is, to convert it from a stable to a metastable state that will allow spontaneous injection during subsequent infection. In T4 this requirement may be met by additional protein cleavages. In λ addition of gpD to the head may serve the same purpose, since the rare D^- particles that incorporate DNA and acquire a tail are unable to inject following adsorption (Hohn et al., 1974). Hohn has shown how gpD subunits might intercalate into the expanded shell formed by conformational change of gpE subunits (Hohn et al., 1976).

7.8. Remaining Problems and Future Applications

Many problems of complex virus assembly remain to be solved. We know little about the process by which capsid proteins assemble into spherical shells, although a promising in vitro system for approaching this problem has been reported recently (Murialdo and Becker, 1977). We do not understand the mechanisms of the DNA packaging and cutting mechanisms in head assembly, although we can expect rapid progress in this area from further study of already available in vitro systems. We know almost nothing about the nature of the highly stable but almost exclusively noncovalent bonds that hold viral proteins together. This problem may be approached not only biochemically and biophysically, but perhaps also genetically by extending recent analyses that identify protein–protein interactions (e.g., Jarvik and Botstein, 1975; Sternberg, 1976; Bishop and Wood, 1976).

Research on bacteriophage assembly is supported primarily on the grounds that knowledge of this process should lead to new antiviral therapies that interfere with assembly. In this regard, further understanding of the DNA packaging problem seems especially important. Drugs that inhibit packaging could be particularly effective since this process, unlike most of the other biosynthetic and assembly reactions in virus reproduction, may have no analogue in normal host cells. Animal virus studies focused specifically on assembly processes also should be encouraged. Finally, studies on bacteriophage assembly also provide models for approaching problems of macromolecular assembly and morphogenesis in higher organisms, with clear implications both for basic developmental biology and for eventual understanding of both congenital and environmentally caused malformation and degeneracy diseases.

ACKNOWLEDGMENTS

Research from the laboratories of the authors was supported by NIH Grants AI-09238 to W. B. W. and GM-17980 to J. K. This chapter was prepared during the tenure of a Guggenheim Fellowship to W. B. W.

8. REFERENCES

Beckendorf, S. K., 1973, Structure of the distal half of the bacteriophage T4 tail fiber, *J. Mol. Biol.* **73**:37.

Becker, A., and Gold, M., 1975, Isolation of the bacteriophage lambda A-gene protein, *Proc. Natl. Acad. Sci. USA* **72**:581.

Benz, W., and Goldberg, E. B., 1973, Interaction between phage T4 absorption intermediates and the bacterial envelope, *Virology* **53**:225.

Berget, P. B., and Warner, H. R., 1975, Identification of P48 and P54 as components of bacteriophage T4 baseplates, *J. Virol.* **16**:1669.

Bijlenga, R. G. L., Aebi, U., and Kellenberger, E., 1976, Properties and structure of a gene 24-controlled T4 giant phage, *J. Mol. Biol.* **103**:469.

Bishop, R. J., and Wood, W. B., 1976, Genetic analysis of T4 tail fiber assembly. I. A gene 37 mutation that allows bypass of gene 38 function, *Virology* **72**:244.

Bishop, R. J., Conley, M. P., and Wood, W. B., 1974, Assembly and attachment of bacteriophage T4 tail fibers, *J. Supramol. Struct.* **2**:196.

Black, L., 1974, Bacteriophage T4 internal protein mutants: Isolation and properties, *Virology* **60**:180.

Boklage, C. E., Chun-ti Wong, E., and Bode, V. C., 1974, Functional abnormality of lambda phage particles from complemented *FII*-mutant lysates, *Virology* **61**:22.

Botstein, D., Chan, R. K., and Waddell, C. H., 1972, Genetics of bacteriophage P22. II. Gene order and gene function, *Virology* **49**:268.

Botstein, D., Waddell, C. H., and King, J., 1973, Mechanism of head assembly and DNA encapsulation in *Salmonella* phage P22. I. Genes, proteins, structures, and DNA maturation, *J. Mol. Biol.* **80**:669.

Branton, D., and Klug, A., 1975, Capsid geometry of bacteriophage T2. A freeze-etching study, *J. Mol. Biol.* **92**:559.

Campbell, A., 1961, Sensitive mutants of bacteriophage λ, *Virology* **14**:22.

Casjens, S., 1974, Bacteriophage lambda *FII* gene protein: Role in head assembly, *J. Mol. Biol.* **90**:1.

Casjens, S., and Hendrix, R., 1974a, Comments on the arrangement of the morphogenetic genes of bacteriophage lambda, *J. Mol. Biol.* **90**:20.

Casjens, S., and Hendrix, R. W., 1974b, Locations and amounts of the major structural proteins in bacteriophage lambda, *J. Mol. Biol.* **88**:535.

Casjens, S., and King, J., 1974, P22 morphogenesis. I. Catalytic scaffolding protein in capsid assembly, *J. Supramol. Struct.* **2**:202.

Casjens, S., and King, J., 1975, Virus assembly, *Annu. Rev. Biochem.* **44**:555.

Caspar, D. L. D., and Klug, A., 1962, Physical principles in the construction of regular viruses, *Cold Spring Harbor Symp. Quant. Biol.* **27**:1.

Celis, J. E., Smith, J. D., and Brenner, S., 1973, Correlation between genetic and translational maps of gene 23 in bacteriophage T4, *Nature (London) New Biol.* **241**:130.

Conley, M. P., and Wood, W. B., 1975, Bacteriophage T4 whiskers: A rudimentary environment-sensing device, *Proc. Natl. Acad. Sci. USA* **72**:3701.

Coombs, D. H., and Eiserling, F. A., 1977, Studies on the structure, protein composition and assembly of the neck of bacteriophage T4, *J. Mol. Biol.* **116**:375.

Crane, H. R., 1950, Principles and problems of biological growth, *Sci. Monthly* **70**:376.

Crick, F. H. C., and Watson, J. D., 1957, Virus structure: General principles, in: *The Nature of Viruses*, Ciba Foundation Symposium (G. E. W. Wolstenholme and E. C. P. Millar, eds.), p. 5, Churchill, London.

Cummings, D. J., Chapman, V. A., DeLong, S. S., and Couse, N. L., 1973, Structural aberrations in T-even bacteriophage. III. Induction of "lollipops" and their partial characterization, *Virology* **54**:245.

Dawes, J., and Goldberg, E. B., 1973, Functions of baseplate components in bacteriophage T4 infection. II. Products of genes 5, 6, 7, 8, and 10, *Virology* **55**:391.

DeRosier, D. J., and Klug, A., 1972, Structure of the tubular variants of the head of bacteriophage T4 (polyheads). I. Arrangement of subunits in some classes of polyheads, *J. Mol. Biol.* **65**:469.

Dickson, R. C., 1973, Assembly of bacteriophage T4 tail fibers. IV. Subunit composition of tail fibers and fiber precursors, *J. Mol. Biol.* **79**.633.

Dickson, R. C., Barnes, S. L., and Eiserling, F. A., 1970, Structural proteins of bacteriophage T4, *J. Mol. Biol.* **53**:461.

Doermann, A. H., Eiserling, F. A., and Boehner, L. A., 1973, Genetic control of capsid length in bacteriophage T4. I. Isolation and preliminary description of four new mutants, *J. Virol.* **12**:374.

Earnshaw, W., Casjens, S., and Harrison, S. C., 1976, Assembly of the head of bacteriophage P22: X-ray diffraction from heads, proheads, and related structures, *J. Mol. Biol.* **104**:387.

Earnshaw, W., Goldberg, E. B., and Crowther, R. A., 1979, The distal half fibre of bacteriophage T4: Rigidly linked domains and cross-β structure, *J. Mol. Biol.* (in press).

Edgar, R. S., and Lielausis, I., 1965, Serological studies with mutants of phage T4D defective in genes determining tail fiber structure, *Genetics* **52**:1187.

Edgar, R. S., and Lielausis, I., 1968, Some steps in the assembly of bacteriophage T4, *J. Mol. Biol.* **32**:263.

Edgar, R. S., and Wood, W. B., 1966, Morphogenesis of bacteriophage T4 in extracts of mutant-infected cells, *Proc. Natl. Acad. Sci. USA* **55**:498.

Eiserling, F. A., and Dickson, R. C., 1972, Assembly of viruses, *Annu. Rev. Biochem.* **41**:467.

Emmons, S. W., 1974, Bacteriophage lambda derivatives carrying two copies of the cohesive and site, *J. Mol. Biol.* **83**:511.

Enholm, C., and Zilversmit, D. B., 1973, Exchange of various phospholipids and of cholesterol between liposomes in the presence of highly purified phospholipid exchange protein, *J. Biol. Chem.* **248:**1719.

Epstein, R. H., Bolle, A., Steinberg, C. M., Kellenberger, G., Boy de la Tour, E., Chevalley, R., Edgar, R. S., Susman, M., Denhardt, G. H., and Lielausis, I., 1963, Physiological studies of conditional lethal mutants of bacteriophage T4D, *Cold Spring Harbor Symp. Quant. Biol.* **28:**375.

Erickson, H. P., 1974, Assembly of microtubules from preformed, ring-shaped protofilaments and 6S tubulin, *J. Supramol. Struct.* **2:**393.

Fairbanks, C., Levinthal, C., and Reeder, R. H., 1965, Analysis of C^{14}-labeled proteins by disc electrophoresis, *Biochem. Biophys. Res. Commun.* **20:**393.

Floor, E., 1970, Interactions of morphogenetic genes in bacteriophage T4, *J. Mol. Biol.* **47:**293.

Fraenkel-Conrat, H., and Williams, R. C., 1955, Reconstitution of active tobacco mosaic virus from its inactive protein and nucleic acid components, *Proc. Natl. Acad. Sci. USA* **41:**690.

Frankel, F. R., Batcheler, M. L., and Clark, C. K., 1971, The role of gene 49 in DNA replication and head morphogenesis in bacteriophage T4, *J. Mol. Biol.* **62:**439.

Geisselsoder, J., Chidambaram, M., and Goldstein, R., 1978, Transcriptional control of capsid size in the P2 : P4 bacteriophage system, *J. Mol. Biol.* **126:**447.

Georgopoulos, C. P., and Eisen, H., 1974, Bacterial mutants which block phage assembly, *J. Supramol. Struct.* **2:**349.

Giri, J. G., McCullough, J. E., and Champe, S. P., 1976, Identification of gene products required for *in vitro* formation of the internal peptides of bacteriophage T4, *J. Virol.* **18:**894.

Hagen, E. W., Reilly, B. E., Tosi, M. E., and Anderson, D. L., 1976, Analysis of gene function of bacteriophage φ29 of *Bacillus subtilis*: Identification of cistrons essential for viral assembly, *J. Virol.* **19:**501.

Hartman, R., Schwaner, R. C., and Hermans, J., 1974, Beta poly(L-lysine): A model system for biological self-assembly, *J. Mol. Biol.* **90:**415.

Hendrix, R. W., and Casjens, S. R., 1974a, Protein fusion: A novel reaction in bacteriophage λ head assembly, *Proc. Natl. Acad. Sci. USA* **71:**1451.

Hendrix, R. W., and Casjens, S., 1974b, Protein cleavage in bacteriophage λ tail assembly, *Virology* **61:**156.

Hendrix, R. W., and Casjens, S., 1975, Assembly of bacteriophage lambda heads: Protein processing and its genetic control in petit λ assembly, *J. Mol. Biol.* **91:**187.

Hoffman, B., and Levine, M., 1975, Bacteriophage P22 virion protein which performs an essential early function. II. Characterization of the gene 16 function, *J. Virol.* **16:**1547.

Hohn, B., 1975, DNA as substrate for packaging into bacteriophage lambda, *in vitro*, *J. Mol. Biol.* **98:**93.

Hohn, B., and Hohn, T., 1974, Activity of empty, headlike particles for packaging of DNA of bacteriophage λ *in vitro*, *Proc. Natl. Acad. Sci. USA* **71:**2372.

Hohn, B., Wurtz, M., Klein, B., Lustig, A., and Hohn, T., 1974, Phage lambda DNA packaging *in vitro*, *J. Supramol. Struct.* **2:**302.

Hohn, T., and Katsura, I., 1977, Structure and assembly of bacteriophage lambda, *Curr. Top. Microbiol. Immunol.* **78:**69.

Hohn, T., Flick, H., and Hohn, B., 1975, Petit λ, a family of particles from coliphage lambda infected cells, *J. Mol. Biol.* **98:**107.

Hohn, T., Wurtz, M., and Hohn, B., 1976, Capsid transformation during packaging of bacteriophage lambda DNA, *Philos. Tr. Roy. Soc.* **276**:143.

Hosoda, J., and Cone, R., 1970, Analysis of T4 phage proteins. I. Conversion of precursor proteins into lower molecular weight peptides during normal capsid formation, *Proc. Natl. Acad. Sci. USA* **66**:1275.

Hosoda, J., and Levinthal, C., 1968, Protein synthesis by *Escherichia coli* infected with bacteriophage T4D, *Virology* **34**:709.

Hsaio, C. L., and Black, L. W., 1977, DNA packaging and the pathway of bacteriophage T4 head assembly, *Proc. Natl. Acad. Sci. USA* **74**:3652.

Ishii, T., and Yanagida, M., 1976, Molecular organization of the shell of the T-even bacteriophage head, *J. Mol. Biol.* **97**:655.

Israel, J. V., Anderson, T. F., and Levine, M., 1967, *In vitro* morphogenesis of phage P22 from heads and base-plate parts, *Proc. Natl. Acad. Sci. USA* **57**:284.

Israel, V., 1976, Role of the bacteriophage P22 tail in the ealy stages of infection, *J. Virol.* **18**:361.

Iwashita, S., and Kanegasaki, S., 1973, Smooth specific phage adsorption: Endorhamnosidase activity of tail parts of P22, *Biochem. Biophys. Res. Commun.* **55**:403.

Jara, L., and Murialdo, H., 1975, Isolation of nonsense mutants in the morphogenetic region of the bacteriophage lambda chromosome, *Virology* **64**:264.

Jarvik, J., and Botstein, D., 1975, Conditional-lethal mutations that suppress genetic defects in morphogenesis by altering structural proteins, *Proc. Natl. Acad. Sci. USA* **72**:2738.

Kaiser, A. D., and Masuda, T., 1973, *In vitro* assembly of bacteriophage lambda heads, *Proc. Natl. Acad. Sci. USA* **70**:260.

Kaiser, A. D., Syvanen, M., and Masuda, T., 1974, Processing and assembly of the head of bacteriophage lambda, *J. Supramol. Struct.* **2**:318.

Kaiser, A. D., Syvanen, M., and Masuda, T., 1975, DNA packaging steps in bacteriophage lambda head assembly, *J. Mol. Biol.* **91**:175.

Katsura, I., 1976, Morphogenesis of bacteriophage lambda tail: Polymorphism in the assembly of the major tail protein, *J. Mol. Biol.* **107**:307.

Katsura, I., and Kühl, P. W., 1974, A regulator protein for the length determination of bacteriophage lambda tail, *J. Supramol. Struct.* **2**:239.

Katsura, I., and Kühl, P. W., 1975a, Morphogenesis of the tail of bacteriophage λ. II. *In vitro* formation and properties of phage particles with extra long tails, *Virology* **63**:238.

Katsura, I., and Kühl, P. W., 1975b, Morphogenesis of the tail of bacteriophage λ. III. Morphogenetic pathway, *J. Mol. Biol.* **91**:257.

Kellenberger, E., 1969, Studies on the morphopoiesis of the head of phage T4. VII. Polymorphic assemblies of the same major virus protein subunit, in: *Symmetry and Function of Biological Systems at the Macromolecular Level*, Nobel Symposium II (A. Engström and B. Strandberg, eds.), p. 349, Wiley, New York.

Kellenberger, E., and Edgar, R. S., 1971, Structure and assembly of phage particles, in: *The Bacteriophage* λ (A. D. Hershey, ed.), p. 271, Cold Spring Harbor Press, Cold Spring Harbor, N.Y.

Kellenberger, E., and Kellenberger-van der Kamp, C., 1970, On a modification of the gene product 23 according to its use as a subunit of either normal capsids of phage T4 or of polyheads, *FEBS Lett.* **8**:140.

Kellenberger, E., Bolle, A., Boy de la Tour, E., Epstein, R. H., Franklin, N. C., Jerne, N. K., Reale-Scafati, A., Séchaud, J., Bendet, S., Goldstein, D., and Lauffer, M.

A., 1965, Functions and properties related to the tail fibers of bacteriophage T4, *Virology* **26**:419.

Kells, S. S., and Haselkorn, R., 1974, Bacteriophage T4 short tail fibers are the product of gene 12, *J. Mol. Biol.* **83**:473.

Kemper, B., and Brown, D. T., 1976, Function of gene 49 of bacteriophage T4. II. Analysis of intracellular development and the structure of very fast-sedimenting DNA, *J. Virol.* **18**:1000.

Kerr, C., and Sadowski, P. D., 1974, Packaging and maturation of DNA of bacteriophage T7 *in vitro*, *Proc. Natl. Acad. Sci. USA* **71**:3545.

Kikuchi, Y., and King, J., 1975a, Genetic control of bacteriophage T4 baseplate morphogenesis. I. Sequential assembly of the major precursor, *in vivo* and *in vitro*, *J. Mol Biol.* **99**:645.

Kikuchi, Y., and King, J., 1975b, Genetic control of bacteriophage T4 baseplate morphogenesis. II. Mutants unable to form the central part of the baseplate, *J. Mol. Biol.* **99**:673.

Kikuchi, Y., and King, J., 1975c, Genetic control of bacteriophage T4 baseplate morphogenesis. III. Formation of the central plug and overall assembly pathway, *J. Mol. Biol.* **99**:695.

King, J., 1968, Assembly of the tail of bacteriophage T4, *J. Mol. Biol.* **32**:231.

King, J., 1971, Bacteriophage T4 tail assembly: Four steps in core formation, *J. Mol. Biol.* **58**:693.

King, J., and Casjens, S., 1974, Catalytic head assembling protein in virus morphogenesis, *Nature (London)* **251**:112.

King, J., and Laemmli, U. K., 1971, Polypeptides of the tail fibres of bacteriophage T4, *J. Mol. Biol.* **62**:465.

King, J., and Laemmli, U. K., 1973, Bacteriophage T4 tail assembly: Structural proteins and their genetic identification, *J. Mol. Biol.* **75**:315.

King, J., and Mykolajewycz, N., 1973, Bacteriophage T4 tail assembly: Proteins of the sheath, core, and base plate, *J. Mol. Biol.* **75**:339.

King, J., and Wood, W. B., 1969, Assembly of bacteriophage T4 tail fibers: The sequence of gene product interaction, *J. Mol. Biol.* **39**:583.

King, J., Lenk, E., and Botstein, D., 1973, Mechanism of head assembly and DNA encapsulation in *Salmonella* phage P22. II. Morphogenetic pathway, *J. Mol. Biol.* **80**:697.

King, J., Hall, C., and Casjens, S., 1978, Control of the synthesis of phage P22 scaffolding protein is coupled to capsid assembly, *Cell* **15**:551.

Kirschner, M . W., and Williams, R. C., 1974, The mechanism of microtubule assembly *in vitro*, *J. Supramol. Struct.* **2**:412.

Klug, A., 1972, Assembly of tobacco mosaic virus, *Fed. Proc.* **31**:30.

Kozloff, L. M., and Lute, M., 1977, Zinc, an essential component of the base plates of T-even bacteriophages, *J. Biol. Chem.* **252**:7715.

Kozloff, L. M., Lute, M., Crosby, L., K., Rao, N., Chapman, V. A., and De Long, S. S., 1970a, Bacteriophage tail components. I. Pteroyl polyglutamates in T-even bacteriophages, *J. Virol.* **5**:726.

Kozloff, L. M., Verses, C., Lute, M., and Crosby, L. K., 1970b, Bacteriophage tail components. II. Dihydrofolate reductase in T4D bacteriophage, *J. Virol.* **5**:740.

Kozloff, L. M., Lute, M., and Baugh, C. M., 1973, Bacteriophage tail components. V. Complementation of T4D gene 28⁻-infected bacterial extracts with pteroyl hexaglutamate, *J. Virol.* **11**:637.

Kozloff, L. M., Crosby, L. K., Lute, M., and Hall, D. H., 1975a, Bacteriophage T4 base plate components. II. Binding and location of bacteriophage-induced dihydrofolate reductase, *J. Virol.* **16**:1401.

Kozloff, L. M., Crosby, L. K., and Lute, M., 1975*b*, Bacteriophage T4 base plate components. III. Location and properties of the bacteriophage structural thymidylate synthetase, *J. Virol.* **16**:1409.

Kühl, P. W., and Katsura, I., 1975, Morphogenesis of the tail of bacteriophage λ. *In vitro* intratail complementation, *Virology* **63**:221.

Laemmli, U. K., 1970, Cleavage of structural proteins during the assembly of the head of bacteriophage T4, *Nature (London)* **227**:680.

Laemmli, U. K., 1975, Characterization of DNA condensates induced by poly(ethylene oxide) and polylysine, *Proc. Natl. Acad. Sci. USA* **72**:4288.

Laemmli, U. K., and Favre, M., 1973, Maturation of the head of bacteriophage T4. I. DNA packaging events, *J. Mol. Biol.* **80**:575.

Laemmli, U. K., and Quittner, S. F., 1974, Maturation of the head of bacteriophage T4. IV. The proteins of the core of the tubular polyheads and *in vitro* cleavage of the head proteins, *Virology* **62**:483.

Laemmli, U. K., Beguin, F., and Gujer-Kellenberger, G., 1970*a*, A factor preventing the major head protein of bacteriophage T4 from random aggregation, *J. Mol. Biol.* **47**:69.

Laemmli, U. K., Mölbert, E., Showe, M., and Kellenberger, E., 1970*b*, Form-determining function of the genes required for the assembly of the head of bacteriophage T4, *J. Mol. Biol.* **49**:99.

Laemmli, U. K., Paulson, J. R., and Hitchins, V., 1974, Maturation of the head of bacteriophage T4, V. A possible DNA packaging mechanism: *In vitro* cleavage of the head proteins and the structure of the core of the polyhead, *J. Supramol. Struct.* **2**:276.

Laemmli, U. K., Amos, L. A., and Klug, A., 1976, Correlation between structural transformation and cleavage of the major head protein of T4 bacteriophage, *Cell* **7**:191.

Lengyel, J. A., Goldstein, R. N., Marsh, M., and Calendar, R., 1974, Structure of the bacteriophage P2 tail, *Virology* **62**:161.

Lenk, E., Casjens, S., Weeks, J., and King, J., 1975, Intracellular visualization of precursor capsids in phage P22 mutant infected cells, *Virology* **68**:182.

Luftig, R. B., Wood, W. B., and Okinaka, R., 1971, Bacteriophage T4 head morphogenesis: on the nature of gene 49-defective heads and their role as intermediates, *J. Mol. Biol.* **57**:555.

MacHattie, L. A., Ritchie, D. A., and Thomas, C. A., 1967, Terminal repetition in permuted T2 bacteriophage DNA molecules, *J. Mol. Biol.* **23**:355.

Male, C. J., and Kozloff, L. M., 1973, Function of T4D structural dihydrofolate reductase in bacteriophage infection, *J. Virol.* **11**:840.

Matsuo-Kato, H., and Fujisawa, H., 1975, Studies on bacteriophage T3. III. Characterization of capsids as intermediates of the T3 head assembly, *Virology* **63**:105.

Mendez, E., Ramirez, G., Salas, M., and Vinuela, E., 1971, Structural proteins of bacteriophage φ29, *Virology* **45**:567.

Minagawa, T., and Ryo, Y., 1978, Substrate specificity of gene 49-controlled deoxyribonuclease of bacteriophage T4: Special reference to DNA packaging, *Virology* **91**:222.

Mindich, L., Sinclair, J. F., and Cohen, J., 1976, The morphogenesis of bacteriophage φ6: Particles formed by nonsense mutants, *Virology* **75**:224.

Moody, M. F., 1965, The shape of the T-even bacteriophage head, *Virology* **26**:567.

Moody, M. F., 1967, Structure of the sheath of bacteriophage T4. II. Rearrangement of the sheath subunits during contraction, *J. Mol. Biol.* **25**:201.

Moody, M. F., 1973, Sheath of bacteriophage T4. III. Contraction mechanism deduced from partially contracted sheaths, *J. Mol. Biol.* **80**:613.

Murialdo, H., and Becker, A., 1977, Assembly of biologically active proheads of bacteriophage lambda *in vitro*, *Proc. Natl. Acad. Sci. USA* **74**:906.

Murialdo, H., and Becker, A., 1978, Head morphogenesis of complex double-stranded deoxyribonucleic acid bacteriophages, *Microbiol. Rev.* **42**:529.

Murialdo, H., and Ray, P. N., 1975, Model for arrangement of minor structural proteins in head of bacteriophage λ, *Nature (London)* **257**:815.

Murialdo, H., and Siminovitch, L., 1972a, The morphogenesis of bacteriophage lambda. IV. Identification of gene products and control of the expression of the morphogenetic information, *Virology* **48**:785.

Murialdo, H., and Siminovitch, L., 1972b, The morphogenesis of phage lambda. V. Form-determining function of the genes required for the assembly of the head, *Virology* **48**:824.

Nelson, R. A., Reilly, B. E., and Anderson, D. L., 1976, Morphogenesis of bacteriophage ϕ29 of *Bacillus subtilis:* Preliminary isolation and characterization of intermediate particles of the assembly pathway, *J. Virol.* **19**:518.

O'Farrell, P. Z., Gold, L. M., and Huang, W. M., 1973, The identification of prereplicative bacteriophage T4 proteins, *J. Biol. Chem.* **248**:5499.

Olmstead, J. B., and Borisy, G. G., 1973, Microtubules, *Annu. Rev. Biochem.* **42**:507.

Onorato, L., and Showe, M. K., 1975, Gene 21 protein-dependent proteolysis *in vitro* of purified gene 22 product of bacteriophage T4, *J. Mol. Biol.* **92**:395.

Ortin, J., Vasquez, C., Vinuela, E., and Sals, M., 1971, DNA-protein complex in circular DNA from phage ϕ29, *Nature (London) New Biol.* **234**:275.

Parkinson, J. S., 1968, Genetics of the left arm of the chromosome of bacteriophage lambda, *Genetics* **59**:311.

Paulson, J. R., Lazaroff, S., and Laemmli, U. K., 1976, Head length determination of bacteriophage T4: The role of the core protein P22, *J. Mol. Biol.* **103**:155.

Paulus, H., and Alpers, J. B., 1971, Preconditioning: An obligatory step in the biosynthesis of oligomeric enzymes and its promotion by allosteric ligands, *Enzyme* **12**:385.

Poteete, A., and Botstein, D., 1976, Functions of p1, p2, and p3 in P22 DNA packaging *in vitro*, Abstract, 5th Biennial Conference on Bacteriophage Assembly, Snowbird, Utah.

Poteete, A. R., and King, J., 1977, Functions of two new genes in bacteriophage P22 assembly, *Virology* **76**:725.

Pruss, G., Barrett, K., Lengyel, J., Goldstein, R., and Calendar, R., 1974, Phage head size determination and head protein cleavage *in vitro*, *J. Supramol. Struct.* **2**:337.

Pruss, G. J., Wang, J. C., and Calendar, R., 1975, *In vitro* packaging of covalently closed circular monomers of bacteriophage DNA, *J. Mol. Biol.* **98**:465.

Pulitzer, J. F., and Yanagida, M., 1971, Inactive T4 progeny virus formation in a temperature-sensitive mutant of *Escherichia coli* K12, *Virology* **45**:539.

Ray, P., and Murialdo, H., 1975, The role of gene *Nu3* in bacteriophage lambda head morphogenesis, *Virology* **64**:247.

Ray, P., and Pearson, M. L., 1974, Evidence for posttranscriptional control of the morphogenetic genes of bacteriophage lambda, *J. Mol. Biol.* **85**:163.

Revel, H. R., Herrmann, R., and Bishop, R. J., 1976, Genetic analysis of T4 tail fiber assembly. II. Bacterial host mutants that allow bypass of T4 gene 57 function, *Virology* **72**:255.

Revel, H. R., Stitt, B. L., Lielausis, I., and Wood, W. B., 1979, The role of the host cell in bacteriophage T4 development I: Characterization of mutants that block T4 head assembly, *J. Virol.* (in press).

Richards, K. E., Williams, R. C., and Calendar, R., 1973, Mode of DNA packing within bacteriophage heads, *J. Mol. Biol.* **78**:255.

Ritchie, D. A., Thomas, C. A., Jr., MacHattie, L. A., and Wensink, P. C., 1967, Terminal repetition in nonpermuted T3 and T7 bacteriophage DNA molecules, *J. Mol. Biol.* **23**:365.

Roeder, G. S., and Sadowski, P. D., 1977, Bacteriophage T7 morphogenesis: Phage-related particles in cells infected with wild type and mutant T7 phage, *Virology* **76**:263.

Russell, W. C., and Winters, W. D., 1975, Assembly of viruses, *Progr. Med. Virol.* **19**:1.

Saigo, K., and Uchida, H., 1974, Connection of the right-hand terminus of DNA to the proximal end of the tail in bacteriophage lambda, *Virology* **61**:524.

Serwer, P., 1975, Buoyant density sedimentation of macromolecules in sodium iothalamate density gradients, *J. Mol. Biol.* **92**:433.

Serwer, P., 1976, The internal proteins of bacteriophage T7, *J. Mol. Biol.* **107**:271.

Shore, D., Deho, G., Tsipis, J., and Goldstein, R., 1978, Determination of capsid size by satellite bacteriophage P4, *Proc. Natl. Acad. Sci. USA* **75**:400.

Showe, M. K., and Black, L. W., 1973, Assembly core of bacteriophage T4: An intermediate in head formation, *Nature (London) New Biol.* **242**:70.

Showe, M. K., and Kellenberger, E. K., 1975, Control mechanisms in virus assembly, in: *Control Processes in Viral Multiplication* (D. C. Burke and W. C. Russell, eds.), p. 407, Cambridge University Press, Cambridge.

Showe, M. K., and Onorato, L., 1978, Kinetic factors and form determination of the head of bacteriophage T4, *Proc. Natl. Acad. Sci. USA* **75**:4165.

Showe, M. K., Isobe, E., and Onorato, L., 1976, T4 prehead proteinase: Identification and characterization of the purified enzyme and its cleavage from the T4 gene 21 protein, Abstract, 5th Biennial Conference on Bacteriophage Assembly, Snowbird, Utah.

Silverstein, J. L., and Goldberg, E. B., 1976a, T4 DNA injection. I. Growth cycle of a gene 2 mutant, *Virology* **72**:195.

Silverstein, J. L., and Goldberg, E. B., 1976b, T4 DNA injection. II. Protection of entering DNA from host exonuclease V, *Virology* **72**:212.

Simon, L. D., 1972, Infection of *Escherichia coli* by T2 and T4 bacteriophages as seen in the electron microscope: T4 head morphogenesis, *Proc. Natl. Acad. Sci. USA* **69**:907.

Simon, L. D., and Anderson, T. F., 1967a, The infection of *Escherichia coli* by T2 and T4 bacteriophages as seen in the electron microscope. I. Attachment and penetration, *Virology* **32**:279.

Simon, L. D., and Anderson, T. F., 1967b, The infection of *Escherichia coli* by T2 and T4 bacteriophages as seen in the electron microscope. II. Structure and function of the baseplate, *Virology* **32**:298.

Simon, L. D., Snover, D., and Doermann, A. H., 1974, Bacterial mutation affecting T4 phage DNA synthesis and tail production, *Nature (London)* **252**:451.

Simon, L. D., McLaughlin, T. J. M., Snover, D., Ou, J., Grisham, C., and Loeb, M., 1975, *E. coli* membrane lipid alteration affecting T4 capsid morphogenesis, *Nature (London)* **256**:379.

Skalka, A., Poonian, M., and Barth, P., 1972, Concatemers in DNA replication: Electron microscopic studies of partially denatured intracellular lambda DNA, *J. Mol. Biol.* **64**:541.

Snopek, T. J., Wood, W. B., Conley, M. P., Chen, P., and Cozzarelli, N. R., 1977, Bacteriophage T4 RNA ligase is gene 63 product, the protein that promotes tail fiber attachment to the baseplate, *Proc. Natl. Acad. Sci. USA* **74**:3355.

Stahl, F. W., and Murray, N. E., 1966, The evolution of gene clusters and genetic circularity in microorganisms, *Genetics* **53**:569.

Sternberg, N., 1976, A genetic analysis of bacteriophage lambda head assembly, *Virology* **71**:568.

Steven, A. C., Couture, E., Aebi, U., and Showe, M. K., 1976, Structure of T4 polyheads. II. A pathway of polyhead transformation as a model for T4 capsid maturation, *J. Mol. Biol.* **106**:187.

Streisinger, G., Emrich, J., and Stahl, M. M., 1967, Chromosome structure in phage T4. III. Terminal redundancy and length determination, *Proc. Natl. Acad. Sci. USA* **57**:292.

Studier, F. W., 1972, Bacteriophage T7, *Science* **176**:367.

Studier, F. W., and Maizel, J. F., Jr., 1969, T7-directed protein synthesis, *Virology* **39**:575.

Syvanen, M., 1975, Processing of bacteriophage lambda DNA during its assembly into heads, *J. Mol. Biol.* **91**:165.

Takahashi, H., Coppo, A., Manzi, A., Martire, G., and Pulitzer, J. F., 1975, Design of a system of conditional lethal mutations (*tab/k/com*) affecting protein–protein interactions in bacteriophage T4-infected *Escherichia coli*, *J. Mol. Biol.* **96**:563.

Terzaghi, B. E., Terzaghi, E., and Coombs, D., 1979, Mutational alteration of the T4D tail fiber attachment process, *J. Mol. Biol.* **127**:1.

Terzaghi, E., 1971, Alternative pathways of tail fiber assembly in bacteriophage T4? *J. Mol. Biol.* **59**:319.

Tsugita, A., Black, L. W., and Showe, M. K., 1975, Cleavage during virus assembly: Characterization of cleavage in T4 phage, *J. Mol. Biol.* **98**:271.

Tye, B.-K., Huberman, J. A., and Botstein, D., 1974, Non-random circular permutation of phage P22 DNA, *J. Mol. Biol.* **85**:501.

Vanderslice, R. W., and Yegian, C. D., 1974, The identification of late bacteriophage T4 proteins on sodium dodecyl sulfate polyacrylamide gels, *Virology* **60**:265.

Wake, R. G., Kaiser, A. D., and Inman, R. B., 1972, Isolation and structure of phage λ head-mutant DNA, *J. Mol. Biol.* **64**:519.

Walsby, A. E., 1972, Structure and function of gas vacuoles, *Bacteriol. Rev.* **36**:1.

Wang, J. C., and Kaiser, A. D., 1973, Evidence that the cohesive ends of mature λ DNA are generated by the gene *A* product, *Nature (London) New Biol.* **241**:16.

Ward, S., and Dickson, R. C., 1971, Assembly of bacteriophage T4 tail fibers. III. Genetic control of the major tail fiber polypeptides, *J. Mol. Biol.* **62**:479.

Ward, S., Luftig, R. B., Wilson, J. H., Eddleman, H., Lyle, H., and Wood, W. B., 1970, Assembly of bacteriophage T4 tail fibers. II. Isolation and characterization of tail fiber precursors, *J. Mol. Biol.* **54**:15.

Watson, J. D., 1976, *Molecular Biology of the Gene*, 3rd ed., p. 247, Benjamin, Menlo Park, Calif.

Williams, R. C., and Richards, K. E., 1974, Capsid structure of bacteriophage lambda, *J. Mol. Biol.* **88**:547.

Wirtz, K. W. A., 1974, Transfer of phospholipids between membranes, *Biochim. Biophys. Acta* **344**:95.

Wood, W. B., 1973, Genetic control of bacteriophage T4 morphogenesis, in: *Genetic Mechanisms of Development* (F. H. Ruddle, ed.), p. 29, Academic Press, New York.

Wood, W. B., and Bishop, R. J., 1973, Bacteriophage T4 tail fibers: Structure and assembly of a viral organelle, in: *Virus Research* (C. F. Rox and W. S. Robinson, eds.), p. 303, Academic Press, New York.

Wood, W. B., and Conley, M. P., 1979, Attachment of tail fibers in bacteriophage T4 assembly. Role of the phage whiskers, *J. Mol. Biol.* **127**:15.

Wood, W. B., and Henninger, M., 1969, Attachment of tail fibers in bacteriophage T4 assembly: Some properties of the reaction *in vitro* and its genetic control, *J. Mol. Biol.* **39**:603.

Wood, W. B., and Revel, H. R., 1976, The genome of bacteriophage T4, *Bacteriol. Rev.* **40**:847.

Wood, W. B., Conley, M. P., Lyle, H., and Dickson, R. C., 1977, Attachment of tail fibers in bacteriophage T4 assembly. II. Purification, properties, and site of action of the accessory protein coded by gene *63p*, *J. Biol. Chem.* **253**:2437.

Wurtz, M., Kistler, J., and Hohn, T., 1976, Surface structure of *in vitro* assembled bacteriophage lambda polyheads, *J. Mol. Biol.* **101**:39.

Yamamoto, M., and Uchida, H., 1975, Organization and function of the tail of bacteriophage T4. II. Structural control of tail contraction, *J. Mol. Biol.* **92**:207.

Zachary, A., Simon, L. D., and Litwin, S., 1976, Lambda head morphogenesis as seen in the electron microscope, *Virology* **72**:429.

Zweig, M., and Cummings, D. J., 1973a, Structural proteins of bacteriophage T5, *Virology* **51**:443.

Zweig, M., and Cummings, D. J., 1973b, Cleavage of head and tail proteins during T5 assembly: Selective host involvement in the cleavage of a tail protein, *J. Mol. Biol.* **80**:505.

Index